Thieme

Operative Fundamentals in Neurological Surgery

Nitin Agarwal, MD
Associate Professor, Neurological Surgery and Bioengineering
Director, Minimally Invasive Spine and Robotics Surgery
Associate Program Director, Neurological Surgery Residency
Co-Director, Complex and Minimally Invasive Spine Deformity Fellowship
Department of Neurological Surgery
University of Pittsburgh Medical Center
Pittsburgh, Pennsylvania, USA

Hanna N. Algattas, MD
Assistant Professor
Department of Neurosurgery
University at Buffalo
Williamsville, New York, USA

Edward G. Andrews, MD
Assistant Professor
Department of Neurological Surgery
University of Pittsburgh Medical Center
Pittsburgh, Pennsylvania, USA

Kamil W. Nowicki, MD, PhD
Assistant Professor
Department of Neurological Surgery
Columbia University
New York, New York, USA

Xiaoran Zhang, MD, MS
Neurosurgeon
Department of Neurosurgery
Sutter West Bay Medical Group
Danville, California, USA

310 illustrations

Thieme
New York • Stuttgart • Delhi • Rio de Janeiro

Library of Congress Cataloging-in-Publication Data is available from the publisher.

Thieme Medical Publishers, Inc.
333 Seventh Avenue, 18th Floor,
NY 10001 New York, USA
www.thieme.com
https://customerservice.thieme.com

Cover design: © Thieme
Cover image source: Cover illustration created by Carol Hrejsa, MS, CMI / © Thieme
Typesetting by TNQ Tech Private Limited, India

Printed in India by Replika Press Pvt. Ltd.

DOI: 10.1055/b000000825

ISBN: 978-1-68420-561-5 5 4 3 2 1

Also available as an e-book:
eISBN (PDF): 978-1-68420-562-2
eISBN (epub): 978-1-68420-563-9

Important note: Medicine is an ever-changing science undergoing continual development. Research and clinical experience are continually expanding our knowledge, in particular our knowledge of proper treatment and drug therapy. Insofar as this book mentions any dosage or application, readers may rest assured that the authors, editors, and publishers have made every effort to ensure that such references are in accordance with **the state of knowledge at the time of production of the book.**

Nevertheless, this does not involve, imply, or express any guarantee or responsibility on the part of the publishers in respect to any dosage instructions and forms of applications stated in the book. **Every user is requested to examine carefully** the manufacturers' leaflets accompanying each drug and to check, if necessary in consultation with a physician or specialist, whether the dosage schedules mentioned therein or the contraindications stated by the manufacturers differ from the statements made in the present book. Such examination is particularly important with drugs that are either rarely used or have been newly released on the market. Every dosage schedule or every form of application used is entirely at the user's own risk and responsibility. The authors and publishers request every user to report to the publishers any discrepancies or inaccuracies noticed. If errors in this work are found after publication, errata will be posted at www.thieme.com on the product description page.

Some of the product names, patents, and registered designs referred to in this book are in fact registered trademarks or proprietary names even though specific reference to this fact is not always made in the text. Therefore, the appearance of a name without designation as proprietary is not to be construed as a representation by the publisher that it is in the public domain.

Thieme addresses people of all gender identities equally. We encourage our authors to use gender-neutral or gender-equal expressions wherever the context allows.

MIX
Paper | Supporting responsible forestry
FSC™ C016779
www.fsc.org

To my family for the unconditional support. To my colleagues for helping me carry the message. To my mentors for educating me in the art of neurosurgery. To my patients for teaching me on a daily basis.

Nitin Agarwal, MD

For my entire loving and supportive family, Amanda, Ava, Cora, and Zeus!

Hanna N. Algattas, MD

To Lucy, Alex, and Rosie: This journey has only been possible with you by my side through the highs and the lows. You are my calm in the storm.

To David, Sarah, Erin, and Molly: Your unwavering guidance and support have molded me into the person I am today.

Edward G. Andrews, MD

I would like to dedicate this book to my wife, Meredith, who has always supported me in residency and in all of my endeavors. You have always made every mountain easier to climb and turned every storm into a passing breeze.

I would also like to thank my family and friends, especially my fellow co-authors, without whom residency would have been a much lonelier and less exciting journey. You were, and always will be, my fellow brothers-in-arms.

Lastly, I would like to dedicate this book to all students and residents who wish to embark upon a journey in this unique and humbling field. Remember, if you can dream it, you can do it!

Kamil W. Nowicki, MD, PhD

To my wife, Nupur, who has been there every step of the way.

To my parents, John and Lina, who gave me the freedom to figure out my passion in life.

To my Pitt Neurosurgery family, with whom I spent the most amazing 7 years of my life.

Xiaoran Zhang, MD, MS

Contents

Part IV: Spine Surgery

Videos

Video 3.1 Parasagittal craniotomy, including interhemispheric dissection and transcallosal approach into the lateral ventricle to the foramen of Monroe with subsequent placement of an external ventricular drain.

Video 4.1 Surgical video (from Synaptive Modus X robotic exoscope) from a case of redo temporal craniotomy for brain tumor resection.

Video 4.2 Narrative video from a left temporal arteriovenous malformation case.

Video 5.1 Fronto-orbital craniotomy for a lesion located at the interface of the anterior fossa and the orbit.

Video 7.1 The modified lateral orbitotomy approach to a cavernous malformation in the mesial temporal lobe.

Video 8.1 An surgical video demonstrating a supracerebellar infratentorial approach resection of a pineal region mass in the sitting position (Chapter 8). The transtentorial dural incision is demonstrated (1:33) in the case of a supracerebellar transtentorial approach (Chapter 9).

Video 10.1 Operative video demonstrating the telovelar approach for resection of metastasis within the fourth ventricle.

Video 11.1 This surgical video demonstrates the translabyrinthine approach for resection of a left internal auditory canal soft tissue mass with extension into the cerebellopontine angle, with pathology confirming a vestibular schwannoma. The illustrated steps include drilling the mastoid with extensive skeletonization of the tegmen, sinodural angle, and sigmoid sinus; identification of the facial nerve; labyrinthectomy; removal of retrofacial air cells; decompression of the middle and posterior fossa dura; identification of the endolymphatic sac and ligation of the duct; skeletonization of the internal auditory canal with deepening of superior and inferior troughs; opening of the posterior fossa and IAC dura; removal of tumor; and layered closure including obliteration of the eustachian tube and repair of the dural defect.

Video 13.1 Case illustration of a foramen magnum meningioma resection using the far lateral approach.

Video 16.1 Demonstration of the transpterygoid approach used in the endonasal resection of a craniocervical junction chordoma (No Audio).

Video 18.1 A 65-year-old woman with an incidentally found clival lesion, biopsy-proven conventional type chordoma. An endoscopic endonasal resection was performed to achieve gross total resection, with no residual disease at 7 months postoperatively.

Video 21.1 Example case, from the interventionalist's perspective, demonstrating the key technical steps of the transradial approach for neuroendovascular procedures. (Used with permission from Barrow Neurological Institute, Phoenix, Arizona.)

Video 23.1 Procedural implementation for transcarotid artery revascularization (TCAR).

Video 24.1 Narrated surgical exposure of the supraclavicular brachial plexus. (Used with permission of Mayo Foundation for Medical Education and Research, all rights reserved.)

Video 25.1 Narrated surgical exposure of the infraclavicular brachial plexus. (Used with permission of Mayo Foundation for Medical Education and Research, all rights reserved.)

Video 26.1	Submuscular ulnar nerve transposition. (Copyright of Susan Mackinnon, A. Lee. Washington University.)
Video 27.1	Median nerve decompression at the proximal forearm for pronator and anterior interosseous nerve syndromes.
Video 28.1	Posterior interosseous nerve decompression.
Video 29.1	Carpal tunnel release.
Video 33.1	A discussion of the expert tips and tricks for performing an occipitocervical fusion.
Video 34.1	Goel's technique of atlantoaxial fixation.
Video 35.1	Surgical video describing the LMS and CPS placement in a patient with cervical deformity.
Video 35.2	Surgical video describing the surgical setup, positioning, and technique of CPS placement for cervicothoracic deformity correction.
Video 37.1	Transpedicular approach for decompression of ventral thoracic epidural abscess.
Video 38.1	Demonstrating exposure of the lateral vertebral body from a side view with the lamina intact.
Video 38.2	Demonstrating exposure of the lateral vertebral body.
Video 38.3	Disarticulating the rib head using a Cobb elevator.
Video 41.1	Identification of the sacroiliac joint (SIJ) starting point.
Video 41.2	Confirmation of no bony breach after crossing the sacroiliac joint (SIJ) and tapping of screw trajectory.
Video 41.3	Tapping a parallel secondary trajectory and inspecting for bony breach.
Video 41.4	Two fixation points across the sacroiliac joint are required for fusion.
Video 41.5	Placing the second implant medial to the first.
Video 41.6	Implant with tulip head offering bone ongrowth and through growth.
Video 42.1	Step-by-step demonstration of anterior cervical discectomy and fusion (ACDF), including exposure, discectomy, endplate preparation, graft placement, and plate fixation, with key techniques to optimize outcomes and reduce complications.
Video 43.1	Anterior odontoid fixation uses one or two screws to facilitate fusion for odontoid fractures (**Fig. 43.7**). In contrast to C1–C2 fusions, the goal is to restore spinal stability without compromising the atlantoaxial range. In order to perform this procedure, the patient should be positioned supine with the head extended and biplanar fluoroscopy is necessary (**Fig. 43.2**). If possible, the fracture is reduced before surgical access. The surgery makes use of a transverse incision and an anterior cervical spinal exposure. Following exposure and retraction, the surgeon should create an entry point at the anteroinferior lip of the C2 body (i.e., the C2 endplate). The sequence of steps for screw insertion are as follows: the drill guide is placed first, after which an initial trajectory is drilled (**Fig. 43.4**). The surgeon next inserts a K-wire into the drilled trajectory, advancing to the tip of the odontoid (**Fig 43.5**). Finally, a cannulated, partially threaded lag screw is placed (**Fig. 43.6**). A second screw may be inserted in the same fashion, unless the odontoid diameter is too small to accommodate two screws (as in **Fig. 43.7**).

Video 46.1 OLIF approach (No Audio). (Copyright of Neel Anand).

Video 46.2 Retractor placement (No Audio). (Copyright of Neel Anand).

Video 46.3 OLIF disc access (No Audio). (Copyright of Neel Anand).

Video 46.4 OLIF disc preparation (No Audio). (Copyright of Neel Anand).

Video 46.5 OLIF interbody placement (No Audio). (Copyright of Neel Anand).

Video 50.1 Single-level endoscopic transforaminal lumbar interbody fusion (TLIF) with fluoroscopy-based instrument tracking. A 62-year-old woman with a history of hypertension and hyperlipidemia presented with significant pain in the lower back, left leg in the buttock, and posterior thigh in addition to numbness and tingling. The neurological examination was grossly normal, even though the patient relied on a cane for ambulation and exhibited poor patient-reported pain scores. Imaging depicted an unstable grade 1 L4–L5 spondylolisthesis with central and lateral recess stenosis and bilateral facet hypertrophy. The patient underwent a transforaminal endoscopic lumbar interbody fusion at L4–L5 with tracking fluoroscopy assistance. Postoperatively, reduction of the spondylolisthesis was achieved, as evidenced by imaging, and the patient's pain and mobility substantially improved.

Video 51.1 Overview of frame placement for stereotactic Gamma Knife radiosurgery and expert pearls from Dr. L. Dade Lunsford.

Video 52.1 Frameless Gamma Knife stereotactic radiosurgery case.

Video 54.1 Operative video demonstrating the use of robotics (ROSA, Zimmer Biomet, Warsaw, IN) in the placement of stereoelectroencephalography electrodes for medically refractory epilepsy.

Video 56.1 Operative video demonstrating ROSA-assisted stereotactic implantation for deep brain stimulation, including patient preparation and Leksell frame fixation under conscious sedation, intraoperative imaging for registration and trajectory planning, microelectrode recording and macrostimulation for target verification, lead placement, and closure.

Video 57.1 This video reviews stereotactic laser amygdalohippocampotomy (SLAH) as a minimally invasive alternative to open temporal lobe surgery for medically refractory epilepsy. The discussion highlights LITT's lower complication rates and superior neuropsychiatric outcomes despite lower seizure freedom rates compared to open surgery. The video then outlines available LITT systems (Visualase and NeuroBlate) and stereotactic platforms used for laser probe placement. Trajectory planning considerations for mesial temporal epilepsy are discussed, followed by a step-by-step overview of SLAH using the ClearPoint SmartFrame and Visualase laser probe. The workflow includes patient positioning, probe placement, MR thermography-guided ablation, and postoperative imaging to confirm ablation.

Foreword

It is said, "He who works with his hands is a laborer; he who works with his hands and his head is a craftsman; and he who works with his hands, his head, and his heart is an artist." Neurosurgery is, indeed, an art form that requires the hand, the head, and the heart.

In 1972, Peter Jannetta invited me, fresh out of residency, to assist him in forming the first department of neurosurgery at the University of Pittsburgh. He told me that three qualities were essential for an academic neurosurgeon: (1) demonstrated research capabilities, (2) competent administrative skills, and (3) surgical ability. He emphasized the "sine qua non" (without which nothing) for a neurosurgeon is to be a skilled operative surgeon and an empathetic physician. Operative competence has remained a primary focus at the University of Pittsburgh for over five decades.

In this book, Dr. Nitin Agarwal and his colleagues have compiled and synthesized the absolute essence of neurosurgical procedures and techniques. Clifton Hillegass, in 1958, introduced "Cliff Notes." Initially, these were a series of study guides used to simplify understanding of more complex works and designed to provide the main points without all the details. It is now expanded to hundreds of works. This book serves as a unique compilation of neurosurgical "cliff notes" to help residents and faculty quickly, understandably, and efficiently acquire knowledge of the essential elements required for the most frequent operations performed by a neurosurgeon. It provides the neurosurgical student, at all levels, with a concise and understandable overview of what to prepare for and how to perform procedures from carpal tunnel operations to the most complex skull base surgery.

Traditional learning methods and static didactics are no longer sufficient in an era of rapidly advancing neuroguidance, surgical tools, and increasingly complex operative approaches. No practical, handy reference exists for real-time use in clinical settings. This operative handbook has been thoughtfully crafted to address the demands of contemporary neurosurgical education, providing clear, concise explanations and focused procedural guidance.

It is highly recommended for all those seeking what will become the "Cliff Notes" for operative neurosurgery. Embrace this resource as a meaningful step forward on your path to becoming a capable, confident, and thoughtful operative neurosurgeon.

Joseph C. Maroon, MD, FACS
Clinical Professor and Vice Chairman
Department of Neurological Surgery
Heindl Scholar in Neuroscience
University of Pittsburgh Medical Center
Neurological Consultant, The Pittsburgh Steelers
Neurological Consultant, WWE
Pittsburgh, Pennsylvania, USA

Preface

Developed with the practical demands of neurosurgical training in mind, this handbook is intended to provide clarity, structure, and confidence in the operating room. It serves as a hands-on guide for trainees as they begin building their technical foundation during the early stages of their careers. At the same time, it is designed to function as a concise, high-yield refresher for anyone involved in neurosurgical education, regardless of their experience level, offering a reliable reference at any given point in time.

Operative Fundamentals in Neurological Surgery offers a procedure-specific reference that is both portable and user-friendly. Each chapter presents a focused snapshot of a single operative approach, summarizing key anatomical landmarks, positioning, steps, and technical considerations necessary for safe and effective execution. This handbook was developed to act as a go-to resource on the day of surgery, at the scrub sink, or during moments between cases.

The handbook is organized according to major subdivisions: cranial, spinal, peripheral nerve, endovascular, and stereotactic and functional procedures. The structure reflects the breadth of cases encountered during residency while maintaining a sharp focus on the most essential technical details. Each section is intentionally concise, allowing the reader to rapidly internalize critical information.

As surgical training continues to evolve, *Operative Fundamentals in Neurological Surgery* stands as a modern response to the growing need for streamlined, high-yield operative education. We hope it becomes a trusted companion for trainees, ready at hand, practical in tone, and deeply aligned with the demands of clinical learning.

Nitin Agarwal, MD
Hanna N. Algattas, MD
Edward G. Andrews, MD
Kamil W. Nowicki, MD, PhD
Xiaoran Zhang, MD, MS

Acknowledgments

Our utmost gratitude goes to all our colleagues who contributed to this book. We would like to thank the Department of Neurological Surgery at the University of Pittsburgh for the exceptional residency training program that the editors had the honor and privilege to complete. To our families, friends, and mentors, thank you for your unwavering support and sponsorship. We are grateful to the entire Thieme editorial team, especially Karen Edmonson, for championing efforts to expand educational opportunities for medical students, advanced practice providers, residents, and fellows in neurological surgery. Finally, we extend our sincere thanks to the Spine Computational Outcomes Learning Institute (SCOLI) team for moving this project across the finish line.

Nitin Agarwal, MD
Hanna N. Algattas, MD
Edward G. Andrews, MD
Kamil W. Nowicki, MD, PhD
Xiaoran Zhang, MD, MS

Contributors

Hussam Abou-Al-Shaar, MD
Cerebrovascular and Skull Base Surgery Fellow
Vivian L. Smith Department of Neurosurgery
McGovern Medical School
The University of Texas Health Science Center at Houston
Houston, Texas, USA

Nancy Abu-Bonsrah, MD
Resident
Department of Neurological Surgery
Johns Hopkins University
Baltimore, Maryland, USA

Nitin Agarwal, MD
Associate Professor, Neurological Surgery and Bioengineering
Director, Minimally Invasive Spine and Robotics Surgery
Associate Program Director, Neurological Surgery Residency
Co-Director, Complex and Minimally Invasive Spine Deformity Fellowship
Department of Neurological Surgery
University of Pittsburgh Medical Center
Pittsburgh, Pennsylvania, USA

Prateek Agarwal, MD, MBA
Resident Physician
Department of Neurosurgery
University of Pittsburgh Medical Center
Pittsburgh, Pennsylvania, USA

Hasan S. Ahmad, MD
Resident
Department of Neurosurgery
University of Pennsylvania
Philadelphia, Pennsylvania, USA

A. Karim Ahmed, MD
Neurosurgery Resident
Department of Neurosurgery
Johns Hopkins University School of Medicine
Baltimore, Maryland, USA

Hanna N. Algattas, MD
Assistant Professor
Department of Neurosurgery
University at Buffalo
Williamsville, New York, USA

Nima Alan, MD
Assistant Clinical Professor
Department of Neurological Surgery
University of California, San Francisco
San Francisco, California, USA

Anthony M. Alvarado, MD
Assistant Professor
Department of Neurosurgery
University of Kansas Health System
Kansas City, Kansas, USA

Neel Anand, MD, MChOrth, FAAOS
Professor
Department of Orthopaedics
Cedars Sinai Medical Center
Los Angeles, California, USA

Joseph P. Antonios, MD, PhD
Physician
Department of Neurosurgery
Yale University School of Medicine
New Haven, Connecticut, USA

Ayush Arora, BS
Medical Student
Department of Orthopaedic Surgery
University of California, San Francisco
San Francisco, California, USA

Bhargav Ayloo, BS
Medical Student Research Fellow
Department of Neurosurgery
Columbia University Irving Medical Center
New York City, New York, USA;
Medical Student
Wayne State University School of Medicine
Detroit, Michigan, USA

Ammad A. Baig, MD
Physician
Department of Neurosurgery
University of Illinois Chicago
Chicago, Illinois, USA

Mustafa Kemal Baskaya, MD
Robert J. Dempsey Professor in Neurological Surgery
Department of Neurological Surgery
University of Wisconsin School of Medicine and Public Health
Madison, Wisconsin, USA

Alexander Becker, MD
Resident Physician
Department of Neurosurgery
University at Buffalo
Buffalo, New York, USA

Andrew Becker, MD, MPH
Faculty, Clinical Instructor
Department of Anesthesiology, Perioperative, and Pain Medicine
Harvard Medical School
Boston, Massachusetts, USA

Greg Bednarz, PhD
Medical Physicist
Department of Radiation Oncology
University of Pittsburgh Medical Center
Pittsburgh, Pennsylvania, USA

Stephen M. Bergin, MD, PhD
Neurological Surgery Resident
Department of Neurosurgery
Duke University
Durham, North Carolina, USA

Sigurd Berven, MD
Professor in Residence, Chief of Spine Service
Department of Orthopaedic Surgery
University of California, San Francisco
San Francisco, California, USA

Meghana Bhimreddy, BA
Medical Student
Department of Neurosurgery
Johns Hopkins University School of Medicine
Baltimore, Maryland, USA

Salil Bhole, MD, BS
Student
Department of Neurosurgery
Washington University in St. Louis
St. Louis, Missouri, USA

Othman Bin-Alamer, MBBS
Research Fellow
Center for Image-Guided Neurosurgery, Department of Neurological Surgery
University of Pittsburgh Medical Center
Pittsburgh, Pennsylvania, USA

Michael T. Bounajem, MD
Resident Physician
Department of Neurosurgery
University of Utah
Salt Lake City, Utah, USA

Alexandros Bouras, MD
Senior Research Scientist
Department of Neurosurgery
University of Pittsburgh Medical Center
Pittsburgh, Pennsylvania, USA

Mehdi Bouslama, MD, MSc
Neuroendovascular Surgery and Vascular Neurology
Department of Neurology
Broward Health
Fort Lauderdale, Florida, USA

Karol P. Budohoski, MD, PhD
Assistant Professor
Department of Neurosurgery
University of Utah
Salt Lake City, Utah, USA

David T. Fernandes Cabral, MD
Assistant Professor
Department of Neurological Surgery
University of Pittsburgh School of Medicine;
Director of Resident Education
Department of Neurological Surgery
University of Pittsburgh Medical Center
Pittsburgh, Pennsylvania, USA

Joshua S Catapano, MD
Assistant Professor
Department of Neurosurgery
University of Pennsylvania
Philadelphia, Pennsylvania, USA

Maria Jose Cavagnaro, MD
Resident
Department of Neurosurgery
Stanford University
Palo Alto, California, USA

Andrew K. Chan, MD
Assistant Professor
Director, Minimally Invasive Scoliosis Surgery
Director, Neurosurgical Spine Research
Department of Neurological Surgery
Columbia University Irving Medical Center
New York, New York, USA

Veronica L. Chiang, MD
Professor
Department of Neurosurgery
Yale University School of Medicine
New Haven, Connecticut, USA

Serah Choi, MD, PhD
Associate Professor
Department of Radiation Oncology
University of Pittsburgh Medical Center
Pittsburgh, Pennsylvania, USA

Dean Chou, MD
Bennett M. Stein Professor
Spine Division Chief
Vice Chair of Neurosurgery
Columbia University/Och Spine
New York, New York, USA

Ryan T. Cleary, MD
Assistant Professor
Department of Neurosurgery
Virginia Commonwealth University
Richmond, Virginia, USA

William T. Couldwell, MD, PhD
Professor and Chair
Department of Neurosurgery
University of Utah
Salt Lake City, Utah, USA

Andrew T. Coxon, MD, MSCI
Resident Physician
Department of Neurosurgery
Barnes-Jewish Hospital/Washington University in St. Louis
St. Louis, Missouri, USA

Jesus G. Cruz-Garza, PhD
Research Scientist
Department of Neurosurgery
Houston Methodist
Houston, Texas, USA

Jason Davies, MD, PhD
Associate Professor
Department of Neurosurgery and Biomedical Informatics
University at Buffalo
Buffalo, New York, USA

Hansen Deng, MD
Fellow
Department of Neurosurgery
University of Pittsburgh Medical Center
Pittsburgh, Pennsylvania, USA

Anthony M. DiGiorgio, DO, MHA, FAANS
Assistant Professor
Department of Neurological Surgery
UC San Francisco
San Francisco, California, USA

Andrew F. Ducruet, MD
Professor
Department of Neurosurgery
Barrow Neurological Institute
Phoenix, Arizona, USA

Charles C. Duncan, MD
Emeritus Professor
Senior Research Scientist
Director of Human Anatomy Program
Departments of Neurosurgery and Education
Yale School of Medicine
New Haven, Connecticut, USA

Margaret I. Engelhardt, MD
Fellow
Department of Otolaryngology-Head & Neck Surgery
University of Pittsburgh Medical Center
Pittsburgh, Pennsylvania, USA

Ufuk Erginoglu, MD
Neurosurgeon – Medical Scientist
Department of Neurological Surgery
University of Wisconsin School of Medicine and Public Health
Madison, Wisconsin, USA

Amir H. Faraji, MD, PhD
Director of Functional Neurosurgery
Department of Neurosurgery
Houston Methodist
Houston, Texas, USA

Richard G. Fessler, MD, PhD
Professor
Department of Neurological Surgery
Rush University Medical Center
Chicago, Illinois, USA

Brandon M. Fox, MD, PhD
Resident Physician
Department of Neurosurgery
Barrow Neurological Institute
Phoenix, Arizona, USA

Paul A. Gardner, MD
Professor and Peter J. Jannetta Endowed Chair
Department of Neurological Surgery
University of Pittsburgh School of Medicine
Pittsburgh, Pennsylvania, USA

Peter Carlos Gerszten, MD, MPH, FACS
Peter E. Sheptak Professor of Neurological Surgery and Radiation Oncology
Vice Chairman for Quality Improvement
Department of Neurological Surgery
University of Pittsburgh Medical Center
Pittsburgh, Pennsylvania, USA

Yohannes Ghenbot, MD, MS
Resident
Department of Neurosurgery
Hospital of the University of Pennsylvania
Philadelphia, Pennsylvania, USA

Atul Goel, MCh
Professor and Head
Department of Neurosurgery
Lilavati Hospital and Research Center;
Professor and Head
Department of Neurosurgery
K. J. Somaiya Medical College and Hospital
Mumbai, Maharashtra, India

Phoebe Greenwald, MD
Resident
Department of Pediatrics
University of Washington
Seattle, Washington, USA

Mehmet Sabri Gurbuz, MD
Associate Professor
Department of Neurological Surgery
University of Wisconsin School of Medicine & Public Health-Madison
Madison, Wisconsin, USA;
Associate Professor
Department of Neurosurgery
İstanbul Medeniyet University
Istanbul, Turkey

Constantinos G. Hadjipanayis, MD, PhD
L. Dade Lunsford Professor of Neurosurgery
Executive Vice-Chair of Neurological Surgery
Director, Center for Image-Guided Neurosurgery
Co-Director, UPMC Brain Tumor Program
University of Pittsburgh School of Medicine
University of Pittsburgh Medical Center (UPMC)
Chair, AANS/CNS Joint Section on Tumors
Director, Brain Tumor Nanotechnology Laboratory, Hillman Cancer Center
University of Pittsburgh Medical Center
Center for Image-Guided Neurosurgery, Department of Neurological Surgery
University of Pittsburgh Medical Center
Pittsburgh, Pennsylvania, USA

Daniel M. Hafez, MD, PhD
Assistant Professor
Department of Neurosurgery
Washington University
St. Louis, Missouri, USA

D. Kojo Hamilton, MD
Professor
Residency Program Director
Director of Neurological Surgery Spine Services
Co-Director of Neurological Surgery Spine Fellowship Program
Department of Neurological Surgery
University of Pittsburgh Medical Center
Pittsburgh, Pennsylvania, USA

Kimberly Harbaugh, MD
Professor
Department of Neurosurgery
Penn State University
Hershey, Pennsylvania, USA

Brynn Alison Hathaway, MD
Resident
Department of Plastic Surgery
Oregon Health and Science University
Portland, Oregon, USA

Ryan M. Hebert, MD
Assistant Professor
Department of Neurosurgery
Yale University School of Medicine
New Haven, Connecticut, USA

Daniel J. Hoh, MD, MBA
Professor
Dunspaugh - Dalton Endowed Professorship
Division Chief, Spine
Department of Neurosurgery
University of Florida
Gainesville, Florida, USA

Steven Blake Housley, MD, MS
Physician-Neurosurgeon
Department of Neurosurgery
Neurosurgical Associates, P.C.
Knoxville, Tennessee, USA

Judy Huang, MD, FAANS
Irving J. & Florence Sherman Professor,
Vice Chair & Program Director
Department of Neurosurgery
Johns Hopkins University School of Medicine
Baltimore, Maryland, USA

Joseph Hudson, MD
Chief Resident
Department of Neurosurgery
University of Pittsburgh Medical Center
Pittsburgh, Pennsylvania, USA

Sakibul Huq, MD
Neurosurgery Resident
Department of Neurological Surgery
University of Pittsburgh Medical Center
Pittsburgh, Pennsylvania, USA

Wataru Ishida, MD
Chief Resident
Department of Neurosurgery
Johns Hopkins Hospital
Baltimore, Maryland, USA

Andrew S. Jack, MD, MSc, FRCSC
Assistant Clinical Professor
Department of Neurosurgery
University of Alberta
Edmonton, Alberta, Canada

Line Jacques, MD, MSc, FRCSC
John Adams Endowed Professorship in
Peripheral Nerve and Pain Management
Professor and Vice Chair
Director of Peripheral Nerve and Pain
Surgery
Department of Neurological Surgery
University of California, San Francisco
San Francisco, California, USA

Kelly Jiang, MS
Medical Student
Department of Neurosurgery
Johns Hopkins School of Medicine
Baltimore, Maryland, USA

Jacob R. Joseph, MD
Associate Professor
Department of Neurosurgery
University of Michigan
Ann Arbor, Michigan, USA

Gregory M Mundis, Jr, MD
Professor
Department of Orthopedic Surgery
Scripps Clinic
La Jolla, California, USA;
President
San Diego Spine Foundation
San Diego, California, USA

Anita Kalluri, BA
Medical Student
Department of Neurosurgery
Johns Hopkins School of Medicine
Baltimore, Maryland, USA

Rafid Kasir, MD
Spine Surgeon
Department of Orthopedic Spine Surgery
San Diego Orthopedic Institute
San Diego, California, USA

Abdullah Keles, MD
Scientist I
Department of Neurological Surgery
University of Wisconsin School of Medicine and Public Health
Madison, Wisconsin, USA

Wasiq Khawar, BA
Research Associate
Department of Neurosurgery
Buffalo General Medical Center
Buffalo, New York, USA;
Medical Student
SUNY Upstate Medical University
Syracuse, New York, USA

Harmon S. Khela, BS
Medical Student
Department of Neurosurgery
Perelman School of Medicine at the University of Pennsylvania
Philadelphia, Pennsylvania, USA

Nora C. Kim, MD
Resident Physician
Department of Neurosurgery
NYU Grossman School of Medicine
New York, New York, USA

Andrew B. Koo, MD
Neurosurgery Resident
Department of Neurosurgery
Yale University School of Medicine
New Haven, Connecticut, USA

Jay I. Kumar, MD
Fellow
Department of Spine Surgery
San Diego Spine Foundation
San Diego, California, USA

Rohit Prem Kumar, MD
Resident
Department of Neurological Surgery
University of Pittsburgh Medical Center
Pittsburgh, Pennsylvania, USA

Rosalind Lai, MD
Assistant Professor
Department of Neurosurgery
University at Buffalo Neurosurgery
Williamsville, New York, USA

Katriel E. Lee, MD
Resident
Department of Neurosurgery
Barrow Neurological Institute
Phoenix, Arizona, USA

Philip S. Lee, MD, PhD, FAANS
Director of Functional Neurosurgery
Department of Neurosurgery
Geisinger Health System
Danville, Pennsylvania, USA

Andrew Legarreta, MD
Chief Resident
Department of Neurosurgery
University of Pittsburgh Medical Center
Pittsburgh, Pennsylvania, USA

Elad I. Levy, MD, MBA
L. Nelson Hopkins Chair, Distinguished Professor, and Professor and Chair
Department of Neurosurgery
Professor
Department of Radiology
Jacobs School of Medicine and Biomedical Sciences
University at Buffalo
Buffalo, New York, USA

Yuping Derek Li, MD
Physician/Surgeon
Department of Neurosurgery
Washington University in St. Louis
St. Louis, Missouri, USA

Jaims Lim, MD
Clinical Endovascular Fellow
Department of Neurosurgery
Jacobs School of Medicine and Biomedical Sciences
University at Buffalo;
Clinical Endovascular Fellow
Department of Neurosurgery
Gates Vascular Institute at Kaleida Health
Buffalo, New York, USA

Joseph R. Linzey, MD, MS
Neurosurgery Resident
Department of Neurosurgery
University of Michigan
Ann Arbor, Michigan, USA

L. Dade Lunsford, MD
Professor
Department of Neurological Surgery;
Director Emeritus
Center for Image-Guided Neurosurgery
University of Pittsburgh School of Medicine
Pittsburgh, Pennsylvania, USA

Mohamed Macki, MD, MPH
Spine Surgeon
Department of Neurosurgery
Cleveland Clinic Foundation
Cleveland, Ohio, USA

Susan E. Mackinnon, MD
Minot Packer Fryer Professor of Plastic Surgery
Director of the Center for Nerve Injury and Paralysis
Department of Plastic and Reconstructive Surgery
Washington University School of Medicine
St. Louis, Missouri, USA

Sonia S. Majid, MD, MPH
Resident
Department of Neurological Surgery
Penn State Milton S. Hershey Medical Center
Hershey, Pennsylvania, USA

Arka N. Mallela, MD, MS
Assistant Professor
Department of Neurological Surgery
Rush University Medical Center
Chicago, Illinois, USA

Charles C. Matouk, MD
Professor
Department of Neurosurgery
Department of Radiology
Yale University School of Medicine
New Haven, Connecticut, USA

Andrew A. McCall, MD
Associate Professor
Vice Chair of Education
Department of Head and Neck Surgery
University of California, Los Angeles
Los Angeles, California, USA

Matthew J. McPheeters, MD, MBA
Neurosurgeon
Department of Surgery
Hennepin Healthcare
Minneapolis, Minnesota, USA

Kaitlyn Melnick, MD
Resident
Department of Neurosurgery
University of Florida
Gainesville, Florida, USA

Aditya M. Mittal, MD
Resident Physician
Department of Neurosurgery
Clinical Neurosciences Center
University of Utah
Salt Lake City, Utah, USA

Andre Monteiro, MD
Resident
Department of Neurological Surgery
University at Buffalo
Jacobs School of Medicine and Biomedical Sciences
Gates Vascular Institute at Kaleida Health
Buffalo, New York, USA

Oliver Mrowczynski, MD, PhD
Resident
Department of Neurosurgery
Penn State
Hershey, Pennsylvania, USA

Debraj Mukherjee, MD, MPH
Associate Professor
Department of Neurosurgery
Johns Hopkins University School of Medicine
Baltimore, Maryland, USA

Ria Mulherkar, MD
Resident Physician
Department of Radiation Oncology
UPMC Hillman Cancer Center
Pittsburgh, Pennsylvania, USA

Jeffrey P. Mullin, MD, MBA
Associate Professor
Director of Spinal Deformity Surgery
Department of Neurosurgery
University at Buffalo
Buffalo, New York, USA

Jonathan Munoz, MD
Resident
Department of Emergency Medicine
University of Florida
Gainesville, Florida, USA

Rijul Nanda, BS
Medical Student
Department of Neurosurgery
Texas A&M School of Engineering Medicine;
Medical Student
Department of Neurosurgery
Houston Methodist Hospital
Houston, Texas, USA

Krishna P. Nayak, BS
Medical Student
Department of Neurosurgery
University of Pittsburgh School of Medicine
Pittsburgh, Pennsylvania, USA

Ajay Niranjan, MD
Professor
Department of Neurological Surgery;
Associate Director
Center for Image-Guided Neurosurgery
University of Pittsburgh
Pittsburgh, Pennsylvania, USA

Kamil W. Nowicki, MD, PhD
Assistant Professor
Department of Neurological Surgery
Columbia University
New York, New York, USA

Enyinna L. Nwachuku, MD
Assistant Professor
Department of Neurological Surgery
Penn State Milton S. Hershey Medical Center
Hershey, Pennsylvania, USA

John Ogunlade, DO
Associate Professor
Taylor Family Department of Neurosurgery
Washington University in St. Louis
St. Louis, Missouri, USA

Luke K. O'Neill, BS
Neurosurgery Research Coordinator
Department of Neurosurgery
Barrow Neurological Institute
Phoenix, Arizona, USA

Paul Park, MD
Professor
Department of Neurosurgery
Semmes-Murphey/University of Tennessee
Memphis, Tennessee, USA

Mitch Paro, MD
Neurosurgery Resident
Department of Neurosurgery
Penn State Health
Hershey, Pennsylvania, USA

Vijay A. Patel, MD
Assistant Professor
Department of Otolaryngology-Head & Neck Surgery
Rady Children's Hospital/UC San Diego
San Diego, California, USA

Neel Patel, MD
Neurosurgeon
Department of Neurosurgery
Doctors Hospital at Renaissance
McAllen, Texas, USA

Rachael M. Payne, MD
Hand Surgery Fellow
Department of Orthopedic Surgery
Baylor College of Medicine
Houston, Texas, USA

Philip L. Perez, MD
Assistant Professor
Department of Otolaryngology-Head & Neck Surgery
University of Pittsburgh Medical Center
Pittsburgh, Pennsylvania, USA

Tritan Plute, BS
Medical Student
Department of Neurological Surgery
University of Pittsburgh
Pittsburgh, Pennsylvania, USA

Sean P. Polster, MD
Assistant Professor
Department of Neurosurgery
University of Chicago
Chicago, Illinois, USA

Sibi Rajendran, MD
Resident
Department of Neurosurgery
Houston Methodist Neurological Institute
Houston, Texas, USA

Kunal P. Raygor, MD
Endovascular Neurosurgery Fellow
Department of Neurosurgery
Jacobs School of Medicine and Biomedical Sciences
University at Buffalo
Buffalo, New York, USA;
Assistant Professor
Department of Neurological Surgery
Vanderbilt University Medical Center
Nashville, Tennessee, USA

Matthew J. Recker, MD
Resident Physician
Department of Neurosurgery
Jacobs School of Medicine and Biomedical Sciences
University at Buffalo
Buffalo, New York, USA;
Assistant Professor
Department of Neurological Surgery
University of Washington
Seattle, Washington, USA

Azeem A. Rehman, MD
Director of Minimally Invasive Spine Surgery
Department of Neurosciences
Intent Medical Group
Arlington Heights, Illinois, USA

Daniela Renedo, MD
Neurosurgery Fellow
Department of Neurosurgery
Yale University School of Medicine
New Haven, Connecticut, USA

Robert C. Rennert, MD
Assistant Professor
Department of Neurosurgery
University of Utah
Salt Lake City, Utah, USA

Jheremy S. Reyes, MD
Research Scholar
Center for Image-Guided Neurosurgery
Department of Neurosurgery
University of Pittsburgh Medical Center
Pittsburgh, Pennsylvania, USA

Renee Reynolds, MD, FAANS, FCNS
Kevin and Janet Gibbons Endowed Chair of Neurosurgery
Department of Neurosurgery
University at Buffalo
Buffalo, New York, USA

Jonathan Riley, MD, MS
Assistant Professor
Department of Neurosurgery
University at Buffalo
Buffalo, New York, USA

Daniel Rivera, BS
Research Scholar
Department of Neurosurgery
University of Pittsburgh Medical Center
Pittsburgh, Pennsylvania, USA;
Medical Student
Department of Neurosurgery
Icahn School of Medicine at Mount Sinai
New York, New York, USA

Elias Rizk, MD, PhD
Professor
Department of Neurosurgery
University of Texas at Austin
Austin, Texas, USA

Benjamin Rodriguez, MD
Resident
Department of Neurosurgery
Barrow Neurological Institute
Phoenix, Arizona, USA

Nicholas R. Rowan, MD
Associate Professor
Department of Otolaryngology-Head and Neck Surgery
Johns Hopkins University School of Medicine
Baltimore, Maryland, USA

Christopher R. Roxbury, MD, MBA
Director, NeuroRhinology and Advanced Endoscopic
Sinus Surgery Fellowship
Department of Otolaryngology
Integrated Surgical Institute
Cleveland Clinic Foundation
Cleveland, Ohio, USA

Joanna M. Roy, MBSS
Postdoctoral Research Fellow
Department of Neurological Surgery
Thomas Jefferson University Hospital
Philadelphia, Pennsylvania, USA

Ryan Sadjadi, MPhil, BA
Medical Student
Department of Orthopaedic Surgery
University of California, San Francisco
San Francisco, California, USA

Shailen G. Sampath, MS
Medical Student
Department of Neurosurgery
Columbia University
New York, New York, USA

Sydney Scanlon, MSc
Department of Neurosurgery
University of Pittsburgh Medical Center
Pittsburgh, Pennsylvania, USA

Henry W.S. Schroeder, MD, PhD
Professor and Chairman
Department of Neurosurgery
University Medicine Greifswald
Greifswald, Germany

Anthony J. Schulien, MD
Resident Physician
Department of Neurological Surgery
University of Pittsburgh
Pittsburgh, Pennsylvania, USA

Bao Y. Sciscent, MD
Department of Neurosurgery
Penn State Milton S. Hershey Medical Center
Hershey, Pennsylvania, USA

Abhidha Shah, MCh
Additional Professor
Department of Neurosurgery
Seth GS Medical College and KEM Hospital;
Consultant Neurosurgeon
Department of Neurosurgery
K.J. Somaiya Hospital and Research Center
Mumbai, Maharashtra, India

Jay Kaushik Shah, DO, MBA
Attending Spine Surgeon
Department of Orthopedic Spine Surgery
New York Presbyterian
New York, New York, USA

Alexander Shin, MD
Orthopedic Surgeon
Department of Orthopedic Surgery
Mayo Clinic
Rochester, Minnesota, USA

Adnan H. Siddiqui, MD, PhD
Professor
Department of Neurosurgery
Jacobs School of Medicine and Biological Sciences
University at Buffalo
Buffalo, New York, USA

Zaid Siddiqui, MD
Assistant Professor
Department of Radiation Oncology
Baylor College of Medicine
Houston, Texas, USA

Isuru Somawardana, BS
Medical Student
Department of Neurosurgery
Texas A&M School of Engineering Medicine;
Medical Student
Department of Neurosurgery
Houston Methodist Hospital
Houston, Texas, USA

Omar Sorour, MD
Resident Physician
Department of Neurosurgery
Tufts Medical Center
Boston, Massachusetts, USA

Robert J. Spinner, MD
Burton M. Onofrio Chair of Neurosurgery
Professor of Neurosurgery, Orthopedics, and Anatomy
Former Chairman of the Department of Neurosurgery
Department of Neurosurgery
Mayo Clinic
Rochester, Minnesota, USA

John C. Flickinger Sr, MD
Professor
Department of Radiation Oncology
University of Pittsburgh School of Medicine
Pittsburgh, Pennsylvania, USA

Shaarada Srivatsa, MD
Resident Physician
Department of Neurosurgery
Cleveland Clinic Foundation
Cleveland, Ohio, USA

Michael J. Strong, MD, PhD
Neurosurgeon
Department of Neurosurgery
Wellstar
Austell, Georgia, USA

Nanthiya Sujijantarat, MD
Assistant Professor
Department of Neurosurgery
Yale University School of Medicine
New Haven, Connecticut, USA

Ali Reza Tafreshi, MD
Resident
Department of Neurosurgery
Geisinger Health System
Danville, Pennsylvania, USA

Khaled Taghlabi, MD
Clinical Research Fellow
Department of Neurosurgery
Houston Methodist Hospital
Houston, Texas, USA

Lee A. Tan, MD
Assistant Professor
Department of Neurological Surgery
University of California, San Francisco
San Francisco, California, USA

Ruby L. Taylor, MD
Research Fellow
Division of Plastic and Reconstructive Surgery
Washington University
St. Louis, Missouri, USA;
Resident Physician
Division of Plastic and Reconstructive Surgery
Oregon Health and Science University
Portland, Oregon, USA

Kelsey Templeton, MD
Resident
Department of Neurosurgery
Yale University School of Medicine
New Haven, Connecticut, USA

Hannah L. Tetreault, BS
Medical Student
Department of Neurosurgery
University of Pittsburgh School of Medicine
Pittsburgh, Pennsylvania, USA

Khoi D. Than, MD
Professor
Department of Neurosurgery
Duke University
Durham, North Carolina, USA

Brianna Carusillo Theriault, MD, PhD
Physician
Department of Neurosurgery
Yale University School of Medicine
New Haven, Connecticut, USA

Erin Thomson, MPAS, PA-C
Physician Assistant
Department of Neurosurgery
University of Pittsburgh Medical Center
Pittsburgh, Pennsylvania, USA

Benjamin Harris Timmins, MD, MS
Surgeon
Department of Plastic and Reconstructive Surgery
Portland VA Medical Center
Portland, Oregon, USA

Ryan C. Turner, MD, PhD
Assistant Professor
Department of Neurosurgery
West Virginia University School of Medicine
Morgantown, West Virginia, USA

Spencer Twitchell, MD
Resident
Department of Neurosurgery
University of Utah
Salt Lake City, Utah, USA

Juan S. Uribe, MD
Professor and Vice Chair, Department of Neurosurgery
Chief, Division of Spinal Disorders
Volker K. H. Sonntag Chair of Spine Research
Department of Neurosurgery
Barrow Neurological Institute
Phoenix, Arizona, USA

Ayesha Akbar Waheed, MBBS
Principal Research Fellow
Director, Undergraduate Intern Program
Department of Neurological Surgery
University of Pittsburgh School of Medicine
Pittsburgh, Pennsylvania, USA

Ayobami Ward, MD, ScM
Resident Physician
Department of Neurosurgery
University of Michigan
Ann Arbor, Michigan, USA

Zachary A. Warren, MD
Associate Professor
Department of Otolaryngology-Head and Neck Surgery
Department of Rhinology
Kaiser Permanente
Houston, Texas, USA

Jon T. Willie, MD, PhD
Associate Professor
Department of Neurological Surgery
Washington University School of Medicine
St. Louis, Missouri, USA;
Associate Professor
Department of Neurosurgery
University of Texas at Austin Dell Medical School
Austin, Texas, USA

Kitty Y. Wu, MD, MSc, FRCSC
Assistant Professor
Division of Plastic Surgery
Mayo Clinic
Rochester, Minnesota, USA

Jang Won Yoon, MD, MSc
Neurosurgeon
Department of Neurosurgery
University of California, San Francisco
San Francisco, California, USA

Xiaoran Zhang, MD, MS
Neurosurgeon
Department of Neurosurgery
Sutter West Bay Medical Group
Danville, California, USA

Pascal O. Zinn, MD, PhD, FAANS
Associate Professor of Neurological Surgery
Director Adult Neurosurgical Oncology
Department of Neurosurgery
UPMC Hillman Cancer Center
Pittsburgh, Pennsylvania, USA

Part I

Cranial

I

1 Convexity Craniotomy

Tritan Plute, Arka N. Mallela, Hussam Abou-Al-Shaar, and Pascal O. Zinn

1.1 Background

- Convexity craniotomies are a principal approach for lesions of various types located on the cerebral convexity.
- Accessible lesions with this approach include supratentorial lesions of any type including extra-axial or intra-axial neoplasms, vascular malformations, intracranial abscesses, epileptic tissue, intracranial hemorrhage, depressed skull fractures, and traumatic bleeds such as subdural or epidural hematomas.
- The convexity craniotomy is a well-utilized approach for various lesions occurring both superficially and deep along the cerebral convexities.
- For the purposes of this chapter, the cerebral convexity is defined as the faces of the frontal, parietal, temporal, and occipital lobe facing the calvarium and not contained in the sylvian fissure or parasagittal regions.[1] It can be performed using both awake and asleep craniotomy procedures and shares some overlap with the parasagittal approach.
- Additionally, craniotomy sizing is widely adjustable from keyhole incisions to larger, hemispheric openings, depending on the pathology and indications.
- The convexity approach is bounded medially by the parasagittal region of the cerebrum that flanks the superior sagittal sinus and defines the parasagittal approach, whereas the inferior limitation of this approach lies at the floor of the middle cranial fossa anteriorly and the tentorium posteriorly.[2]
- The layers of the scalp are crucial to identify as they often provide useful planes for dissection or serve as landmarks. The five layers of the scalp, from superficial to deep, include the overlying skin, a layer of connective tissue, the galea or aponeurosis, a loose connective tissue, and the underlying periosteum.[3] Identification of each layer is critical for the surgeon, as neurovascular structures course through specific layers and oftentimes dictate the plane of optimal dissection.
- Similar to the layers of the scalp, familiarity with the dural layers and their navigation is critical to control operative complications. Tightly adhered to the periosteum is the periosteal layer of the dura, whereas the meningeal layer lies underneath, just above the arachnoid.[4] The distinction between these two layers of dura is critical as they come together to form the dural venous sinuses, which must be carefully avoided during dissection to reduce the risk of intraoperative complications. Also of note, the middle meningeal artery, which arises from the internal maxillary artery, courses over the periosteal dura and serves as the blood supply of the convexity meninges.[5] This is an important anatomical consideration as injury of the middle meningeal artery is a common source of epidural hematoma and can lead to operative complications or be an operative indication itself.
- Intracranially lie numerous cortical and vascular structures that serve as landmarks for the surgeon. On the surface, the sylvian fissure separates the frontal and parietal lobes from the temporal lobe and also serves as the exit point for the M4 branches of the middle cerebral artery (MCA).[2,6] The remaining cortical vasculature of note includes the branches of the M4, and the dural bridging veins that drain the superior sagittal sinus, as injury to these structures can lead to avoidable complications.
- Another important consideration when operating within the convexity is the venous system. A thorough understanding of the cerebral venous system is imperative to avoiding operative morbidity. Concerning the convexity, the two most important veins are the veins of Trolard and Labbé. Both veins arise from the superior sylvian vein that courses through the sylvian fissure.[7] The vein of Labbé typically runs across the temporal lobe and under the occiput, whereas the vein of Trolard courses superiorly over the parietal lobe and terminates in the midline.[7] Both veins may be present in duplicates or exhibit anatomical variations, but the identification and sparing of them is crucial

for one to prevent postoperative complications and intact venous draining.

1.2 Indications and Contraindications

- The convexity craniotomy approach is indicated when a lesion that lies along the cerebral convexity (▶ Fig. 1.1) causes focal neurological deficits, mass effect, or edema that threatens epileptogenicity.[8]
- These lesions typically include supratentorial neoplasms, vascular malformations, epileptic tissue, and spontaneous and traumatic bleeds (▶ Fig. 1.2). The convexity approach may also be utilized to reach deep lesions within the sylvian fissure.

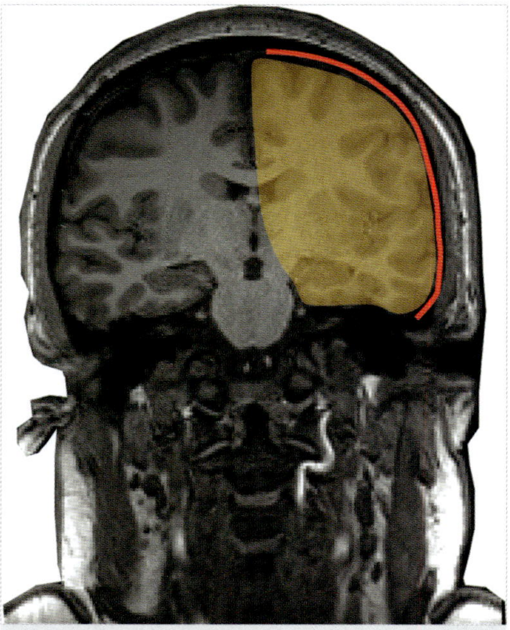

Fig. 1.1 Exposure to access gained for convexity craniotomy.

1.3 Patient Preparation

- The personnel required for this approach include the standard operating room staff of an attending surgeon, a co-surgeon or resident/fellow, a scrub nurse, a circulating nurse, an attending anesthesiologist, a nurse anesthetist, and neurophysiology monitoring personnel. Standard materials for craniotomy are required along with any additional tools needed for treatment of the specific lesion (e.g., operating microscope, neuronavigation, ultrasonic aspiration, stimulator probe, Dopplers, ultrasound, indocyanine green, etc.).
- Following positioning, the navigation system is registered and crossed-checked to the patient as well as neurophysiological monitoring electrodes depending on the desired monitoring technique needed for the procedure.
- The patient's head should be shaved, and the incision area demarcated and infiltrated with a local anesthetic. The area is prepped and draped in a sterile fashion. Once the cranium has been exposed, both visible landmarks and

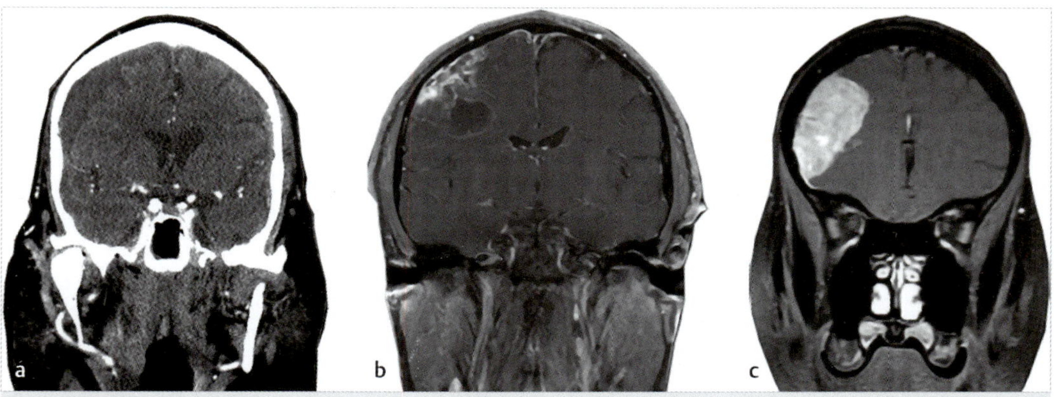

Fig. 1.2 Convexity approach can facilitate access to **(a)** bleeds and **(b, c)** supratentorial tumors.

neuronavigation (if utilized) should be used in conjunction to accurately visualize cortical veins before burr hole sites are planned.

- Landmarks for this approach are primarily useful for identifying the midline and lobes. For example, the coronal suture marks the frontoparietal junction, and the lambdoid suture is useful for identification of the parieto-occipital border.[1] Additionally, the sagittal suture serves as an approximation of the midline.[1] In some cases, the temporalis muscle will have to be reflected downward to perform the craniotomy.

1.4 Patient Positioning

- Patient positioning varies on how anterior/posterior and medial/lateral the lesion is. In general, frontal lesions can be approached in a supine position with varying degrees of head flexion/extension and head turn. Occipital lesions can be approached from a prone position. Intermediate regions, such as the parietal or temporal convexities, can be accessed with the patient in a supine position with head turn or in the lateral position.[8] Head fixation can be achieved either with the Mayfield head holder (or other rigid fixation) or a horseshoe head holder as is dictated by operative needs.

1.5 Technique

- Once the incision lines have been drawn, the craniotomy may be performed in a variety of ways, and similarly dural opening can be variable in the form of a C-shaped, linear, or cruciate opening. This is followed by retraction and dural fixation using tack-up sutures. If phase reversal is deemed necessary, a grid is placed to obtain phase reversal and/or direct cortical stimulation using a probe is performed. If the lesion is at the cortical level, then resection can proceed as normal with careful attention paid to the cortical vasculature and any structures engulfed by the lesion or just inferior to it. For deeper intracerebral lesions, additional tools such as retractors or port-based systems may be required with or without direct subcortical stimulation. The utilization of intraoperative ultrasound is of a great utility in deep-seated lesions, especially smaller ones.
- Once the lesion of interest has been addressed and meticulous hemostasis is achieved, closure is performed according in the standard manner. Drains may be utilized as needed.
- Following closure of the dura, the resected bone flap is fixated to titanium plates and adhered back onto the skull with standard screws. This step must be completed with care to achieve adequate cosmesis of the overlying scalp. The bone flap must be level with the surrounding cranium, particularly in cosmetically sensitive areas such as the forehead or in patients with posterior hairlines.

1.6 Complications

- Complications of the convexity craniotomy can arise at numerous stages of the procedure and can be grouped into several distinct categories.
- Intraoperatively, direct brain injury can occur if one is operating on or near the eloquent cortex; however, vascular complications are more common.
- Arterial injury could involve damage to the anterior, middle, or posterior cerebral artery branches or smaller cortical arteries, while venous injuries can occur on the cortex or around the superior sagittal sinus, potentially leading to air embolism.
- Postoperative complications include stroke, wound infections, abscess formation, and meningitis.
- Common postoperative medical complications include seizure, pulmonary embolism or deep vein thrombosis, postoperative hematoma, and cerebrospinal fluid leak/pseudomeningocele.[8]

1.7 Management Pearls

- This approach is suitable for lesions along the cerebral convexity (see above). For lesions within the sylvian fissure, pterional approaches may be more appropriate, while for those near the midline, the parasagittal or intrahemispheric approach may be better indicated. Posterior fossa lesions may require other approaches as described in other chapters.
- The craniotomy and dural opening can be carried out in a variety of ways so long as care is

taken to prevent injury to the underlying vasculature. Once the brain has been exposed, surface-level lesions may be resected with care taken to avoid vascular injury, excess tissue resection, or traversing of the eloquent cortex. Deeper lesions may require additional dissection or port-based approaches as described in subsequent chapters. Complications include seizure, vascular injury, neurological deficits, air embolus, deep vein thrombosis, pulmonary embolism, and infection, among others.

References

[1] Rhoton AL, Jr. The cerebrum. Neurosurgery. 2002; 51(4) Suppl:S1–S51

[2] Chandra A, Li WA, Stone CR, Geng X, Ding Y. The cerebral circulation and cerebrovascular disease I: anatomy. Brain Circ. 2017; 3(2):45–56

[3] Sharman AM, Kirmi O, Anslow P. Imaging of the skin, subcutis, and galea aponeurotica. Semin Ultrasound CT MR. 2009; 30(6):452–464

[4] Kiliç T, Akakin A. Anatomy of cerebral veins and sinuses. Front Neurol Neurosci. 2008; 23:4–15

[5] Bonasia S, Smajda S, Ciccio G, Robert T. Middle meningeal artery: anatomy and variations. AJNR Am J Neuroradiol. 2020; 41(10):1777–1785

[6] Chauhan P, Rathawa A, Jethwa K, Mehra S. The Anatomy of the Cerebral Cortex. In: Pluta R, ed. Cerebral Ischemia. Brisbane, Australia: Exon Publications; 2021

[7] Rhoton AL, Jr. The cerebral veins. Neurosurgery. 2002; 51(4) Suppl:S159–S205

[8] Asthagiri A, Shaikhouni A, Lonser RR. Surgical management of parasagittal and convexity meningiomas. In: Operative Neurosurgical Techniques. 7th ed. Philadelphia, PA: Elsevier; 2022:267–277

2 Frontotemporal (Pterional) Craniotomy

Aditya M. Mittal, Kamil W. Nowicki, and Xiaoran Zhang

2.1 Background

- Frontotemporal (FT) craniotomy is a workhorse skull base approach for accessing lesions in the anterior and middle cranial fossae, including most anterior circulation aneurysms and some posterior circulation aneurysms, anterior or middle fossa skull base tumors, tumors in the suprasellar cistern, frontal and temporal lobe tumors, arteriovenous malformations (AVMs), and temporal lobe epilepsy.[1]
- This approach is used with patients in the supine position with variable head turning based on target location. Preoperative imaging is necessary to understand the lesion and for tailoring the approach. Potential complication includes frontalis palsy, injury to the temporomandibular joint, temporalis atrophy, cerebrospinal fluid leak, infection, and hemorrhage.

2.2 Indications and Contraindications

- The FT approach is appropriate for most anterior circulation aneurysms and can be appropriate for some posterior circulation aneurysm such as basilar apex aneurysms. Lesions located in the suprasellar cistern and frontal and temporal lobes can be readily accessed using FT.[2]
- FT craniotomy is a versatile approach with very few anatomical contraindications. As with most neurosurgical procedures, preoperative evaluation is needed to ensure the patient's suitability to undergo anesthesia from a cardiopulmonary perspective.[3]

2.3 Patient Preparation

- Preoperative workup is dependent on the type of lesion being treated. For most tumors, a brain magnetic resonance imaging (MRI) with and without intravenous (IV) contrast is the minimum imaging required. For lesions involving eloquent brain, functional MRI or diffusion tensor imaging fiber tracking can be utilized. For skull base tumor, a computed tomography (CT) angiogram can be useful for evaluating the relationship of the lesion to major vessels. In our experience, a high-definition CT scan often provides the best accuracy for neuronavigation and can be useful for the cases where precise neuronavigation is needed. CT is particularly useful for avoidance of frontal sinus violation. For vascular lesions such as aneurysms and AVMs, a catheter-based diagnostic angiogram can be useful to better understand lesion structure and flow dynamics.
- If patients have a history or physical examination findings suggestive of cervical spine stenosis, consider a preoperative cervical MRI and/or preposition neural monitoring to decrease the risk of spinal cord injury from head positioning.
- Anesthesiologists with neurological experience are preferred for all neurosurgical procedures. Neurophysiological monitoring including somatosensory evoked potentials (SSEPs) and motor evoked potentials (MEPs) can be used when appropriate.
- A FT craniotomy can be performed either under general anesthesia with endotracheal intubation or under monitored anesthesia care (MAC) with local scalp blocks for awake craniotomies.
- At a minimum, adequate IV access in the form of two 16- or 18-gauge IV lines and continuous blood pressure monitoring (i.e., arterial line) are required.
- Additional adjuncts such as defibrillator pacer pads, central lines, and femoral catheter sheath are utilized on an as needed basis. Brain relaxation can be achieved via hyperventilation, diuresis with mannitol and/or furosemide, or through release of CSF.

2.4 Patient Positioning

- The patient is positioned supine with 15 to 20 degrees of reverse Trendelenburg to allow for effective venous drainage. Head fixation is accomplished using a rigid head clamp (such as a Mayfield head holder).
- The head is then placed in gentle extension and rotated contralateral to the lesion.

- Rotation can be anywhere between 15 and 45 degrees dependent on location of the lesion. Minimal (15 degrees) rotation is needed for midline lesions such as anterior communicating artery aneurysms, where more (45 degrees) rotation is needed for lateral lesions such as middle cerebral artery aneurysms.
- In patients with immobile cervical spine or with cervical stenosis, shoulder rolls can be used to achieve the necessary rotation at the cost of potentially elevating the shoulder into the operative zone.

2.5 Technique

- A curvilinear incision is marked extending from the widow's peak to 1 cm in front of the tragus at the level of the zygoma. The incision can be on or behind the hairline depending on surgeon preference and the posterior extent of the lesion.
- For the cases where frontal sinus violation is expected or likely, a pericranial flap should be harvested (▶ Fig. 2.1a). After skin incision, the temporalis muscle and scalp flap can be retracted away together as a single myocutaneous flap or as a differential flap via the subfascial or interfascial approach.
- The single myocutaneous flap can be retracted using fish hook retractors anteriorly.
- The interfascial approach requires incision of the temporal fascia at the upper edge of the fat pad, which can then mobilize the superficial layer of the temporal fascia with the facial nerve branches.
- The subfascial technique elevates the deep surface of the temporal fascia, allowing mobilization of the superficial, deep temporalis fascia and fat pad.
- All three approaches aim to prevent injury to the frontalis branch of the facial nerve, which travels within the areolar tissue to prevent frontalis palsy.
- Differential flaps allow for added downward retraction of the temporalis muscle, allowing for improved anterior exposure and skull base visualization (▶ Fig. 2.1b, c).
- Preservation of the superficial temporal artery (STA) is important in preserving the blood supply to the scalp and help with postoperative healing but can be sacrificed if necessary.
- An FT craniotomy is started with at least one burr hole placed at the pterion. Additional burr holes can be placed on the frontal and temporal bones if there is concern for dura adhesions. The bone flap is made using a craniotome that follows the temporalis incision posteriorly and varies in extent depending on location of the pathology to be treated (▶ Fig. 2.1d). For lesions requiring a subfrontal approach, the sphenoid wing can be thinned with a diamond burr to improve subfrontal visualization. It is important to preserve the dura during the craniotomy. A curvilinear incision is made on the dura, which is then reflected. Additional brain relaxation can be achieved at this point by following the frontal dura toward the suprasellar cistern and opening the cistern to allow for CSF egress.

2.6 Postoperative Care

- Following the procedure, patients should be admitted into the neurosurgical intensive care unit. Patient length of stay (LOS) can vary depending on the severity of their pathology. Elective treatment of tumors or aneurysms generally report a LOS of up to 3 days postoperatively.
- In case a patient's aneurysm ruptures intraoperatively or postoperatively, the patient's LOS may reach up to 1 month and require close neurological monitoring for vasospasm, delayed cerebral infarction, or other complications because of subarachnoid hemorrhage.[4]

2.7 Complications

- Complications can vary and are largely dependent on the pathology being treated. Treatment of an aneurysm risks intraoperative or postoperative aneurysmal rupture. Other complications are not unique to the FT approach and include infection, stroke, seizure, and anesthetic complications.

2.8 Management Pearls

- The FT craniotomy is a workhorse skull base approach for accessing lesions in the anterior and middle cranial fossa.

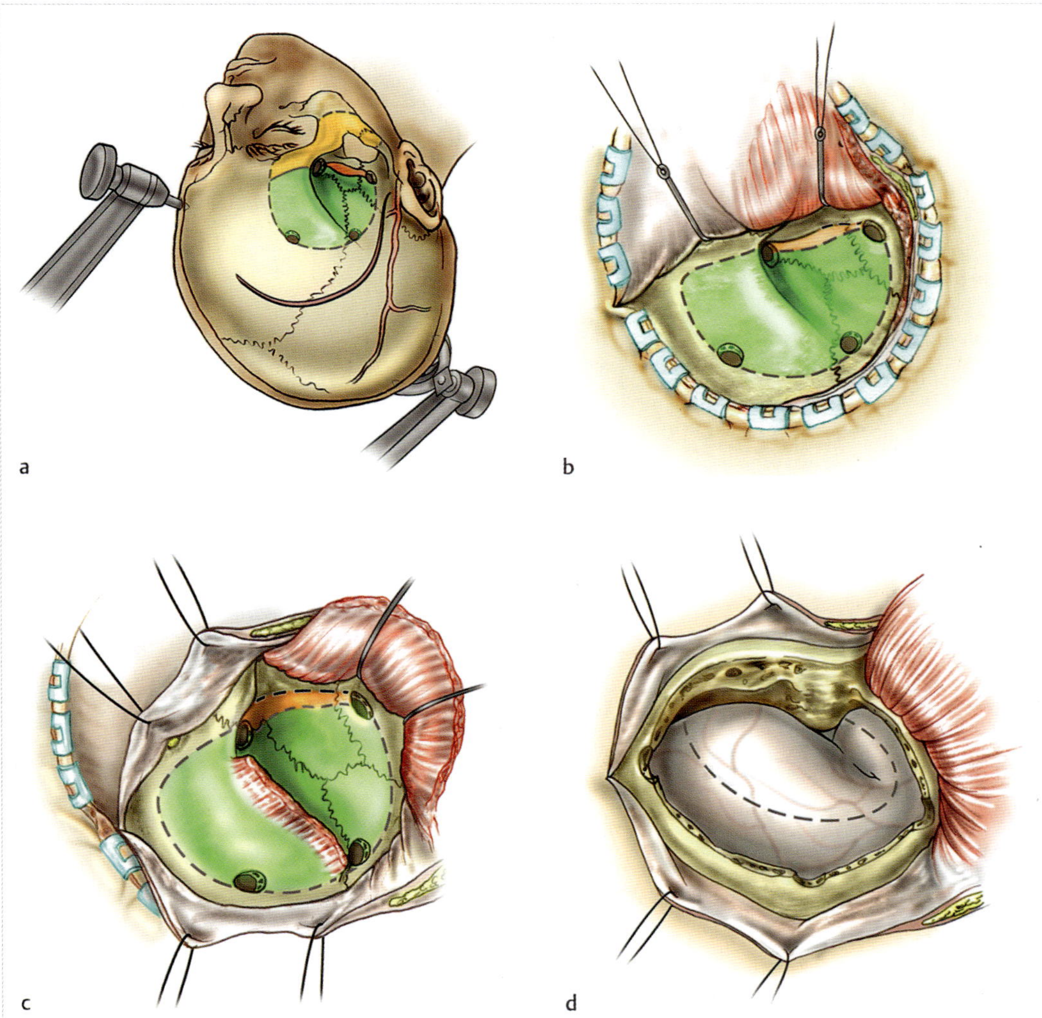

Fig. 2.1 **(a)** Standard pterional approach (*green*) with orbitozygomatic extension (*yellow*). **(b)** Standard pterional approach with muscle retraction and burr holes. **(c)** Standard pterional approach with a more anterior and inferior reflection of the muscle. **(d)** Dural incision. (Reproduced from Eddleman CS, Rahme RJ, Aoun SG, Fishman AJ, Batjer HH, Bendok BR. Clipping of Complex and Giant Aneurysms. In: Bendok B, Naidech A, Walker M, Batjer H, ed. Hemorrhagic and Ischemic Stroke: Medical, Imaging, Surgical and Interventional Approaches. 1st Edition. New York: Thieme; 2011. Illustration by Jennifer Pryll.)

- Head rotation, temporalis dissection, and the amount of sphenoid wing drilling should be tailored to patient's specific pathology to achieve optimal exposure.
- Possible complications from a FT approach include injury to the frontalis branch of the facial nerve, injury to the temporomandibular joint, frontal sinus violation, and cosmetic defect from temporalis atrophy.
- As the FT approach requires dissection of the temporalis muscle, patients may have difficulty with mastication or temporalis atrophy following the procedure.[5] Injury to the temporomandibular joint is also a possibility. The frontalis branch of the facial nerve along with the STA can be damaged during the procedure, resulting in frontalis palsy or suboptimal wound healing with possible dehiscence, respectively.[6,7,8]

References

[1] Yasargil MG, Fox JL. The microsurgical approach to intracranial aneurysms. Surg Neurol. 1975; 3(1):7–14

[2] Bernardo A, Evins AI. Anterolateral routes to the skull base-the frontotemporal approaches and exposure of the sellar and parasellar regions. World Neurosurg. 2023; 172:131–145

[3] Sivanaser V, Manninen P. Preoperative assessment of adult patients for intracranial surgery. Anesthesiol Res Pract. 2010; 2010

[4] Keegan J, Hwang D. Principles of neurocritical care. In: Salardini A, Biller J, eds. The Hospital Neurology Book. New York, NY: McGraw-Hill Education; 2016

[5] Kadri PA, Al-Mefty O. The anatomical basis for surgical preservation of temporal muscle. J Neurosurg. 2004; 100(3): 517–522

[6] Aoki N. Incision of facial nerve branch at aneurysm surgery. J Neurosurg. 1987; 66(3):482

[7] Ammirati M, Spallone A, Ma J, Cheatham M, Becker D. Preservation of the temporal branch of the facial nerve in pterional-transzygomatic craniotomy. Acta Neurochir (Wien). 1994; 128(1–4):163–165

[8] Ammirati M, Spallone A, Ma J, Cheatham M, Becker D. An anatomicosurgical study of the temporal branch of the facial nerve. Neurosurgery. 1993; 33(6):1038–1043, discussion 1044

3 Parasagittal Craniotomy

Kelsey Templeton, Brianna Carusillo Theriault, Charles C. Duncan, and Veronica L. Chiang

3.1 Background

- This chapter will explore the techniques used for parasagittal craniotomies for lesions in the parafalcine, interhemispheric, and intra- or paraventricular regions. We will also discuss the preoperative, intraoperative, and postoperative considerations.

3.2 Indications and Contraindications

3.2.1 Indications

- Parafalcine tumors (▶ Fig. 3.1)—most typically meningioma but also including lesions such as dural-based lesions arising from the linings of the superior sagittal sinus (SSS).
- Access to the interhemispheric space—most commonly for falcine meningiomas but also for medial hemispheric lesions—tumors, vascular lesions, abscesses, subdural hemorrhage, or placement of monitoring grids for epilepsy.
- Extracerebral approach to intra-/paraventricular tumors of the lateral and third ventricles (▶ Fig. 3.2).

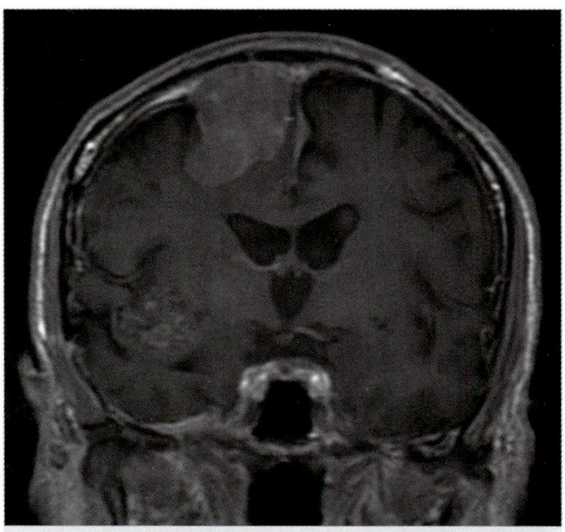

Fig. 3.1 Coronal postcontrast T1-weighted MRI depicting a medially located meningioma.

3.2.2 Contraindications

- Tumors with possible involvement or invasion of the SSS.
- The lesion demonstrates extensive invasion of the overlying bone.

3.3 Informed Consent: Expected Benefits and Potential Complications To Be Mentioned

- Risk of venous injuries or infarctions associated with the manipulation of the SSS and its associated venous structures.
- Risk of venous drainage removal leading to a venous infarction.
- Risk for serious complications that may permanently alter a patient's ability to perform everyday tasks (including disconnection syndrome from callosotomy, anterograde amnesia from forniceal injury, or akinetic mutism from cingulate injury).

3.4 Instruments

- High-speed drill.
- Frameless stereotaxy.
- Mayfield head holder.
- Yasargil bar and Greenberg retractor.
- Headlight.
- Loupes.
- Bipolar cautery and Bovie cautery.
- Microscope.
- Precordial Doppler—if opening is across the SSS.
- Neuromonitoring if the lesion is along the middle third of the anterolateral plane.

3.5 Patient Preparation

- Computed tomography (CT) of the head without contrast for overlying bony involvement to determine the necessity of the craniotomy.
- Magnetic resonance imaging (MRI) with and without contrast should be obtained to define

the tumor and visualize relevant anatomy (► Fig. 3.3 and ► Fig. 3.4).

- MR venography (MRV) or CT venography (CTV) to look at SSS occlusion/involvement, cortical and venous displacement, or cortical or scalp venous collateral drainage.
- A surgeon may also consider CT angiography (CTA) or digital subtraction angiography (DSA) for this as well as evaluating the feeding arterial supply and venous drainage profile, especially for surgical targets of vascular pathologies (► Fig. 3.5).
- Anesthesia should have the following prepared: standard antibiotics, dexamethasone, mannitol, furosemide, levetiracetam, and hydration.

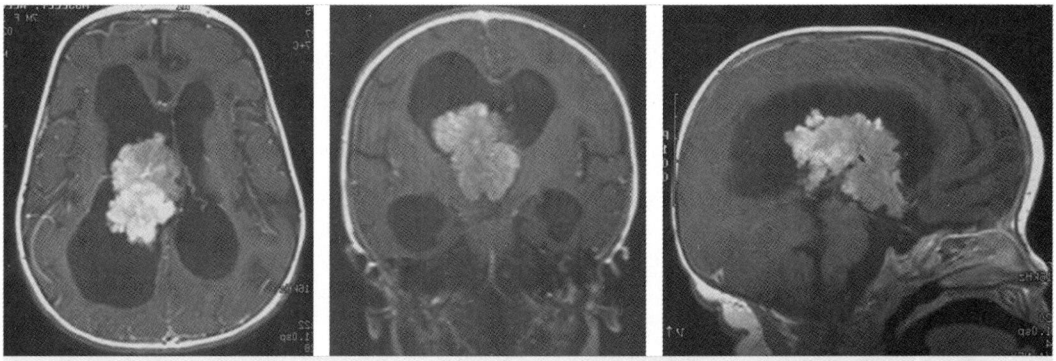

Fig. 3.2 Postcontrast T1-weighted MR images depicting large intraventricular mass with associated ventriculomegaly.

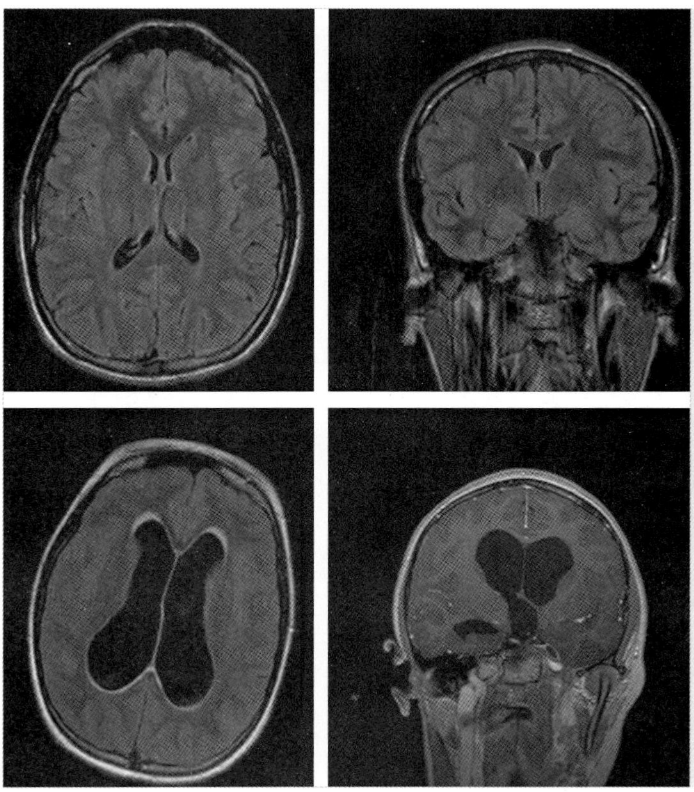

Fig. 3.3 Top panel: Axial and coronal views of T1-weighted MRI sequences demonstrating lateral and third ventricles of typical caliber for a healthy adult. The bottom panel images demonstrate significant ventriculomegaly of the lateral and third ventricles. The anterior and posterior interhemispheric approaches may be used to access the ventricular system in the absence of ventriculomegaly.

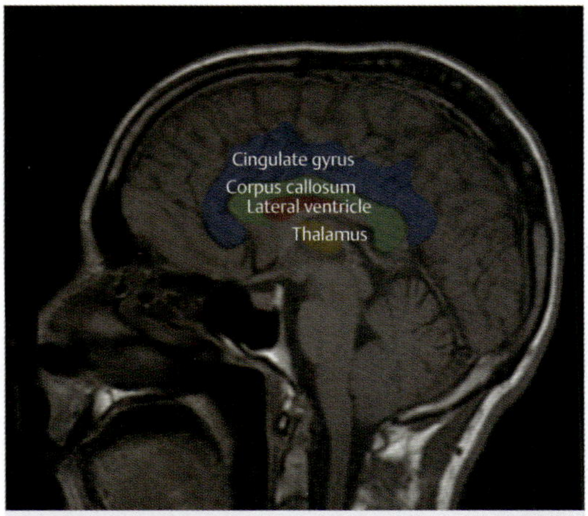

Fig. 3.4 Midline, sagittal T1-weighted MRI with highlighted cingulate gyrus, corpus callosum, lateral ventricle, and thalamus as relevant anatomy to the interhemispheric transcallosal approach to intraventricular lesions.

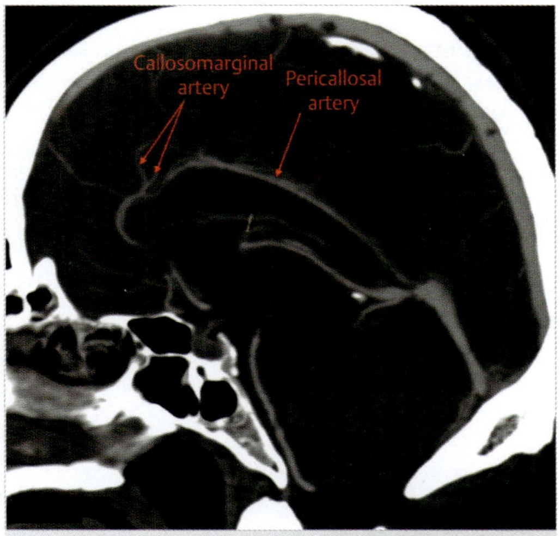

Fig. 3.5 Sagittal CT angiogram depicting midline vascular structures, including the pericallosal and callosomarginal arteries.

3.6 Patient Positioning

- Stereotactic navigation can be used to assist with positioning and planning of the incision by defining the margin of the lesion, as well as the SSS (**Video 3.1**).
- Lesions within the anterior third of the anteroposterior plane:
  - Incision should be in front of the coronal suture.
  - The patient should be positioned supine with the head neutral, or with slight flexion for a bicoronal incision.
- Lesions in the middle third:
  - A **U**-shaped skin incision is made with the base ipsilateral to tumor, with incision extending at least 2 cm across the midline while centered on the tumor over a region between displaced draining veins.
  - The patient should be positioned in the semi-sitting position or the lateral position with the vertex raised and the tumor side down to allow the brain to fall away from the tumor to decrease necessary brain retraction.
- Lesions in the posterior third:
  - A **U**-shaped incision is made suboccipitally, with a flap that has a width exceeding 1.5 times the height. A vascularized pedicle should always be maintained.
  - The patient can be positioned prone with head neutral or three-fourths prone with the head lateral.
- The head should be secured with a fixed head frame with at least three points of fixation to the skull. One point of fixation should be on the ipsilateral temple to minimize interference of the frame while also ensuring the side holding more weight of the head has a higher number of points of fixation.

3.7 Technique

- Bone flap (**Video 3.1**):
  - For complete resection, the bone will need to be removed as anywhere that bone bleeds excessively is likely to be fed by the tumor.
  - If there is no excessive bleeding, but there is hyperostosis, plan a flap based on the surgical approach only and drill off the inner table prior to replacement of the bone flap.
  - Use of neuronavigation should ensure the bone flap extends at least 2 cm beyond dural tails.
  - If the frontal sinus will likely be opened, a pericranial flap will be needed for closure.

- Tumors that do not invade the sinus:
  - Two or three burr holes can be made directly over the sinus, with one to two burr holes placed on the lateral side of the bone flap.
  - The dura or tumor can then be sharply dissected from the bone to ensure that the tumor is not torn from its underlying vascularity.
- Tumors that invade the sinus:
  - Two to three burr holes should be placed on either side of the SSS and one to two burr holes lateral to the tumor plus one to two burr holes on the contralateral side to expose the contralateral side of the sinus.
  - The craniotomy should be removed in two or three pieces, with the lateral portions removed first, followed by the portion over the sinus.
  - The last bony cuts of the craniotomy should be those directly over the sinus to allow for quick elevation of the bone flap in the event of bleeding.
  - Copious irrigation and Gelfoam should be ready to place over the sinus to control hemorrhage and avoid potential air emboli.
- Dural opening:
  - It should be **C**-shaped, starting furthest away from the SSS.
  - The dura should be opened 1 cm beyond the outer edge of the tumor. The dural resection medially occurs at the edge of the SSS, if the SSS is not to be resected.
  - The edge of the sinus can be sutured closed using running 4–0 Nurolon.
- Surgical resection:
  - Internal debulking of the tumor initially with concomitant use of bipolar electrocautery and suction, or with the Cavitron Ultrasonic Surgical Aspirator (CUSA), followed then by separation of the tumor from the surrounding brain.
  - If only the portion of tumor outside the SSS is being removed, then neuronavigation should be used to ensure that the dural plane is not crossed.
  - If the planning is to sacrifice the SSS, then the dura will also need to be opened on the contralateral side in a small **C**-shaped fashion and dissection down the contralateral falx is needed to expose the region of the SSS to be removed.
  - Upon completion, the dural opening can be closed with a dural patch, followed by possible mesh cranioplasty or replacement of the original bone flap with the inner table shaved down.

3.8 Postoperative Care

- The patient should be monitored postoperatively in the neurointensive care unit for observation particularly for venous injury.
- Postoperative imaging with a head CT should be obtained and venous injury should be suspected if CT shows progressively worsening edema or hemorrhage into adjacent brain.
- If venous injury is suspected, MRV or CTV is utilized for diagnosis. The patient should be kept hydrated with a hematocrit goal above 30 and low-dose mannitol at 30 mL/h.
- The patient should be monitored for 2 to 4 days during the window of risk of venous injury or infarct.
- Steroids may be administered for managing vasogenic edema.
- Antiseizure medications are often used depending on the location and pathology of the lesion.
- Hypertension or hypotension should be avoided, as well as overmedication with sedatives such as narcotics that would affect the ability to follow a patient's neurological examination.

3.9 Complications

- Venous injuries or infarctions associated with the manipulation of the SSS and its associated venous structures.
- Injury to the SSS.
- Venous drainage removal leading to a venous infarction.
- Arterial injury.
- Subdural or epidural hematoma.
- Bone flap infection.
- Seizures—depending on the location and pathology of the lesion.

3.10 Management Pearls

- It is imperative to notify anesthesia prior to removal of the bone so that they may lower the head if needed and monitor for cardiovascular instability.
- In the event of injury to the sinus, avoid the use of bipolar electrocautery as it will cause dural edges to shrink and expand the tear.

4 Temporal Craniotomy

Jheremy S. Reyes, Krishna P. Nayak, Anita Kalluri, Sydney Scanlon, Kelly Jiang, Othman Bin-Alamer, Meghana Bhimreddy, Benjamin Rodriguez, Nancy Abu-Bonsrah, Sakibul Huq, Judy Huang, and Constantinos G. Hadjipanayis

4.1 Background

- Temporal craniotomy is a workhorse neurosurgical approach through the temporal bone of the skull that provides access to the temporal lobe, mesial temporal structures, lateral aspect of the thalamus, and basal cisterns.[1,2,3,4] Its counterpart, the subtemporal craniotomy, provides additional access to the middle fossa floor, upper clivus, and basal cisterns.

4.2 Indications and Contraindications

- Extra-axial tumors (e.g., meningiomas and schwannomas).
- Intra-axial tumors (e.g., gliomas; **Video 4.1**).
- Vascular lesions (e.g., cavernous malformations, arteriovenous malformations, aneurysms, and intraparenchymal hemorrhages; **Video 4.2**).
- Epilepsy (with multiple possible approaches, such as temporal lobectomy or selective amygdalohippocampectomy).[4,5,6,7,8,9,10,11,12,13,14]
- Trauma.
- Extensions to the temporal approach may be utilized to gain access to additional areas:
  - Pterional craniotomy for lesions extending superior to the sylvian fissure.
  - Extended middle fossa approach for lesions that extend deep into the middle fossa, such as those in the internal auditory canal, and to access the prepontine clivus and superior cerebellopontine angle.
  - Lateral orbitotomy for lesions in the dorsal, anterior, lateral, or inferior aspects of the orbit.
- Consider patient functional status, medical comorbidities, radiological findings, anatomical variants, expectations, and anticipated outcomes; multidisciplinary discussion involving neuroradiology, radiation oncology, and neuro-oncology may be beneficial to determine the best treatment plan for a given patient.[7,13,15]

4.3 Instruments

- Mayfield clamp.
- Perforator or other drill.
- Kerrison punches or rongeurs.
- Penfield 3.
- Craniotome.
- No. 15 blade.
- Metzenbaum or tenotomy scissors.
- Bipolar cautery and hemostatic agents.
- Titanium plating systems.
- Depending on the indication for surgery, intraoperative adjuncts such as the microscope or exoscope, neuronavigation, neurophysiological monitoring including subcortical motor mapping, ultrasound, and fluorescence guidance are used.

4.4 Patient Preparation

- Functional magnetic resonance imaging (MRI) scan or a magnetoencephalogram (MEG) can help determine language dominance and localization of Wernicke's area involving the superior temporal gyrus. For lesions in close proximity to the eloquent cortex, preoperative resting-state or task-based functional MRI can be used for functional mapping, the latter of which can help in understanding language dominance.
- Diffusion tensor imaging (DTI) and tractography can help localize adjacent medial corticospinal motor tracts traveling through the posterior limb of the internal capsule and optic radiations involving the posterior temporal lobe.
- Comprehensive assessment of all arterial and venous structures along the surgical trajectory should be performed to avoid vascular injury.
- In select instances, cerebrospinal fluid (CSF) diversion can be considered to promote brain relaxation, minimize need for brain retraction, and facilitate intra- and extradural dissection; this is typically accomplished through lumbar drain placement and external ventricular drainage.[13,14,15,16]

- Perioperative medications include the following:
  - Dexamethasone for neuroprotection and to minimize postoperative edema.
  - Mannitol for osmotic diuresis to achieve temporal lobe relaxation.
  - Seizure prophylaxis (most commonly with levetiracetam).
  - Antibiotic prophylaxis (most commonly with cefazolin).

4.5 Patient Positioning

- The patient is placed supine with a bump under the ipsilateral shoulder and hip to minimize neck strain (▶ Fig. 4.1a, b).
- The head is turned away from the surgical site and positioned in three-point fixation with the Mayfield clamp with a slight downward tilt to facilitate gravity retraction and venous drainage.
- Avoid nonphysiologic neck rotation, as this may compromise venous return and increase postoperative pain.
- Upper extremities should be padded to minimize pressure injuries and draped over the torso or by the patient's ipsilateral side.
- Lateral rather than supine positioning should be considered for older patients, patients with a large body habitus, and patients with cervical spondylosis.

4.6 Technique

- Skin incision is planned based on the required surgical access to the temporal lobe (anterior, middle, or posterior temporal lobe lesions) and middle fossa (▶ Fig. 4.1c, d):
  - Access to the superior or middle temporal gyri necessitates a small curvilinear incision; in these cases, the lower limb starts anterior to the tragus and the curve starts directly above the pinna, the superior end of the curve reaches the superior temporal line, and the anterior end reaches the hairline (▶ Fig. 4.1c).

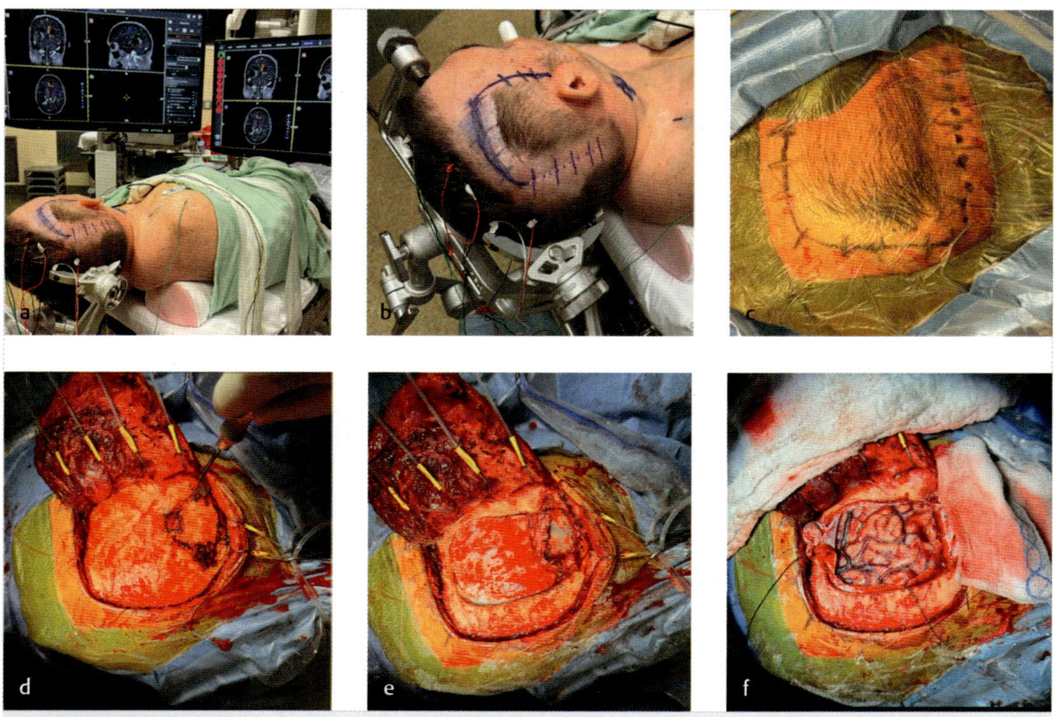

Fig. 4.1 **(a, b)** Patient positioning for redo temporal craniotomy. Exoscope monitors are placed in ergonomically favorable positions for the surgeon. **(c)** Horseshoe-shaped skin incision. **(d)** Elevation of myocutaneous flap. **(e)** Completion of craniotomy. **(f)** Dural opening and tack-up to facilitate temporal lobe visualization.

  - Cases requiring access to the temporal pole may benefit from a reverse question mark incision.[17,18,19,20]
  - For lesions involving the middle or posterior temporal lobe, a trapdoor incision is beneficial; it is centered over the external auditory canal.
- At least one burr hole is made with a perforator or other drill bit just above the root of the zygoma. Multiple other burr holes may be made as desired to facilitate careful dural dissection, especially with a trapdoor incision. Burr hole(s) can be extended with Kerrison punches or rongeurs (▶ Fig. 4.1e).
- The dura is dissected off the inner table of the calvarium using a Penfield 3 (▶ Fig. 4.1f).
- A craniotome is used to complete the craniotomy and subsequent bone flap elevation.
- The dura is carefully incised with a no. 15 blade and subsequently opened in the desired fashion using Metzenbaum or tenotomy scissors.
- Dural closure is ideally performed in a watertight fashion using a running suture when possible; for inadequate dural closure, use of dural substitutes for onlays or duraplasties may be considered.
- Bone flap is replaced and secured using titanium plating systems. Bone grafts or other sealant materials may be added if desired. If the mastoid air cells are exposed, they must be waxed to avoid a CSF leak.
- Incision is then reapproximated in layers, with careful approximation of the muscle, fascia, galea, and skin, to promote wound healing and satisfactory cosmetic outcome.[12,19,20,21,22,23,24,25,26,27]
- Use of a subgaleal drain or headwrap may be considered based on surgeon preference.

4.7 Postoperative Care

- Surgical site infection is avoided through strict aseptic and antiseptic technique, and prophylactic antibiotics (typically cefazolin or a similar agent with gram-positive coverage).[11,28,29,30,31,32]
- Patients may be initially monitored in the intensive care unit prior to transfer to the neurosurgical ward.
- Patients should be kept well hydrated to avoid venous infarction and vasospasm and placed on seizure prophylaxis with antiepileptic drugs for at least 1 week postoperatively.

4.8 Complications

- Injury may occur from damage to the superficial temporal artery (STA) or facial nerve during surgery. If the STA is affected, the risk of a wound-healing problem rises due to loss of the main blood supply of the myocutaneous flap.
- Sacrifice of veins should be avoided when possible to avoid venous infarcts.
- Care must be taken to avoid any injury to the vein of Labbe, which courses into the transverse sinus. Gelatin sponges or cottonoids can be placed on this vein in order to protect it.[3]
- If a dural sinus injury is encountered, it can be managed with packing, tamponade, and/or primary repair.
- Temporal lobe retraction should be minimized with a preference for gravity retraction. Fixed retraction should be avoided if possible.
- The temporal lobe contains the eloquent cortex involved with language in the perisylvian region and medially is adjacent to eloquent white matter tracts and hippocampal structures that should be carefully considered in approach planning to minimize postoperative neuropsychologic and visual deficits.
- Intraoperative neuromonitoring is critical for detecting and preventing inadvertent neural injuries; this may include some combination of somatosensory and motor evoked potentials, and in cases of awake craniotomy, language mapping.
- After execution of the procedure, there is potential for CSF leakage. Placing adipose tissue as a barrier during closure can prevent this complication.
- Thromboembolic complications are mitigated through early mobilization, sequential compression devices, and chemical prophylaxis.[33,34,35]
- Other general postsurgical complications include bone flap infection, soft tissue infections, empyema, extradural abscesses, cosmetic disfigurement, malocclusion, and trismus.[1]

4.9 Management Pearls

- The root of the zygoma is where the zygoma connects to the squamous part of the temporal bone; this key landmark is an external reference for the middle fossa floor.

- With each skin incision, the STA should be considered and preserved through careful dissection above the superficial temporal fascia. The STA typically lies one fingerbreadth anterior to the tragus, runs above the superficial temporal fascia, and bifurcates into its frontal and parietal branches approximately 5 cm above the zygoma.[1,11] The STA travels over the posterior zygomatic root before dividing into anterior and posterior branches, which run along the superficial temporal fascia with the corresponding vein and auriculotemporal nerve.
- The facial nerve is an important consideration during exposure; branches of the facial nerve course over the zygoma and under the superficial temporal fascia.[10,12]
- The vein of Labbe, also known as the inferior anastomotic vein, is the largest superficial vein on the lateral surface of the brain that connects the sylvian venous system to the transverse sinus. Its identification on preoperative imaging and intraoperative preservation are essential,[12,13,14] and special care should be taken to avoid it. It will usually be visualized at the posterior margin of the craniotomy.[1] This is particularly relevant in the cases requiring posterior subtemporal exposure.[16,17,18]
- In the cases where the dominant posterior superior temporal gyrus is involved, an awake craniotomy can be considered for language mapping with direct cortical stimulation.

References

[1] Rao D, Le RT, Fiester P, Patel J, Rahmathulla G. An illustrative review of common modern craniotomies. J Clin Imaging Sci. 2020; 10:81

[2] Cohen-Gadol AA. Temporal/Subtemporal Craniotomy. In: Neurosurgical Atlas

[3] Greenberg MS. Temporal craniotomy. In: Handbook of Neurosurgery. 8th ed. New York, NY: Thieme; 2020:1456–1459

[4] Nader R, Gragnaniello C, Berta S, Sabbagh A, Levy M, eds. Neurosurgery Tricks of the Trade: Cranial. New York, NY: Thieme; 2014

[5] Peraud A, Ibel R. Controversies in the treatment of arachnoid cysts with special emphasis on temporal arachnoid cysts. In: Advances and Technical Standards in Neurosurgery. Cham: Springer International Publishing; 2023:175–192

[6] Swanson J, Oetojo W, Uram Z, et al. Treatment of tegmen dehiscence using a middle fossa approach and autologous temporalis fascia graft: outcomes from a single center. Clin Neurol Neurosurg. 2022; 219(107331):107331

[7] Shenoy VS, Sekhar LN. Orbitozygomatic transsylvian and subtemporal transzygomatic approaches for clipping of basilar tip aneurysms: 2-dimensional operative video. Oper Neurosurg (Hagerstown). 2023; 25(1):e23–e24

[8] Soto JM, Feng D, Sun H, et al. Novel decompressive hemicraniectomy technique for traumatic brain injury: technical note. World Neurosurg. 2021; 146:15–19[Internet]

[9] Schwam ZG, Mavrommatis M, Gidumal S, et al. The role of lumbar drains in the perioperative management of primary spontaneous temporal lobe encephaloceles and cerebrospinal fluid leaks. Otol Neurotol. 2024; 45(4):404–409

[10] Sindou M, Guenot M. Surgical anatomy of the temporal lobe for epilepsy surgery. In: Advances and Technical Standards in Neurosurgery. Vienna: Springer; 2003:315–343

[11] Kim YB, Lee KS. Subtemporal approach. In: July J, Wahjoepramono E, eds. Neurovascular Surgery. Singapore: Springer; 2019

[12] Chaddad-Neto F, Silva da Costa MD. Surgical anatomy of the temporal lobe. In: Microneuroanatomy and Surgery. Cham: Springer International Publishing; 2022:55–103

[13] Lau R, Malhotra AK, McAndrews MP, Kongkham P. Subcortical language localization using sign language and awake craniotomy for dominant posterior temporal glioma resection in a hearing-impaired patient. Acta Neurochir (Wien). 2023; 165(6):1665–1669

[14] Graziano F, Scalia G, Paolini F, et al. "The double S" technique: subfascial dissection and temporalis muscle splitting to prevent cerebrospinal fluid leak and maximize surgical exposure. J Craniofac Surg. 2023; 34(3):1067–1070

[15] Seçer M, Çam İ, Gökbel A, et al. Effects of modified osteoplastic pterional craniotomy on temporal muscle volume and frontal muscle nerve function. J Neurol Surg B Skull Base. 2021; 83(5): 554–558

[16] Sarmento SA, Rabelo NN, Figueiredo EG. Minimally invasive technique (nummular craniotomy) for mesial temporal lobe epilepsy: a comparison of 2 approaches. World Neurosurg. 2020; 134:e636–e641]

[17] Hyakutake Y, Shibahara I, Toyoda M, et al. Frontotemporal craniotomy with skin incision along the superior temporal line outside the hairline in bald male patients with temporal gliomas. Neurosurg Rev. 2023; 46(1):296

[18] Rai SKR, Gajbhiye NKS, Mahore A, et al. Anchoring the temporalis muscle with an intact fascial layer along the superior temporal line in pterional craniotomy: a technical note. World Neurosurg. 2022; 164:388–392

[19] Finger G, Kaul VF, Adunka OF, Prevedello DM. Subfascial dissection and extended temporal muscle detachment for middle fossa approach. Acta Neurochir (Wien). 2023; 165 (11):3473–3477

[20] Figueroa J, Morell A, Bowory V, et al. Minimally invasive keyhole temporal lobectomy approach for supramaximal glioma resection: a safety and feasibility study. J Clin Neurosci. 2020; 72:57–62

[21] Rindler RS, Soriano RM, Elsherbini MM, et al. Exoscopic en bloc carotid-sparing total temporal bone resection: feasibility study and operative technique. World Neurosurg. 2022; 160: e1–e8

[22] de Oliveira Manduca Palmiero H, Ribas EC, Teixeira MJ, Figueiredo EG. Anatomic evaluation of the posterior temporal approach via the Heschl's gyrus to the thalamus, internal capsule, and atrium. Acta Neurochir (Wien). 2023; 165(2): 517–523

[23] Zanaty M, Choutka O. Minimally invasive double-barrel superficial temporal artery: middle cerebral artery bypass. World Neurosurg. 2022; 168:154

[24] Frisoli FA, Baranoski JF, Catapano JS, Lang MJ, Lawton MT. Contralateral supracerebellar-transtentorial approach for

posterior mediobasal temporal cavernous malformation resection. World Neurosurg. 2022; 158:166
[25] Pilipenko Y, Abramyan A. Temporal aneurysmorrhaphy technique for the management of complex middle cerebral artery aneurysm: a video case. World Neurosurg. 2021; 148:196–197
[26] Nouri M, Schneider JR, Shah KA, Katz JM, Dehdashti AR. Sphenoid wing meningioma with surgical revascularization of an injured anterior temporal artery. World Neurosurg. 2020; 140:192
[27] Sponton LS, Archavlis E, Conrad J, et al. Variants of the anterior subtemporal approach to the gasserian ganglion and related structures: an anatomical study with relevant implications for keyhole surgery. World Neurosurg. 2023; 176:e587–e597
[28] Sastry RA, Poggi J, King VA, et al. Superficial temporal artery injury and delayed post-cranioplasty infection. Neurochirurgie. 2023; 69(2):101422
[29] Arivazhagan A, Sinha S, Rao MB. Avoidance of pitfalls and complications during surgery for temporal lobe epilepsy. In: Acta Neurochirurgica Supplement. Cham: Springer International Publishing; 2023:109–119
[30] Garneau JC, Laitman BM, Cosetti MK, Hadjipanayis C, Wanna GB. Repair of a temporal bone encephalocele with the surgical exoscope. Otol Neurotol. 2020; 41(4):561
[31] Symms JT, Dabecco R, Ballard D, Yu A, Chen D, Hillman T. Fibrin glue–coated collagen complex patch: a novel material for surgical repair of spontaneous temporal bone cerebrospinal fluid leak and encephalocele. Otol Neurotol. 2023; 44(5):469–477
[32] Welling LC, Rabelo NN, Figueiredo EG. The mini-pterional approach and the atrophy of the temporal muscle. Neurosurg Rev. 2022; 45(2):1811
[33] Jarc N, Scheiwe C, Plachta DTT, Schmoor C, Gierthmuehlen PC, Gierthmuehlen M. Assessment of postoperative pain, dysesthesia, and weather sensitivity after pterional and temporal neurosurgical approaches. J Neurosurg. 2023; 140 (5):1406–1413
[34] Yamashiro K, Adachi K, Omi T, et al. Risk of postoperative scalp necrosis in the occipital artery region after posterior cranial fossa surgery. Neurosurg Rev. 2023; 46(1):277
[35] Sayer FT, Alanezi AK, Zaidan SN. Spontaneous chronic subdural hematoma associated with arachnoid cyst in a child: a case report and critical review of the literature. Surg Neurol Int. 2022; 13(156):156

5 Technical Nuances of the Fronto-Orbital Craniotomy

Spencer Twitchell, Karol P. Budohoski, Robert C. Rennert, and William T. Couldwell

5.1 Background

- Lesions that can be treated using this approach include all tumors of the sellar and suprasellar compartments; tumors of the clinoid and sphenoid wing; aneurysms in the cavernous sinus, anterior circulation, and basilar apex (when the craniotomy is combined with removal of the temporal bone); lesions of the roof and lateral wall of the orbit; and intraorbital lesions located between the superior and lateral rectus muscles.[1]

5.2 Indications and Contraindications

- The fronto-orbital craniotomy is used to gain access to lesions along the anterior fossa floor, sella, and paraclinoid regions, as well as the anterior middle fossa floor and superolateral orbit.[2,3]

5.3 Informed Consent

- The patient should be advised about all of the details of their surgery and should provide informed consent to proceed.

5.4 Instruments

- The patient is positioned supine on the operative table. A Mayfield three-point head holder is used for stabilization. A shoulder roll is placed under the ipsilateral shoulder for positioning.
- Depending on the lesion being treated, intraoperative neuromonitoring can be utilized. Stereotactic image guidance may be used as well per surgeon preference.

5.5 Patient Preparation

- Total intravenous anesthesia with endotracheal intubation is the standard method for anesthetizing patients undergoing cranial procedures.
- Intraoperative neuromonitoring, although not mandatory, is commonly used for procedures involving intracranial tumors or vascular lesions to increase the safety of the procedure. Electroencephalograms, somatosensory evoked potentials, and motor evoked potentials are monitored in these cases. Monitoring of cranial nerves III to VI can be performed but is not routine at our institution.
- Perioperative corticosteroids are administered alongside hyperosmolar therapy to facilitate brain relaxation.
- Antiepileptic drug administration is controversial and is often dictated by the pathology and surgeon preference.

5.6 Patient Positioning

- The patient is positioned supine. The contralateral shoulder can be elevated depending on the mobility of the neck.
- Mayfield three-point fixation is standard, with the single pin at the contralateral frontal bossa ("widows peak") and the double-pin posterior to the ear, below the equator of the head and above the insertion of the suboccipital musculature (▸ Fig. 5.1).
- The operating table is reflexed to allow the hips to sit lower, with the head and legs elevated to facilitate venous drainage. Once the table position is secured, the neck is rotated to the contralateral side and extended to allow the malar eminence to be the uppermost projection; the Mayfield frame is then fixed in place.
- The degree of head turn is dictated by the location of the pathology but typically varies from 10 to 45 degrees. All pressure points are padded.

5.7 Technique

- A curvilinear incision is planned.
- The inferior portion of the incision overlies the root of the zygoma, one fingerbreadth anterior to the tragus on the ipsilateral side. The incision curves superiorly and anteriorly behind the hairline and terminates at the midline or just contralateral to the midline just behind the hairline.

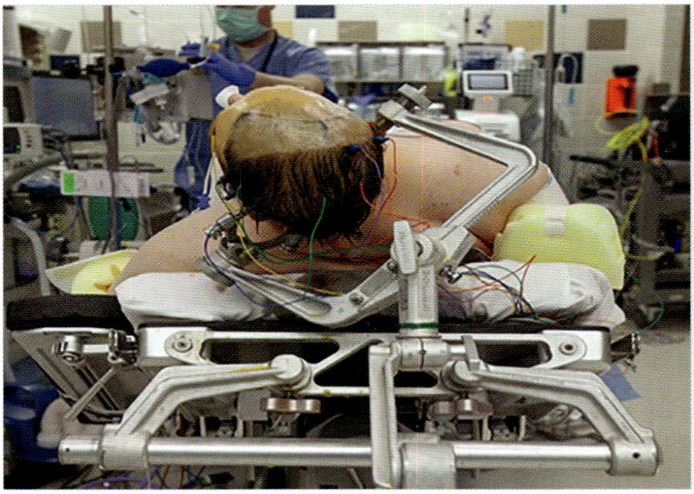

Fig. 5.1 Patient positioning for a right fronto-orbital craniotomy.

- The incision is reflexed away from the forehead to avoid tearing of the skin toward the patient's forehead and should be planned to preserve hair-bearing areas when possible (▶ Fig. 5.2).
- For a standard pterional craniotomy, the authors prefer to use a myocutaneous flap, which provides the best protection for the temporal branch of the facial nerve. However, when the roof of the orbit needs to be removed, as in the fronto-orbital craniotomy, an interfascial or subfascial dissection and retraction of the temporal muscles inferiorly is required to gain access to the inferior orbital fissure.
- For the subfascial dissection, the initial skin flap is elevated off the temporalis fascia. Once the root of the zygoma is palpable, the superficial temporalis fascia is incised along the line coursing about 2 cm posterior to the zygomatic process of the frontal bone toward the keyhole.[4]
- The nerve lies superficial to the superficial temporalis fascia and therefore the interfascial dissection under the superficial fat pad is sufficient to preserve the facial nerve, but the subfascial dissection is equally good and often easier.
- The skin flap, along with the fat pad, is elevated medially until the anterolateral orbital rim and the superior zygomatic arch are exposed.
- The orbital rim is freed using periosteal dissectors.
- If the supraorbital nerve is encased in bone, a small notch may be cut out along the nerve to free it from the frontal bone and allow retraction with the rest of the skin flap.
- The temporalis muscle is cut superiorly, preserving a cuff of muscle and fascia overlying the superior temporal line, and posteriorly down to the zygoma.
- The muscle is dissected off the temporal bone and retracted inferiorly, exposing the inferior orbital fissure on the lateral orbital wall.
- The periorbita is stripped from the superior and lateral orbit, exposing the lateral margin of the inferior orbital fissure and extending to the supraorbital notch medially (▶ Fig. 5.3).
- The size of the craniotomy is determined based on the underlying pathology and the desired exposure. In particular, the craniotomy can be taken to the contralateral side to allow for access into the frontal sinus and interhemispheric fissure or a more direct approach to the area of the olfactory groove or interoptic window. Similarly, the temporal extension of the craniotomy can be tailored to the pathology and need to access the middle fossa and/or the sylvian fissure.
- The fronto-orbital craniotomy can be done as a single-piece or a two-piece craniotomy.[5] The authors prefer a single-piece craniotomy because of the ease of later reconstruction and cosmetic result.
- For the single-piece fronto-orbital exposure, the MacCarty burr hole is created with a high-speed drill to allow for tailoring of the size of the burr hole. The MacCarty burr hole is located 1 cm

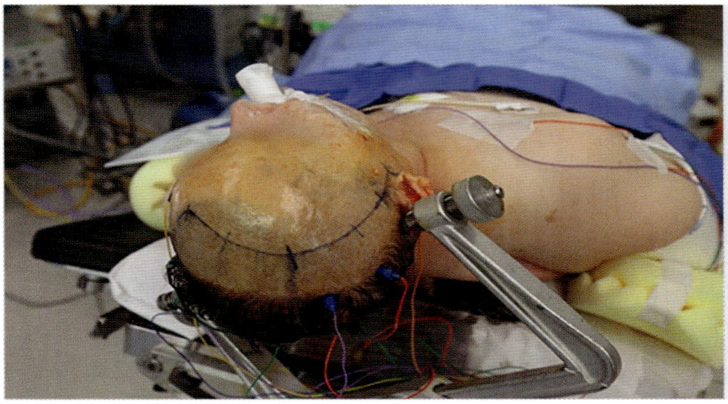

Fig. 5.2 Planned incision and positioning.

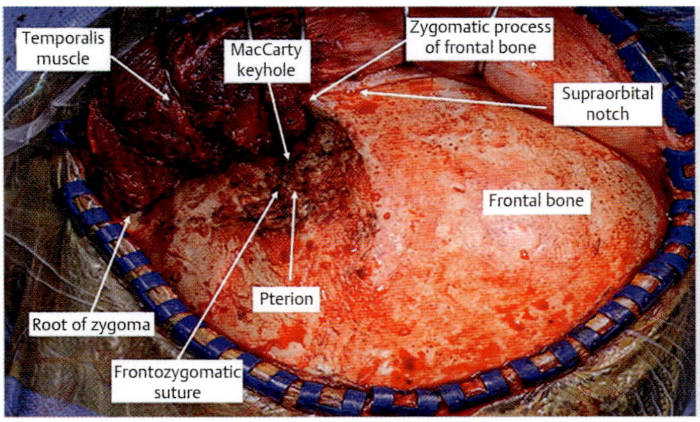

Fig. 5.3 Left fronto-orbital craniotomy exposure and myocutaneous flap elevation. (© Department of Neurosurgery, University of Utah.)

posterior to the frontozygomatic junction and is centered over the roof of the orbit, exposing the orbit anteriorly and the middle fossa dura posteriorly. The temporal burr hole position depends on the need for temporal extension of the craniotomy and can be skipped altogether if only the subfrontal view is required.

- Six cuts are required for removal of the fronto-orbital craniotomy flap (▶ Fig. 5.4a, b):
  - A standard cut using the footplate of the craniotome from the temporal burr hole over the temporal and frontal bones toward the supraorbital groove/notch. This cut can be done from the anterior fossa component of the keyhole burr hole in the cases where gaining temporal and/or middle fossa exposure is not required.
  - A cut made using the footplate of the craniotome from the temporal to the keyhole burr hole, mimicking the standard inferior cut in the pterional craniotomy. This can be omitted in the cases where the temporal burr hole is not used.
  - A cut made using the footplate of the craniotome from the orbital part of the keyhole burr hole inferiorly to the lateral margin of the inferior orbital fissure. The authors prefer to dissect the periorbita from the lateral orbital wall and perform this cut using direct visualization and/or a malleable brain retractor as protection for the intraorbital contents.
  - A cut made using the footplate of the craniotome extending from the end of the third cut in the inferior orbital fissure out to the inferior part of the frontal process of the zygomatic bone. Direct visualization and a malleable brain retractor are used for this in a fashion similar to cut no. 3.
  - A cut made using the B5 tip or the oscillating saw extending from the orbital rim posteriorly in a straight line, cutting the orbital roof. The

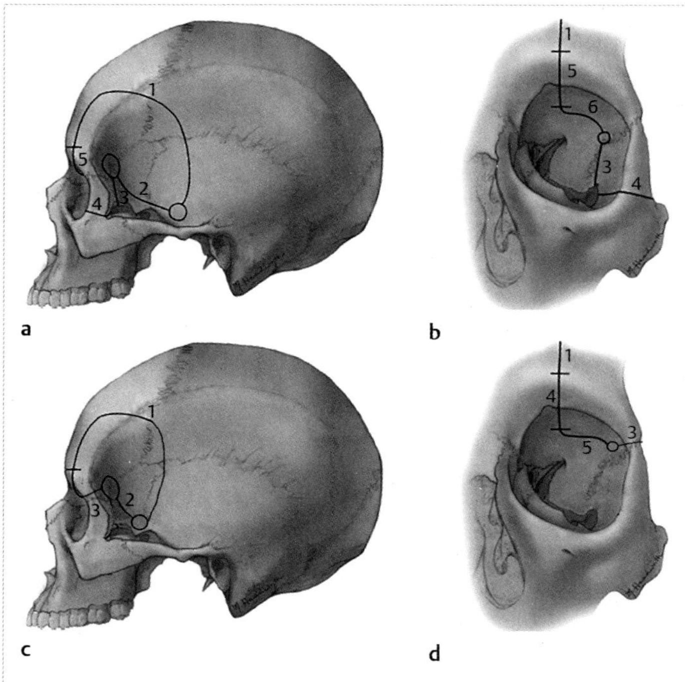

Fig. 5.4 (a, b) Illustrations showing traditional planned burr holes and craniotomy for the fronto-orbital approach. **(c, d)** Illustrations showing modifications to traditional craniotomy. (© Department of Neurosurgery, University of Utah.)

posterior extent of this cut is variable and is dictated by the available space within the orbit for visualization. In the authors' experience, the posterior extent is not relevant because the most posterior portion of the orbital roof is easy to remove once the craniotomy flap has been turned.

- The final cut involves making a lateral-to-medial cut in the roof of the orbit from the keyhole to the fifth cut described above. The authors prefer to perform this using a narrow chisel, which can fit into the keyhole burr hole. The orbital roof is made of thin bone, and typically a few gentle taps with the mallet will free up the bone flap.

- A simple modification to the traditional craniotomy described above eliminates the temporal portion of the craniotomy. Rather than dissecting and carrying the craniotomy inferior to the inferior orbital fissure, the craniotomy is carried directly from the MacCarty keyhole through the lateral orbital wall. This approach allows for access to the superior part of the orbit, the anterior clinoid process, and the optic canal, but does not allow uninhibited access to the lateral orbit for intraconal pathologies and lesions extending through the inferior orbital fissure.
- Nevertheless, the reduced dissection associated with this modification allows decreased operative time and provides adequate exposure for most cases located at the interface of the anterior fossa and orbit (**Video 5.1**). Five cuts are required for this modified craniotomy.
  - A standard cut using the footplate of the craniotome from the temporal burr hole over the anterior temporal and frontal bones toward the supraorbital groove/notch.
  - A cut made connecting the burr hole at the junction of the squamosal temporal bone and sphenoid to the MacCarty keyhole burr hole.
  - A cut made using the footplate of the craniotome from the orbital part of the keyhole burr hole laterally through the lateral wall of the orbit. The authors prefer to dissect the periorbita from the lateral orbital wall and perform this cut using direct visualization and/or a malleable brain retractor as protection for the periorbita. This cut exits just below the frontozygomatic suture.
  - A cut made using the B5 tip or the oscillating saw extending from the orbital rim posteriorly in a straight line, cutting the orbital roof. The posterior extent of this cut is variable and is dictated by the available space within the orbit

for visualization. In the authors' experience, the posterior extent is not relevant because the most posterior portion of the orbital roof is easy to remove once the craniotomy flap has been turned.
  - The final cut involves making a lateral-to-medial cut in the roof of the orbit from the keyhole to the fourth cut described above. The authors prefer to perform this using a narrow chisel, which can fit into the keyhole burr hole. The orbital roof is made of thin bone, and typically a few gentle taps with the mallet will free up the bone flap.
- Once the bone flap is removed, the sphenoid is drilled if necessary and if a temporal bone flap has been incorporated. Inspection at this point enables the identification of the extent of additional removal of the lateral orbital wall and orbital roof required by the specific pathology.
- The orbital removal is typically done with a combination of the rongeurs, cutting burr, and diamond burr, and every effort is made to protect the periorbita. Injury to the periorbita invariably leads to significant protrusion of intraorbital fat and makes further bone removal harder. Orbital wall removal can be taken as far posteriorly as the anterior clinoid, which can be easily removed using this approach (▸ Fig. 5.4c, d). The middle fossa and sphenoid ridge should be exposed to allow a safe anterior clinoidectomy, a step that necessitates a degree of temporal bone removal and should be taken into consideration when planning the bone flap.
- A detailed description of extradural anterior clinoidectomy exceeds the scope of this chapter, and the reader is directed to the studies by Otani et al[6] and Abou-Al-Shaar et al.[7]
- A curvilinear dural opening is the norm. The extent of dural opening is determined by the size of the craniotomy performed. The dura is typically flapped anteriorly or laterally and secured with stay stiches to the Leyla retractor bar. Stay stitches are valuable to significantly tension the dura over the orbital contents, depressing the latter to allow a more inferior-to-superior trajectory to intracranial pathologies. Tacking stitches can be placed if epidural bleeding is seen, but are often unnecessary for small bony openings.
- The fronto-orbital craniotomy allows for subfrontal access to the anterior fossa floor, optic nerves, anterior circulation, and sellar and suprasellar compartment (▸ Fig. 5.5). If exposure of the cavernous sinus and middle fossa is required, the fronto-orbital craniotomy benefits from a temporal component and flattening of the sphenoid. Brain relaxation can be readily achieved by release of cerebrospinal fluid from the opticocarotid cistern. The same approach allows for significant extradural work around the periorbita and orbit as well as the lateral cavernous sinus.
- Following the achievement of adequate hemostasis, primary dural closure can typically be attempted; however, should the dura have shrunk or the pathology dictated significant dural resection, duraplasty may be performed using a variety of autologous or synthetic grafts as needed (▸ Fig. 5.6). Typically, the pericranium saved during the approach or the temporalis fascia can be used for this purpose. Careful

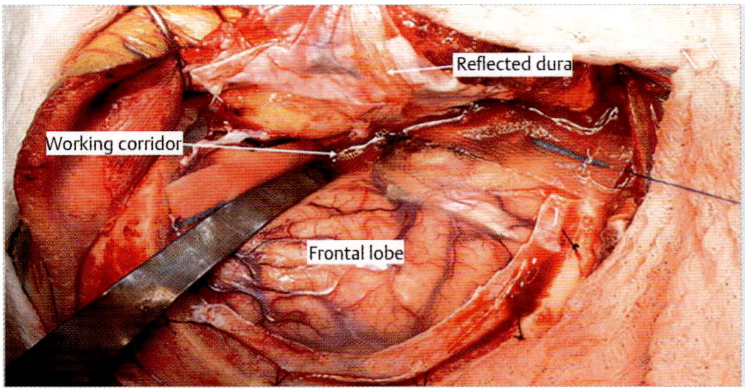

Fig. 5.5 Left fronto-orbital craniotomy with dural opening demonstrating the typical working corridor. (© Department of Neurosurgery, University of Utah.)

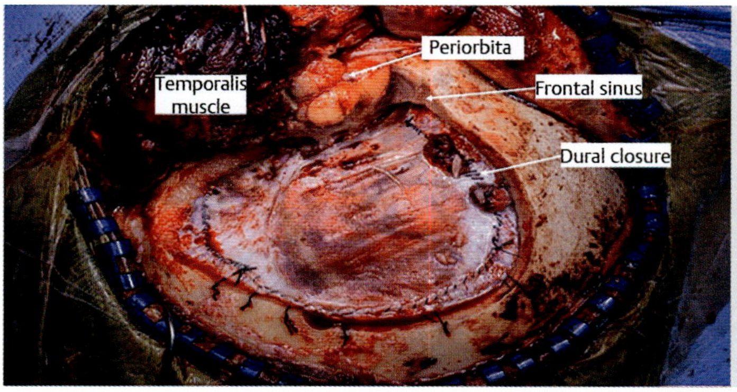

Fig. 5.6 Left fronto-orbital craniotomy dural closure with several muscle patches for watertight closure. (© Department of Neurosurgery, University of Utah.)

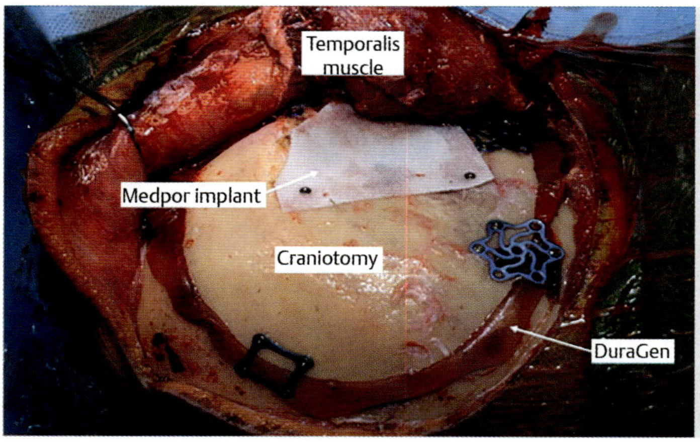

Fig. 5.7 Left fronto-orbital craniotomy following dural closure, with onlay DuraGen, titanium plate fixation, and subtemporalis Medpor implant for cosmesis. (© Department of Neurosurgery, University of Utah.)

consideration should be paid to the paranasal sinuses. In the case of breach into the paranasal sinuses, the authors recommend aggressive removal of mucosa and obliteration of the sinus with fat and closure with pericranial flaps and fibrin glue.

- The bone flap may then be replaced using a combination of titanium plates and screws. The benefits of a single-piece craniotomy are cosmesis on closure and easier re-approximation of bone edges. The single-piece craniotomy follows the technique of a standard pterional craniotomy with the addition of a titanium plate over the frontozygomatic junction (▶ Fig. 5.7).

5.8 Postoperative Care

- Patients are typically observed in the intensive care unit for close postoperative monitoring including regular blood pressure checks and neurological examination.
- Depending on the indication for surgery, special considerations should be given to monitoring vision if the operation involved optic nerve decompression and/or manipulation.
- Postoperative imaging will depend on pathology undergoing treatment and may involve head CT and/or MRI with and without contrast (e.g., meningioma) or CT angiography (e.g., aneurysm).
- In some cases, antiepileptic medications or a short course of steroids may be indicated.

5.9 Complications

- Proper patient positioning, meticulous skin incision, bone flap creation, dural opening, and brain exposure are crucial for achieving optimal outcomes.

- Potential complications of the fronto-orbital approach, which are rarely seen in the standard frontal and frontotemporal craniotomies, include cosmetic deformity affecting the eye and forehead, enophthalmos from excessive drilling of the orbital wall, external oculomotor muscle damage with resultant diplopia, and blindness from injury to the optic nerve. Therefore, the orbital component of the frontal or frontotemporal craniotomy should be used judiciously in indicated cases.

5.10 Management Pearls

- An interfascial or subfascial dissection and retraction of the temporal muscles inferiorly is required to gain access the inferior orbital fissure.
- The authors prefer a single-piece craniotomy over a two-piece craniotomy because of the ease of later reconstruction and cosmetic result.
- A simple modification to the traditional craniotomy eliminates the temporal portion of the craniotomy, which allows for access to the superior part of the orbit, the anterior clinoid process, and the optic canal with shorter operative time, but does not allow uninhibited access to the lateral orbit for intraconal pathologies and lesions extending through the inferior orbital fissure.
- Primary dural closure can typically be attempted, but duraplasty may be performed using autologous grafts, such as the pericranium saved during the approach or the temporalis fascia, or synthetic grafts as needed.
- The risks specific to this approach include cosmetic deformities, risk to the optic nerve and orbital contents, and postoperative anosmia resulting from manipulation or damage to the olfactory nerves.

5.11 Special Risks

- Other than the usual risks of infection, bleeding, cerebrospinal fluid leak, seizures, hematoma formation, and those associated with anesthesia, the risks specific to this approach include cosmetic deformities resulting from the repair of the craniotomy (visible scarring, asymmetry, deformity of the forehead or orbital area).
- Additionally, there is risk to the optic nerve and orbital contents during the surgery and removal of overlying bone. There is also the potential for postoperative anosmia resulting from manipulation or damage to the olfactory nerves.

References

[1] Frazier CHI. I. An approach to the hypophysis through the anterior cranial fossa. Ann Surg. 1913; 57(2):145–150

[2] McArthur LL. An aseptic surgical access to the pituitary body and its neighborhood. JAMA. 1912; 58(26):2009–2011

[3] Jane JA, Park TS, Pobereskin LH, Winn HR, Butler AB. The supraorbital approach: technical note. Neurosurgery. 1982; 11(4):537–542

[4] Coscarella E, Vishteh AG, Spetzler RF, Seoane E, Zabramski JM. Subfascial and submuscular methods of temporal muscle dissection and their relationship to the frontal branch of the facial nerve. Technical note. J Neurosurg. 2000; 92(5):877–880

[5] Andaluz N, van Loveren HR, Keller JT, Zuccarello M. The one-piece orbitopterional approach. Skull Base. 2003; 13 (4):241–245

[6] Otani N, Muroi C, Yano H, Khan N, Pangalu A, Yonekawa Y. Surgical management of tuberculum sellae meningioma: role of selective extradural anterior clinoidectomy. Br J Neurosurg. 2006; 20(3):129–138

[7] Abou-Al-Shaar H, Krisht KM, Cohen MA, et al. Cranio-orbital and orbitocranial approaches to orbital and intracranial disease: eye-opening approaches for neurosurgeons. Front Surg. 2020; 7:1

6 Supraorbital Approach

Michael T. Bounajem, Robert C. Rennert, Karol P. Budohoski, Henry W.S. Schroeder, and William T. Couldwell

6.1 Background

- In 1982, the supraorbital approach was formally described by Jane et al[1] as a method for obtaining access to lesions of the frontal skull base and superior orbit, as well as aneurysms of the anterior communicating artery (ACoA) while minimizing brain retraction. Using this approach, Jane et al[1] reported successful treatment of ACoA aneurysms, sellar/parasellar/suprasellar tumors, and olfactory groove meningiomas.
- The supraorbital approach has undergone many iterations, and, depending on the mediolateral and superior extent of the craniotomy, may be referred to as the lateral supraorbital, superior orbital, or superior frontotemporal approach.

6.2 Indications and Contraindications

- The supraorbital approach can be used to treat pathologies located in the anterior cranial fossa, sphenoid wing, anterior clinoid, sellar/parasellar/suprasellar areas, superior orbit, orbital apex, and medial sylvian fissure.
- Such lesions include but are not limited to ACoA aneurysms, sellar/parasellar/suprasellar tumors, clinoidal meningiomas, medial frontal lobe tumors, parafalcine meningiomas, planum sphenoidale meningiomas, and olfactory groove meningiomas.
- The inclusion of an orbitotomy in a supraorbital craniotomy can be selectively applied, which affords better exposure of the orbital apex, thereby expanding the use of the supraorbital approach to include a greater proportion of intraorbital pathologies. This also allows for enhanced rostral visualization for high-riding ACoA aneurysms or lesions with significant suprasellar extent.
- Although there are not necessarily strict contraindications to the supraorbital approach, the extent of visualization afforded by the supraorbital craniotomy defines its limits of appropriate use. Lesions extending inferior to the sellar and parasellar area can be challenging to visualize because the sphenoid wing limits the surgeon's ability to look inferiorly.

6.3 Informed Consent

- The patient should be advised about all of the details of their surgery and should provide informed consent to proceed.

6.4 Instruments

- Requisite equipment in general consists of an adjustable operating table with ample patient straps to allow for rotation/angling of the table, head clamp for stable fixation, high-speed drill (potentially requiring diamond drill bits), operative microscope, cranial plating system, bipolar and monopolar electrocautery, and microdissection instruments.
- Pathology-specific equipment may also be necessary, such as aneurysm clips, ultrasonic aspirator, and a neuronavigation system. An endoscope can also be used in specific cases for better visualization and access to deeper/hidden structures.

6.5 Patient Preparation

- Pathology-specific preoperative imaging is crucial for operative planning (e.g., vascular imaging for aneurysm ligation, magnetic resonance imaging with and without contrast for tumor resection).
- Thin-cut computed tomography (CT) scans without contrast are also useful to visualize the characteristics of surrounding sinuses, such as the lateral extent of the frontal sinus, and pneumatization of the anterior clinoid, as well as for neuronavigation.
- General anesthesia, commonly with intraoperative neuromonitoring, is used for the supraorbital approach.

6.6 Patient Positioning

- As is the case with most keyhole approaches, positioning of the patient's head is vital to the success of the surgery.
- The head is first clamped in a Mayfield head holder to prepare for positioning. For target lesions in the ipsilateral frontotemporal area, minimal rotation of the patient's head (10–20 degrees) is necessary, but for lesions of the parasellar region and those extending further contralateral/anterior, greater rotation may be needed (20–40 and 40–60 degrees, respectively).[2]
- The neck is also extended to allow the frontal lobe to fall away from the skull base, thus allowing for minimal use of retractors.

6.7 Technique

- The modern supraorbital approach has been tailored to be a less invasive, keyhole-style approach (▶ Fig. 6.1).[3]
- The prior bicoronal incision has, in most cases, been replaced by a transciliary eyebrow incision, which has the obvious benefit of a much less morbid scalp dissection while still maintaining satisfactory cosmesis.[4] The eyebrow incision generally starts just lateral to the supraorbital nerve and is extended to the lateral extent of the eyebrow.
- The temporalis fascia can be incised along the superior temporal line and the muscle reflected laterally, while the frontalis fascia is incised from its connection with the superior temporal line and reflected inferiorly.[3]
- It is critical to avoid injuring the frontalis branch of the facial nerve as it courses superomedially over the temporal fossa.
- Care should be taken with the temporalis muscle because damage can contribute to unnecessary postoperative pain and discomfort with mastication.
- Hook retractors arranged radially on the soft tissue opening can be used to maximize bony exposure.
- The craniotomy is then performed, beginning with a burr hole often directly inferior to the superior temporal line such that it will be covered by the temporalis muscle at the conclusion of the case and remain invisible on the forehead.
- The craniotomy can then be turned with a high-speed craniotome and footplate to protect the underlying dura. The size of the craniotomy can be tailored to specific needs relative to the pathology, but generally it is 2 to 3.5 cm in width and 1.5 to 2 cm in height.[3]
- Entrance into the frontal sinus is normally avoided (by mapping with neuronavigation and/or transillumination), thus eliminating the need for a pericranial flap and decreasing the chance of postoperative cerebrospinal fluid (CSF) leak or mucocele formation.
- Although the supraorbital notch has been suggested as a landmark for the lateral aspect of the frontal sinus, the sinus often extends laterally beyond it, making it an unreliable marker.[5] Further, the orbital rim is not necessarily removed with the bone flap. Instead, the inferior cut is carried along the superior margin of the orbital rim, and the inner cortical surface of the frontal bone is drilled down to facilitate greater maneuverability of microinstruments.[3]
- The durotomy can be tailored to specific needs of the operation. For many intradural pathologies, the dura is opened in a **C**-shaped fashion with a base along the roof of the orbit, allowing for a subfrontal operative corridor as the brain falls away from the anterior skull base (▶ Fig. 6.2).
- Closure is performed in a layered fashion, with low-profile plates to fix the bone to minimize postoperative visibility. The skin is closed with a subcuticular absorbable or fine nonabsorbable running suture that is removed within 5 to 7 days. A temporary lumbar drain or lumbar puncture can be used to minimize the risk of postoperative CSF leak.
- The supraorbital approach is a prime example of a craniotomy that lends itself well to the addition of endoscopy.
- Arnaout et al[6] demonstrated no significant differences in visualized area between the microscope and endoscope alone, suggesting that the endoscope could potentially be used as a standalone system when performing the supraorbital approach. Berhouma et al[7] described their technique for conducting the fully endoscopic supraorbital approach: a standard transciliary incision followed by creation of a burr hole posterior to the superior

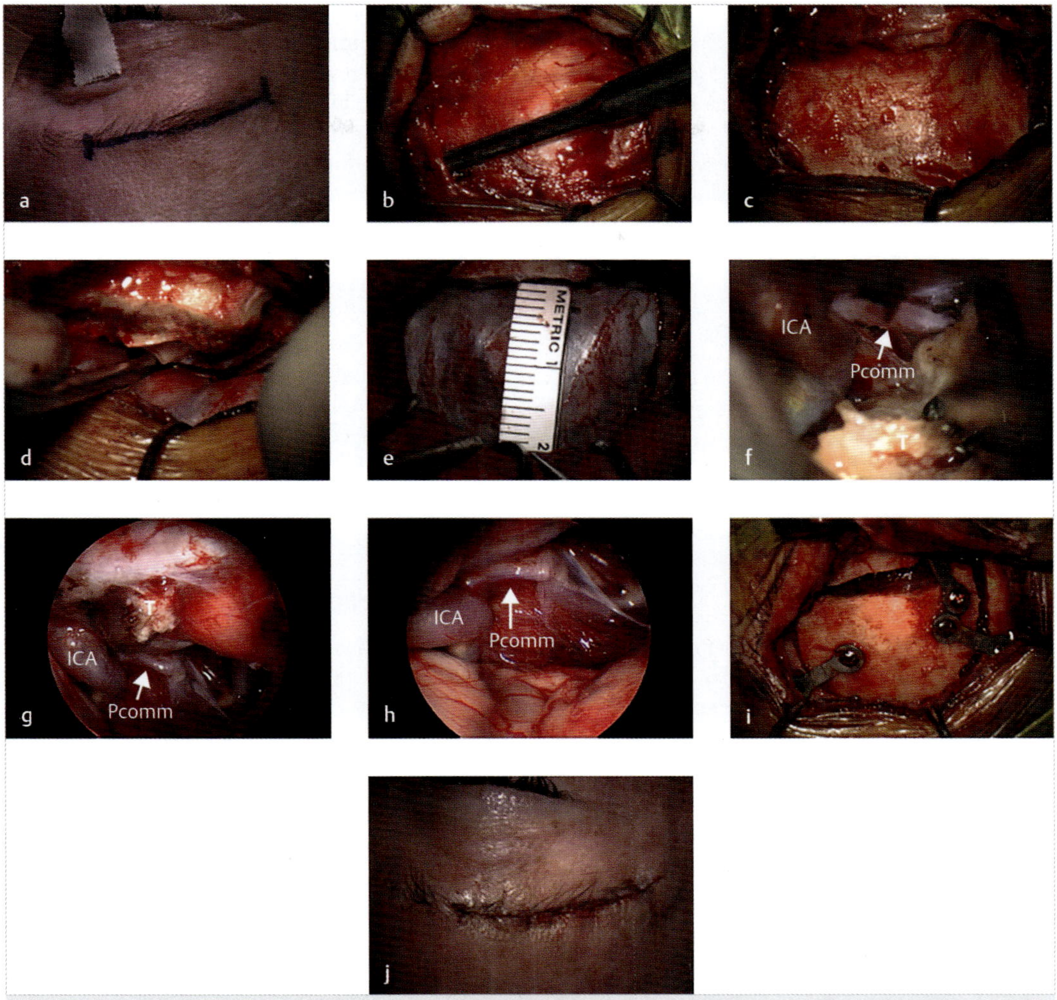

Fig. 6.1 Supraorbital approach for resection of a right tuberculum sella meningioma. **(a)** An eyebrow incision is marked from just lateral to the supraorbital nerve and extending to the lateral extent of the eyebrow. **(b)** Hook retractors are placed, and a subfascial dissection is used to preserve a pericranial flap, which is elevated inferiorly. **(c–e)** A frontal craniotomy is performed, and the floor of the anterior fossa is drilled flush. **(f)** After dural opening, subfrontal dissection allows direct visualization of the anterior skull base for detachment and devascularization of the tumor. **(g, h)** Endoscopic assistance allows for enhanced visualization of surrounding critical structures, and to check the extent of tumor resection. **(i, j)** The bone is replated, and the incision is closed in a layered fashion. ICA, internal carotid artery; Pcomm, posterior communicating artery; T, tumor.

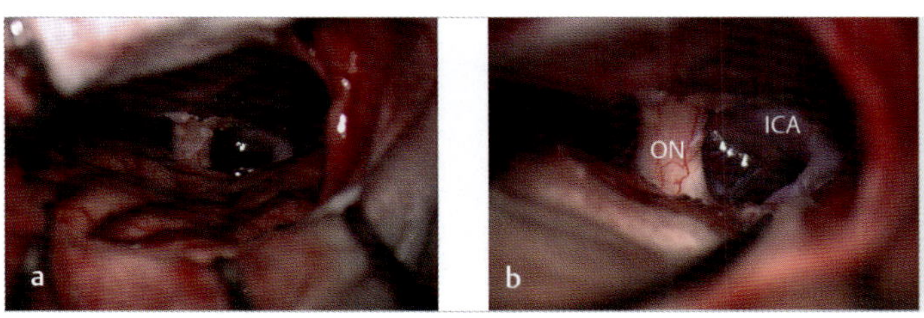

Fig. 6.2 View of the opticocarotid triangle via a supraorbital approach. **(a, b)** Subfrontal dissection allows for direct corridor to access lesions in and around the opticocarotid triangle and anterolateral skull base. ICA, internal carotid artery; ON, optic nerve.

temporal line and a 2-cm craniotomy. The dura is incised and reflected toward the orbital roof, and a rigid 4-mm 0-degree endoscope is introduced into the field and secured in its holding arm.
- At the conclusion of the intradural portion of the procedure, the dura can be closed in standard fashion, and the bone replated with titanium miniplates and screws.

6.8 Postoperative Care

- Patients are typically observed in the intensive care unit for close postoperative monitoring. Special attention must be paid to potential swelling of the frontal lobe, given the retraction of the frontal lobe that may be necessary to access the target pathology during surgery.
- A short course of corticosteroids is often used for this reason, as well as prophylactic antiepileptic medication.
- Postoperative imaging will depend on target pathology (e.g., magnetic resonance imaging with and without contrast after tumor resection).

6.9 Complications

- Possible complications that are not specific to the supraorbital approach but are generally applicable for its target pathology include hypopituitarism, injury to the optic or olfactory nerves, and vascular injury (anterior or middle cerebral artery territory).
- Potential risks specific to the supraorbital approach include entrance into the frontal sinus and associated mucocele formation or persistent CSF leak, injury to the frontalis nerve, and injury to the orbital contents.

6.10 Management Pearls

- The supraorbital approach is a minimally invasive, cosmetically optimal, yet versatile and tailorable method for accessing lesions of the anterior cranial fossa, as well as the sellar/parasellar/suprasellar, orbital, and select sylvian/middle fossa regions.
- The supraorbital approach can be modified depending on the pathology, with the potential addition of orbital osteotomies or the adjunctive use of endoscopy.
- The surgical incision can be hidden in the eyebrow for satisfactory cosmesis; however, care must be taken to ensure close apposition between the craniotomy flap and surrounding skull during closure.
- Entrance into the frontal sinus can be avoided depending on the target pathology; however, if entrance is necessary, care must be taken to prevent future mucocele formation or persistent CSF leakage (using, e.g., cranialization of sinus, use of vascularized pericranial flap, or fat graft).

Acknowledgments

- We thank Kristin Kraus and Cortlynd Olsen for editorial assistance.

References

[1] Jane JA, Park TS, Pobereskin LH, Winn HR, Butler AB. The supraorbital approach: technical note. Neurosurgery. 1982; 11(4):537–542

[2] van Lindert E, Perneczky A, Fries G, Pierangeli E. The supraorbital keyhole approach to supratentorial aneurysms: concept and technique. Surg Neurol. 1998; 49(5):481–489, discussion 489–490

[3] Mori K. Keyhole concept in cerebral aneurysm clipping and tumor removal by the supraciliary lateral supraorbital approach. Asian J Neurosurg. 2014; 9(1):14–20

[4] Ziai K, Shah S, Daggubati LC, Zacharia BE, Lighthall JG. The supraorbital approach via an eyebrow incision: analysis of cosmetic outcomes using the Scar Cosmesis Assessment Rating Scale. J Craniofac Surg. 2022; 33(1):307–311

[5] Ostergard TA, Glenn CA, Dekker SE, Bambakidis NC. Is the supraorbital notch a reliable landmark to avoid the frontal sinus? Oper Neurosurg (Hagerstown). 2019; 16(3):360–367

[6] Arnaout MM, Luzzi S, Galzio R, Aziz K. Supraorbital keyhole approach: pure endoscopic and endoscope-assisted perspective. Clin Neurol Neurosurg. 2020; 189:105623

[7] Berhouma M, Jacquesson T, Jouanneau E. The fully endoscopic supraorbital trans-eyebrow keyhole approach to the anterior and middle skull base. Acta Neurochir (Wien). 2011; 153(10): 1949–1954

7 Lateral Orbital Approach

Robert C. Rennert, Michael T. Bounajem, Karol P. Budohoski, and William T. Couldwell

7.1 Background

- The lateral orbital approach (LOA) is a keyhole approach best suited to provide targeted access to small- to medium-sized lesions involving the orbital apex (OA), superior orbital fissure (SOF), cavernous sinus (CS), and middle cranial fossa (MCF) as well as lesions of the anterolateral to posterolateral orbit, with full-thickness removal of the anterior aspect of the lateral orbital wall.[1]
- The modified lateral orbital approach (mLOA) provides similar access with less orbital manipulation and lower risk to critical intraorbital structures through preservation of the medial aspect of the lateral orbital wall.[1]
- Endoscopic lateral orbital and transorbital techniques have also been reported to access the OA, SOF, CS, and MCF,[2,3,4] although these commonly involve traversing the orbit with compression of the intraorbital contents.
- Pathologies addressed or diagnosed with the LOA and mLOA from prior reports include meningiomas, cavernomas, esthesioneuroblastomas, lymphomas, chordomas, Ewing's sarcomas, squamous cell carcinomas, and smooth muscle tumors.[1,5]

7.2 Indications and Contraindications

- Suitable goals of surgery with an LOA or mLOA range from a gross total resection for discrete lesions that fall within the anatomical boundaries to a diagnostic biopsy with or without symptom palliation from neurovascular decompression for more extensive spheno-orbital disease or lesions within the CS (▶ Fig. 7.1, ▶ Fig. 7.2, and **Video 7.1**).[5,6]

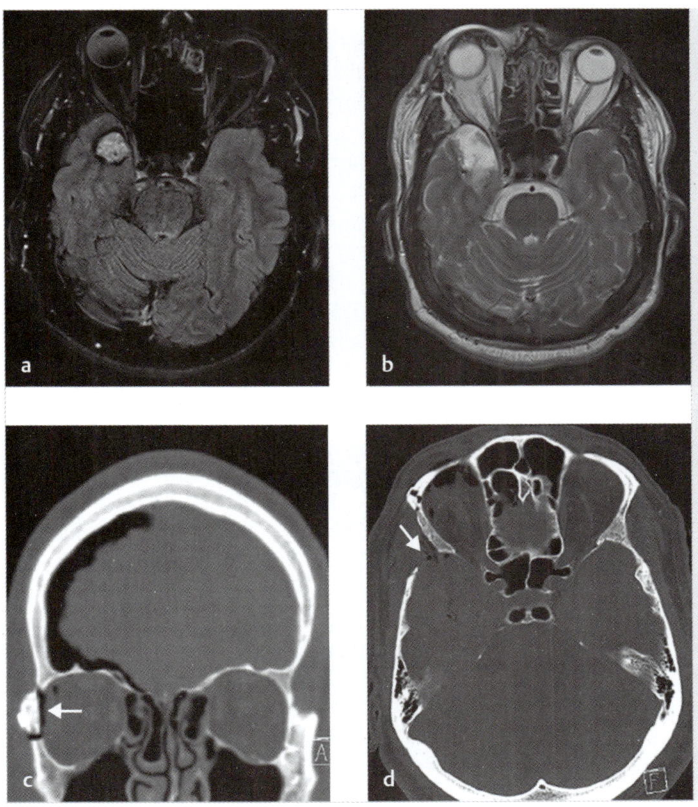

Fig. 7.1 A 58-year-old man had a 2-cm right mesial temporal cavernous malformation causing medically refractory seizures. **(a)** Axial fluid-attenuated inversion recovery (FLAIR) MRI. He underwent a successful right modified lateral orbital approach for complete cavernoma resection. **(b)** Axial T2-weighted MRI. **(c)** Coronal and **(d)** Axial CT images demonstrate the replated lateral orbital rim and the operative corridor through the drilled sphenoid wing, with preservation of the medial aspect of the lateral orbital rim. The patient was seizure free and neurologically stable on follow-up. This case has been reported previously.[14]

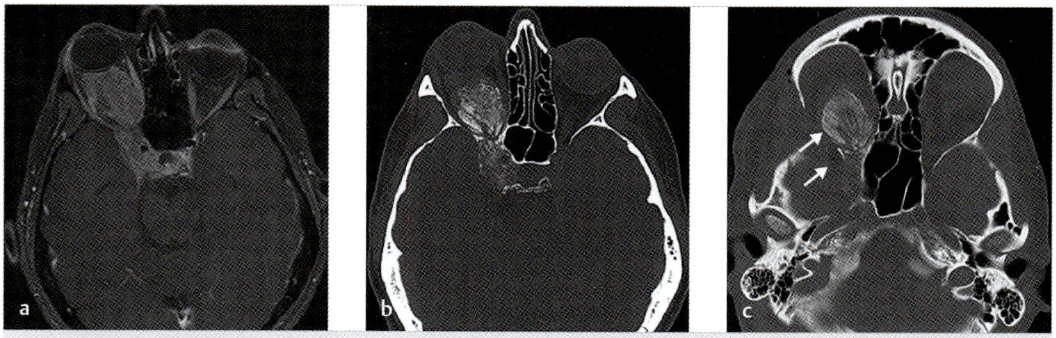

Fig. 7.2 **(a)** Postcontrast axial T1-weighted MRI and **(b)** axial CT image of a 37-year-old woman with a growing, invasive right optic nerve sheath meningioma who had undergone irradiation of the tumor was recommended for tissue sampling to identify possible targeted therapies as well as to decompress the lateral orbit/orbital apex (OA), superior orbital fissure (SOF), and cavernous sinus (CS). She underwent a successful right lateral orbital approach, including biopsy of the tumor within the CS and bony decompression of the SOF and lateral orbit/OA. **(c)** Axial MRI, with *arrows* highlighting bony decompression and CS access site. On follow-up examination, she had improved exophthalmos, stable vision, and slightly worsened cranial nerve VI paresis and was identified to be a candidate for clinical trials.

- The LOA is also ideal for lesions with symptomatic lateral to medial compression of the orbit because it allows for targeted decompression of this site.
- An LOA or mLOA can also be combined with other approaches to expand the operatively accessible area based on patient-specific pathologies and surgical goals. For example, combining an LOA with a supraorbital approach can extend visualization medially to the contralateral optic nerve while also providing access to the anterior cranial fossa and allowing for removal of the anterior clinoid process.[5]
- Alternatively, transorbital endoscopic approaches use the orbit as an operative corridor and can be combined with transnasal, transmaxillary, transpetrosal, or supraorbital approaches to access a wider anatomical area extending from the posterior fossa/clivus inferiorly to the suprasellar region superiorly.[2,7,8,9,10,11,12]
- Standard open (frontotemporal, orbitozygomatic, or combined) approaches are nonetheless generally preferred, because of their expanded operative corridors and preservation of two-handed microsurgical technique, for larger lesions or those with multicompartment extension when the surgical goal is a maximal safe resection.
- The accessible skull base anatomical limits of these approaches are bounded by the floor of the middle fossa inferiorly, the ipsilateral optic nerve medially, the orbital roof and anterior clinoid process superiorly, the foramen spinosum laterally, and Meckel's cave posteriorly.[5,6]
- Aside from the anatomic constraints of the LOA and mLOA, an additional limitation of the LOA is the risk of injury to the orbital contents with medial retraction or drilling, which can result in transient or permanent vision defects or diplopia.[5,13]
- This risk is minimized with the mLOA and preservation of the medial aspect of the lateral orbital wall, but the modifications result in a slightly narrowed (yet adequate) operative corridor.
- The key is to thin the wall to the medial cortical bone without violation of the orbit.

7.3 Informed Consent

- The patient should be advised about all of the details of their surgery and should provide informed consent to proceed.

7.4 Instruments

- Relevant equipment includes an operative microscope, drill with diamond bits, and neuronavigation. An endoscope can also be used to aid assessment of difficult-to-visualize sites.

7.5 Patient Preparation

- Pathologies in the anterior and middle skull base and orbit are typically best visualized through a combination of brain and/or orbit magnetic resonance imaging (MRI), with and without contrast.
- Thin-cut computed tomography (CT; with or without vessel imaging [CT angiography]) is useful to assess for bony reactive changes and for intraoperative neuronavigation.
- A thorough neurologic examination and a neuro-ophthalmology evaluation are crucial to understand any baseline neurologic and/or visual changes that may inform surgical planning.
- General anesthesia is used for the LOA and mLOA, with neuromonitoring for cases requiring intracranial access.

7.6 Patient Positioning

- The patient is positioned supine on the operating room table, with the bed flexed and the patient padded and secured.
- The head is secured in three-point fixation with the neck slightly extended. The head is rotated appropriately for the operative target and the desired surgical trajectory, with no rotation when targeting the MCF; 15 to 20 degrees of contralateral rotation when targeting the OA, SOF, or CS; and additional contralateral rotation as needed when targeting increasingly anterior aspects of the orbit.
- The eye is lubricated and protected with a corneal shield.

7.7 Technique

- The general considerations and basic operative steps of the LOA and mLOA have been described previously.[1,5,6,15] Here we provide additional step-by-step details of the mLOA as performed by the senior author, with commentary on how this is modified from the LOA.
- Neuronavigation is registered, because it is useful for confirming relevant anatomy within the small operative corridor of the keyhole approach, especially during bony removal and lesion targeting. Baseline neuromonitoring signals are obtained (most commonly motor and somatosensory evoked potentials), as is standard with skull base surgical approaches.
- For the mLOA, an incision is marked in the lateral third of the upper eye crease, with a temporal extension no more than 1 cm lateral to the orbital rim, and a short medial fork toward the superior eyelid.
- This incision centers the opening over the lateral orbit and provides maximal exposure along the surgical trajectory while also using natural skin creases to maximize cosmetic outcomes. The lateral canthus is not disrupted, and the incision and soft tissue dissection avoid the frontal branch of the facial nerve to maintain eye positioning and facial motor symmetry. Local injection of anesthetic and dilute epinephrine is used to assist with incisional pain and hemostasis.
- An alternative linear incision for the LOA has been described to extend 1.5 cm laterally from the lateral commissure and includes division of the lateral canthus to facilitate a wide bony exposure.[5] In the authors' experience, however, the incision described for the mLOA provides a similar exposure and can be used for either approach with a smaller soft tissue disruption.
- A no. 15 blade is used to sharply open the planned incision down to the level of the periosteum of the lateral orbital rim and zygoma, including opening the orbicularis oculi but preserving the underlying orbital septum and lateral canthal tendon medially.
- Monopolar electrocautery is used to elevate the temporalis muscle laterally away from the lateral aspect of the orbital rim and the lateral orbital wall, exposing the keyhole region. The periorbita is elevated in a subperiosteal fashion from the medial aspect of the orbital rim using a Freer elevator or Penfield no. 1 instrument. A self-retaining retractor is placed under the temporalis muscle, centered over the exposed lateral orbital rim.
- An approximately 1.5-cm segment of the lateral orbital rim is targeted for removal, extending from above the frontozygomatic suture to just above where the frontal process joins with the body of the zygoma. A C1 drill bit is used to make an inferior and superior cut in the orbital rim, followed by a controlled fracture of the underlying lateral orbital wall using heavy rongeurs.

- After the C1 cuts and before fracture removal of the rim, thin titanium bone fixation plates can be secured to the segment of the rim that will be removed, and pilot screw holes can be drilled with the C1 bit medially and laterally on the orbital rim to ensure a cosmetic rim reconstruction during closure.
- After orbital rim removal, additional exposure can be gained with hook retraction of the temporalis muscle in the lateral direction.
- The lateral orbital wall is visualized, and anatomy is confirmed with neuronavigation. With enhanced visualization from the microscope, the lateral aspect of the orbital wall, greater sphenoid wing, and sphenoid ridge are drilled as needed, based on the operative target, using a diamond drill bit under irrigation.
- Critically, the medial cortical wall is preserved to avoid exposure or damage to the periorbita or underlying orbital structures. Liberal use of neuronavigation can be helpful during bony removal for surgeons who are inexperienced with this approach.
- The preservation of the medial cortical wall is the main difference between the mLOA and the LOA, with the latter approach involving complete removal of the lateral orbital wall and retraction of the orbital contents to maximize the operative corridor.
- To access the SOF and CS, the meningo-orbital band is exposed and divided and the dura propria is elevated from the lateral wall of the CS. CS entry is often achieved with this approach through the anteromedial triangle; the anterolateral, infratrochlear, and supratrochlear triangles can also be accessed.
- To address lesions of the MCF, lateral orbital wall thinning is followed by more focal drilling of the greater sphenoid wing overlying the target; a 2 cm^2 bone opening can be made to provide adequate access to the anterior and medial temporal region.
- Finally, for targets within the OA, in addition to drilling of the sphenoid ridge/wing as needed, all layers of the lateral orbital wall overlying the lesion are removed. To limit manipulation of the anterior orbit while accessing the OA, the more superficial aspect of the orbital wall is thinned but the medial cortex is preserved, as with approaches to deeper targets.
- After the targeted lesion is addressed, closure is tailored to the operative anatomy encountered. If the lesion is entirely extradural or confined to the orbit, cerebrospinal fluid leak may not be encountered.
- Watertight dural closure is generally not achievable when the dura is opened, but a dural substitute combined with liquid/cut Gelfoam is typically adequate for deep closure in the absence of a sinus breach because there is limited tissue disruption and potential space creation associated with this approach.
- If the nasal sinuses are entered, autologous fat with or without fascia grafts is used to prevent a spinal fluid leak. The orbital rim is replated using the predrilled pilot holes to optimize cosmesis. The wound is closed in a layered fashion with interrupted absorbable sutures for the deep tissues, and a subcuticular absorbable suture and Steri-Strips for the dermis. A lumbar puncture or temporary lumbar drainage can be performed to bolster the closure and decrease risk of cerebrospinal fluid leak.

7.8 Postoperative Care

- Patients are typically observed in the intensive care unit postoperatively, with close neurologic monitoring and standard postoperative imaging.

7.9 Complications

- Complications from orbital compression are likely minimized with an mLOA. Dural closure is difficult when accessing the intradural space with an LOA or mLOA, and a lumbar drain is useful in cases with concern for a cerebrospinal fluid leak.
- Corneal injury is a concern when operating near the eye. A corneal protector with lubricant is placed to avoid abrasions, followed by preparation with 5% povidone-iodine.

7.10 Management Pearls

- The LOA is a keyhole technique that can be used to directly access lesions of the orbit and OA, as well as the SOF, CS, and MCF.
- As with any skull base approach, a thorough understanding of the involved anatomy and

prior cadaveric dissection is critical to successful implementation.

- The use of the microscope facilitates bimanual microsurgical technique with a small surgical footprint, with endoscopic supplementation as needed for difficult-to-visualize areas.
- The recently described mLOA also limits orbital manipulation and risk to critical structures through preservation of the lateral orbital wall.

References

[1] Bounajem MT, Rennert RC, Budohoski KP, Azab M, Karsy M, Couldwell WT. Modified lateral orbitotomy approach to lesions of the orbital apex, superior orbital fissure, cavernous sinus, and middle cranial fossa. Oper Neurosurg (Hagerstown). 2023; 24(5):514–523

[2] Vural A, Carobbio ALC, Ferrari M, et al. Transorbital endoscopic approaches to the skull base: a systematic literature review and anatomical description. Neurosurg Rev. 2021; 44(5): 2857–2878

[3] Lyson T, Sieskiewicz A, Rogowski M, Mariak Z. Endoscopic lateral orbitotomy. Acta Neurochir (Wien). 2014; 156(10): 1897–1900

[4] Kong DS, Young SM, Hong CK, et al. Clinical and ophthalmological outcome of endoscopic transorbital surgery for cranioorbital tumors. J Neurosurg. 2018; 131(3):667–675

[5] Chabot JD, Gardner PA, Stefko ST, Zwagerman NT, Fernandez-Miranda JC. Lateral orbitotomy approach for lesions involving the middle fossa: a retrospective review of thirteen patients. Neurosurgery. 2017; 80(2):309–322

[6] Alzhrani GA, Gozal YM, Sherrod BA, Couldwell WT. A modified lateral orbitotomy approach to the superior orbital fissure: a video case report and review of anatomy. Oper Neurosurg (Hagerstown). 2019; 16(6):685–691

[7] Ciporen JN, Moe KS, Ramanathan D, et al. Multiportal endoscopic approaches to the central skull base: a cadaveric study. World Neurosurg. 2010; 73(6):705–712

[8] Noiphithak R, Yanez-Siller JC, Revuelta Barbero JM, Otto BA, Carrau RL, Prevedello DM. Quantitative analysis of the surgical exposure and surgical freedom between transcranial and transorbital endoscopic anterior petrosectomies to the posterior fossa. J Neurosurg. 2018; 131(2):569–577

[9] Lubbe DE, Douglas-Jones P, Wasl H, Mustak H, Semple PL. Contralateral precaruncular approach to the lateral sphenoid sinus—a case report detailing a new, multiportal approach to lesions, and defects in the lateral aspect of well-pneumatized sphenoid sinuses. Ear Nose Throat J. 2020; 99(1):62–67

[10] Raza SM, Quinones-Hinojosa A, Lim M, Boahene KD. The transconjunctival transorbital approach: a keyhole approach to the midline anterior skull base. World Neurosurg. 2013; 80(6):864–871

[11] Dallan I, Sellari-Franceschini S, Turri-Zanoni M, et al. Endoscopic transorbital superior eyelid approach for the management of selected spheno-orbital meningiomas: preliminary experience. Oper Neurosurg (Hagerstown). 2018; 14(3):243–251

[12] Jeon C, Hong SD, Woo KI, et al. Use of endoscopic transorbital and endonasal approaches for 360° circumferential access to orbital tumors. J Neurosurg. 2020; 135(1):103–112

[13] Mariniello G, Maiuri F, de Divitiis E, et al. Lateral orbitotomy for removal of sphenoid wing meningiomas invading the orbit. Neurosurgery. 2010; 66(6 Suppl Operative):287–292, discussion 292

[14] Rennert RC, Bounajem MT, Budohoski KP, Mortimer VR, Couldwell WT. Modified lateral orbitotomy approach for resection of anterior temporal cavernous malformation. Surg Neurol Int. 2022; 13:389

[15] Cohen MA, Couldwell WT. Resection of cavernous sinus meningioma via lateral orbitotomy approach: 2-dimensional operative video. Oper Neurosurg (Hagerstown). 2020; 18(5):E164

8 Supracerebellar Infratentorial Approach

Matthew J. Recker, Jaims Lim, Joanna M. Roy, Bao Y. Sciscent, Steven Blake Housley, Adnan H. Siddiqui, and Renee Reynolds

8.1 Background

- The supracerebellar infratentorial (SCIT) approach allows access to various pathologies in the pineal region, posterior third ventricle, dorsal midbrain, tectum, and medial thalamus, including neoplasms, cavernous malformations, dural arteriovenous fistulas (AVFs), arteriovenous malformations (AVMs), and distal superior cerebellar artery aneurysms.
- This approach can be used with the patient in a sitting, prone, or park bench lateral position. A preoperative imaging evaluation is necessary for understanding the regional anatomy, specifically the tentorial angle; precise location, size, and degree of infiltration of the lesion; and the adjacent vascular anatomy, such as the size of the transverse sinuses bilaterally, and the distance from the foramen magnum to the tentorial angle and the venous sinuses.
- Potential complications include infection, cerebrospinal fluid (CSF) leak, hemorrhage, venous injury, and venous air embolism.

8.2 Indications and Contraindications

- The SCIT approach is appropriate for lesions located in the pineal region, including lesions of the posterior third ventricle, dorsal midbrain, and along the tentorium. Neoplastic processes seen in this region include germ cell tumors, pineoblastomas, astrocytomas and other gliomas, meningiomas, and epidermoid tumors.[1,2,3,4] This approach can also be used to target vascular lesions in this region, such as tentorial AVFs and AVMs, as well as distal superior cerebellar artery aneurysms. In particular, straight sinus dural AVFs can be easily visualized.[5,6,7]
- Patient-specific factors can pose challenges for the SCIT approach. A steep tentorial angle makes visualization and working angles at the depth of this operative corridor difficult.[8,9] Posterior displacement of the deep venous structures by the pathology may preclude the use of this approach. Obesity, a short neck, and poor neck flexion will compound this challenge and sway the surgeon to choose a sitting position. The sitting position poses increased risk for venous air embolism, particularly in patients with a history of pulmonary hypertension or right ventricular dysfunction.[10,11] A ventriculoatrial shunt and a right-to-left cardiac shunt are absolute contraindications to this positioning.[12]

8.3 Instruments

- All equipment utilized for a standard craniotomy should be available, including electrocautery, appropriate retractors, and a high-speed drill.
- A Mayfield head clamp (Integra LifeSciences) is required for fixation of the patient in the chosen operative position.
- Neuronavigation can be utilized to identify venous sinuses and provide guidance to the location of the pathology.
- An adjustable operating table is important to manipulate viewing angles intraoperatively.
- For this reason, the patient should be well secured to the operating table with tape and straps.
- In the park bench lateral position, an axillary roll should be placed to avoid blockage of venous drainage in the bottom arm.
- A full array of microsurgical instruments are required.
- Based on surgeon preference, an operating microscope or endoscope will be utilized after dural opening.
- If the sitting position is chosen, appropriate support of the surgeon's arm is critical to prevent fatigue.
- Options include using a surgical chair with armrests or using the head of the operating table as an armrest.
- Depending on the particular lesion being targeted, a combination of brainstem auditory evoked response testing, somatosensory evoked potential testing, motor evoked potential testing, and electroencephalography may be utilized for neurophysiologic monitoring.

8.4 Patient Preparation

- Preoperative imaging should include high-quality computed tomography (CT) and magnetic resonance imaging (MRI) with and without contrast administration to visualize the pathology in order to determine the optimal approach. Many centers will include a stereotactic imaging protocol for registration to an intraoperative neuronavigation system. Depending on the particular pathology, a formal catheter-based angiogram may be necessary to fully understand the vascular anatomy with particular attention to the deep venous structures. If the lesion is a pineal region tumor, laboratory studies may be conducted preoperatively to identify biological markers such as alpha fetoprotein, placental alkaline phosphatase, and human chorionic gonadotropin.[13]
- For neoplastic processes, the tumor's enhancement pattern, mass effect, and degree of infiltration, and the relative location of the venous anatomy surrounding the lesion should be studied. Because many pineal region tumors often displace the venous anatomy, it is imperative to evaluate the locations of the deep veins, including the internal cerebral veins, vein of Galen, basal vein of Rosenthal, and venous sinuses.[14] For vascular pathologies such as dural AVFs and AVMs, a diagnostic cerebral angiogram is the "gold standard" for identifying feeding arteries and draining veins.
- An anesthesia team well versed in neuroanesthesia is preferred for all craniotomies. The choice of anesthetic agents requires consideration of the intraoperative neurophysiologic monitoring chosen, and total intravenous anesthesia may be preferred. Vital sign monitoring, oxygen saturation monitoring, electrocardiography, intra-arterial blood pressure monitoring, and temperature probe and Foley catheter placement are standard. Prior to incision, prophylactic intravenous antibiotics (such as cefazolin) should be administered. Depending on the pathology, intravenous steroids (e.g., dexamethasone) and mannitol may be utilized perioperatively, at a dose determined at the discretion of the surgeon. At the end of the procedure, prophylactic use of labetalol may be considered to attenuate hypertension occurring during emergence from anesthesia and postoperative hemorrhage.[10,15]
- If the sitting position is chosen, intraoperative monitoring for venous air embolism is essential. Options include precordial Doppler ultrasonography and transesophageal echocardiography. A central venous catheter terminating at the superior vena cava–right atrial junction should be placed for aspiration in case of an air embolism.[16]

8.5 Patient Positioning

- The patient may be positioned in a Concorde prone, park bench, or sitting position. Measurement of the tentorial angle is an important consideration in the determination of an optimal approach. The tentorial angle can be measured on MRI by various methods. One method involves measuring the angle between the line joining the nasion with the tuberculum sellae and tentorium in the midsagittal plane.[17,18] A steep tentorial angle (> 55 degrees) makes the SCIT approach more challenging. In this circumstance, the paramedian variant and/or the sitting position may be preferred, and consideration should be given to an occipital transtentorial approach instead of an SCIT approach.[8]
- If the surgeon chooses to utilize a sitting position during the operation, a patent foramen ovale must be ruled out as this is a contraindication to this position. Echocardiography (transthoracic or transesophageal; with or without a bubble study) or transcranial Doppler imaging with a bubble study can be performed to assess for a patent foramen ovale.
- The sitting position offers the advantage of a clearer surgical field due to the drainage of CSF and blood by gravity. Additionally, there is less need to retract the cerebellum away from the tentorium in the sitting position; however, this position carries increased risk of air embolism and hemodynamic instability and is scarcely used at many centers.[19]
- Patients in the park bench or lateral oblique position are turned on their side, with an axillary roll underneath. The head is flexed and turned slightly toward the downward shoulder to increase the angle between the atlas and the

foramen magnum. The upward shoulder is taped forward and toward the feet, away from the operative field. Pillows are placed between the legs and arms. Pressure points are protected with gel pads or foam cushions. Tape and belts are used to secure the patient to the operating table to allow rotation and dynamic positioning to best visualize the operative corridor.

- Image guidance is registered if it is being utilized. The transverse and sigmoid venous sinuses are identified using image guidance or based on anatomical landmarks. The top of the mastoid notch or the asterion is used to localize the transverse–sigmoid junction.
- If there is concern for obstructive hydrocephalus, an external ventricular drain (EVD) entry site should be marked, prepared, and draped into the surgical field should emergency intracranial pressure management be required. The surgeon may consider the placement of an EVD preoperatively or at the beginning of the case, but judicious drainage of CSF is advisable until the mass is decompressed. If no concern exists for obstructive hydrocephalus, the surgeon may choose to place a lumbar drain preoperatively for use during the case to relax the brain.

8.6 Technique

- **Midline SCIT approach**:
  - A midline vertical incision is made from approximately 1 to 2 cm above the inion to the C2 spinous process. The soft tissues are dissected in the midline avascular plane and retracted with self-retaining retractors to expose the occipital bone below the inion. The lateral extent of dissection should be adequate to accommodate the planned craniotomy. Several techniques for craniotomy exist. Burr holes may be created just underneath the transverse sinus with a high-speed drill. A B1 drill bit with a footplate can be utilized to turn a wide craniotomy flap. Bony removal generally does not need to extend down to the foramen magnum. Use of the footplate over the transverse sinus should be avoided. Once the flap has been turned, the craniotomy can be extended superiorly in layers after the dura is stripped to reveal the transverse sinus to allow for mobilization of the sinus after dural opening. Regardless of the technique chosen for the craniotomy, at least the inferior edge of the transverse sinus must be exposed to allow sufficient dural retraction. A curvilinear incision is used to open the dura. Tack-up sutures along the dural opening and tentorium should be placed to gently elevate and rotate the torcula and transverse sinus.[20] The adhesions between the cerebellum and the tentorium are dissected, allowing the cerebellum to fall away toward the foramen magnum. Midline bridging veins are cauterized and divided on the cerebellar side. The precentral vein can be coagulated and divided. A deeper, thick layer of arachnoid is encountered and divided, revealing the vein of Galen complex and adjacent anatomical structures. The microsurgical technique is utilized to address the patient's specific pathology.
- **Paramedian SCIT approach**:
  - The side of the paramedian approach should be determined by the location of the patient's pathology and the venous anatomy. An approach from the side of the nondominant transverse sinus should be favored. A vertical paramedian incision is made, extending one-third above and two-thirds below the transverse sinus. Its mediolateral position is determined according to the optimal trajectory to the lesion, which can be planned with the assistance of neuronavigation. A burr hole is made at the inferior edge of the transverse sinus and a bone flap spanning the width of the transverse sinus is elevated. The bony opening is extended superiorly to expose the transverse sinus, as described above. A curvilinear dural incision toward the sinus is utilized, and tack-up sutures are placed to elevate the tentorium and transverse sinus. Paramedian bridging veins are coagulated and cut on the cerebellar side and arachnoid adhesions are released. The trochlear nerve (cranial nerve IV) should be visualized and protected.[21] The microsurgical technique is employed to address the patient's specific pathology.
- For either technique, after hemostasis has been achieved, the dura is closed in a watertight fashion. A synthetic dural substitute or pericranial graft may be utilized. The bone flap is then replaced using cranial plates and the

muscle is approximated, followed by fascial and skin closure.

- The relevant anatomy is included in **Video 8.1**.

8.7 Postoperative Care

- The patient is typically extubated in the operating room unless there is concern raised by the surgeon or anesthesiologist about the patient's readiness for extubation. A neurological examination is performed in the operating room once the patient emerges from anesthesia. The patient is transferred to the intensive care unit, where the vital signs and neurological examination are closely monitored.
- An EVD may be left postoperatively to monitor intracranial pressure and drain CSF as needed. Some patients with obstructive hydrocephalus will require permanent CSF diversion. Steroids are often prescribed postoperatively to treat edema and reduce the risk of aseptic meningitis. Any change in neurological status or vital signs should prompt immediate evaluation and neuroimaging. After 24 to 48 hours, if the patient is doing well, the Foley catheter and arterial line can be removed and the patient can be started on chemoprophylaxis for deep vein thrombosis.
- The patient can be transferred to a neurosurgical step-down unit or other appropriate lower level of care with emphasis on ambulation and dietary intake and regular examination for signs of CSF leak, wound infection, or neurological deficits.
- Depending on the pathology treated, a postoperative MRI of the brain with and without contrast administration or postoperative formal cerebral angiography may be warranted. Most patients are discharged to home and scheduled for appropriate follow-up.
- For patients with postoperative deficits due to iatrogenic complications or the primary pathology, physical therapy and occupational therapy evaluation and outpatient follow-up are critical for maximal recovery and functional rehabilitation.[22]

8.8 Complications

- Venous air embolism may occur due to relatively low pressure in the cranial veins when the head is positioned above the level of the heart. Patients in the sitting position are at higher risk of air embolism.[23] Monitoring for venous air embolism is mandatory in the sitting position. Should venous air embolism occur, one of the first signs is a dramatic decrease in end-tidal CO_2. Preoperative placement of a central venous catheter at the cavoatrial junction is imperative to allow for aspiration of air in the event of an air embolism. Hypotension may also occur more frequently in the sitting position due to pooling of blood in the lower extremities, and thus the legs should be elevated and wrapped preoperatively to prevent venous pooling.
- The development of a postoperative hematoma in the posterior fossa can lead to brainstem compression and obstruct CSF flow causing obstructive hydrocephalus. Although bridging veins are not usually preserved during surgery, cerebellar congestion or venous infarction has been reported in those rare cases in which bridging veins were sacrificed.[24] Prolonged retraction of the cerebellum may also contribute to injury and postoperative swelling. Retraction and manipulation of the venous sinuses can lead to venous sinus thrombosis.[25] Thus, the length of time of static retraction, if used, should be considered and the use of dynamic manual retraction may be preferred by the surgeon. A postoperative CSF leak is possible given the location of the operation low in the cranium. The risk of CSF leak is higher in patients with hydrocephalus. Meningitis and surgical site infections are also possible in the postoperative period.

8.9 Management Pearls

- The SCIT approach provides access to the pineal region, posterior third ventricle, dorsal midbrain, tectum, and medial thalamus.
- The SCIT approach can be subdivided into midline and paramedian approaches, which may be variably used based on surgeon preference, the pathology, and patient-specific anatomy.
- Preoperative understanding of the location of the pathology and the relationship to surrounding vascular anatomy is vital to determining the optimal operative approach.

- Potential complications from the SCIT approach include venous air embolism (particularly in the sitting position), venous injury or infarction, hematoma, CSF leak, and infection.
- Bridging veins may have to be sacrificed while operating on lesions situated in the pineal region or near the posterior part of the third ventricle. This could lead to venous cerebellar infarction.[24]
- The paramedian variant of the SCIT approach is less likely to require sacrifice of bridging veins because fewer bridging veins cross the surgical field.[26] Resection of lesions located in proximity to the brainstem can result in neurological deficits due to damage to cranial nerve nuclei. In particular, resection of cavernous malformations can lead to hemorrhage, which may worsen neurological deficits.[27,28]

References

[1] Abbassy M, Aref K, Farhoud A, Hekal A. The supracerebellar infratentorial approach in pineal region tumors: technique and outcome in an underprivileged setting. Alex J Med. 2018; 54(4):725–729

[2] Zhao X, Belykh E, Przybylowski CJ, et al. Surgical treatment of falcotentorial meningiomas: a retrospective review of a single-institution experience. J Neurosurg. 2019; 133(3): 630–641

[3] Papadimitriou K, Cossu G, Hewer E, Diezi M, Daniel RT, Messerer M. Endoscope-assisted extreme lateral supracerebellar infratentorial approach for resection of superior cerebellar peduncle pilocytic astrocytoma: technical note. Children (Basel). 2022; 9(5):640

[4] Choudhri O, Chang SD. Supracerebellar infratentorial sitting craniotomy for a pinealoblastoma. Neurosurg Focus. 2016; 40 Video, Suppl 1:2016.1-.FocusVid.15417

[5] Tyler Patterson T, Webb M, Wallace DJ, Caron JL, Mascitelli JR. Suboccipital, supracerebellar, infratentorial approach for microsurgical clipping of a ruptured tentorial, straight sinus type dural arteriovenous fistula. World Neurosurg. 2020; 142:131–135

[6] Rutkowski MJ, Jian B, Lawton MT. Surgical management of cerebral dural arteriovenous fistulae. Handb Clin Neurol. 2017; 143:107–116

[7] Vishteh AG, David CA, Marciano FF, Coscarella E, Spetzler RF. Extreme lateral supracerebellar infratentorial approach to the posterolateral mesencephalon: technique and clinical experience. Neurosurgery. 2000; 46(2):384–388, discussion 388–389

[8] Syed HR, Jean WC. A novel method to measure the tentorial angle and the implications on surgeries of the pineal region. World Neurosurg. 2018; 111:e213–e220

[9] Nemir J, NjiriÄ N, IvankoviÄ D, et al. Tentorial alignment and its relationship to cisternal dimensions of the pineal region: MRI anatomical study with surgical implications using the new clivotentorial method. Clin Neurol Neurosurg. 2018; 172:99–104

[10] Slbin MS, Babinski M, Maroon JC, Jannetta PJ. Anesthetic management of posterior fossa surgery in the sitting position. Acta Anaesthesiol Scand. 1976; 20(2):117–128

[11] Black S, Ockert DB, Oliver WC, Jr, Cucchiara RF. Outcome following posterior fossa craniectomy in patients in the sitting or horizontal positions. Anesthesiology. 1988; 69(1): 49–56

[12] Jagannathan S, Krovvidi H. Anaesthetic considerations for posterior fossa surgery. Contin Educ Anaesth Crit Care Pain. 2014; 14(5):202–206

[13] Zaazoue MA, Goumnerova LC. Pineal region tumors: a simplified management scheme. Childs Nerv Syst. 2016; 32 (11):2041–2045

[14] Giordano M, Lüdemann WO, Stieglitz L, et al. Identification of venous variants in the pineal region with three-dimensional preoperative magnetic resonance imaging navigation in patients harbouring tumors in this area: significance for surgical approach to the lesion. Clin Neurol Neurosurg. 2011; 113(5):387–392

[15] Himes BT, Mallory GW, Abcejo AS, et al. Contemporary analysis of the intraoperative and perioperative complications of neurosurgical procedures performed in the sitting position. J Neurosurg. 2017; 127(1):182–188

[16] Al-Afif S, Elkayekh H, Omer M, et al. Analysis of risk factors for venous air embolism in the semisitting position and its impact on outcome in a consecutive series of 740 patients. J Neurosurg. 2021; 137(1):258–265

[17] Kao SC, Waziri MH, Smith WL, Sato Y, Yuh WT, Franken EA, Jr. MR imaging of the craniovertebral junction, cranium, and brain in children with achondroplasia. AJR Am J Roentgenol. 1989; 153(3):565–569

[18] Hasegawa M, Yamashita J, Yamashima T. Anatomical variations of the straight sinus on magnetic resonance imaging in the infratentorial supracerebellar approach to pineal region tumors. Surg Neurol. 1991; 36(5):354–359

[19] Sanai N, Mirzadeh Z, Lawton MT. Supracerebellar-supratrochlear and infratentorial-infratrochlear approaches: gravity-dependent variations of the lateral approach over the cerebellum. Neurosurgery. 2010; 66(6) Suppl Operative:264–274, discussion 274

[20] Rey-Dios R, Cohen-Gadol AA. A surgical technique to expand the operative corridor for supracerebellar infratentorial approaches: technical note. Acta Neurochir (Wien). 2013; 155(10):1895–1900

[21] La Pira B, Sorenson T, Quillis-Quesada V, Lanzino G. The paramedian supracerebellar infratentorial approach. Acta Neurochir (Wien). 2017; 159(8):1529–1532

[22] Bartolo M, Zucchella C, Pace A, et al. Early rehabilitation after surgery improves functional outcome in inpatients with brain tumours. J Neurooncol. 2012; 107(3):537–544

[23] Grady MS, Bedford RF, Park TS. Changes in superior sagittal sinus pressure in children with head elevation, jugular venous compression, and PEEP. J Neurosurg. 1986; 65(2): 199–202

[24] Smrcka M, Navratil O. What is the risk of venous cerebellar infarction in the supracerebellar infratentorial approach? Neurosurg Rev. 2021; 44(2):897–900

[25] Kodera T, Bozinov O, Sürücü O, Ulrich NH, Burkhardt JK, Bertalanffy H. Neurosurgical venous considerations for tumors of the pineal region resected using the infratentorial supracerebellar approach. J Clin Neurosci. 2011; 18(11): 1481–1485

[26] Ueyama T, Al-Mefty O, Tamaki N. Bridging veins on the tentorial surface of the cerebellum: a microsurgical anatomic study and operative considerations. Neurosurgery. 1998; 43 (5):1137–1145
[27] Rutledge C, Raper DMS, Rodriguez Rubio R, Winkler EA, Abla AA. Supracerebellar infratentorial infratrochlear trans-quadrangular lobule approach to pontine cavernous malformations. Oper Neurosurg (Hagerstown). 2021; 20 (3):268–275
[28] de Oliveira JG, Lekovic GP, Safavi-Abbasi S, et al. Supracerebellar infratentorial approach to cavernous malformations of the brainstem: surgical variants and clinical experience with 45 patients. Neurosurgery. 2010; 66 (2):389–399

9 Supracerebellar Transtentorial Approach

Jaims Lim, Matthew J. Recker, Bao Y. Sciscent, Joanna M. Roy, Steven Blake Housley, Adnan H. Siddiqui, and Renee Reynolds

9.1 Background

- The supracerebellar transtentorial (SCTT) approach is indicated for pathology of the medial and posterior temporal region including tentorial meningiomas, intraparenchymal lesions (such as gliomas, cavernous malformations and arteriovenous malformations [AVMs], and distal posterior cerebral artery [PCA] aneurysms).
- This approach can be performed in the sitting or lateral (park bench) position.
- Preoperative imaging evaluation, including computed tomography (CT), digital subtraction angiography (DSA), magnetic resonance (MR) imaging, and MR angiography, is key to a safe and successful procedure and understanding of the regional anatomy.
- It is important to be aware of the location of the transverse and sigmoid sinuses as they can have varied courses and positions, and the angle of the tentorium should be considered.
- A steep tentorial angle can provide a limited view of lesions in the medial temporal lobe.
- Complications include infarction, cerebrospinal fluid (CSF) leak, venous injury or infarction, posterior fossa hemorrhage, infection, and venous air embolism.

9.2 Indications and Contraindications

- As mentioned, the SCTT approach can be used to treat various pathologies in the medial and posterior temporal region including tentorial meningiomas, distal PCA aneurysms, medial temporal AVMs, cavernous malformations, and mesiobasal temporal epilepsy.[1,2,3,4,5,6] This approach provides a window to reach the mesiobasal region of the temporal lobe from the uncus to the posterior medial temporal lobe.[3,4,7] It is minimally invasive as it involves a small posterior fossa craniotomy and does not require significant retraction of the temporal or occipital lobe. However, the operating corridor is deep and narrow so lesions that are large or extend too far lateral or anterior may require an alternative or a combined approach that includes a temporal or frontotemporal craniotomy.[8]
- Anatomical considerations and patient factors may pose contraindications to the SCTT approach. The SCTT approach can be performed in either the sitting or the park bench position. The sitting position increases the risk of venous air embolism and the presence of a ventriculoatrial shunt and a right-to-left cardiac shunt are contraindications to this positioning.[9] Drainage of the basal vein of Rosenthal into the channels of the tentorium can be seen and increases the risk for venous infarction postoperatively.[1] A steep tentorial angle may be a contraindication to this approach if a significant amount of retraction on the cerebellum is necessary after opening the tentorium to access the medial temporal region. The approach may be deemed suboptimal for obese patients with a short neck and poor neck flexion. Absence of a vein-free corridor along the supracerebellar space may be a contraindication as the sacrifice of such veins can cause cerebellar infarct, venous engorgement, and obstruction of the deep veins (including the basal vein of Rosenthal).

9.3 Instruments

- A Mayfield head holder (Integra LifeSciences) and equipment for a standard craniotomy should be available. Positioning adjuncts such as an axillary roll, tape, and pillows are required and should be available. Correct orientation and functioning of the bed should be checked before positioning the patient on the bed because significant manipulation of the bed may be required intraoperatively to obtain the proper viewing angles. Equipment specific to the SCTT approach may include a lumbar drain and a self-retaining retractor. A lumbar drain may facilitate cerebellar decompression and improve the tentorial viewing angle, increase the working space between the cerebellar surface and tentorium, and prevent excessive retraction on the cerebellum. Neuronavigation can be utilized to identify the transverse sinus. Based on the location and nature of the pathology, a combination of somatosensory evoked potential testing, brainstem auditory evoked response testing, motor evoked potential testing, and electroencephalography monitoring may be utilized.

9.4 Patient Preparation

- CT and MR imaging with and without contrast enhancement are utilized to visualize the pathology and adjacent anatomical structures in order to determine the optimal approach to the lesion. Careful examination of preoperative venous phase imaging obtained as part of the CT and MR angiography (i.e., CT venography, MR venography) or DSA helps the surgeon to appreciate the course and dominance of the venous sinuses and the orientation of the deep veins to minimize the risk of bleeding and venous infarction. In particular, the petrosal and tentorial veins must be located because they drain a significant portion of the blood supply from the posterior fossa; and if there are a significant number of veins along the tentorium on the side of the lesion, an SCTT approach should not be considered.[1]
- For neoplastic mass lesions, the lesion's size, mass effect, and adherence to nearby structures should also be studied. Because this approach uses a narrow operative window, the distance from the incision to the mesiotemporal region and the angle to the posterior structures should be measured.[10] Cerebral DSA can also be performed to identify any feeding arteries and draining veins. It is also important to know the proximity of these vessels to major vessels, including the PCA. If major branches of the PCA are located in between the operative corridor and the mass, the SCTT approach may not be optimal as the risk of ischemic injury is high.
- Preoperative stereotactic imaging may be obtained and used for intraoperative neuronavigation. If the surgeon chooses to utilize a sitting position during surgery, preoperative evaluation using transthoracic echocardiography with or without a bubble study should be performed to determine whether the patient has a patent foramen ovale.

9.5 Patient Positioning

- The patient can be placed in the sitting position or the lateral park bench position based on surgeon preference, and the decision is made on a case-by-case scenario. The sitting position may provide a clearer surgical field and operative corridor with the help of gravity facilitating CSF and blood drainage. In addition, there is less need for cerebellar retraction in the sitting position with the aid of gravity.[11]
- However, it is important to be aware of the additional risks of air embolism and hemodynamic instability associated with the sitting position.[12] This position may provide clear viewing angles, albeit at the expense of surgeon comfort due to neck strain and reach.[13]
- Patients in the lateral park bench position are turned on their side with an axillary roll underneath. The head is flexed and turned slightly downward to increase the angle of the atlas and the foramen magnum. The upward shoulder is taped forward toward the feet to provide greater degree of mobility of the surgeon's hands and equipment around the surgical site. The patient's legs and arms are padded appropriately to prevent iatrogenic nerve injury and venous pooling. The patient should be secured to the operating table with tape and straps to ensure safety when turned and tilted during the operation, allowing the surgeon to obtain optimal viewing angles throughout the case.
- Once the patient is positioned, the head is fixed in the Mayfield head holder and rotated contralateral to the lesion.

9.6 Technique

- **Anesthesia**:
    - An anesthesia team with experience in posterior fossa craniotomies is preferred for the SCTT approach. A similar protocol is followed for all posterior fossa craniotomies. The procedure is performed preferably with total intravenous anesthesia with propofol when neurophysiologic monitoring will be

utilized. Monitoring of vital signs and use of Foley catheters, arterial lines, oxygen saturations, and peripheral intravenous lines are standard. If the patient is placed in the sitting position, intraoperative monitoring for venous air embolism is crucial with precordial Doppler imaging or transesophageal echocardiography.[14,15] It is also important to consider that during tentorial manipulation, a temporary arrhythmia due to the trigeminal vagal pathway may occur.[2]
  - Prior to surgical incision, prophylactic antibiotics of the surgeon's choice should be administered. Steroids and mannitol, depending on the lesion, vasogenic edema, mass effect, and brain shift, can be administered perioperatively.
- **Technique**:
  - If preoperative imaging raises concern for obstructive hydrocephalus, an external ventricular drain (EVD) site, usually at Keen's point for the SCTT approach, should be marked and prepared in case urgent management of intracranial pressure (ICP) is necessary intraoperatively. Based on the surgeon's judgement relative to the patient's preoperative images and the size of the lesion, an EVD may be placed preoperatively either at Keen's point or at Kocher's point. Preoperative placement may aid in CSF drainage and brain relaxation.
  - A paramedian vertical linear incision on the side of the lesion is made between the inion and asterion with one-third of the incision above and two-thirds of the incision below the transverse sinus. Alternatively, a hockey stick incision may be made with its vertical component along the midline, and the horizontal aspect of the incision positioned one-quarter above and three-quarters below the transverse sinus.
  - After meticulous soft tissue dissection, a unilateral burr hole is made above the transverse sinus. It is imperative to make sure the sinus is carefully stripped off the overlying bone with a Woodson elevator or another means for flat dissection and that it is not violated. A craniotomy is created to remove the bone overlying the transverse sinus as well as inferior to the sinus with a drill and Kerrison rongeurs.
  - This is where preoperative evaluation of the transverse sinuses and awareness of the dominant side of the sinus are key. Meticulous hemostasis after each stage of the opening is key for adequate visualization and quick and efficient intracranial dissection. The dura is opened using a curvilinear incision 15 mm below the transverse sinus and in a **U** shape, and retraction sutures are placed along the tentorium to facilitate elevation of the transverse sinus superiorly.
  - Careful dissection of the arachnoid adhesions can reveal the cisterna magna toward the inferior pole of the cerebellum and CSF can be released for relaxation of the cerebellum.[16] Bridging veins that drain the basal aspect of the occipital lobe are sacrificed as they cross the tentorial surface. Care must be taken to avoid sacrificing the midline tentorial bridging vein and the petrosal vein. The quadrigeminal cisterns are exposed, and arachnoid granulations are dissected to visualize the mid-distal segments of the PCA and the trochlear nerve (cranial nerve IV). The tentorium is cut with care to prevent injury to the trochlear nerve as it passes along the free edge of the tentorial incisura. A lateral to medial incision is usually easier than in a medial to lateral direction due to the steep upward angulation of the tentorium.[2]
  - The tentorial opening can be performed in a linear or **T**-shaped fashion based on the specific lesion to be targeted, and the assistance of neuronavigation is valuable in planning this opening intraoperatively (see **Video 8.1**). The cut edges of the tentorium can be mobilized and retracted with sutures on either side. Bleeding from the tentorium is controlled using bipolar coagulation or clips. Once the tentorium is opened, the surgeon gains access to the posterior, medial temporal lobe.
  - When operating in the mediobasal temporal region, extreme care must be taken to visualize and expose the trochlear nerve in order to avoid accidental injury to this nerve. The trochlear nerve arises from the dorsal region of the brainstem in the posterior incisural space and courses through the ambient cistern around the midbrain. It passes through the gap between the PCA and the

superior cerebellar artery and along the free edge of the tentorium.[2,17] When incising the tentorium during the SCTT approach and making progress toward the mediotemporal region, it is important to be mindful that the trochlear nerve courses along the free edge of the tentorium. Stereotactic image guidance or intraoperative fluorescence, such as is achieved with an indocyanine green injection, can aid navigation of the operative corridor and visualization of important nerves and vasculature.
  - Advantages of the SCTT approach include early devascularization of lesions, such as tumors, that lie adjacent to the tentorium by making small incisions and subsequently coagulating the tentorium with bipolar electrocautery around these lesions from which blood supply is frequently recruited. This provides the surgeon with a relatively bloodless operative field and surgery. Although the SCTT approach requires a long operative corridor, the approach allows minimal manipulation and disruption of actual brain parenchyma compared to a transcortical approach to the mediotemporal region.
  - Once the goal of the surgical procedure has been accomplished (depending on the pathology treated), achieving meticulous hemostasis is imperative. The cavity is irrigated with fluid to remove residual air. Watertight closure of the dura is performed, and the bone flap is replaced. Multilayered closure of the subcutaneous fascia and skin is then performed.

9.7 Postoperative Care

- Barring any intraoperative complications or airway issues, the patient should be extubated at the end of the case after the anesthesia wears off. The patient is transferred to an intensive care unit for close postoperative monitoring of ICP.
- An EVD (if placed preoperatively or intraoperatively) may be left postoperatively for ICP monitoring.
- Steroids can be used to treat vasogenic edema and reduce the risk of aseptic meningitis.
- Any change in neurological status or vital signs should prompt immediate evaluation and neuroimaging.
- After 24 to 48 hours, if the patient is doing well, the Foley catheter and arterial line can be removed and deep vein thrombosis chemoprophylaxis can be initiated to prevent thromboembolic complications.
- The patient is transferred to a neurosurgical step-down unit or other appropriate level of care with emphasis on ambulation, dietary intake, and regular examination for signs of CSF leak, wound infection, or neurological deficits.
- Depending on the pathology treated, postoperative MR imaging of the brain with and without contrast enhancement or postoperative formal cerebral angiography may be warranted.

9.8 Complications

- There is a higher risk of venous air embolism and postoperative hematoma when the SCTT approach is performed in the sitting position.[18] Monitoring for venous air embolism is mandatory in that position. Heightened precautions should be taken by both the neurosurgery and anesthesia teams with specific attention to the end-tidal CO_2, which will precipitously decline in the event of a venous air embolism. A right central ventral venous line ending at the atrium will help aspirate air in the event of an embolism. Hypotension may also occur during the sitting position due to venous pooling in the lower extremities.
- Venous congestion, edema, thrombosis, ischemia, and retraction injury can occur due to prolonged retraction on the cerebellum and venous sinuses. Sacrificing the midline tentorial bridging veins or the petrosal veins during surgery can compromise venous drainage and lead to cerebellar venous congestion and should be avoided.[1,2] In the case of venous sinus thrombosis, the patient may be started on heparin therapy after careful evaluation of the risks and benefits in the setting of recent surgery. The patient's clinical examination should also be considered, and intensive care unit monitoring and serial imaging of the venous sinuses are critical to monitor for propagation of clot. Preservation of as many veins as possible during the operation is recommended to lower the risk of venous complications. The use of

retractors with fixed blades can also increase the risk of ischemic injury. Dynamic retraction can mitigate this risk as there is intermittent retraction along the cerebellum and vasculature.[19]

- A postoperative CSF leak is possible given the location of the operation. The risk of CSF leak is higher in patients at risk of hydrocephalus. Meningitis and surgical site infections are also possible in the postoperative period. Although not a complication, postoperative pain is a common sequelae after this operation and can be minimized by the use of a midline incision that allows for subperiosteal dissection of paravertebral muscles.[17] Postoperative benzodiazepines such as diazepam might also help ease the pain.

9.9 Management Pearls

- The SCTT approach provides access to the medial posterior temporal and parahippocampal regions at the level of the cerebral peduncle and posterior to the temporal uncus.
- The SCTT approach provides good working angles but through a long working distance, making awareness of its indications and limitations critical.
- Pathologies amenable to this approach include superiorly oriented tentorial meningiomas, distal PCA aneurysms, mesiotemporal AVMs, cavernous malformations, and medically intractable mesiobasal temporal epilepsy.
- Careful review of preoperative imaging, including CT, MR imaging, and MR angiography or DSA, is imperative to planning and completion of a low-risk operation.
- Complications of the SCTT approach include venous air embolism (particularly in the sitting position), venous injury or infarction, CSF leak, infection, postoperative hematoma, and venous congestion.
- Bradycardia and arrhythmia may occur due to stimulation of the trigeminal nerve during inadvertent retraction and manipulation while the tentorium is being incised.[2] Large venous lakes or sinuses encountered during incision of the tentorium must be closed with titanium clips or coagulated to minimize air exposure, which could result in venous air embolism. This risk is higher in children due to the presence of more venous lakes in the tentorium.[5] Preoperative venous angiography and image guidance can help identify these sinuses to prevent injury during surgery.

References

[1] Türe U, Harput MV, Kaya AH, et al. The paramedian supracerebellar-transtentorial approach to the entire length of the mediobasal temporal region: an anatomical and clinical study. Laboratory investigation. J Neurosurg. 2012; 116(4): 773–791

[2] Yonekawa Y, Imhof HG, Taub E, et al. Supracerebellar transtentorial approach to posterior temporomedial structures. J Neurosurg. 2001; 94(2):339–345

[3] de Oliveira JG, Lekovic GP, Safavi-Abbasi S, et al. Supracerebellar infratentorial approach to cavernous malformations of the brainstem: surgical variants and clinical experience with 45 patients. Neurosurgery. 2010; 66(2):389–399

[4] Voigt K, Yaşargil MG. Cerebral cavernous haemangiomas or cavernomas. Incidence, pathology, localization, diagnosis, clinical features and treatment. Review of the literature and report of an unusual case. Neurochirurgia (Stuttg). 1976; 19 (2):59–68

[5] Weil AG, Middleton AL, Niazi TN, Ragheb J, Bhatia S. The supracerebellar-transtentorial approach to posteromedial temporal lesions in children with refractory epilepsy. J Neurosurg Pediatr. 2015; 15(1):45–54

[6] Uchiyama N, Hasegawa M, Kita D, Yamashita J. Paramedian supracerebellar transtentorial approach for a medial tentorial meningioma with supratentorial extension: technical case report. Neurosurgery. 2001; 49(6):1470–1473, discussion 1473–1474

[7] Matsushima K, Yagmurlu K, Kohno M, Rhoton AL, Jr. Anatomy and approaches along the cerebellar-brainstem fissures. J Neurosurg. 2016; 124(1):248–263

[8] Teton ZE, Hendricks BK, Marotta DA, Cohen-Gadol A. Transtentorial approach to parahippocampal lesions: a technically challenging approach for preserving temporal lobe structures. World Neurosurg. 2020; 142:626–635

[9] Jagannathan S, Krovvidi H. Anaesthetic considerations for posterior fossa surgery. Contin Educ Anaesth Crit Care Pain. 2014; 14(5):202–206

[10] Coca A, Ganau M, Todeschi J, et al. Endoscopic-enhanced supra-cerebellar trans-tentorial (SCTT) approach to temporo-mesial region: a multicenter study. Neurosurg Rev. 2022; 45 (6):3749–3758

[11] Moftakhar R, Izci Y, BaÅkaya MK. Microsurgical anatomy of the supracerebellar transtentorial approach to the posterior mediobasal temporal region: technical considerations with a case illustration. Neurosurgery. 2008; 62(3) Suppl 1:1–7, discussion 7–8

[12] Sanai N, Mirzadeh Z, Lawton MT. Supracerebellar-supratrochlear and infratentorial-infratrochlear approaches: gravity-dependent variations of the lateral approach over the cerebellum. Neurosurgery. 2010; 66(6) Suppl Operative: 264–274, discussion 274

[13] Villanueva P, Louis RG, Cutler AR, et al. Endoscopic and gravity-assisted resection of medial temporo-occipital lesions through a supracerebellar transtentorial approach: technical notes with case illustrations. Oper Neurosurg (Hagerstown). 2015; 11(4): 475–483

[14] Al-Afif S, Elkayekh H, Omer M, et al. Analysis of risk factors for venous air embolism in the semisitting position and its impact on outcome in a consecutive series of 740 patients. J Neurosurg. 2021; 137(1):258–265
[15] Abramov I, Scherschinski L, Labib MA, et al. Supracerebellar infratentorial approach for a malignant pineal region tumor mimicking a cavernous malformation. World Neurosurg. 2022; 167:122
[16] Cohen-Gadol AA. The paramedian supracerebellar approach: a less disruptive and more flexible operative corridor to the pineal and posterior upper brainstem regions. World Neurosurg. 2020; 143:647–657
[17] Ansari SF, Young RL, Bohnstedt BN, Cohen-Gadol AA. The extended supracerebellar transtentorial approach for resection of medial tentorial meningiomas. Surg Neurol Int. 2014; 5:35
[18] Grady MS, Bedford RF, Park TS. Changes in superior sagittal sinus pressure in children with head elevation, jugular venous compression, and PEEP. J Neurosurg. 1986; 65(2): 199–202
[19] Kodera T, Bozinov O, Sürücü O, Ulrich NH, Burkhardt JK, Bertalanffy H. Neurosurgical venous considerations for tumors of the pineal region resected using the infratentorial supracerebellar approach. J Clin Neurosci. 2011; 18(11): 1481–1485

10 Telovelar and Transvermian Approaches

Matthew J. Recker, Jaims Lim, Bao Y. Sciscent, Joanna M. Roy, Steven Blake Housley, Adnan H. Siddiqui, and Renee Reynolds

10.1 Background

- The transvermian and telovelar approaches allow access to pathologies located in the region of the fourth ventricle including ependymomas, medulloblastomas, hemangioblastomas, cavernous malformations, arteriovenous malformations, choroid plexus papillomas, gliomas, and brain metastases. This approach is typically performed in the prone (Concorde) or park bench position. Preoperative imaging with computed tomography (CT) and magnetic resonance imaging (MRI) is necessary to determine whether the pathology in question is amenable to these approaches. Potential complications including posterior fossa syndrome (PFS), brainstem and cranial nerve (CN) injury, hydrocephalus, hemorrhage, and postoperative edema may occur.

10.2 Indications and Contraindications

- These approaches are indicated to address pathologies of the fourth ventricle and surrounding structures, such as ependymomas, medulloblastomas, hemangioblastomas, cavernous malformations, arteriovenous malformations, choroid plexus papillomas, gliomas, and brain metastases.[1,2,3,4] The transvermian approach is the traditional route to address pathology in this region, although the telovelar approach has more recently become the predominant approach at many centers. Some argue that splitting the vermis leads to increased rates of postoperative complications such as nystagmus, gait disturbance, truncal ataxia, and cerebellar mutism.[3,5,6] The transvermian approach may be favored for large lesions that extend rostrally within the fourth ventricle. However, anatomical studies comparing the two approaches have found similar rostral access with the addition of a C1 laminectomy to the telovelar approach.[7] The telovelar approach provides improved access and visualization of the lateral recess of the fourth ventricle and some data suggest it carries lower risk of PFS compared to a transvermian approach.[2,4]
- Although there are no absolute contraindications to these approaches, several factors should be considered. Adherence and invasion of the lesion to the floor of the fourth ventricle adds complexity to the case and may limit the ability to safely achieve a gross total resection. Lesions that extend laterally beyond the foramen of Luschka may not be fully visualized by these approaches. Deep rostral tumor attachment may also present a specific limitation to the telovelar approach.[2]

10.3 Instruments

- The usual equipment for a suboccipital craniotomy is required. This includes a Mayfield head holder (Integra LifeSciences), high-speed drill, cerebellar self-retaining retractors, and monopolar and bipolar electrocautery. Neuronavigation can be used to identify the transverse sinus and guide intracranial dissection. Equipment that may be used for positioning includes an axillary roll, tape, bed straps, and pillows. An operative microscope is utilized for the intracranial portion of the surgery. Neuromonitoring using electromyography, somatosensory evoked potentials, motor evoked potentials, brainstem auditory evoked potentials, and stimulation mapping of CN nuclei are commonly utilized surgical adjuncts in procedures that involve the fourth ventricle.

10.4 Patient Preparation

- Preoperative noninvasive imaging with CT and MRI with and without contrast administration is necessary to visualize the pathology and guide operative planning. The location and size of the lesions play a role in selecting either the transvermian or the telovelar approach.[7] The location and course of the posteroinferior cerebellar arteries should be visualized either on dedicated blood vessel imaging or on the T2-weighted MRI sequences. The surgeon should pay careful attention to the location of the lesion relative to regional anatomy and note any possible adherence to the floor of the fourth ventricle or other surrounding structures. The MRI may also show whether the patient has a patent occipital sinus, which is more common in children.[8] Cerebral angiography may be performed in patients with vascular lesions such as hemangioblastomas. If intraoperative neuronavigation will be utilized, an image using stereotactic protocols should be obtained. A detailed baseline CN examination should be documented preoperatively.[3,9]

10.5 Patient Positioning

- The patient is positioned for a midline suboccipital craniotomy in the prone or park bench position with flexion of the neck to facilitate expansion of the space between the craniovertebral junction. The prone position offers the surgeon greater versatility to comfortably access both the medial intraventricular space, as well as the lateral recess.[10] Some surgeons feel the park bench position is more comfortable and offers better working angles for the primary surgeon. The patient is placed in a Mayfield head holder with pins at the superior temporal line. Care should be taken to avoid over-flexion of the neck, which can cause kinking of the endotracheal tube.

10.6 Technique

- **Anesthesia**:
  - An anesthesia team with considerable neuroanesthesia experience is optimal for these approaches. If neurophysiologic monitoring is used, total intravenous anesthesia may be appropriate. Intraoperative identification and mapping of CN nuclei may also be performed.[11,12] As the patient's head will be fixed in a head holder and manipulated to achieve optimal viewing angles, the endotracheal tube should be carefully positioned and well secured. Routine intraoperative monitoring includes pulse oximetry, electrocardiography, intra-arterial blood pressure monitoring, and temperature probe. A Foley catheter is also placed. Steroids (e.g., dexamethasone) and mannitol may be administered, depending on the pathology. Prophylactic antibiotics should be given, most commonly intravenous cefazolin.
- **Technique**:
  - Image guidance is registered if being used. The expected courses of the transverse and sigmoid sinuses are marked anatomically or with the aid of neuronavigation. A midline linear incision is made extending from just below the inion to the spinous process of the C2 vertebra. Soft tissue dissection is performed in the midline avascular plane to minimize bleeding and postoperative pain and carried down to expose the occipital bone and posterior arch of the C1 vertebra. A suboccipital craniotomy is performed with a high-speed drill. A laminectomy may be performed at the level of C1 to gain a better trajectory to the rostral fourth ventricle.[13]
  - A Y-shaped dural incision is performed and the dura is tacked up using retention sutures. Some surgeons suggest that the inferior aspect of the dura should be opened first to allow for cerebrospinal fluid (CSF) egress and assist in decompression prior to complete dural opening when raised posterior fossa pressure is encountered after the craniotomy is performed. If present, the midline occipital sinus should be coagulated during the dural opening. The arachnoid membrane overlying the cisterna magna is opened to visualize the cerebellar tonsils and spinal cord, and care is taken to visualize and protect the branches of the posteroinferior carotid artery.[1]
  - If there is concern for obstructive hydrocephalus, an external ventricular drain (EVD) entry site is marked, prepared, and draped into the surgical field in case emergency intracranial pressure management is required intraoperatively. The surgeon may consider use of an EVD in advance, but judicious drainage of CSF is advisable until the mass is decompressed. If there is no concern for obstructive hydrocephalus, the surgeon may choose to place a lumbar drain before positioning the patient to relax the brain during the case.

- At this point, the fourth ventricle can be accessed via the transvermian approach or the telovelar approach.
- *Transvermian approach:*
  - The vermis is split inferiorly to a variable distance depending on the pathology to be addressed. The vermian incision typically involves the uvula, pyramid, tuber, and folium. Risk of postoperative sequelae increases the further rostral that the vermian incision extends, and as such, limiting the vermian split to the smallest size possible is recommended. The two halves of the inferior vermis are retracted, and an incision is made in the tela choroidea and the inferior medullary velum to access the fourth ventricle.[4]
- *Telovelar approach*:
  - Sharp dissection is carried out in the cerebellomedullary fissure and uvulotonsillar space to allow mobilization of the tonsils away from the uvula and expose the tela choroidea and inferior medullary velum. The tela choroidea and inferior medullary velum are divided to access the fourth ventricle. The tonsils may be retracted or resected to facilitate exposure. Retraction of the uvula may be necessary to increase the operative field of view. Resection provides a wider corridor to access the lateral recesses of the fourth ventricle.[13]

- For either technique, once access to the fourth ventricle is achieved, microsurgical techniques are utilized to address the specific lesion. Caution should be exercised when working around the floor of the fourth ventricle and manipulation should be minimized. A neurosurgical pattie can be placed over the floor of the fourth ventricle to protect it from injury.
- Once the goal of the procedure is complete (depending on the pathology treated), hemostasis is obtained and the dura is closed in a watertight fashion. A synthetic dural substitute or pericranial graft—harvested from above the craniotomy site—may be used to assist in dural closure. The bone flap may be replaced depending on surgeon preference and patient-specific factors. Suboccipital muscles are approximated and fascial closure is performed followed by dermal and skin closure.[13]
- Relevant anatomy is detailed in **Video 10.1**.

10.7 Postoperative Care

- Once the patient awakens, a neurological examination is performed in the operating room. Antiemetics and steroids are prophylactically administered. The decision to extubate is made after assessing respiratory function. The patient is then transported to the intensive care unit for close monitoring. An EVD may be left in place for 2 to 3 days to monitor intracranial pressure.[9] Arterial blood gas monitoring may be performed at regular intervals, especially if there is concern for decreased respiratory drive. Swallowing function should be formally assessed postoperatively before the patient is allowed to eat or drink to minimize risk of aspiration. Based on the patient's specific pathology, postoperative MRI with or without contrast administration or another imaging modality may be indicated.
- After 24 to 48 hours, a patient who is neurologically stable may be ready for transfer to the neurosurgical step-down unit or floor.[3] The arterial line and Foley catheter can be removed and deep vein thrombosis chemoprophylaxis initiated. The incision is monitored for signs of CSF leak or infection and regular neurological examinations are performed. Diet should be advanced in accordance with the patient's swallowing function. The patient is generally able to be discharged to home with appropriate follow-up or to rehabilitation if any postoperative neurological deficits are present.

10.8 Complications

- General complications relevant to the suboccipital craniotomy have been described in previous subsections, including postoperative edema, hematoma, infection, CSF leak, pseudomeningocele formation, and aseptic meningitis. Complications specific to approaches to the fourth ventricle are related to injury to the adjacent structures and include PFS, pseudobulbar palsy, ophthalmoplegia and other CN deficits, intractable vomiting, and cerebellar signs such as ataxia, dysmetria, nystagmus, and tremor.[2,3]
- Complications specific to approaches involving the fourth ventricle include mutism, swallowing deficits, emotional lability, and cognitive

changes. These symptoms are commonly referred to as PFS or cerebellar mutism and are more often reported after the transvermian approach.[3] The exact pathophysiology of this condition is poorly understood but injury to the dentato-rubro-thalamic tract may play a role.[14]

10.9 Management Pearls

- Both the transvermian and telovelar approaches provide access to the fourth ventricle and adjacent structures, each having particular nuances and advantages.
- The precise location of the lesion and degree of invasion of the floor of the fourth ventricle must be considered in surgical planning to avoid injury to the brainstem.
- Potential complications from these approaches include postoperative edema, hematoma, hydrocephalus, PFS, and brainstem injury.

References

[1] Matsushima T, Rhoton AL, Jr, Lenkey C. Microsurgery of the fourth ventricle: part 1. Microsurgical anatomy. Neurosurgery. 1982; 11(5):631–667

[2] Tomasello F, Conti A, Cardali S, La Torre D, Angileri FF. Telovelar approach to fourth ventricle tumors: highlights and limitations. World Neurosurg. 2015; 83(6):1141–1147

[3] Ferguson SD, Levine NB, Suki D, et al. The surgical treatment of tumors of the fourth ventricle: a single-institution experience. J Neurosurg. 2018; 128(2):339–351

[4] Tanriover N, Ulm AJ, Rhoton AL, Jr, Yasuda A. Comparison of the transvermian and telovelar approaches to the fourth ventricle. J Neurosurg. 2004; 101(3):484–498

[5] Holmes G. The Croonian Lectures on the clinical symptoms of cerebellar disease and their interpretation. Lecture II. 1922. Cerebellum. 2007; 6(2):148–153, discussion 141

[6] Han S, Wang Z, Wang Y, Wu A. Transcerebellomedullary fissure approach to lesions of the fourth ventricle: less is more? Acta Neurochir (Wien). 2013; 155(6):1011–1016

[7] Deshmukh VR, Figueiredo EG, Deshmukh P, Crawford NR, Preul MC, Spetzler RF. Quantification and comparison of telovelar and transvermian approaches to the fourth ventricle. Neurosurgery. 2006; 58(4) Suppl 2:ONS-202–ONS-206, discussion ONS-206–ONS-207

[8] Cavalheiro S, Yagmurlu K, da Costa MD, et al. Surgical approaches for brainstem tumors in pediatric patients. Childs Nerv Syst. 2015; 31(10):1815–1840

[9] Tomasello F, Conti A, Angileri FF, Cardali S. Telo-velar approach to fourth-ventricle tumours: how I do it. Acta Neurochir (Wien). 2015; 157(4):607–610

[10] Jittapiromsak P, Sabuncuoglu H, Deshmukh P, Spetzler RF, Preul MC. Accessing the recesses of the fourth ventricle: comparison of tonsillar retraction and resection in the telovelar approach. Neurosurgery. 2010; 66(3) Suppl Operative:30–39, discussion 39–40

[11] Lee CC, Lin CF, Yang TF, et al. Telovelar approach for choroid plexus papilloma in the foramen of Luschka: a safe way using a neuromonitor. Clin Neurol Neurosurg. 2012; 114(3): 249–253

[12] Jagannathan S, Krovvidi H. Anaesthetic considerations for posterior fossa surgery. Contin Educ Anaesth Crit Care Pain. 2014; 14(5):202–206

[13] Liu JK, Dodson VN. Telovelar approach for microsurgical resection of fourth ventricular subependymoma arising from rhomboid fossa: operative video and technical nuances. Neurosurg Focus Video. 2019; 1(2):V5

[14] Ghali MGZ. Telovelar surgical approach. Neurosurg Rev. 2021; 44(1):61–76

11 Translabyrinthine Approach

Margaret I. Engelhardt, Philip L. Perez, and Andrew A. McCall

11.1 Background

- The translabyrinthine approach is used to expose tumors of the cerebellopontine angle (CPA) via lateral dissection through the temporal bone. This technique provides a direct route to the CPA with a wide area of exposure while avoiding the temporal lobe retraction and narrower corridor of the middle fossa approach and the cerebellar retraction of the retrosigmoid approach.[1,2] It allows for identification of the facial nerve at a consistent anatomical location.[1,3] All drilling is extradural and the entirety of the internal auditory canal (IAC) from the porus to the fundus can be fully exposed.[2]
- The translabyrinthine approach can be used for resection of tumors of the CPA, including vestibular schwannomas, meningiomas, tumors of the facial nerve, endolymphatic sac tumors, lipomas, glomus tumors, epidermoid cysts, and choroid plexus papillomas.[2] Rarely, primary malignant tumors and metastases may arise in this location.

11.2 Indications and Contraindications

- The decision on surgical approach for vestibular schwannoma resection is based on tumor size and location, preoperative hearing thresholds, outlook for hearing preservation during surgery, and surgeon expertise and familiarity.[2,3] The translabyrinthine approach is typically indicated for tumors of any size in patients with poor functional hearing on the operative side.[1,2]
- Performing the translabyrinthine approach on an only hearing ear is a contraindication since doing so would render a patient bilaterally deafened. The presence of active infection, such as otitis media, should also be considered an absolute contraindication to avoid creation of a direct route for intracranial spread of infection.[1]

11.3 Instruments

- Standard neurotologic and neurosurgical microdissection instruments, operating microscope, high-speed drill, suction/continuous irrigation setup, stereotactic localization, and neurophysiologic monitoring system are utilized.

11.4 Patient Preparation

- Preoperative imaging consists of magnetic resonance imaging (MRI) with and without gadolinium and noncontrast computed tomography (CT) imaging of the temporal bone with fine cuts of the IAC and CPA, typically with protocols enabling intraoperative stereotactic localization.
- All patients should have a preoperative audiogram to assess hearing in the operated ear and to confirm functional hearing on the contralateral side given the hearing sacrifice in the operated ear with the translabyrinthine approach.
- General anesthesia with endotracheal intubation is used. Neurophysiologic monitoring of cranial nerves (V–XI) is performed, with particular emphasis on facial electromyography.
- The use of long-acting muscle relaxants, such as rocuronium, is avoided to allow for intraoperative nerve monitoring.[2] If a long-acting paralytic is required for induction, a reversal agent should be given prior to drilling in the vicinity of the facial nerve.

11.5 Patient Positioning

- The patient is positioned supine with the head rotated toward the contralateral side and the bed turned 90 or 180 degrees from the anesthesiologist. A curved **C**-shaped incision is fashioned approximately 4 to 6 cm behind the postauricular sulcus.

11.6 Technique

- This incision is carried through the subcutaneous tissue until the superficial temporal fascia is encountered. An anteriorly-based musculoperiosteal flap is then fashioned by incising transversely along the linea temporalis posteriorly to the sinodural angle and then anteroinferiorly to the mastoid tip.

- Care should be taken to offset this incision from the overlying skin incision to reduce the incidence of wound dehiscence and postoperative cerebrospinal fluid (CSF) egress.
- A periosteal elevator is used to raise the soft tissue from the underlying cortical bone until the spine of Henle and external auditory canal are reached anteriorly. Superficial temporal fascia and portions of the temporalis or sternocleidomastoid muscle can be taken for future packing material. Fish hooks or temporary sutures are placed anteriorly to retract the musculoperiosteal layer and ear to aid in exposure.
- A cortical mastoidectomy is then performed with a suction-irrigator and a large cutting burr with removal of the mastoid air cells and identification of the tegmen mastoideum, external auditory canal, and sigmoid sinus (▶ Fig. 11.1).
- The mastoid antrum is opened until the lateral semicircular canal and short process of the incus are identified. These landmarks allow identification of the facial nerve in the proximal vertical segment including drilling of the facial recess between the facial nerve and chorda tympani (▶ Fig. 11.2).
- If substantial inferior extension is needed, the vertical facial nerve is skeletonized to the digastric ridge with removal of the retrofacial air cells. Additional bone is removed to decompress the middle fossa dura, sigmoid sinus (a thin, mobile bony plate is often left overlying the anterior sigmoid sinus to protect the sigmoid from the rotating shaft of the burr during deeper drilling), sinodural angle, and posterior fossa dura.
- A labyrinthectomy is then performed with removal of the lateral, posterior, and superior semicircular canals (▶ Fig. 11.3).
- The lateral canal is drilled posteriorly until the posterior canal is identified, which can then be

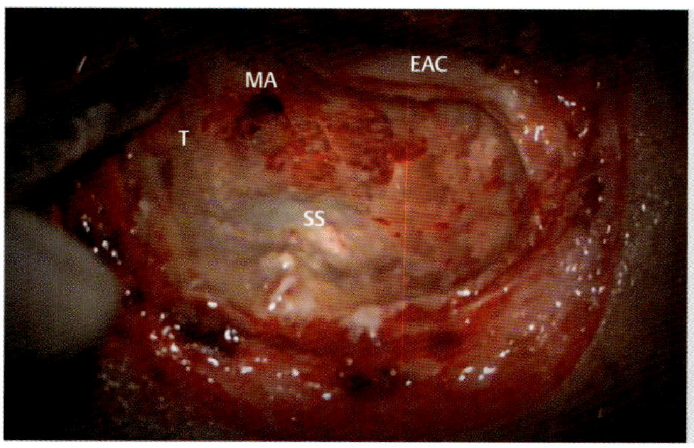

Fig. 11.1 Cortical mastoidectomy (right side) is performed with removal of air cells over the tegmen (T), sigmoid sinus (SS), and external auditory canal (EAC). MA, mastoid antrum.

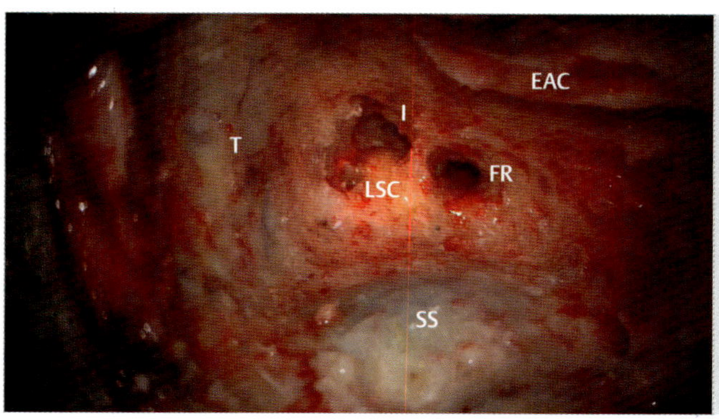

Fig. 11.2 The mastoid antrum is drilled to visualize the short process of the incus (I) and lateral semicircular canal (LSC), which are used as landmarks for the facial nerve. The facial recess (FR) can then be drilled into the tympanic cavity, allowing for the stapedial tendon and incudostapedial joint to be visualized. The thin bone of the incus buttress separates the mastoid antrum and facial recess. EAC, external auditory canal; SS, sigmoid sinus; T, tegmen.

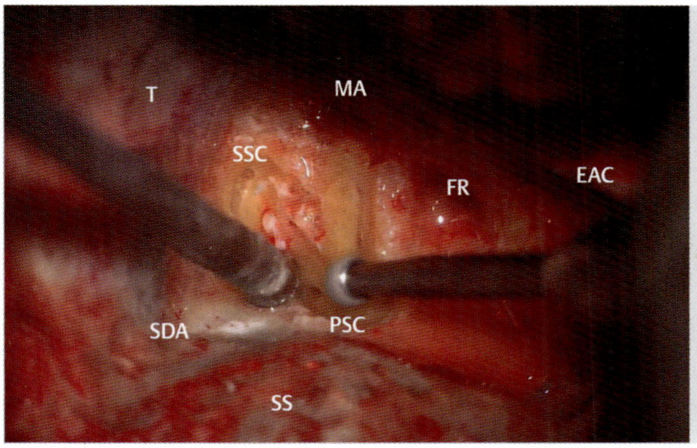

Fig. 11.3 Labyrinthectomy is performed with drilling of the lateral semicircular canal (LSC) until the posterior semicircular canal (PSC) is found posteriorly, which can then be traced to its common crus to the superior semicircular canal (SSC). EAC, external auditory canal; FR, facial recess; MA, mastoid antrum; SDA, sinodural angle; SS, sigmoid sinus; T, tegmen.

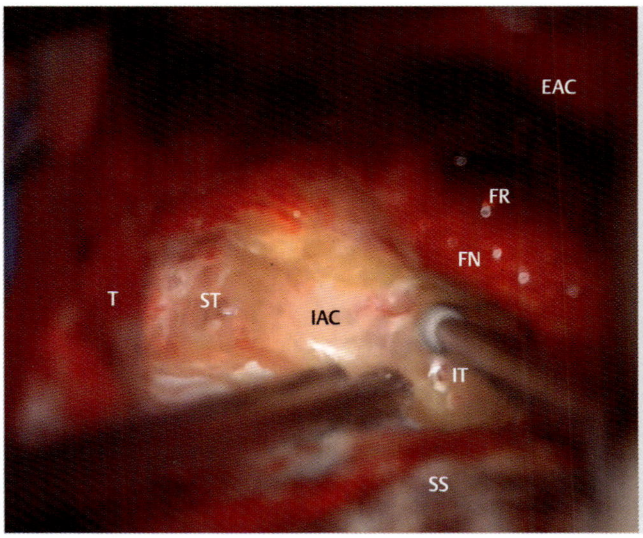

Fig. 11.4 Access to the internal auditory canal (IAC) is facilitated by drilling the superior (ST) and inferior (IT) troughs until 270 degrees of exposure are achieved. The suction-irrigator is used to keep the sigmoid sinus (SS) away from the working burr. EAC, external auditory canal; FN, facial nerve; FR, facial recess; T, tegmen.

followed via its common crus to the superior semicircular canal and its ampullated end anteriorly.

- The anterior ampullated ends of the lateral and superior semicircular canals should be left in place as a landmark for the IAC and to prevent injury to the facial nerve. The vestibule is opened widely, noting that the facial nerve lies immediately lateral to it. The ampullated end of the posterior semicircular canal courses medial to the facial nerve to join the vestibule as well, so skeletonizing the posterolateral aspect of the facial nerve at the second genu is of critical importance to provide access while avoiding damage to the nerve.
- Dissection continues with drilling of the bone superior, inferior, and posterior to the IAC to an eggshell thickness. The endolymphatic duct is identified and transected. The retrofacial air cells inferior to the labyrinth are drilled and the jugular bulb identified. The cochlear aqueduct is identified further medially between the IAC and the jugular bulb and can be opened to allow egress of CSF.
- Drilling is not performed inferior to the cochlear aqueduct to avoid injury to the lower cranial nerves in the jugular foramen.
- Bone removal continues to the porus acusticus medially with formation of troughs superior and inferior to the IAC until there is approximately 270 degrees of exposure at the porus and tapered toward the fundus (▶ Fig. 11.4 and ▶ Fig. 11.5). The dura of the IAC is opened.

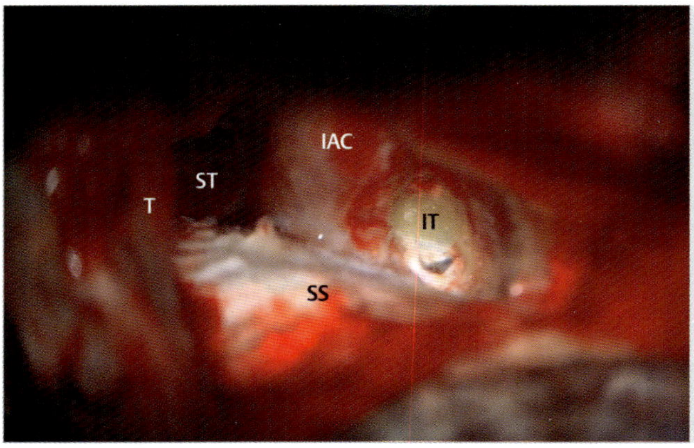

Fig. 11.5 Completed drilling of the internal auditory canal (IAC) prior to opening of the dura. IT, inferior trough; SS, sigmoid sinus; ST, superior trough; T, tegmen.

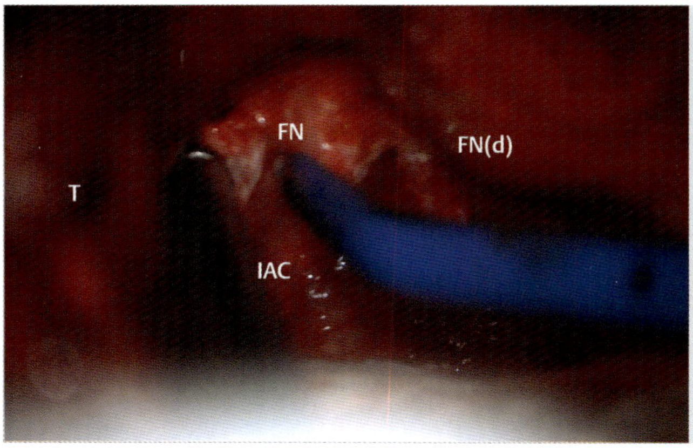

Fig. 11.6 After opening the dura of the internal auditory canal (IAC), the meatal or canalicular segment of the facial nerve (FN) can be located medial to the superior vestibular nerve and Bill's bar and confirmed with the use of a nerve stimulator. FN(d), descending segment of the facial nerve; T, tegmen.

- At the IAC fundus, the superior and inferior vestibular nerves are separated by the transverse crest. Superiorly, the facial nerve is separated from the superior vestibular nerve by the vertical crest ("Bill's bar"). Once the facial nerve has been identified, tumor is dissected in a lateral to medial fashion (▶ Fig. 11.6). The posterior fossa dura is then opened sharply medial to the sigmoid sinus allowing for drainage of CSF from the lateral cistern, which can result in relaxation of the cerebellum and increased working space.
- Debulking of a tumor can be helpful prior to dissecting a plane between the tumor and the adjacent cranial nerves and brainstem.
- The facial nerve can be confirmed electrophysiologically throughout the dissection, including identification at the brainstem. After complete dissection and tumor removal, meticulous hemostasis is achieved followed by obliteration of the mastoid cavity with fat harvested from the abdomen. The previously harvested fascia and muscle are used to pack the eustachian tube orifice.
- Removal of the incus and dividing the tensor tympani tendon facilitates access to the eustachian tube.
- The defect is then closed in layers with re-approximation of the musculoperiosteal layer and closure of the subcutaneous tissue and skin.[1,2,3,4,5,6]
- The accompanying video to this chapter (**Video 11.1**) shows an example of a translabyrinthine approach for resection of a left IAC mass with mild extension into the CPA, which was confirmed pathologically to be a vestibular schwannoma.

11.7 Postoperative Care

- Initial postoperative care is in the intensive care unit, typically for one night followed by transfer to a floor bed. Use of perioperative corticosteroids is variable. A mastoid pressure dressing is typically used for several days after surgery.[2] Postoperative dizziness is common and patients typically work with physical therapy to improve balance function.

11.8 Complications

- CSF leak is the most common postoperative complication, occurring in about 1 to 17% of patients.[2,7] Typically, this presents as unilateral rhinorrhea or less likely an incisional leak. CSF leak can lead to increased hospital length of stay or rehospitalization, meningitis, and need for lumbar drain placement or revision operation. Conservative treatment includes bed rest, avoidance of straining, and pressure dressings. Complete loss of hearing in the operative ear is an expected sequela of total labyrinthectomy.[1] Additional complications include facial nerve injury, CPA hematoma, and postoperative meningitis.[2,7,8,9]
- The patient's anatomy and otologic history should be reviewed to assess the feasibility of the translabyrinthine approach. Anterior positioning of the sigmoid sinus narrows the operative window to the IAC requiring significant retraction on the sinus and additional posterior fossa drilling. A high-riding jugular bulb similarly narrows the operative window and may make drilling of the inferior aspect of the IAC difficult. Perforations of the tympanic membrane should be addressed prior to proceeding with a translabyrinthine approach or tympanomastoid obliteration should be performed with oversewing of the ear canal. Similarly, patients with a preexisting canal wall down mastoid cavity require tympanomastoid obliteration and oversewing.[1]

11.9 Management Pearls

- *Anatomy*:
  - Key to the success of this approach is familiarity with the positioning of the contents of the IAC. This relationship is most consistent at the fundus with the facial nerve in the anterosuperior quadrant and superior vestibular nerve in the posterosuperior quadrant separated by Bill's bar. The cochlear nerve is positioned anteroinferiorly and the inferior vestibular nerve posteroinferiorly with the falciform or transverse crest separating the superior and inferior contents. The presence of a high-riding jugular bulb, course of the facial nerve, and relationship between the tumor and intracranial vasculature should be evaluated on preoperative imaging.
- *Variations*:
  - Various presigmoid approaches beyond the translabyrinthine technique can be utilized based on the location and size of the target lesion. These include the retrolabyrinthine, transotic, and transcochlear routes, which are beyond the scope of this chapter.[10]
  - An additional variation of the translabyrinthine approach involves a partial labyrinthectomy with sacrifice and plugging of one or two semicircular canals with preservation of the remaining labyrinthine structures. These patients can have preservation of their preoperative hearing in contrast to the standard approach.[11]

References

[1] Brackmann DE, Green JD, Jr. Translabyrinthine approach for acoustic tumor removal. 1992. Neurosurg Clin N Am. 2008; 19(2):251–264, vi

[2] Arriaga MA, Lin J. Translabyrinthine approach: indications, techniques, and results. Otolaryngol Clin North Am. 2012; 45 (2):399–415, ix

[3] Bennett M, Haynes DS. Surgical approaches and complications in the removal of vestibular schwannomas. Otolaryngol Clin North Am. 2007; 40(3):589–609, ix–x

[4] Schwam ZG, Cosetti MK, Wanna GB. Translabyrinthine approach for sporadic vestibular schwannoma: patient selection, technical pearls, and patient outcomes. Otolaryngol Clin North Am. 2023; 56(3):483–493

[5] Day JD, Chen DA, Arriaga M. Translabyrinthine approach for acoustic neuroma. Neurosurgery. 2004; 54(2):391–395, discussion 395–396

[6] Lanman TH, Brackmann DE, Hitselberger WE, Subin B. Report of 190 consecutive cases of large acoustic tumors (vestibular schwannoma) removed via the translabyrinthine approach. J Neurosurg. 1999; 90(4):617–623

[7] Mamikoglu B, Wiet RJ, Esquivel CR. Translabyrinthine approach for the management of large and giant vestibular schwannomas. Otol Neurotol. 2002; 23(2):224–227

[8] Sade B, Mohr G, Dufour JJ. Vascular complications of vestibular schwannoma surgery: a comparison of the suboccipital

retrosigmoid and translabyrinthine approaches. J Neurosurg. 2006; 105(2):200–204

[9] Mass SC, Wiet RJ, Dinces E. Complications of the translabyrinthine approach for the removal of acoustic neuromas. Arch Otolaryngol Head Neck Surg. 1999; 125 (7):801–804

[10] Hoz SS, Palmisciano P, Albairmani SS, et al. A proposed classification system for presigmoid approaches: a scoping review. J Neurosurg. 2023; 139(4):965–971

[11] Hirsch BE, Cass SP, Sekhar LN, Wright DC. Translabyrinthine approach to skull base tumors with hearing preservation. Am J Otol. 1993; 14(6):533–543

12 Retrosigmoid Approach

Jaims Lim, Alexander Becker, Steven Blake Housley, Andrew Becker, Andre Monteiro, and Elad I. Levy

12.1 Background

- The retrosigmoid (RS) approach for craniotomy or craniectomy is a neurosurgical staple that allows management of lesions in the cerebellopontine (CP) angle and ventrolateral brainstem, such as vestibular schwannomas, meningiomas, and epidermoid cysts.
- Microvascular decompression of the trigeminal (V), facial (VII), and glossopharyngeal (IX) cranial nerves (CNs) for trigeminal neuralgia, hemifacial spasm, and glossopharyngeal neuralgia, respectively, can also be performed.
- Other vascular lesions, including arteriovenous malformations (AVMs) in the CP angle or brainstem cavernomas, can also be managed.
- The RS approach gives wide access to the CP angle and the CNs in this area, including CNs IV, V, VII, VIII, IX, X, and XI.
- Careful review of preoperative imaging including computed tomography (CT) and magnetic resonance imaging (MRI) is key in planning and conducting a successful operation.
- Possible complications include postoperative wound infection, cerebrospinal fluid (CSF) leak or fistula formation, pneumocephalus, and posterior fossa hemorrhage.

12.2 Indications and Contraindications

- The RS craniotomy is an established route of access to lesions in the CP angle and ventrolateral brainstem. Various neoplastic and vascular pathologies can be treated with the RS approach.
- Vestibular schwannomas,[1] meningiomas,[2] and epidermoid cysts[3] are some of the common neoplastic pathologies. Epidermoid cysts and meningiomas can also occur at the CP angle, in which case an RS approach is favored for access and resection. Other lesions include arachnoid cysts,[4] lipomas,[5] and metastatic tumors.[6]
- The RS approach affords wide access to the CP angle and the CNs in this area including CNs IV, V, VII, VIII, and IX. Trigeminal neuralgia, hemifacial spasm, and glossopharyngeal neuralgia are three conditions attributable to a specific CN in which an RS approach is favored to perform a microvascular decompression.
- Apart from neoplastic lesions in the CP angle and pain syndromes, the RS approach can be helpful to treat various vascular pathologies. The RS approach provides the surgeon with access to the pontomedullary junction of the brainstem. Brainstem lesions such as cavernomas[7,8] and hemangioblastomas[9,10] can be safely resected.
- Once the CNs are safely identified and mobilized, the arachnoid adhesions can be removed to fully visualize the pontomedullary junction. AVMs can also occur in the CP angle cisterns.[11] Although these AVMs are rare, the RS approach may provide a safe corridor for resection and draining vein ligation.
- The RS approach is a workhorse technique in the field of neurosurgery for lesions such as vestibular schwannomas, epidermoid cysts, and meningiomas, and for pathologies such as trigeminal neuralgia and hemifacial spasm. Although there are few to no absolute contraindications to the RS approach, there are several considerations for the aforementioned pathologies in which this approach should be evaluated to determine whether it is the most optimal approach.
- For vestibular schwannomas, the overall size of the mass should be considered. For tumors ≤ 1.5 cm (extrameatal diameter), the middle fossa approach has been found to be superior to the RS approach for hearing preservation.[12] If the vestibular schwannoma is predominantly located in the intracanalicular space, the RS approach is discouraged due to the lack of exposure of the intracanalicular space during that approach; and for such cases, a middle fossa approach is favored.[13] However, if the mass is larger than 1.5 cm and occupies a large proportion of the CP angle space as well as the intracanalicular space, a staged surgery may be needed. An RS approach can be useful for debulking and separation of the mass from the brainstem.[14]
- For CP angle epidermoid cysts that expand across into the petrous apex and Meckel's cave,

an RS craniotomy may not be the most appropriate approach due to the surgeon's lack of reach and visibility superiorly and ventrally into those regions. Thus, in such cases, a middle fossa craniotomy and petrosectomy may be considered.[15] This same thought process and evaluation of the lesion should be taken into consideration for meningiomas as well.
- The RS approach is an optimal approach for microvascular decompression of CNs V and VII. Rather than the type of approach, the indications for this operation should be considered. If no offending vessel is seen in contact with the vessel associated with the respective CN on noninvasive imaging evaluation, the utility of a microvascular decompression as well as other treatment options such as stereotactic radiosurgery and rhizotomy should be discussed.

12.3 Patient Preparation

- For all RS approaches, noninvasive imaging is required to visualize the pathology in question.
- Noncontrast head CT is ideal for assessment of the bony anatomy in the RS operative corridor. The mastoid air cells and pneumatization of the posterior temporal bone can often be appreciated. The sinuses of the frontal bone can be clearly visualized, and they may be very rostral and superior. It is important to note such findings when placing a Mayfield head holder or clamp (Integra LifeSciences) during the operation in order to avoid anterior sinus wall fractures and insecure head holder placement.
- Brain MRI with and without contrast material is also very helpful for all pathologies. The T1 sequence with and without contrast material not only allows visualization of the pathology in question but also often allows visualization of the transverse and sigmoid sinuses.
- In conjunction with CT imaging, a superiorly located transverse sinus or posteriorly displaced sigmoid sinus may be identified, which is critical for surgical planning. The surgeon is also able to determine whether the right or left transverse sinus is dominant (only 37–50% of transverse sinuses are codominant and equally sized).[16,17,18] If the sinus is dominant on the side of the intended surgery, the surgeon may take additional precautions and utilize the StealthStation system (Medtronic) navigation to plan the craniotomy in order to minimize the risk of sinus injury.
- T2 sequences of the mass are very useful for assessing the consistency of a tumor.
- For example, hyperintense tumors are found to be softer and easier to remove with suction aspiration.[19] The T2 Fast Imaging Employing Steady-state Acquisition (FIESTA) sequence is very useful for visualizing the CSF cisterns, including the prepontine and CP angle cisterns.
- It is also very helpful in identifying the different CNs on MRI and their origins and courses pertinent to the pathology of interest. For example, in patients with trigeminal neuralgia, the identification of the superior cerebellar artery, which is the most common culprit for the facial pain, and its course along the trigeminal nerve is key to safely recognize and separate the trigeminal nerve from the superior cerebellar artery.
- This is also true for an RS approach to conduct microvascular decompression of the anteroinferior cerebellar artery for hemifacial spasm.
- When the RS approach is utilized for vestibular schwannomas, preoperative evaluation of the patient's hearing is essential. Thus, a formal hearing evaluation and auditory tests are recommended, including pure tone audiograms and speech discrimination.
- For vascular pathologies such as CP angle cistern AVMs, a catheter-based diagnostic cerebral angiogram should be performed. An angiogram will allow identification of arterial feeders as well as draining veins. Identification of the normal vasculature on the angiogram and correlation with intraoperative findings are important to avoid inadvertent vessel injury or sacrifice causing ischemic injury.
- A trained anesthesiologist with neurological experience is preferred for RS approaches.
- Intraoperative monitoring including somatosensory evoked potentials (SSEPs), brainstem auditory evoked responses (BAERs), motor evoked potentials (MEPs), and facial nerve monitoring is preferred for these approaches. This is to ensure close monitoring of brainstem and CN function.[20]
- The anesthetic considerations for the RS approach follow similar tenets of anesthesia care for craniotomy procedures in the posterior fossa.

In addition to managing ICP and hemodynamics throughout induction, maintenance, and emergence, anesthetic selection is often dictated by the requirements of neuromonitoring.

- Total intravenous anesthesia (TIVA) with propofol and a narcotic infusion is preferred but not necessarily required over the use of volatile anesthetics, especially for patients in whom BAERs are being monitored.
- After intubation, patients receive an arterial line (at 0 pressure and placed nearly level with the circle of Willis) and large-bore IV access. The position of the endotracheal tube should be confirmed multiple times throughout the positioning process and secured judiciously.
- Intraoperatively, patients receive active directed resuscitation and blood products are routinely available in the event of uncontrollable bleeding.[20]

12.4 Patient Positioning

- The patient is placed in the lateral position with the side of pathology facing up, as shown in ▶ Fig. 12.1.
- The contralateral arm can be kept on the bed with an axillary roll, or it can be suspended off the top end of the bed ("park bench" position).
- The head is turned approximately 30 degrees toward the floor, and the vertex is directed downward.
- The head is confirmed to be higher than the chest to facilitate venous drainage. Care is taken to avoid turning or flexing the head and causing strain on the neck and obstructing venous drainage because that might contribute to cerebral edema and lack of brain relaxation during the operation.
- The head is affixed to the bed using a three-point Mayfield head holder.
- The ipsilateral shoulder is taped caudally and anteriorly to allow maximal working room.[21]

12.5 Technique

- No particular equipment or supplies are required other than those used for basic craniotomies.
- A Mayfield head holder is frequently required.
- An adjustable surgical bed is imperative.
- Positioning adjuncts such as laminectomy rolls, an axillary roll, and a beanbag are needed.
- Both monopolar electrocautery and bipolar electrocautery are necessary for hemostasis. A high-speed drill with cutting bits is needed for exposure.
- Finally, a surgical microscope and microsurgical instruments are required during the intradural portion of the case.
- Relevant venous anatomy, including the probable location of the transverse and sigmoid venous sinuses, is approximated using external

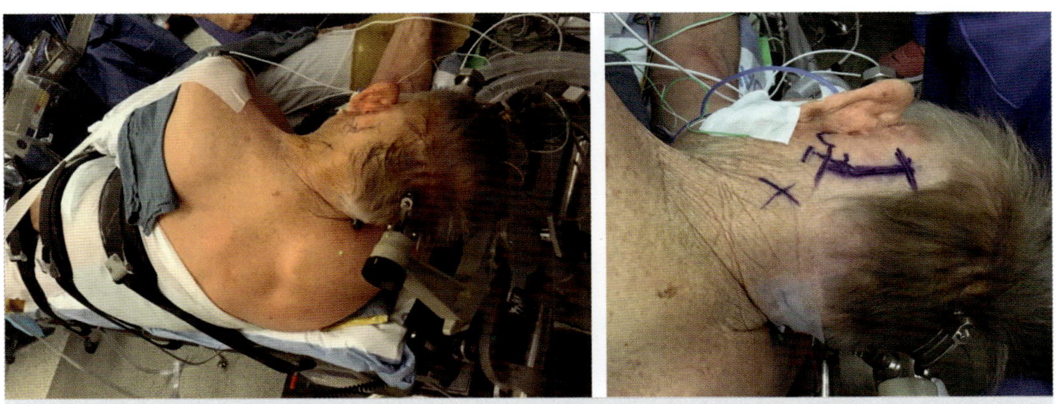

Fig. 12.1 Retrosigmoid positioning and incision. Lateral positioning of a patient for a planned retrosigmoid approach **(left)** with multiple straps and securing tape to allow proper positioning and optimal viewing angles during the arachnoid dissection and work under the microscope. The retroauricular incision behind the ear is also demonstrated **(right)** in the lateral position.

landmarks including the inion, the external auditory meatus, and the digastric groove.

- A theoretical line is drawn from the inion to the zygomatic arch to indicate the transverse sinus.
- The inion–meatal line has also been used to define the location of the transverse sinus.
- Additionally, the junction of the transverse and sigmoid sinuses is traditionally thought to be located near or on the asterion, which is the junction of the parietomastoid, temporomastoid, and lambdoid sutures.
- Using the aforementioned markers indicating the transverse and sigmoid sinuses, a "hockey stick" or curved incision measuring 3 to 5 cm is made and situated approximately 1 cm behind the ear and just posterior to the hairline.
- The incision is extended from the level of the asterion, just above the approximate level of the transverse sinus and down to below the mastoid tip with the final 1 cm of the incision curved anteriorly.
- The hair within the operative field is shaved, and the area is prepared and draped in the typical sterile fashion. In our cases, we utilize the following agents for skin preparation in the order specified: alcohol, chlorhexidine, and betadine.
- The skin is incised using a scalpel.
- The dissection is carried down to the temporomastoid bone, with a slight anterior trajectory toward the digastric groove, using monopolar electrocautery.
- A Penfield no. 1 dissector or similar instrument is used to tease the soft tissue and muscle off of the mastoid bone inferior to where the turn of the skull toward the foramen magnum can be palpated or felt.
- The digastric groove is also identified. A single cerebellar retractor is placed above the bone and the skin, and muscle is retracted.
- Using a pneumatic or electronic drill with a five-round burr, a craniectomy is performed initially away from the transverse and sigmoid sinus.
- This is then extended superiorly and anteriorly using rongeurs and a drill until the bluish hue of the sigmoid and transverse sinuses is identified.
- If mastoid air cells are visualized, they are covered and sealed completely with bone wax.
- The dura is opened in a curved fashion and reflected anteriorly. The flap is retracted using two to four Nurolon sutures (Ethicon).
- The lateral portion of the cerebellum is gently retracted, and arachnoid dissection is performed inferiorly to the cisterna magna.
- At this point, CSF from the cisterna magna is manually drained allowing appropriate relaxation of the cerebellum.
- If the cerebellum appears to be full and gentle light retraction on the cerebellum fails to expose the cisterna magna, the trigeminal cistern can be opened via an arachnoid dissection to drain CSF and create more space for further arachnoid dissection and operation. Patience to allow enough egress of CSF is imperative.
- Using gentle retraction and careful arachnoid dissection (▶ Fig. 12.2), the lower CNs (IX, X, and XI) will be first visualized inferiorly (▶ Fig. 12.3).
- Careful dissection and cutting of the arachnoid adhesions and bands will yield a view of CN VIII (▶ Fig. 12.4) extending into the internal auditory meatus in the middle of the operative field. Commonly, CN VII is hidden behind CN VIII and not easily visualized. Finally, CNs IV and V will be visualized most superiorly.

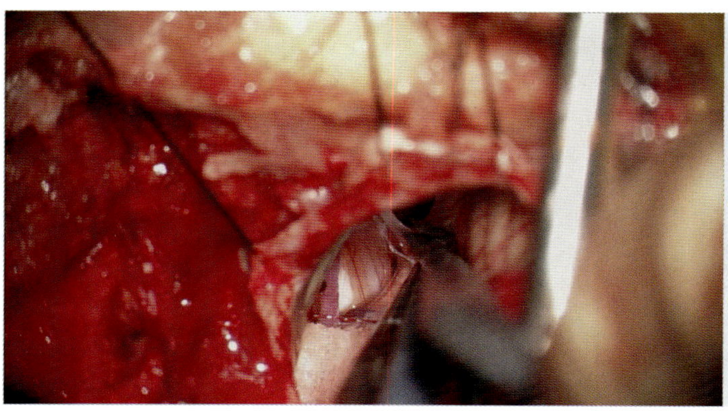

Fig. 12.2 Retrosigmoid arachnoid dissection. Delicate use of microscissors to conduct a clean arachnoid dissection.

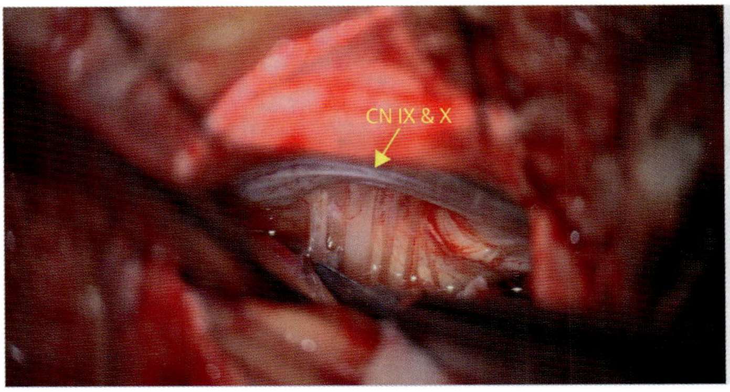

Fig. 12.3 View of cranial nerves (CNs) IX and X from the retrosigmoid approach. After delicate microdissection of the arachnoid, CNs IX and X are clearly visible. Cerebrospinal fluid drainage through the magna cisterna or trigeminal cistern allows good relaxation of the brain and optimal working room for safe dissection.

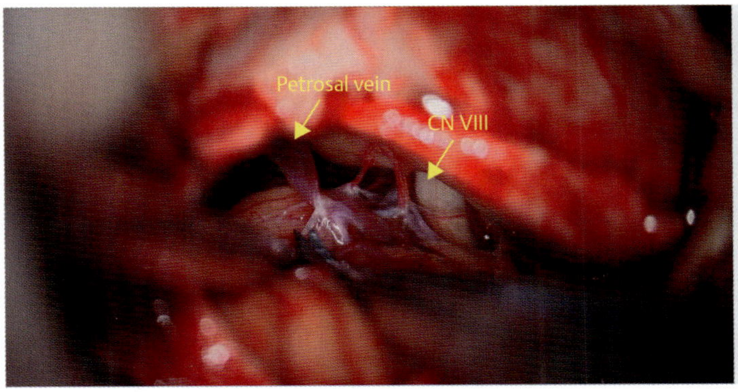

Fig. 12.4 View of cranial nerve (CN) VIII and petrosal vein from a retrosigmoid approach. After careful arachnoid dissection, the superior petrosal vein and CN VIII are visible.

- The remainder of the procedure is dependent on the pathology. During this dissection, the superior petrosal vein is often encountered (▶ Fig. 12.4). Unless this vein is impairing the goal of the operation, it should be preserved and mobilized, if possible, to prevent ischemic injury.
- Once the goal of the procedure is accomplished, a watertight closure of the dura is imperative to avoid CSF leakage and reoperation.
- The dura is closed in a watertight fashion with 4–0 Nurolon sutures (Ethicon-Johnson & Johnson). A sealant of the surgeon's choice is then applied over the dural closure.
- This is followed by a layer of DuraGen (Integra) and a second layer of the sealant. If the bone has been removed and there is no craniotomy flap to replace, a large cranial plate or mesh is placed on top of the DuraGen and secured.
- The cervical muscle and fascia are reapproximated with 0 Vicryl sutures followed by 2–0 Vicryl for the galea.
- The skin is then closed with a monomer permanent suture such as Prolene or nylon.

12.6 Postoperative Care

- Postoperatively, the patient is awakened from anesthesia and extubated in the operating room to allow for a proper neurological examination. The patient is then transported to an appropriate intensive care unit or postanesthesia care unit for additional monitoring and care. An intensive care unit with neurological specialization is preferred. The patient's cervical, retroauricular, and incisional pain is controlled with a combination of IV and oral pain medications. The patient is checked hourly for changes in neurological examination findings by trained nursing staff.
- Imaging is optional with some surgeons preferring to obtain a head CT to ensure no inadvertent pathology is found. In the case of

tumor resections, contrast-enhanced brain MRI is obtained to ensure appropriate tumor removal.

- On postoperative day 1, the patient is moved to the step-down unit for ongoing management. The patient is ambulated early in the day. Pain medications are converted to primarily oral forms. The diet is advanced. The incision is checked daily for signs of a CSF leak. The patient is generally discharged home with family on postoperative day 3 with plans for follow-up in 1 to 2 weeks.

12.7 Complications

- Major complications including death are exceedingly rare in RS cases.
- The primary postoperative complication associated with this procedure is a CSF leak. A 1.5 to 10.3% risk of CSF leak has been estimated, depending on the population examined.
  - This risk can be minimized by judicious watertight closure of the dura with use of a biosynthetic or pericranial graft if needed.
  - Signs of postoperative CSF leak include clear drainage through the incision, significant swelling at the site of operation, a salty taste in the mouth, or rhinorrhea.
  - A CSF leak requires reoperation for definitive control of the leak and possible lumbar drain placement.
  - The CSF should be collected first for analysis to exclude meningitis.
  - If there are no signs of meningitis, a lumbar drain may be initially placed to prevent further CSF leakage and allow self-repair of the leak.
  - If the leak persists after 3 to 5 days of drainage, primary operative repair may be necessary.
  - It is important to ensure that the patient does not have secondary hydrocephalus related to the initial index operation for which permanent CSF diversion may be indicated.
- During the initial craniotomy or dural opening, there is a chance for a sinus injury. With any venous sinus exposure, there is also a risk of an air embolus.
  - Therefore, clear communication with the anesthesia team about monitoring end-tidal CO_2 and vital signs is critical.
  - Vascular clips should also be made available in the room to quickly obtain control of venous bleeding if simple tamponading with thrombin-soaked Gelfoam (Pfizer) is not possible.

12.8 Management Pearls

- The RS craniotomy or craniectomy is a versatile approach for accessing lesions in the CP angle and ventrolateral brainstem.
- Pathological conditions that are addressable through the RS approach include vestibular schwannomas, meningiomas, epidermoid cysts, trigeminal neuralgia, hemifacial spasms, glossopharyngeal neuralgia, brainstem cavernomas or lesions, and CP angle AVMs.
- Careful review of preoperative noninvasive imaging including CT and MRI scans is critical in planning and completing a successful operation. Attention to the MRI characteristics of the mass as well as the surrounding bony and neurovascular anatomy is key.
- Working from a safe to unsafe surgical region is a smart strategy during the bony work for RS craniotomies.
- Possible complications from an RS approach include CSF leak, infection, and hemorrhage. Additional possible complications include sinus injury and air embolus, for which precautions should be taken starting from the initial exposure and craniotomy or craniectomy.
- Special risks to the CNs exist depending on the goal of the RS surgery at hand. With microvascular decompression for trigeminal neuralgia, hearing loss has been reported in approximately 0.59% of cases. Facial nerve palsy is seen in less than 1% of patients and is rarely permanent.[22] Another important consideration is the trigeminal-cardiac reflex, which can manifest as sudden onset hypotension, asystole, arrhythmia, apnea, and gastric hypermotility with stimulation of the afferent sensory fibers of CN V. This stimulation is carried back to the trigeminal nucleus where internuclear fibers connecting to the nucleus of CN X are present that initiate the efferent portion of the reflex.[23]
- In those patients undergoing resection of a vestibular schwannoma, the risk of CN dysfunction is largely dependent on the size of the tumor. In this group, the estimated rate of hearing loss is 44.3 to 71.7%, and the risk of facial nerve dysfunction in this group is approximately 4.0 to 30.2%.[12]

References

[1] Aref M, Kunigelis K, Cass SP, Youssef AS. Retrosigmoid approach for vestibular schwannoma. J Neurol Surg B Skull Base. 2019; 80 Suppl 3:S271

[2] Baroncini M, Thines L, Reyns N, Schapira S, Vincent C, Lejeune JP. Retrosigmoid approach for meningiomas of the cerebellopontine angle: results of surgery and place of additional treatments. Acta Neurochir (Wien). 2011; 153 (10):1931–1940, discussion 1940

[3] Kalani MYS, Couldwell WT. Retrosigmoid craniotomy for resection of an epidermoid cyst of the posterior fossa. J Neurol Surg B Skull Base. 2018; 79 Suppl 5:S411–S412

[4] Jallo GI, Woo HH, Meshki C, Epstein FJ, Wisoff JH. Arachnoid cysts of the cerebellopontine angle: diagnosis and surgery. Neurosurgery. 1997; 40(1):31–37, discussion 37–38

[5] Brodsky JR, Smith TW, Litofsky S, Lee DJ. Lipoma of the cerebellopontine angle. Am J Otolaryngol. 2006; 27(4):271–274

[6] Raza SM, Quinones-Hinojosa A. The extended retrosigmoid approach for neoplastic lesions in the posterior fossa: technique modification. Neurosurg Rev. 2011; 34(1):123–129

[7] Ding D, Starke RM, Crowley RW, Liu KC. Surgical approaches for symptomatic cerebral cavernous malformations of the thalamus and brainstem. J Cerebrovasc Endovasc Neurosurg. 2017; 19(1):19–35

[8] Abla AA, Turner JD, Mitha AP, Lekovic G, Spetzler RF. Surgical approaches to brainstem cavernous malformations. Neurosurg Focus. 2010; 29(3):E8

[9] Lee B, Marquez YD, Giannotta SL. Resection of a cystic brainstem hemangioblastoma via a retrosigmoid approach. Neurosurg Focus. 2014; 36(1) Suppl:1

[10] Persad AR, Khormi YH, van Landeghem F, Chow MM. Unusual case of hemangioblastoma of the cerebellopontine angle. Surg Neurol Int. 2017; 8:264

[11] Nishino K, Hasegawa H, Morita K, et al. Clinical characteristics of arteriovenous malformations in the cerebellopontine angle cistern. J Neurosurg. 2017; 126(1):60–68

[12] Ansari SF, Terry C, Cohen-Gadol AA. Surgery for vestibular schwannomas: a systematic review of complications by approach. Neurosurg Focus. 2012; 33(3):E14

[13] Mangham CA, Jr. Retrosigmoid versus middle fossa surgery for small vestibular schwannomas. Laryngoscope. 2004; 114 (8):1455–1461

[14] Daming C, Yiwen S, Bin Z, et al. Large vestibular schwannoma resection through the suboccipital retrosigmoid keyhole approach. J Craniofac Surg. 2014; 25(2):463–468

[15] Vakharia KV, Naylor RM, Nassiri AM, Driscoll CLW, Link MJ. Microsurgical resection of a petroclival epidermoid cyst using an anterior petrosectomy approach: 2-dimensional operative video. Oper Neurosurg (Hagerstown). 2021; 21 (6):E565

[16] Morris L. Angiography of the superior sagittal and transverse sinuses. Br J Radiol. 1960; 33:606–613

[17] Leach JL, Fortuna RB, Jones BV, Gaskill-Shipley MF. Imaging of cerebral venous thrombosis: current techniques, spectrum of findings, and diagnostic pitfalls. Radiographics. 2006; 26 Suppl 1:S19–S41, discussion S42–S43

[18] Connor SE, Siddiqui MA, Stewart VR, O'Flynn EA. The relationship of transverse sinus stenosis to bony groove dimensions provides an insight into the aetiology of idiopathic intracranial hypertension. Neuroradiology. 2008; 50(12):999–1004

[19] Hoover JM, Morris JM, Meyer FB. Use of preoperative magnetic resonance imaging T1 and T2 sequences to determine intraoperative meningioma consistency. Surg Neurol Int. 2011; 2:142

[20] Butterworth JF, Mackey DC, Wasnick JD. Morgan and Mikhail's Clinical Anesthesiology Cases. New York, NY: McGraw Hill Lange; 2020

[21] Jannetta PJ, McLaughlin MR, Casey KF. Technique of microvascular decompression. Technical note. Neurosurg Focus. 2005; 18(5):E5

[22] McLaughlin MR, Jannetta PJ, Clyde BL, Subach BR, Comey CH, Resnick DK. Microvascular decompression of cranial nerves: lessons learned after 4400 operations. J Neurosurg. 1999; 90 (1):1–8

[23] Meuwly C, Golanov E, Chowdhury T, Erne P, Schaller B. Trigeminal cardiac reflex: new thinking model about the definition based on a literature review. Medicine (Baltimore). 2015; 94(5):e484

13 Far Lateral Approach

Mehmet Sabri Gurbuz, Abdullah Keles, Ufuk Erginoglu, and Mustafa Kemal Baskaya

13.1 Background

- Although the far lateral approach (lateral suboccipital approach) was introduced by Hammon and Kempe in 1972,[1] current descriptions of the far lateral approach were first described by Heros in 1986.[2]
- Heros described an S-shaped paramedian incision combined with a lateral suboccipital craniectomy, C1 laminectomy, and drilling of the occipital condyle.
- Both Hammon and Kempe[1] and Heros[2] began using this approach to treat the aneurysms of the proximal posteroinferior cerebellar artery (PICA), the vertebral artery (VA), and the vertebrobasilar junction.
- Subsequently, the far lateral approach has become widely used for surgical treatment of ventral and ventrolateral foramen magnum tumors, especially meningiomas.

13.2 Indications and Contraindications

- Lesions of the foramen magnum region, such as ventral foramen magnum meningiomas, lower clivus tumors, and aneurysms of the vertebrobasilar junction, should be managed via the far lateral approach.
- When these are approached via traditional suboccipital approaches, the exposure is poor and requires the need to retract neurovascular structures in the craniocervical junction.
- We thus need to approach these lesions with a lateral exposure in order to avoid retraction of the brainstem, the medulla, and the lower cranial nerves.[3]
- Although endonasal and transmaxillary approaches can be alternatives, they have some disadvantages. These include a higher rate of cerebrospinal fluid (CSF) fistula, wound infection, difficulty in reaching lateral limits of the tumor, and a higher depth of surgical field.[4]
- Foramen magnum meningiomas are the most common lesions operated via the far lateral approach (**Video 13.1**). Yasargil et al stated that the origin of foramen magnum meningiomas are around the insertion of the first dentate ligament and where the VA enters the dura.[5]
- Since these structures are located ventrolaterally, the exposure should also be in the same direction. With a lateral exposure, ventral portions of the tumor can be better visualized, and thus gross total resection becomes safer and easier.
- Condylar drilling is particularly useful in exposing aneurysms of the distal VA and vertebrobasilar junction.[6] A lateral angle of view is achieved by drilling the occipital condyle to various degrees depending on the extension of the pathology. However, condylar drilling may come at the cost of the loss of stability, intraoperative injury to the VA and hypoglossal nerve, a longer procedure time, and greater postoperative pain.
- For these reasons, the far lateral approach without condylar drilling has been advocated since it provides adequate exposure to reach the ventral foramen magnum region.[4]

13.3 Informed Consent

- Informed consent for the far lateral approach should include a comprehensive discussion of the surgical risks, including potential cranial nerve deficits, brainstem injury, vascular complications, and the possibility of subtotal resection if the lesion encases critical structures such as the vertebral artery.
- Patients should also be counseled on expected postoperative outcomes, recovery trajectory, and the potential need for postoperative rehabilitation or supportive therapies.

13.4 Instruments

- The far lateral approach for foramen magnum meningioma resection uses standard microneurosurgical instruments in various shapes and sizes under high magnification with an operating microscope.
- A three-pin head clamp ensures stable fixation. Bone removal is performed with a high-speed drill and diamond burrs, and a Cavitron

Ultrasonic Surgical Aspirator (CUSA) is used for tumor debulking when needed.
- Neurophysiological monitoring (somatosensory evoked potentials [SSEPs], motor evoked potentials [MEPs], and cranial nerve monitoring) enhances safety. Neuronavigation is used when available, and hemostatic agents are applied as needed.

13.5 Patient Preparation

- A thorough neurological examination should be performed and baseline deficits, particularly cranial nerve function, gait stability, and signs of myelopathy should be documented.
- Contrast-enhanced magnetic resonance imaging (MRI) of the craniovertebral junction is essential to assess tumor size, location (anterior, lateral, or posterior), dural attachment, compression of the brainstem, and possible encasement of adjacent vascular structures.
- Computed tomography (CT) angiography is essential to identify the relationship between the tumor and vertebral arteries.
- Coordination with neuroanesthesia, neurocritical care, and, when needed, otolaryngology or vascular surgery teams ensures preparedness for intraoperative challenges and comprehensive perioperative care.

13.6 Patient Positioning

- Positioning of the patient and the rest of the operation should be performed under neuromonitoring. The patient may be positioned in a variety of positions including lateral, sitting, semi-sitting, prone, supine and three-quarter positions.
- We prefer a lateral straight position with a slight tilt toward the ipsilateral shoulder, combined with pulling the shoulder down to further open the surgical area. This maneuver brings the head slightly above the level of the heart to make the venous return and CSF drainage easier. This positioning also helps prevent air embolism. Additionally, the axilla of the patient should be adequately padded to avoid brachial plexus injury.

13.7 Technique

- Preoperative radiological images should be carefully assessed, along with the anatomy of the pathology including the surgical anatomy of the foramen magnum and the occipital condyles, and the dominance of the vertebral arteries and venous flow.
- *Incision and muscular phase:* A horse shoe–shaped skin incision starts below the level of the mastoid tip three fingerbreadths medial to the mastoid bone and extends to the level of the external acoustic meatus, and then turns to the midline and goes downward to the level of the spinous process of C2 or lower, depending on the inferior extension of the lesion.
- Suboccipital muscles are dissected in one layer to avoid muscle denervation and atrophy. Sharp dissection is preferred, with electrocautery avoided when approaching the VA.
- The posterior tubercle and the posterior arch of C1 are then exposed by subperiosteal dissection. Following these structures, the sharp edge of the sulcus arteriosus is identified, and the VA is exposed without opening its sheath.[6]
- *Craniotomy:* Bone work consists of three parts—suboccipital craniectomy, C1 laminectomy, and condylar drilling. The suboccipital craniectomy starts from inferior to the transverse sinus and medial to the sigmoid sinus and extends beyond the midline up to the rim of the foramen magnum.
- In addition to this, a C1 laminectomy is performed from the posterior midline to the sulcus arteriosus. This provides a more inferior exposure, thus eliminating the need to retract the cerebellum medially.
- During this phase, bleeding from the peri-vertebral venous plexus might be encountered, which can be easily controlled with basic hemostatic maneuvers.
- *Condylar drilling:* As one proceeds laterally to the rim of the foramen magnum, the bone edge becomes vertical, which prevents a Kerrison rongeur from biting into the bone. This is why high-speed drilling is crucial for this step of the procedure.
- Drilling of the occipital condyle is an important step, particularly for the aneurysms of the distal VA, in order to provide a lateral exposure and provide the ability to reach the ventral and superior parts of the region.[6]

- One-third to one-half of the occipital condyle and the C1 lateral mass is removed in order to expose at least 1 cm beyond the entrance of the VA.[7]
- Effective drilling of the lateral rim of the foramen magnum provides an excellent lateral exposure to reach ventral to the brainstem and the foramen magnum.
- Condylar drilling has been shown to considerably shorten the distance to the anterior foramen magnum and to widen the surgical corridor.[8] In addition, drilling of the jugular tubercle is helpful for aneurysms of the vertebrobasilar junction.[7]
- *Intradural phase:* After completing the bone work, the dura is incised in an oblique fashion extending from the junction of the transverse and sigmoid sinus to the level of C1. The intradural part of this step is completed under the microscope. This enables visualization of the VA, the C1 nerve root, the dentate ligament, the spinal accessory nerve, and other lower cranial nerves.[9] Dentate ligaments may be cut to allow the medulla to fall away by the force of gravity.
- For aneurysm cases, the arterial anatomy must be generously exposed and the location for the placement of a temporary clip must be prepared. If a temporary clip will be applied to the VA, the PICA must be carefully preserved. When the vertebrobasilar junction is targeted, the junction of the tonsil and medulla oblongata must be dissected and exposed.
- For lower basilar artery (BA) aneurysms, the mastoid craniotomy should extend laterally until the sigmoid sinus is visualized and unroofed. Following retraction of the dura of the sigmoid sinus, the lower BA is exposed between the cranial nerves.
- If the vertebrobasilar junction is high and the surgeon must work between cranial nerves IX–X and VII–VIII, one must be extremely gentle since the cranial nerve VII–VIII complex is very sensitive to trauma.
- In cases of arteriovenous malformation, the VA can be visualized starting from its entrance into intradural space up to the vertebrobasilar junction. This exposure provides the surgeon with control of the feeders originating from the VA, PICA, anteroinferior cerebellar artery (AICA) and the BA. The entire configuration of the malformation and the relation of the lesion with the lower cranial nerves can be clearly assessed using this exposure.

13.8 Postoperative Care

- Postoperative management of patients undergoing surgery for foramen magnum meningiomas is critical due to critical neurovascular structures and the risk of complications affecting the lower cranial nerves, brainstem, and upper cervical spinal cord.
- Postoperative care should be conducted in an experienced neurointensive care unit to ensure close monitoring of neurological status, respiratory function, and hemodynamic parameters.
- Close neurological examinations are essential to detect early signs of brainstem compression, cranial nerve involvement, hematoma, or infarction. In the event of any deterioration in cranial nerve function, motor strength, or altered level of consciousness, immediate imaging with CT and MRI is mandatory.
- Early mobilization, when safe, helps reduce the risk of thromboembolic events.
- Given the suboccipital approach, there is a risk of CSF leakage.
- Patients should be monitored for signs of pseudomeningocele, or wound complications. In some cases of leakage, lumbar drainage may be required to facilitate healing. Antibiotic, antiedema, and, if needed, corticosteroids can be used in the short term.
- Postoperative imaging is typically performed within 24 hours to assess the extent of resection and to rule out any hematoma or infarction.

13.9 Complications

- The far lateral approach can be challenging since neurosurgeons rarely use this approach and thus have less experience with its execution. The most important challenge when using this approach is vascular injury when a tumor encases the VA, the BA, the anterior spinal artery, or their perforators. In such cases, the aim should be maximal safe removal.
- When complete tumor removal is not possible, which is common for *en plaque* meningiomas and recurrent cases, the surgeon should not

hesitate to leave a small piece of tumor on the brainstem or other neurovascular structures. Preoperative angiography of the VA should be performed, and its dominance should be noted. If the tumor is in the midline, the side of approach should be from the nondominant side.
- An additional challenge is when there is strong adherence or arachnoid scarring, which are conditions mostly encountered in recurrent cases. In such cases, the lower cranial nerves, brainstem, and vessels should be very carefully preserved. The most common complications are cranial nerve IX and X deficits. Surgical removal in these cases requires experience and patience. Doppler ultrasound can be used for cases of encasement of the major arteries. If radical removal could lead to complications, small remnants should be left behind instead of causing the patient permanent neurological damage.[10]
- A thorough knowledge of the anatomy obtained with laboratory training is of paramount importance for this relatively rarely used surgical approach. Performing cadaver dissections will make the neurosurgeon more familiar with the three-dimensional anatomy of this approach. Laboratory practice of micro-neurosurgical drilling skills, including condylar drilling, will also provide beneficial surgical experience.[11]

13.10 Management Pearls

- Various incisions have been introduced for the far lateral approach including small S-shaped paramedian incisions and relatively large hockey stick incisions.
- We prefer a horse shoe skin incision that begins below the level of the mastoid tip and extends to the level of the external acoustic meatus, and then turns to the midline and goes downward to the spinous process of C2.
- The borders of the suboccipital craniotomy are then the transverse sinus superiorly, the sigmoid sinus laterally, the occipital condyle and foramen magnum inferiorly, and immediately beyond the midline medially.
- In addition to the suboccipital craniotomy, C1 laminectomy begins from the posterior tubercle and goes up to the beginning of the sulcus arteriosus, where the VA makes a turn toward the entrance to the dura (▶ Fig. 13.1).
- The suboccipital muscles can be dissected as either a single layer or layer by layer. However, we prefer elevating the scalp and the superficial

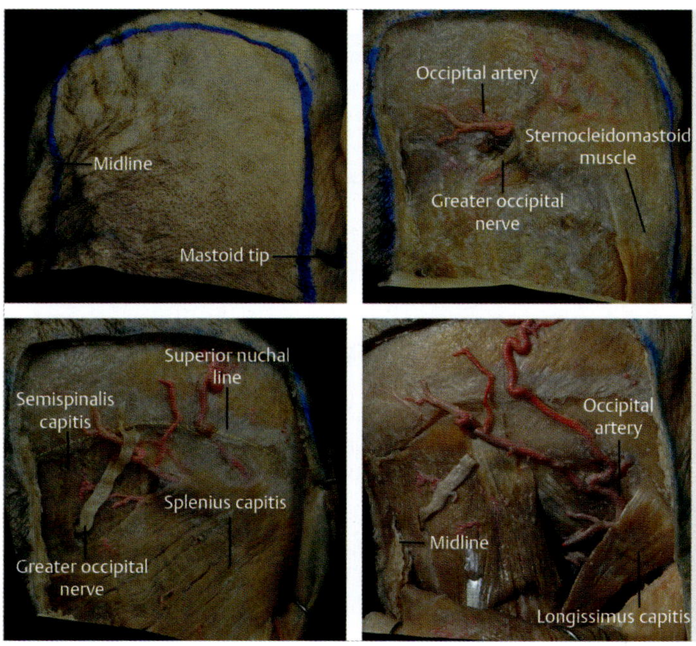

Fig. 13.1 Skin incision and scalp elevation are shown step by step. Following scalp elevation, the most superficial muscle layers become visible. In this cadaver, the scalp incision is higher than normal for teaching and illustration purposes.

muscles in one layer to prevent atrophy. In the final step, a suboccipital triangle is identified with the VA wrapped by its perivertebral venous plexus (▶ Fig. 13.2).
- After opening the dura in a curvilinear fashion, a piece of dura is left behind on the cerebellar hemisphere to prevent its protrusion. This opening enables visualization of the cerebellar tonsil and the lower medulla. Usually, the cerebellomedullary cistern and its contents are not well exposed unless the occipital condyle is drilled (▶ Fig. 13.3). Dissection of the tonsil and opening the cistern then unveils the neurovascular structures. At this time, the intradural segment of the VA, the posterior spinal artery, the spinal accessory nerve, the C1 nerve roots, and the first dentate ligament are then first visualized.

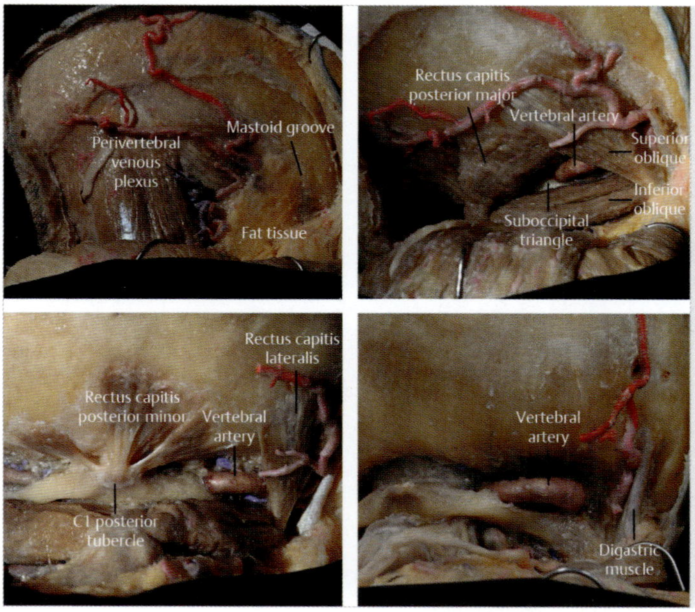

Fig. 13.2 In the upper row, the second layer of musculature and suboccipital triangle are seen. After cleaning the venous plexus and fat, the vertebral artery is seen in the suboccipital triangle. In the lower row, the rectus capitis posterior minor muscles are seen following elevation of the rectus capitis posterior major muscle. After removal of the rectus capitis posterior minor muscles, the vertebral artery and its dural entry at the foramen magnum are visible.

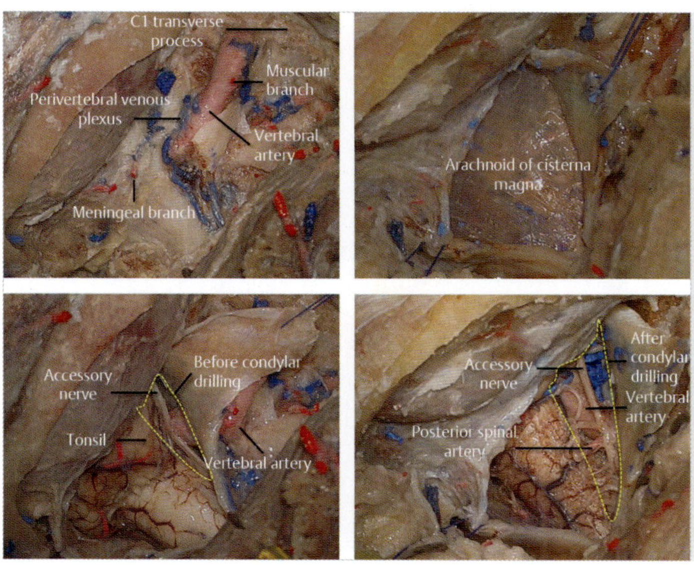

Fig. 13.3 In another cadaver, the upper row reveals entry of the vertebral artery into the dura and dural incision are seen. The dura over the cerebellum is left intact to prevent the cerebellum protruding into the exposure. After dural incision, the arachnoid of the cisterna magna remains intact. In the lower row, the cerebellomedullary cistern and its content are revealed. The *dashed yellow line* outlines the exposures of the cerebellomedullary cistern before and after the condylar drilling. One can notice that after condylar drilling, a flat angle and lateral exposure of the cerebellomedullary cistern are obtained.

- However, when a tumor is present, it already widens the area and thus makes the anatomical structures more accessible. The tumor, while it grows, displaces the VA, the PICA, the lower cranial nerves, and the C1–C2 nerve roots (▶ Fig. 13.4).
- Some tumors encase the VA and PICA, thus making resection more challenging. Following CSF drainage from the cisterna magna and the cerebellomedullary cistern, cranial nerves XII, X, and X, the PICA, the jugular foramen, and the hypoglossal foramen can be visualized. The lateral angle of approach makes it possible to reach the vertebrobasilar junction, the origin of the PICA, the anterior spinal arteries, and the lower BA.[12]

13.11 Conclusion

- The far lateral approach is an ideal approach for both tumoral and vascular lesions of the ventrolateral aspect of the craniocervical junction. Early identification of the VA contributes to safe exposure of the lateral

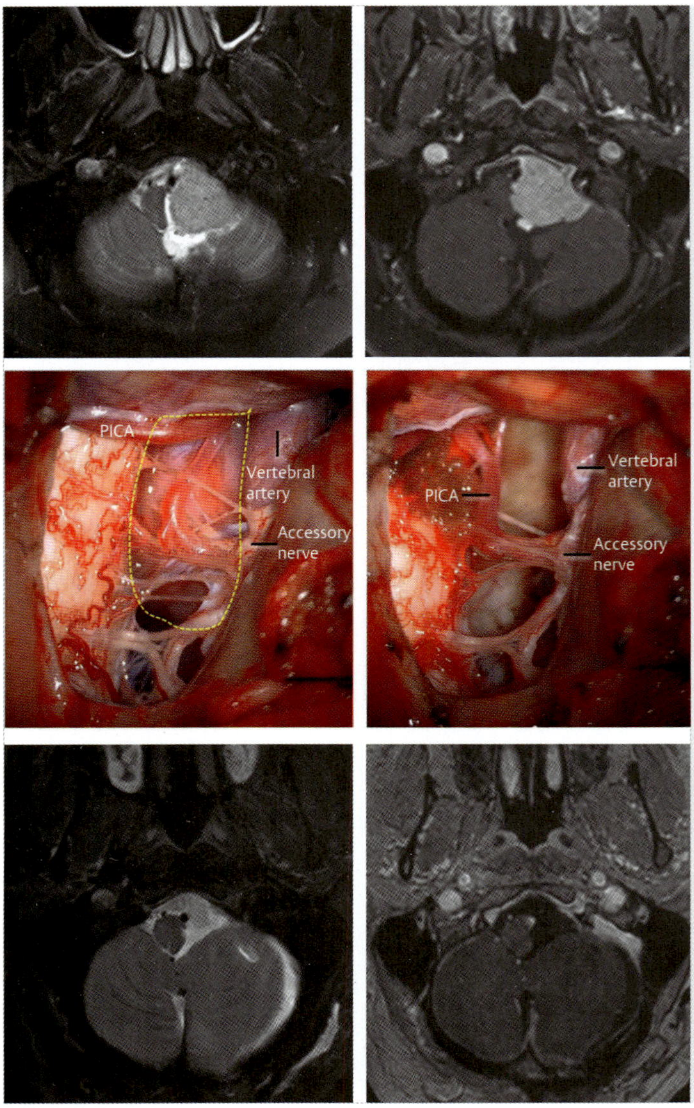

Fig. 13.4 The upper row reveals ventral foramen magnum meningioma immediately after opening the dura and the arachnoid. The *dashed yellow line* outlines the borders of the meningioma. Posteroinferior cerebellar artery (PICA), spinal accessory nerve, C1 nerve roots, and dentate ligament are posteriorly displaced. After tumor removal, all neurovascular structures are seen to be intact. The lower row shows preoperative and postoperative sagittal MR images of the same patient demonstrating gross total removal of the meningioma.

foramen magnum region. Along with the addition of condylar drilling, the far lateral approach provides an excellent exposure of the distal VA and the vertebrobasilar junction.

References

[1] Hammon WM, Kempe LG. The posterior fossa approach to aneurysms of the vertebral and basilar arteries. J Neurosurg. 1972; 37(3):339–347

[2] Heros RC. Lateral suboccipital approach for vertebral and vertebrobasilar artery lesions. J Neurosurg. 1986; 64(4): 559–562

[3] Kratimenos GP, Crockard HA. The far lateral approach for ventrally placed foramen magnum and upper cervical spine tumours. Br J Neurosurg. 1993; 7(2):129–140

[4] Nanda A, Vincent DA, Vannemreddy PS, Baskaya MK, Chanda A. Far-lateral approach to intradural lesions of the foramen magnum without resection of the occipital condyle. J Neurosurg. 2002; 96(2):302–309

[5] Yasargil MG, Mortara RW, Curcic M. Meningiomas of the basal posterior cranial fossa. In: Krayenbuhl H, ed. Advances and Technical Standards in Neurosurgery. Vol. 7. Wien: Springer-Verlag; 1980:1–115

[6] Lanzino G, Paolini S, Spetzler RF. Far-lateral approach to the craniocervical junction. Neurosurgery. 2005; 57(4) Suppl: 367–371, discussion 367–371

[7] Babu RP, Sekhar LN, Wright DC. Extreme lateral transcondylar approach: technical improvements and lessons learned. J Neurosurg. 1994; 81(1):49–59

[8] Açikbaş SC, Tuncer R, Demirez I, et al. The effect of condylectomy on extreme lateral transcondylar approach to the anterior foramen magnum. Acta Neurochir (Wien). 1997; 139(6):546–550

[9] Rhoton AL, Jr. The far-lateral approach and its transcondylar, supracondylar, and paracondylar extensions. Neurosurgery. 2000; 47(3) Suppl:S195–S209

[10] Samii M, Klekamp J, Carvalho G. Surgical results for meningiomas of the craniocervical junction. Neurosurgery. 1996; 39(6):1086–1094, discussion 1094–1095

[11] Arnautović KI, Al-Mefty O, Husain M. Ventral foramen magnum meninigiomas. J Neurosurg. 2000; 92(1) Suppl: 71–80

[12] de Oliveira E, Rhoton AL, Jr, Peace D. Microsurgical anatomy of the region of the foramen magnum. Surg Neurol. 1985; 24 (3):293–352

14 Decompressive Hemicraniectomy

Shaarada Srivatsa, Krishna P. Nayak, and Enyinna L. Nwachuku

14.1 Background

- Usually done in an urgent or emergent setting, decompressive hemicraniectomy (DHC) involves trephination and removal of a unilateral 12- to 17-cm flap of bone and opening of underlying dura mater to relieve underlying intracranial pressure (ICP) and allow for parenchyma to swell outward through the craniectomy defect while preserving surrounding anatomical structures.
- Other names for this procedure include trauma craniectomy, hemicraniectomy, trauma flap, and frontotemporoparietal craniectomy.
- Several studies have been done to ascertain the prognostic and survival benefit of DHC including DECRA, RESCUE-ICP, and RESCUE-ASDH.
- The decision to perform DHC and techniques used to accomplish its goal are ultimately surgeon and context dependent.

14.2 Indications and Contraindications

- Cerebral edema that is refractory to maximal medical management:
  - Traumatic brain injury (TBI) with associated mass lesion or diffuse cerebral edema resulting in midline shift ≥ 5 mm.
  - Large territory middle cerebral artery (MCA) infarct with resultant malignant cerebral edema.
  - Unilateral mass lesion causing elevated ICP.
- Relative contraindications include the following:
  - Advanced age.
  - Presence of a contralateral hemicraniectomy.
  - Low premorbid functional status.
  - Comorbid conditions that preclude general anesthesia.
  - Indicators of poor prognosis such as absence of brainstem reflexes or bilaterally fixed and dilated pupils at the time of patient evaluation.

14.3 Instruments

- "Mayfield" head holder.
- No. 10 blade.
- Monopolar and bipolar cautery.
- "Raney" scalp clips.
- Square- and round-shaped periosteal elevators.
- A high-speed burr and/or perforator drill.
- Penfield no. 1 or no. 3.
- A craniotome.
- A Leksell rongeur or a Kerrison rongeur.
- A dural substitute for the dural closure.
- A 10-mm Jackson-Pratt perforated flat drain.
- Hemostatic agents such as thrombin-soaked gelatin foams or mesh hemostatic sheets.

14.4 Patient Preparation

- Medical optimization of ICP management prior to and during surgery is critical. These measures may include the following:
  - Analgesia.
  - Elevation of the head of the bed.
  - Sedation.
  - Target normothermia.
  - Hyperosmolar therapy (mannitol, hypertonic saline).
  - Hyperventilation to an end-tidal $PaCO_2$ of 30 to 32 mm Hg.
  - Cerebral perfusion pressure (CPP) goal greater than 60 mm Hg.[1]
- ICP and brain PbO_2 monitors may be used to track ICP and brain tissue perfusion in real time, can guide medical management, and can help determine when ICP becomes refractory to nonsurgical treatment. These monitors are used in patients whose neurological examination is difficult to follow or poor (a commonly accepted neurological cutoff is a Glasgow Coma Score of ≤ 8), whether due to the TBI or stroke itself, or other confounders (e.g., metabolic or toxic encephalopathy).

14.5 Patient Positioning

- Supine on the operative table.
- The head should be positioned facing 60 to 90 degrees opposite from the planned craniotomy, either fixed with a three-point "Mayfield" head holder or resting on a "horse shoe" attachment (▶ Fig. 14.1). Care should be taken not to kink

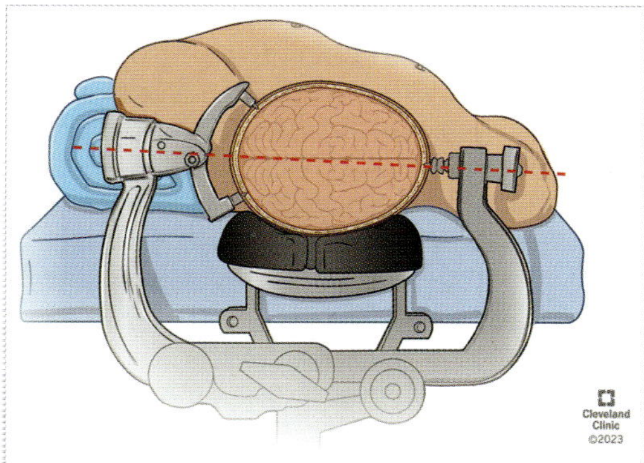

Fig. 14.1 Supine positioning, both with a three-point Mayfield head holder and a horseshoe attachment. (Reprinted with permission, Cleveland Clinic Foundation ©2025. All Rights Reserved.)

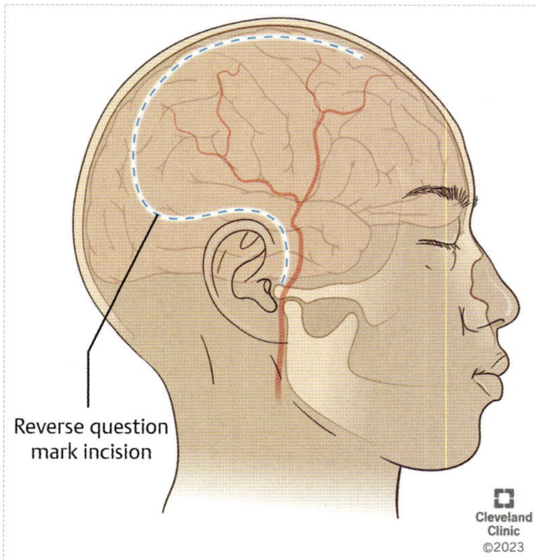

Fig. 14.2 Reverse question mark incision. (Reprinted with permission, Cleveland Clinic Foundation ©2025. All Rights Reserved.)

the internal jugular vein to allow for optimal venous outflow.
- If an ICP monitor is in place, it should be contralateral to the planned incision and tunneled off midline.

14.6 Technique

14.6.1 Incision

- Generally, a no. 10 blade is used to open skin, with monopolar cautery used to achieve hemostasis while opening the subcutaneous tissue. Monopolar and bipolar cautery can be used to expeditiously achieve further hemostasis.
- "Raney" scalp clips can be used to minimize skin bleeding for the duration of the case.
- Once the skin and subcutaneous tissue have been opened, monopolar cautery can be used to incise the temporalis muscle and fascia and the pericranium, following the incision's path.
- The most commonly utilized incision is the reverse question mark (RQM) or question mark (QM) incision depending on the side of surgical approach. The starting point of this incision is 1 cm anterior to the tragus, where the zygomatic arch is palpable. It continues posteriorly, then anteriorly like a "QM" and arches to end at the hairline, just lateral to the midline (▶ Fig. 14.2).

14.6.2 Retractor System

- The periosteum and temporalis muscle are elevated from the skull using a square-shaped and a round-shaped periosteal elevator, respectively.
- The myocutaneous flap that results is retracted anteriorly. In the emergent setting, retraction is typically done using towel clamps or Fisch hooks affixed to drapes or the Mayo stand. In some cases, it is possible to set up a Layla bar system to affix the hooks with elastic.

14.6.3 Burr Holes and Craniotomy

- Commonly used drill bits for creation of the burr holes in hemicraniectomy include a perforator drill bit with an auto-stop function after breach of the inner table, and the acorn drill bit.
- The dura is stripped surrounding the burr holes using a Penfield no. 1 or no. 3.
- The craniotomy itself is achieved using a craniotome.
- Adequate bony exposure should be achieved to place the following burr holes:
  - *MacCarty keyhole*, just posterior to the zygomatic arch of the frontal bone.

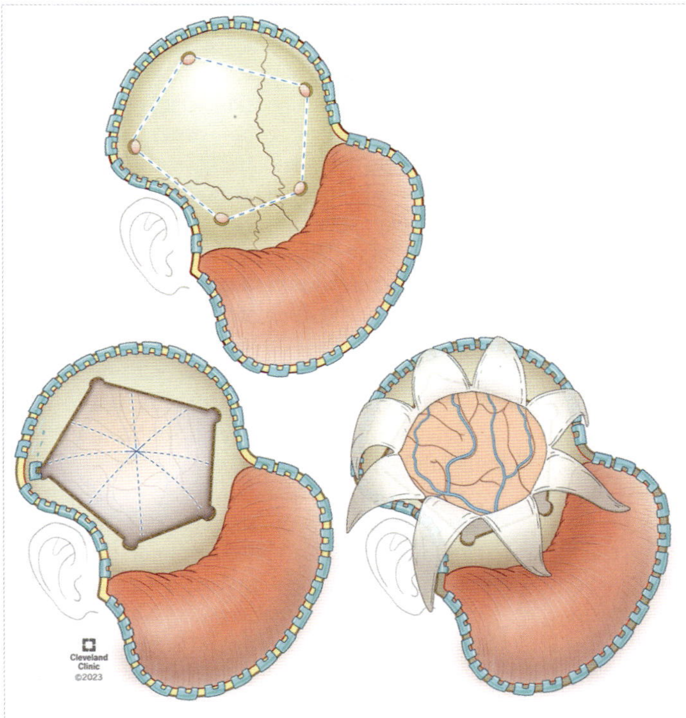

Fig. 14.3 Extent of craniotomy and stellate dural opening. (Reprinted with permission, Cleveland Clinic Foundation ©2025. All Rights Reserved.)

  - Just superior to the root of the zygoma in the squamous temporal bone.
  - *Frontoparietal convexity, 2 to 3 cm lateral to midline:* Commonly, two burr holes are placed at the convexity, with care taken to avoid the superior sagittal sinus (SSS) and its draining veins.
- The goal of this craniotomy is to achieve 15 to 17 cm of exposure anteroposteriorly, extending to the floor of the temporal fossa (▶ Fig. 14.3). Adequate exposure is important, as larger bone flaps have been associated with improved outcomes.[2]
- The bone flap is then elevated from the dura using the periosteal elevator and a Penfield instrument providing counter-leverage, until the sphenoid ridge fractures.
- The flap is carefully separated from any remaining dural attachments.
- It is important at this stage to ensure any remaining squamous temporal bone is adequately removed to maximize temporal lobe decompression. For this step, one can utilize further drilling, Leksell rongeur, or Kerrison rongeur to remove residual bone.

14.6.4 Dural Opening

- The following are the most common dural opening patterns:
  - *Stellate:* A star-shaped dural opening in spokes extending from a center point (▶ Fig. 14.3).
  - ***U-shaped:*** Circumferential opening with the attached base of the “U” at the temporal portion of the craniotomy defect.

14.6.5 Dural Closure

- After the dural opening, if hematoma or blood must be evacuated, it may be done at this stage.
- Once ready to proceed with closure, a flap of pericranium if, still intact, or a dural substitute can be used as on-lay to cover the exposed cortex while allowing room for postoperative swelling and edema.

- The bone flap is not replaced in DHC, and is rather stored sterilely in bone storage for eventual cranioplasty replacement procedure.

14.6.6 Galeal and Skin Closure

- Hemostatic closure of the galea is critical for operative success. This is usually achieved using 2–0 Vicryl sutures to approximate the galeal tissue and the temporalis muscle edges. The galeal closure should be watertight.
- Oftentimes, a 10-mm Jackson-Pratt perforated flat drain is left in the subgaleal space to collect postoperative blood products, with removal around 48 to 72 hours after surgery.
- Skin closure can be performed using skin staples or sutures (typically monofilament suture in a vertical mattress, simple interrupted, or running-locking fashion).
- Clean dressing with or without bacitracin ointment can be applied for 48 to 72 hours.

14.7 Postoperative Care

- The primary considerations should be ICP monitoring and treatment (with hyperosmolar therapy, proper positioning, sedation, and analgesia).
- Liberal systolic blood pressure should be allowed for optimal CPP, especially in patients with preserved autoregulation.
- Infection prevention with nursing hygiene and perioperative prophylactic antibiotics are crucial in the early management of these patients.
- Following the acute postoperative TBI and stroke management, patients commonly spend a period of several days to several months without their bone flap while the cerebral edema equilibrates and improves. Special considerations during this time include post-TBI seizures, wound healing, and ex vacuo hydrocephalus. The specifications and indications of performing the cranioplasty extend past the scope of this chapter.

14.8 Complications

- During exposure with electrocautery, care must be taken not to inadvertently violate the ear canal, given proximity of the lower extent of the incision to the anterior aspect of the external auditory meatus.
- During the course of bony drilling, damage to the frontal sinus anteriorly may increase the patient's risk of infection, CSF leak, and may require more extensive bony repair.
- Damage to the SSS medially can result in life-threatening blood loss, devastating air embolus, postoperative venous strokes, and further worsening refractory cerebral edema.
- Following bony decompression and dural opening, inadvertent injury to the underlying parenchyma and associated vasculature should be avoided.
- Dural sinus injury can occur medially at the SSS due to the size of the craniectomy and the tendency of many surgeons to approach the midline with the craniotomy.
  - Steps to take in the event of this complications include elevation of the head of the bed, copious irrigation, and tamponading of the area of injury or bleeding with a large piece of Gelfoam and/or cottonoids.
  - Avoid the use of more liquid hemostatic agents (such as FloSeal) due to the risk of propagation through the sinus leading to sinus thrombosis, which can result in catastrophic venous injury and infarction.
- Malignant cerebral edema can occur with severely injured or ischemic brain parenchyma and result in immediate swelling of brain tissue outside of the craniectomy defect. This can lead to further ischemic injury at the site of the brain–bone interface and possibly unsalvageable herniation.
  - In this event, it is important to perform all routine ICP-lowering techniques such as head of the bed elevation, use of hyperosmolar therapy (mannitol, hypertonics), use of other diuretics such as Lasix, hyperventilation, further sedation, and drainage via an external ventricular drain (EVD) if one is in place.
  - If these methods are inadequate, in some circumstances, resection of brain tissue via temporal lobectomy can be considered.

14.9 Management Pearls

- Comparison to other procedures:
  - Bifrontal decompressive craniectomy can be performed in cases of bifrontal injury, usually traumatic. This technique, however, is more

rarely performed and reserved almost exclusively for a bifrontal pattern of injury.
  - Hinge or floating craniotomy is another technique that is rarely used to avoid the need to return for cranioplasty at a later date, but limits the extent to which damaged parenchyma may swell postoperatively.
  - Hemicraniotomy with replacement of bone flap at the conclusion of the procedure remains an option when compressive pathology, such as subdural or epidural hematoma, is evacuated without concomitant severe parenchymal injury or intraprocedural swelling.[3]
- Important external landmarks to note prior to incision include the following:
  - *Midline:* For the medial extent of incision. Some surgeons prefer to take the incision to the midline, while others prefer to stop 1 to 2 cm lateral of the midline.
  - *Zygoma:* Marks the inferior extent of the incision and craniectomy.
  - *Location and course of the superficial temporal artery:* Allows for preservation of the vessel for optimal wound healing and skin flap perfusion.
- If possible, the anterior branch of the superficial temporal artery should be preserved to aid in wound healing and skin flap perfusion. The posterior branch can be more commonly sacrificed due to the dual perfusion of the posterior scalp by the occipital and posterior auricular arteries.
- A second, less commonly used incision is the Kempe **T**-shaped incision, wherein the skin is incised along the midline just behind the hairline and through the inion posteriorly. A second incision line is cut from the root of the zygoma through the coronal suture, perpendicular to the midline incision (▶ Fig. 14.4). This incision is used when a future contralateral surgery is likely, cerebral edema that is more posteriorly localized, or in the cases where there is significant facial trauma requiring possible future bicoronal incision for repair.[4] In this chapter, we focus on the RQM and/or the QM approach.
- Following the incision, relevant anatomy includes the following:
  - *Temporalis muscle:* Extending from the superior temporal line to the coronoid process of the mandible. Usually elevated as one myocutaneous flap during the exposure for a DHC.
  - *Root of the zygoma:* Palpable at the inferior extent of the craniectomy.
  - *MacCarty keyhole:* A common location of burr hole that allows access to the anterior cranial fossa floor and the orbit, 7 mm superior and 5 mm posterior to the frontozygomatic suture.
- Following the lifting of the bone flap, relevant anatomy includes the following:
  - Dura mater covering the indicated hemisphere.
  - *Middle meningeal artery:* A branch of the maxillary artery that courses inferosuperiorly along the dura mater and supplies it. It is often cauterized prior to the dural opening.
- In any and all dural opening, care should be taken to leave a substantial area of intact dura off the edge of the craniotomy defect to facilitate later closure.
- Following opening of the dura, relevant anatomy includes the following:
  - *Sylvian fissure:* Oftentimes visible at the lower center of the exposure.
- Literature:
  - Results of the DECRA randomized controlled trial (2011) suggest that decompressive

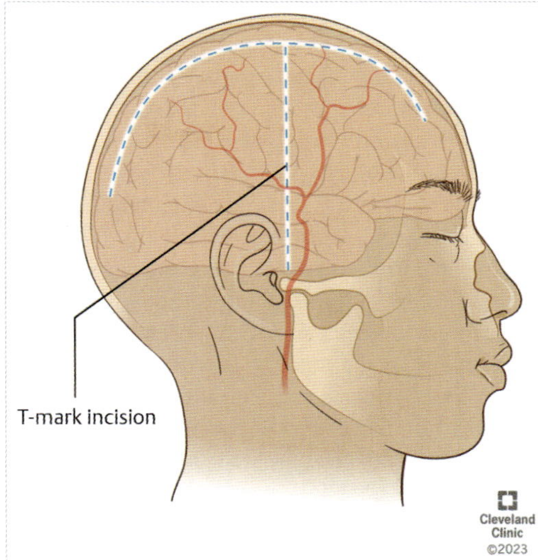

Fig. 14.4 Kempe T-shaped incision. (Reprinted with permission, Cleveland Clinic Foundation ©2025. All Rights Reserved.)

craniectomy for severe TBI does not offer favorable outcomes. The DECRA study concluded that decompressive craniectomy for refractory elevated ICP after TBI resulted in more unfavorable neurological outcomes (vegetative state, upper and lower severe disability on the Extended Glasgow Outcome Scale), but did shorten ICU stay.

- The RescueICP randomized controlled trial data (2016) suggest that decompressive craniectomy does provide favorable neurological outcome.[5,6] The RescueICP data showed surgical intervention for refractory intracranial hypertension after TBI improved mortality, but resulted in higher rates of vegetative state and severe dependency.
- The RESCUE-ASDH randomized controlled trial (2023), compared outcomes after craniotomy versus DHC for traumatic acute subdural hematoma, concluding that disability and quality-of-life outcomes were comparable between the two groups, with more wound complications occurring in the craniectomy group and more reoperation occurring in the craniotomy group.[7]
- Ultimately, the decision to take a patient for hemicraniectomy should be highly individualized.

References

[1] Chesnut R, Aguilera S, Buki A, et al. A management algorithm for adult patients with both brain oxygen and intracranial pressure monitoring: the Seattle International Severe Traumatic Brain Injury Consensus Conference (SIBICC). Intensive Care Med. 2020; 46(5):919–929

[2] Jiang JY, Xu W, Li WP, et al. Efficacy of standard trauma craniectomy for refractory intracranial hypertension with severe traumatic brain injury: a multicenter, prospective, randomized controlled study. J Neurotrauma. 2005; 22(6): 623–628

[3] Kolias AG, Viaroli E, Rubiano AM, et al. The current status of decompressive craniectomy in traumatic brain injury. Curr Trauma Rep. 2018; 4(4):326–332

[4] Abecassis IJ, Young CC, Caldwell DJ, et al. The Kempe incision for decompressive craniectomy, craniotomy, and cranioplasty in traumatic brain injury and stroke. J Neurosurg. 2021; 135(6):1807–1816

[5] Cooper DJ, Rosenfeld JV, Murray L, et al. DECRA Trial Investigators, Australian and New Zealand Intensive Care Society Clinical Trials Group. Decompressive craniectomy in diffuse traumatic brain injury. N Engl J Med. 2011; 364(16): 1493–1502

[6] Hutchinson PJ, Kolias AG, Timofeev IS, et al. RESCUEicp Trial Collaborators. Trial of decompressive craniectomy for traumatic intracranial hypertension. N Engl J Med. 2016; 375(12):1119–1130

[7] Hutchinson PJ, Adams H, Mohan M, et al. British Neurosurgical Trainee Research Collaborative, NIHR Global Health Research Group on Acquired Brain and Spine Injury, and RESCUE-ASDH Trial Collaborators, RESCUE-ASDH Trial Collaborators. Decompressive craniectomy versus craniotomy for acute subdural hematoma. N Engl J Med. 2023; 388(24): 2219–2229

15 Transsellar

Ayesha Akbar Waheed and David T. Fernandes Cabral

15.1 Background

- The sella turcica is the center of the universe in endoscopic skull base surgery. It is located in the midline on the sphenoid bone.[1] To gain access to the sella, general exposure of the nasal cavity must first be completed, which is out of the scope of this chapter.

15.2 Disease Profile

- The most common pathologies treated with transsellar approaches are pituitary adenomas (functioning and nonfunctioning) and Rathke's cleft cysts.

15.3 Preparatory Diagnostics

- A thorough history and physical examination should be performed in all patients. Especial attention should be paid for signs and symptoms of pituitary hormone excess or deficiency as well as any neurological deficits, particularly visual fields due to close relationship of the pituitary gland to the optic chiasm.
- The patient should also be evaluated by the ear, nose, and throat (ENT) team to exclude any active rhinosinusitis and preoperative endoscopic assessment of the nasal anatomy when indicated.
- When possible, all patients should have preoperative thin-cut computed tomography of the head (CTH)/CT angiography (CTA), as well as pituitary magnetic resonance imaging (MRI) with and without contrast. In the cases where MRI is contraindicated, CTH with contrast should be performed. Allergies to contrast can be overcome with a contrast dye allergy protocol prior to scanning.
- Patients should have an endocrinological evaluation with a full pituitary lab workup, and any hormonal deficiency should be treated accordingly.
- If the patient complains of visual symptoms or there is clear compromise of any component of the optic apparatus, a comprehensive ophthalmological evaluation is indicated.
- In cases of growth hormone–producing adenomas, a cardiac workup is warranted.
- At our institution, any patient scheduled for skull base surgery is evaluated by the center for preoperative medicine where a thorough evaluation is performed to minimize complication risks. Additional testing is tailored on an as-needed basis.

15.4 Indications and Contraindications

15.4.1 Indications

- Nonfunctioning adenomas that have shown growth on follow-up images.
- Nonfunctioning adenomas that present with pituitary insufficiency and/or visual disturbances.
- Functional adenomas (especially those causing Cushing's disease or acromegaly).
- Prolactinomas are a subtype of functional adenomas that are usually managed medically with dopamine agonists (bromocriptine or cabergoline). Indications for surgery include contraindication to medical therapy, failure to improve under medical therapy, poor medication tolerance, and/or adverse side effect of dopamine agonist. Women on reproductive age seeking to get pregnant can also consider undergoing surgical resection. Some cystic prolactinomas might require surgical resection.
- Patients presenting with pituitary apoplexy might require urgent surgery if presenting with rapid and sudden onset of vision loss.
- Symptomatic Rathke's cleft cysts.

15.4.2 Contraindications

- Contraindications to undergo to general anesthesia.
- Patients with extensive suprasellar growth might require a craniotomy or a combine approach.

15.5 Informed Consent

- It is the primary surgeon's responsibility to ensure that the patient has provided informed consent before moving forward with the procedure. The history of informed consent reflects an evolving landscape of ethics and legal standards, ensuring up-to-date definitions of patient autonomy.[2]
- The process of informed consent involves educating the patient about the procedure using language and terminology that aligns with their understanding. Components that must always be covered are indications for the procedure, why the patient is a candidate for the surgery, if and why any modifications are being made to the surgery, overview of risks and benefits, complication types and rates, and what to expect during the recovery process.
- While this covers the overarching components of informed consent, much more detail exists in practice. It should be noted that informed consent can only be obtained from an individual with clear decision-making capacity. This must be assessed prior to obtaining consent. If the patient lacks decision-making capacity, their power of attorney (if assigned) or the closest next of kin, as defined by law, will be designated to make decisions on their behalf.

15.6 Instruments

- A 4-mm-diameter endoscope with different degrees: 0, 30, 45, and 70 degrees. We do not use endoscope holders since we apply dynamic endoscopic with two surgeons using four hands.
- Image guidance system.
- Endonasal drills.
- Standard paranasal sinus endoscopic tray.
- Ultrasonic aspirator (more commonly used in fibrous meningiomas).
- Long suctions (Frazier for drilling and Fukushima for tumor resection and microsurgical technique).
- Pistol grip bipolar electrocautery.
- Needle tip Bovie.
- Hemostatic agents.
- Neuropatties.
- Retractable knife blade.
- Feather blade.
- Warmed irrigation.

15.7 Patient Preparation

15.7.1 Anesthesia

- Patients undergo general anesthesia with oral endotracheal intubation. The tube is taped toward the left side of the patient since the surgical team is standing on the right side of the patient.
- It is important to communicate with the anesthesia team the need for stress dose steroids if needed. Similarly, if motor monitoring is planned for cranial nerves, patients might need to undergo total intravenous anesthesia instead of halogenated agents.
- It is critical to place a Foley catheter for strict monitoring of intake and output in case the patient develops intraoperative diabetes insipidus (DI). If there is concern of intraoperative DI, the anesthesia team must check serum sodium level, urine-specific gravity, and osmolarity. The decision of administering desmopressin (DDAVP) must be discussed with the neurosurgeon.
- Another important factor is to keep an open communication regarding estimated blood loss. Some tumors might be extremely bloody and can trigger disseminated intravascular coagulation, which must be addressed immediately. If there is any concern from the surgical or anesthesia team, a coagulation lab panel must be ordered, and abnormal values must be evaluated and corrected as needed.
- We always prep the abdomen in case fat graft is needed, or to harvest rectus muscle to plug as a patch in the event of an internal carotid injury. The external surface of the nose and upper lip is cleaned with Betadine antiseptic solution. For general operating room (OR) setup, please see ▶ Fig. 15.1.

15.8 Patient Positioning

- Once the patient is intubated and lines and catheters are properly placed, we turn the OR table counterclockwise (▶ Fig. 15.1).
- We routinely obtain prepositioning somatosensory evoked potentials (SSEPs) in patients older than 65 years and/or in those with known cervical spondylosis. The patient is positioned supinely in the OR table.

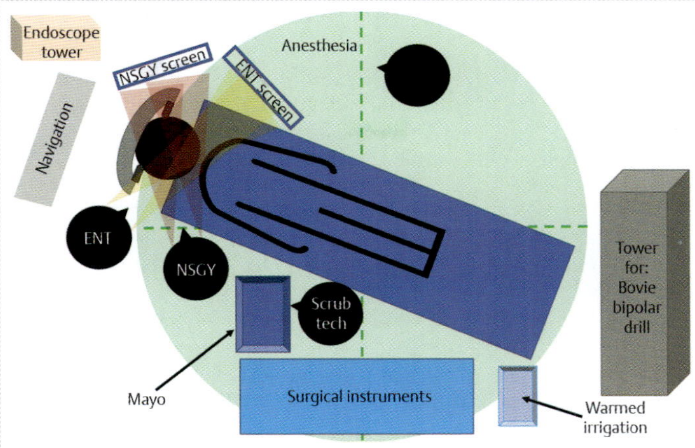

Fig. 15.1 Operating room setup for endoscopic endonasal surgery. The *green circle* and *green dashed lines* have been drawn to work as a reference for the degree of bed rotation. ENT, ear, nose, and throat; NSGY, neurosurgery.

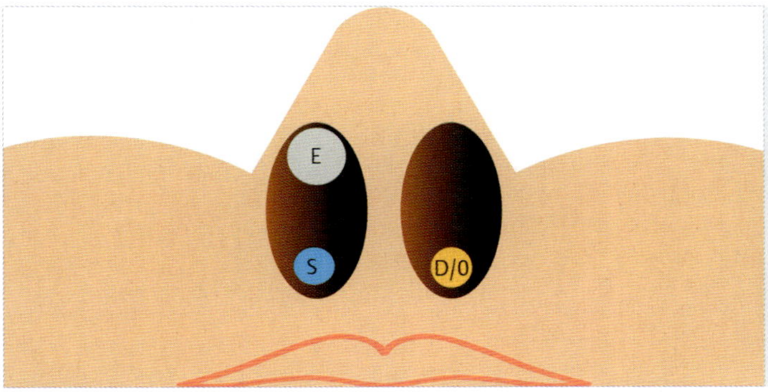

Fig. 15.2 Illustration of instrument positions in the nostrils as seen from below. This represents the most common setup used at our institution. The endoscope (E) is positioned at the 12 o'clock position in the right nostril. The left-hand suction (S) is located at the 6 o'clock position in the right nostril. The left nostril is mostly used for the drill or other instruments (D/O).

- The right arm is paddled and tackled against the trunk. A Mayfield clamp is applied, and the head is positioned by translating upward, gentle extension, rotating toward the right and left lateral flexion.
- The head of the table is elevated up to 15 degrees (more elevation might be needed intraoperatively to increase venous return and decrease bleeding in the surgical field).

15.9 Technique

- We prefer a binarial, two-surgeon, four-hand technique for optimal exposure, dynamic endoscopy, and proper microsurgical techniques (▶ Fig. 15.2).
- Once the nasal cavity exposure is completed by the ENT team, the neurosurgeon comes into the field and starts the drilling of the sphenoid rostrum. The sphenoid septations should be drilled down instead of fracturing them to avoid potential vascular injury to the internal carotid arteries (ICAs).[3,4]
- At this point, the surgeons must take their time to identify the anatomical landmarks available in the sphenoid sinus (see in the next section below). The anterior wall and the floor of the sella is drilled with a 4-mm diamond drill under constant irrigation by the ENT surgeon.
- The drilling for the sellar osteotomy involves making four osteotomies in a square shape, which will be peeled off the dura with the help of a no. 2 Kerrison rongeur or a Cottle nasal dissector. Special attention must be paid when drilling the middle clinoid since a caroticoclinoid ring might exist unilaterally in about 20% of cases and bilaterally in about 6%.[3] This could potentially cause a vascular injury to the ICA.

- Once the bony exposure has been completed and the dura of the sella is exposed, we proceed to open the dura with a retractable blade scalpel, making an inverted "V" incision.
- These initial cuts are extended with the help of a combination of feather blade and curved scissors to the left. It is of upmost importance to avoid dural opening above the middle clinoid to decrease incidental exposure of the suprasellar area that could lead to cerebrospinal fluid (CSF) leak.
- Any dural bleed can be easily controlled with bipolar cautery. After dural opening, the tumor is identified, and a combination of microsurgical technique and 2-Fukushima suctions technique is implemented for tumor resection.
- In cases of cavernous sinus invasion, the use of intraoperative stimulation with a Kartush or suction tip stimulator can be implemented to guide the localization of the oculomotor, trochlear, and abducens nerves when needed.
- After tumor resection has been completed, copious warm irrigation is used to achieve hemostasis. If no CSF leak was encountered, the reconstruction is usually made with a free mucosa flap from the middle turbinate or the nasal floor cavity.
- In cases of CSF leak, this could be also performed with the use of a nasoseptal flap (NSF). In some cases of functioning adenomas in which total resection is not feasible, a piece of fat can be placed as spacer in the sella to protect neural structures from future radiosurgery treatments.

15.10 Relevant Anatomy

- ▶ Fig. 15.3 summarizes the relevant anatomy for transsellar approaches. For more in-depth knowledge, please review the recommended literature.

15.11 Postoperative Care

- The patient should be extubated at the end of the case.
- The head of the bed is elevated above 30 degrees.
- Hormonal replacement is ordered if indicated.
- There should be strict intake and output recording to monitor for DI.
- Early mobilization out of the bed is advised.
- Avoid passage of nasal tubing.
- Counsel patients to avoid use of straws.

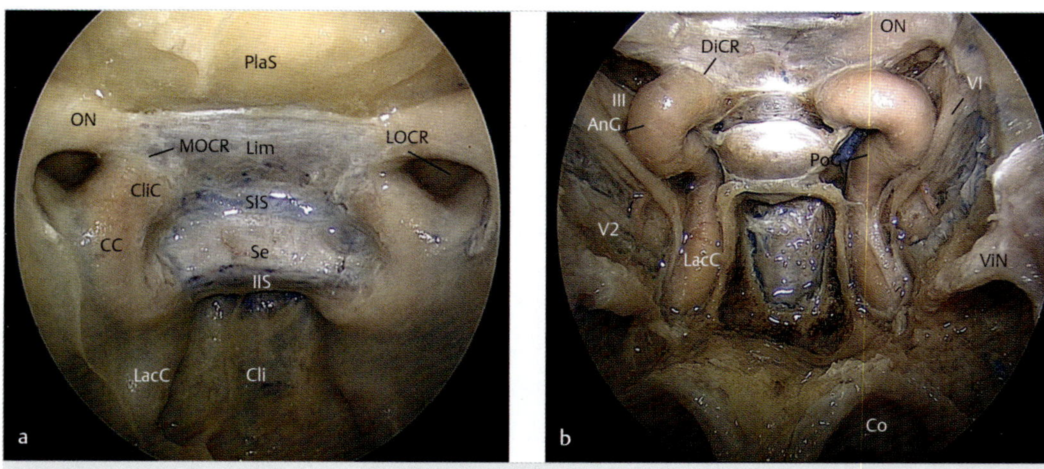

Fig. 15.3 Endoscopic view of **(a)** the sella and parasellar regions and **(b)** the cavernous sinus. AnG, anterior genu; CC, cavernous carotid; Cli, clivus; CliC, clinoidal carotid; DiCR, distal carotid ring; III, third cranial nerve; IIS, inferior intercavernous sinus; LacC, lacerum carotid; Lim, limbus; LOCR, lateral opticocarotid recess; MOCR, medial opticocarotid recess; ON, optic nerve; PlaS, planum sphenoidale; PoG, posterior genu; Se, sella; SIS, superior intercavernous sinus; V2, second trigeminal division; VI, sixth cranial nerve; ViN, vidian nerve. (Reproduced from Anterior cranial base. In: Hanna E, DeMonte F, eds. Comprehensive Management of Skull Base Tumors. 2nd Edition. New York: Thieme; 2021.)

- Sneezing with open mouth should be recommended.
- Avoid use of noninvasive positive pressure ventilation. Use nasal cannula oxygen in patients with obstructive sleep apnea.
- Postoperative pituitary labs can be tailored to individual cases.

15.12 Complications

15.12.1 Intraoperative

- Pin lacerations from inappropriate placement of the Mayfield head holder.
- DI (transient or permanent).
- Panhypopituitarism.
- Hemodynamic instability from inappropriate replacement of steroid in the cases with adrenal insufficiency.
- *Vascular injury:* ICA, intracranial ICA branches, cavernous sinus. Sphenopalatine artery injury on the ipsilateral side of the NSF (if needed).
- Stroke from excessive manipulation of atherosclerotic ICAs.
- *Nerve injury:* Optic nerve injury, optic chiasm injury, and vidian nerve injury. Cranial nerve injury in tumors invading the cavernous sinus.
- CSF leak.

15.12.2 Postoperative

- CSF leak, tension pneumocephalus, DI, hematoma, NSF necrosis or displacement, meningitis, visual loss, cranial nerve palsy, periorbital hematoma (from neurophysiology needles), and anosmia.

15.12.3 Special Risks

- Kissing carotids could cause a narrow corridor toward the sella and are at higher risk of injury.
- Sphenoid septation fracture could lead to ICA injury.
- Middle clinoid ring might limit the sellotomy and the removal of the bone from the cavernous sinus, which could cause ICA injury.
- Opening the dura above the line between both middle clinoids could lead to exposure of the suprasellar space and cause CSF leak.
- Resection of tumor invading the cavernous sinus could lead to cranial nerve injury as well as vascular injury of the ICA or its branches.

15.13 Management Pearls

15.13.1 Expert Pearls

- Make sure to review the preoperative CTH/CTA and look for kissing carotids, caroticoclinoid ring, and sphenoid septations. If the patient is placed in a pin holder, pay extra attention for evidence of prior craniotomies or shunt catheters before pinning.
- Review the dedicated pituitary MRI for adenoma laterality (if any) and cavernous sinus invasion and to identify the normal pituitary gland location.
- If compression of the optic apparatus is present, consider placing a preinduction arterial line and maintain mean arterial pressure elevated above 80 mm Hg.
- Review the pituitary labs and use stress dose steroids if appropriate.
- Review visual fields if available.
- Discuss with your ENT colleague the reconstruction options beforehand.
- Always prep the abdomen for possible abdominal fat harvesting; you never know when you will need it.

References

[1] Sella turcica: an overview | ScienceDirect Topics. Accessed January 2, 2025 at: https://www.sciencedirect.com/topics/neuroscience/sella-turcica

[2] Shah P, Thornton I, Turrin D, Kopitnik NL, Hipskind JE. Informed Consent. Treasure Island, FL: StatPearls Publishing; 2024

[3] Dziedzic T, Koczyk K, Gotlib T, Kunert P, Maj E, Marchel A. Sphenoid sinus septations and their interconnections with parasphenoidal internal carotid artery protuberance: radioanatomical study with literature review. Wideochir Inne Tech Malo Inwazyjne. 2020; 15(1):227–233

[4] Vaz-Guimaraes F, Su SY, Fernandez-Miranda JC, Wang EW, Snyderman CH, Gardner PA. Hemostasis in endoscopic endonasal skull base surgery. J Neurol Surg B Skull Base. 2015; 76(4):296–302

16 Transpterygoid

Hanna N. Algattas and Paul A. Gardner

16.1 Background

- The transpterygoid approach is the transnasal module allowing extension into the coronal (paramedian) plane for pathologies of the central and lateral skull base, nasopharynx, and infratemporal fossa (ITF).
- This allows improved management of multiple midline neoplasms, encephaloceles, cholesterol granulomas, and cerebrospinal fluid (CSF) leaks, which start or extend beyond standard midline (sagittal plane) endonasal corridors.
- Extending from the sphenoid sinus into the maxillary sinus provides access to the pterygopalatine fossa (PPF) and pterygoid bone, which creates the corridor of access to the paramedian skull base.
- Understanding the articulation between the sphenoid and paired palatine bones is the central concept that allows exposure of the pterygoid wedge.
- The sphenoid bone contains two inferiorly projecting pterygoid processes (or plates), medially and laterally, attached to the pterygoid base (▶ Fig. 16.1a). The palatine bones are paired structures made of a perpendicular and horizontal plate. From the former are two processes, the sphenoidal and orbital, which contribute to the sphenopalatine foramen and are situated anterior to the pterygoid base and PPF contents (▶ Fig. 16.1b).
- By meticulously working from medial to lateral, one can systematically disarticulate the bony processes and sacrifice the necessary soft tissue structures to expose the pterygoid "wedge" and eventually the pterygoid base.

16.2 Indications and Contraindications

- The transpterygoid approach is recommended for those lesions approached endonasally with extension within the coronal plane of the skull base and toward the lateral recess of the sphenoid sinus. This includes access to the PPF, Meckel's cave, petrous apex, lateral cavernous sinus, ITF, and more. The approach is also a particularly useful module within the contralateral transmaxillary (CTM) approach.
- Pathologies include, but are not limited to, chordomas, schwannoma, encephaloceles of the lateral recess, meningioma, nasopharyngeal malignancies, and more. Relative contraindications may include intradural pathologies where no viable nasoseptal flap is present on the contralateral side.

16.3 Informed Consent

- For this approach, patients are specifically counseled on risks of vidian nerve injury which can reduce lacrimation and cause nasal dryness.

16.4 Instruments

- Standard endonasal instruments are necessary for the transpterygoid approach, in addition to angled endoscopes if desired.
- Bipolar cautery to manage bleeding and ligation of the sphenopalatine artery (SPA) is essential.
- Coarse, round diamond burrs are preferred for their combined hemostatic effect and careful reduction of bone.

16.5 Patient Preparation

- Patients obtain the necessary preoperative imaging including fine-cut computed tomography (CT) imaging as well as contrasted magnetic resonance imaging (MRI). They are induced and intubated by the anesthesia team in the typical fashion.
- For pathologies that are extensive and require complex reconstructions, patients are briefed on the possibility of fascia lata or fat harvest in addition to lumbar drain placement.

16.6 Patient Positioning

- The patient is positioned in the standard fashion for endoscopic endonasal surgery. The patient is positioned in the three-point Mayfield fixation with slight extension, ipsilateral rotation, and contralateral lateral flexion as previously

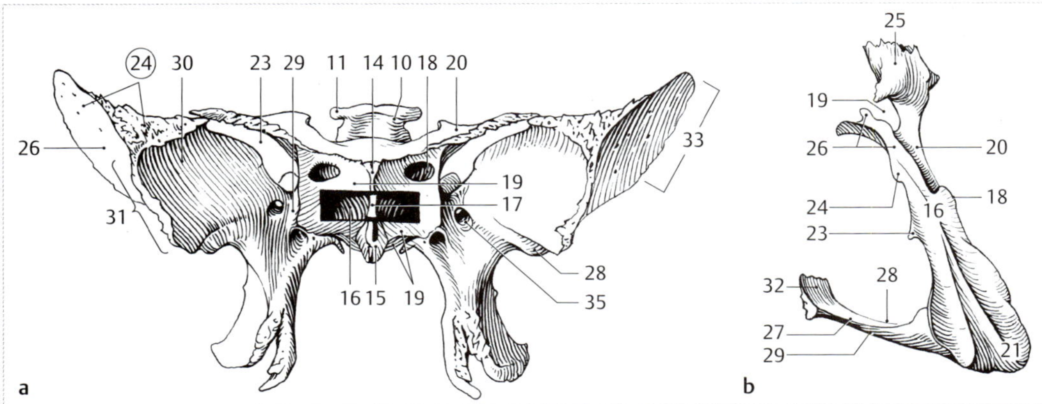

Fig. 16.1 **(a)** Anterior fenestrated view of the sphenoid bone: 10. Dorsum sellae—posterior wall of the sella turcica. 11. Posterior clinoid process—protuberance on both sides of the dorsum sellae. 14. Sphenoidal crest—median bony ridge on the anterior surface of the body of the sphenoid that articulates with the perpendicular plate of the ethmoid. 15. Sphenoidal rostrum—prolongation of the sphenoidal crest inferiorly that articulates with the vomer. 16. Sphenoidal sinus—paired sphenoidal sinuses. 17. Septum of the sphenoidal sinuses—septum that divides the right and left sphenoidal sinuses. 18. Opening of the sphenoidal sinus—anterior opening of the sphenoidal sinus into the sphenoethmoidal recess. 19. Sphenoidal concha—originally a pair of separate, hollow bones, it is united with the body of the sphenoid to form part of the anterior and inferior wall of the sphenoidal sinus. 20. Lesser wing of the sphenoid. 23. Superior orbital fissure—cleft between the greater and lesser wings of the sphenoid for the passage of nerves and the superior ophthalmic vein. 24. Greater wing of the sphenoid. 26. Temporal surface—lateral facing surface of the greater wing of the sphenoid. 28. Infratemporal crest—bony ridge between the (vertical) temporal surface and the (horizontal) infratemporal surface of the greater wing of the sphenoid. 29. Maxillary surface—surface of the greater wing of the sphenoid facing the maxilla. The foramen rotundum opens here. 30. Orbital surface—surface of the greater wing of the sphenoid facing the orbit. 31. Zygomatic margin—border of the greater wing of the sphenoid for articulation with the zygomatic bone. 33. Parietal margin—border of the greater wing of the sphenoid that is united with the parietal bone. 35. Foramen rotundum—foramen that opens anteriorly into the pterygopalatine fossa. It transmits the maxillary nerve. **(b)** Palatine bone: 16. Perpendicular plate of palatine bone—vertical bony plate contributing to the walls of the nasal and maxillary sinuses. 18. Maxillary surface—external surface of the perpendicular plate of the palatine bone. Its posterior part borders with the pterygopalatine fossa from medial, and its anterior part with the maxillary sinus from posterior. 19. Sphenopalatine notch—semi-oval notch between the orbital process and the sphenoidal process of the perpendicular plate of the palatine bone. 20. Greater palatine groove—channel that unites with the greater palatine groove of the maxilla to form the greater palatine canal, which lodges the greater palatine nerve and the descending palatine artery. 21. Pyramidal process—inferoposterior end of the perpendicular plate of the palatine bone, which is inserted in the pterygoid notch. 23. Conchal crest—ridge providing attachment for the posterior end of the inferior nasal concha. 24. Ethmoidal crest—ridge providing attachment for the posterior end of the middle nasal concha. 26. Sphenoidal process—process behind the sphenopalatine notch that borders with the body and the vaginal process of the sphenoid. 27. Horizontal plate of the palatine bone. It forms the posterior third of the hard palate and thus the floor of the nasal cavity. 29. Palatine surface—surface of the horizontal plate that faces the oral cavity. 32. Nasal crest—median bony ridge along the union with the opposing palatine bone. (Reproduced from Dauber W. Pocket Atlas of Human Anatomy. 5th Edition. © 2006 Thieme Publishers, Stuttgart. Illustration created by Professor Gerhard Spitzer.)

described.[1,2] If the fascia lata is planned for harvest, the leg is flexed, padded, and internally rotated with a linear incision planned medial to the iliotibial band.

16.7 Technique

- A nasoseptal flap is elevated on the contralateral side of the intended transpterygoid approach (the posterior nasal and sphenopalatine arteries that supply the flap are typically sacrificed for a transpterygoid approach) and an ipsilateral reverse flap is elevated to protect the exposed septum.[3]
- After sphenoidotomy is complete, an ipsilateral maxillary antrostomy is performed. Only the necessary mucosa is stripped from the posterior wall of the maxillary sinus, anterior to the PPF (▶ Fig. 16.2).

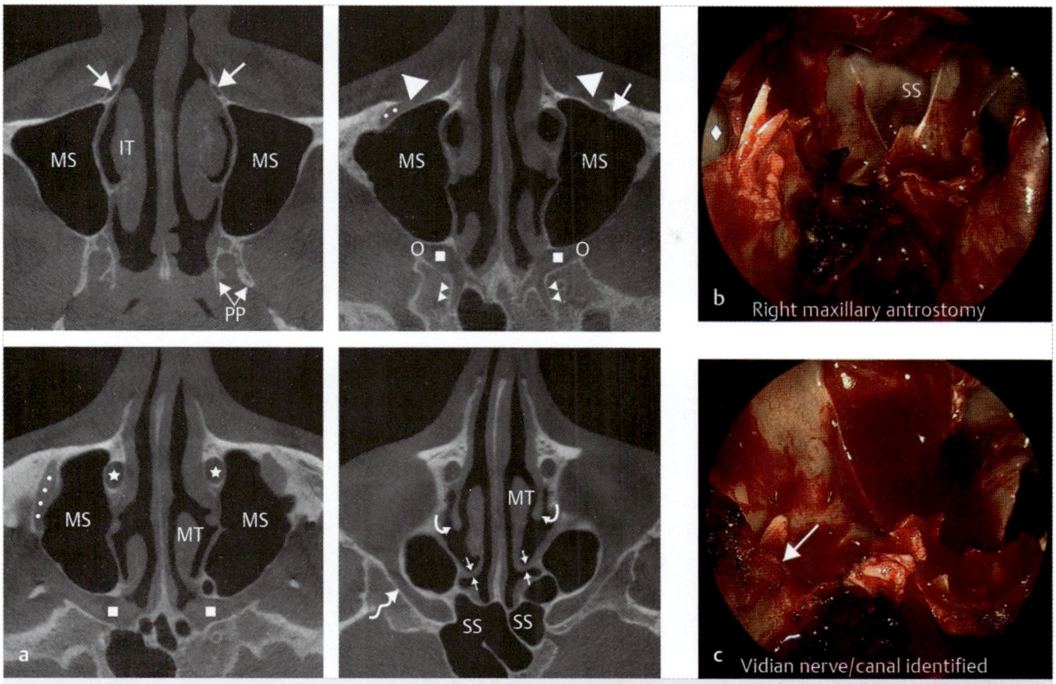

Fig. 16.2 (a) Axial cone beam computed tomography (CBCT) images at the level of the maxillary sinuses. The anterosuperior alveolar canal (*arrow*), infraorbital canal (*dotted line*), infraorbital foramen (*large arrowheads*), pterygopalatine fossa (*square*), pterygomaxillary fissure (*open circle*), vidian canal (*small arrowheads*), nasolacrimal duct (*star*), uncinate process (*small curved arrow*), basal lamella of the middle turbinate (*small opposing arrows*), and inferior orbital fissure (*wavy arrow*) are visible. IT, inferior turbinate; MS, maxillary sinus; MT, middle turbinate; PP, pterygoid plates; SS, sphenoid sinus. (Reproduced from Maroldi R, Borghesi A. Imaging of the maxilla and paranasal sinuses. In: Felisati G, Chiapasco M, eds. Sinonasal Complications of Dental Disease and Treatment: Prevention–Diagnosis–Management. 1st Ed. © 2015 Thieme Publishers, Stuttgart.) **(b)** Intraoperative view after right maxillary antrostomy. *White diamond* = maxillary sinus. The mucosa remains intact anterior to the posterior wall of the maxillary sinus and pterygopalatine fossa. SS, sphenoid sinus. **(c)** Identification of the vidian nerve/canal within the pterygoid wedge.

- Attention is turned medially toward the sphenoid rostrum and sphenoid sinus floor. Moving laterally along the rostrum will first expose the palatovaginal (also known as palatosphenoidal) artery, which is widely coagulated, then ligated.
- Next, the articulation with the sphenoidal process of the palatine bone is seen. Removal of the sphenoidal, and subsequent orbital, process of the palatine bone with either a Kerrison rongeur or high-speed drill will next identify the SPA, which is coagulated widely and cut. After successful ligation, the medial-most contents of the PPF will be exposed and partially released.
- The crista ethmoidalis is identified and the posterior aspect of the maxillary sinus, which is the bone covering the anterior face of the PPF is removed using Kerrison rongeurs, exposing laterally into the maxillary sinus.
- If continued laterally, this exposes the ITF and the internal maxillary (IMAX) artery. If further lateral access is required, the transpterygoid module can be coupled with an anterior transmaxillary, transalisphenoid approach.
- After adequate bone is removed, the PPF can be cautiously bipolar coagulated to retract tissue, facilitate lateralization, and visualize critical landmarks.
- The pterygoid wedge is the bone where the medial pterygoid plate meets the floor of the sphenoid sinus and is the V-shaped medial extension of the base of the pterygoid bone.

Gently mobilizing the PPF further laterally will expose the vidian canal (VC) at the base of the pterygoid wedge "V."
- Depending on the pathology and extent of the transpterygoid approach necessary, the vidian nerve and artery traveling within the canal can be sacrificed, preserving a stump of the nerve as a landmark.
- Of note, sacrificing the nerve in patients with preexisting neuropathy of the ophthalmic division of the trigeminal nerve may increase the risk of postoperative corneal keratopathy and should be avoided in this specific situation when possible.[4]
- The vidian nerve serves as an endonasal landmark approximating the level of the middle fossa floor,[5] but more importantly as a guide to the internal carotid artery (ICA).
- When followed posteriorly, it crosses over the petrous portion of the ICA as well as tracking lateral to the lateral border of the paraclival ICA at the foramen lacerum.[6]
- The sphenoid lingula is the bony process lateral to the lacerum ICA and can be removed to provide additional access and facilitate lateralization of the paraclival ICA, if necessary.
- After sacrifice of the vidian nerve, the next anatomical structures that limit PPF mobilization are the descending greater and lesser palatine nerves.[7]
- Sacrifice of the vidian nerve alone (combined with opening of the bone inferior orbital fissure) suffices to visualize the foramen rotundum (FR) superolateral to the VC.[8]
- The infraorbital nerve, from the maxillary division of the trigeminal nerve, exits the FR and travels from medial to lateral in the roof of the maxillary sinus.
- The maxillary nerve can be divided into three segments, an interdural segment (gasserian ganglion to the proximal maxillary strut), an intracanalicular segment, and a pterygopalatine segment (distal to the maxillary strut).[9]
- The FR can be skeletonized, at the intracanalicular segment of the nerve, by reducing the bone medial to it as well as the maxillary strut between the FR and VC, to expose the nerve. If followed posteriorly, this leads to the middle fossa floor and Meckel's cave. This exposure is much simpler in patients with a highly pneumatized lateral recess as the V2 prominence is often readily evident.
- After exposure is complete, the pterygoid wedge can then be reduced using a high-speed drill with care taken to skeletonize and preserve the stump of the vidian nerve, which serves as the essential landmark to the transition between the petrous and paraclival ICA.
- After identification of the paraclival ICA and foramen lacerum, the ensuant surgical steps are dependent on the pathology.
- For lateral recess CSF leaks, the dural defect is identified for repair.
- For schwannomas of the middle fossa and cranial nerve V (CN V), Meckel's cave is exposed prior to resection.
- For chordoma, chondrosarcoma, and sinonasal adenocarcinomas, additional modules may be required for adequate exposure, including extension into the petrous apex, which can be facilitated by the addition of the CTM approach.[10]

16.8 Case Example

- A 12-year-old girl presented for definitive removal of an extensive craniocervical junction and lower clival chordoma. This was first identified 4 years prior when she complained of occipital and neck pain. Given her young age, the tumor was biopsied, which revealed a poorly differentiated chordoma.
- She first underwent serial chemotherapy with multiple agents; the initial response was promising, but eventually, the tumor began to progress. She continued to have neck pain but no focal neurological deficits or cranial neuropathies.
- Imaging demonstrated an extensive chordoma with significant involvement of the craniocervical junction with extension into the right occipital condyle, abutting the right vertebral artery, as well as anterolateral displacement of the right petrous carotid artery (▶ Fig. 16.3a–d).
- A staged procedure was planned for complete resection given the demonstrated survival benefit of gross total resection (GTR). Given significant involvement of the right lateral mass and the right vertebral artery, a three-staged approach was taken.
- First, an endonasal resection performed for removal of the majority of the tumor and then

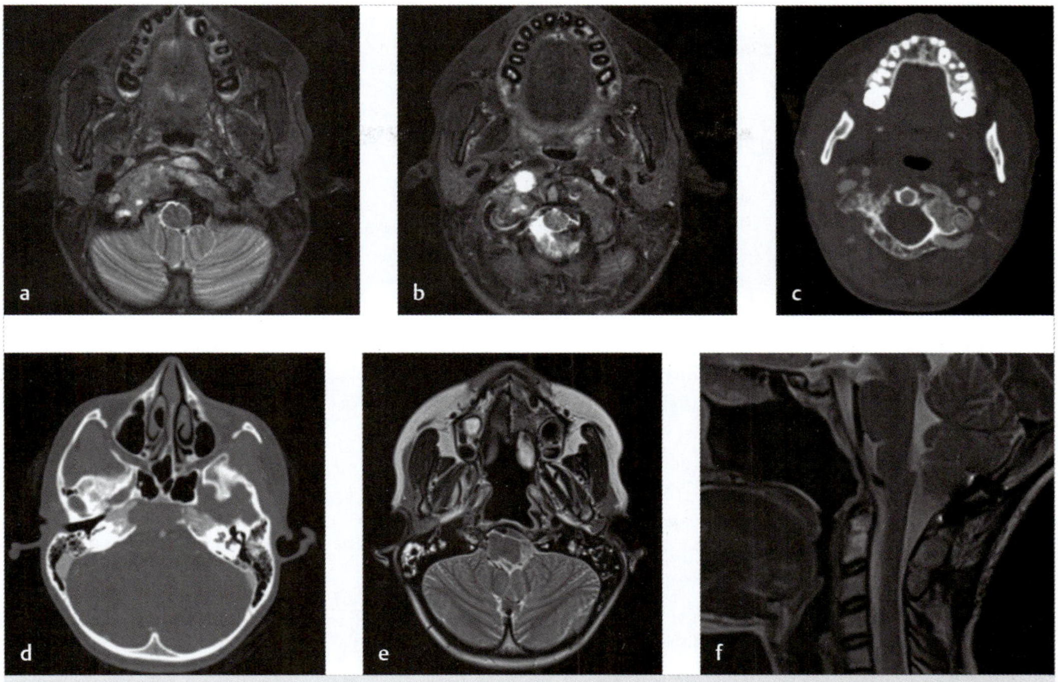

Fig. 16.3 **(a)** Axial T2-weighted MRI demonstrating a hyperintense lesion centered around the craniocervical junction but eccentric with involvement of jugular tubercle. **(b)** Axial T2-weighted MRI again showing a hyperintense lesion with involvement of the right occipital condyle. Flow void showing the V3 segment of the vertebral artery is noted with tumor abutting the vessel. **(c)** Axial CT imaging with arterial contrast noting bony erosion of the right lateral mass of C1 with hypodense changes along the right C1 anterior and posterior arches concerning for tumor involvement. **(d)** Axial CT imaging with arterial contrast noting involvement of the lower and middle segments of the clivus with anterolateral displacement of the petrous carotid artery on the right. **(e)** Axial T2 postoperative MRI with no concern for residual tumor. **(f)** Sagittal T2 postoperative MRI with no concern for residual tumor.

an extreme far lateral approach with mobilization of the vertebral artery was utilized for resection of the remaining lateral tumor.
- After resection, a third stage with occipitocervical fixation was done given the instability at the craniocervical junction after the extensive resection.
- The endonasal resection required extensive exposure; however, most essential was a right transpterygoid approach, which allowed access to the right petrous apex and the jugular tubercle as well as gaining control of the right petrous and paraclival carotid artery (**Video 16.1**).
- Postoperatively the patient did well without added neurological deficits or morbidity. She underwent all three stages of surgery and was discharged on postoperative day 11.

16.9 Postoperative Care

- Patients may be managed in the intensive care unit if procedures are more extensive, but it is not a necessity. Lumbar drainage may be used for lateral recess encephaloceles or CSF leak repairs. Patients are mobilized early to prevent venous thromboembolism.

16.10 Complications

- Special complications more unique to the transpterygoid approach include those from manipulation of the contents of the PPF.
- These include palatal numbness, maxillary numbness or pain (related to injury to the maxillary division of the trigeminal nerve), lack

of emotional tearing (in the case of vidian nerve sacrifice related to the approach), and of course CSF leak.

16.11 Management Pearls

- The endonasal transpterygoid approach is a useful module that unlocks the endonasal coronal plane via the maxillary sinus and creates an extended nasal working corridor for management of several pathologies.
- Increased lateral access beyond the standard midline transnasal corridor is provided with serial sacrifice of the SPA and vidian nerve, if necessary.
- Midline or paramedian tumors, which extend into the lateral cavernous sinus, petrous apex, petroclival junction, Meckel's cave, or middle fossa, can all be accessed by using this approach.
- If needed, the transpterygoid approach can be coupled with a CTM approach for deep-seated lesions of the petrous apex, jugular tubercle, and ITF.

References

[1] Algattas HN, Wang EW, Zenonos GA, Snyderman CH, Gardner PA. Endoscopic endonasal surgery for anterior cranial fossa meningiomas. J Neurosurg Sci. 2021; 65(2):118–132

[2] Algattas H, Setty P, Goldschmidt E, et al. Endoscopic endonasal approach for craniopharyngiomas with intraventricular extension: case series, long-term outcomes, and review. World Neurosurg. 2020; 144:e447–e459

[3] Caicedo-Granados E, Carrau R, Snyderman CH, et al. Reverse rotation flap for reconstruction of donor site after vascular pedicled nasoseptal flap in skull base surgery. Laryngoscope. 2010; 120(8):1550–1552

[4] Lin PY, Cheng CY, Wu CC, et al. Bilateral neurotrophic keratopathy complicating vidian neurectomy. Am J Ophthalmol. 2001; 132(1):106–108

[5] Prevedello DM, Pinheiro-Neto CD, Fernandez-Miranda JC, et al. Vidian nerve transposition for endoscopic endonasal middle fossa approaches. Neurosurgery. 2010; 67(2) Suppl Operative:478–484

[6] Wang WH, Lieber S, Mathias RN, et al. The foramen lacerum: surgical anatomy and relevance for endoscopic endonasal approaches. J Neurosurg. 2018; 131(5):1571–1582

[7] Geltzeiler M, Turner M, Rimmer R, et al. Endoscopic nasopharyngectomy combined with a nerve-sparing transpterygoid approach. Laryngoscope. 2020; 130(10): 2343–2348

[8] Karkas A, Zimmer LA, Theodosopoulos PV, Keller JT, Prades JM. Endonasal endoscopic approach to the pterygopalatine and infratemporal fossae. Eur Ann Otorhinolaryngol Head Neck Dis. 2021; 138(5):391–395

[9] Abhinav K, Panczykowski D, Wang WH, et al. Endoscopic endonasal interdural middle fossa approach to the maxillary nerve: anatomic considerations and surgical relevance. Oper Neurosurg (Hagerstown). 2017; 13(4):522–528

[10] Snyderman CH, Gardner PA, Wang EW, Fernandez-Miranda JC, Valappil B. Experience with the endoscopic contralateral transmaxillary approach to the petroclival skull base. Laryngoscope. 2021; 131(2):294–298

17 Transcribriform

Ayesha Akbar Waheed and David T. Fernandes Cabral

17.1 Background

- The transcribriform approach is a surgical technique used to access the anterior cranial fossa and olfactory groove region. This minimally invasive transnasal route is predominantly employed for managing lesions such as esthesioneuroblastomas and olfactory groove meningiomas. By avoiding open craniofacial approaches, this technique significantly reduces morbidity associated with frontal lobe retraction while ensuring direct access to the target site. In the case of olfactory groove meningiomas, it provides early access to the ethmoidal arteries that provide blood supply to the tumor.[1,2,3] Refer to ▶ Fig. 17.1 to see the exact location of the transcribriform approach relative to other endonasal approaches.
- The transcribriform approach is indicated for various pathological conditions involving the anterior skull base and cribriform plate.[4] These include benign and malignant pathologies as well as structural defects.
  - **Esthesioneuroblastomas:** Malignant tumors of the olfactory neuroepithelium.
  - **Sinonasal carcinomas:** Locally aggressive epithelial tumors invading the cribriform plate.
  - **Meningiomas:** Slow-growing benign tumors of the anterior skull base.
  - **Cerebrospinal fluid (CSF) leaks:** Resulting from trauma, prior surgery, or spontaneous etiologies.
  - **Inflammatory and infectious conditions:** Cases refractory to medical management, such as fungal sinusitis.

17.1.1 Preparatory Diagnostics

- A comprehensive set of preoperative diagnostics is employed to evaluate the extent and classification of disease, assess patient and anatomical feasibility of a case, and prepare for case-based potential complications.[5,6]
- **History and physical examination:** Physicians and specialists must pay special attention to this

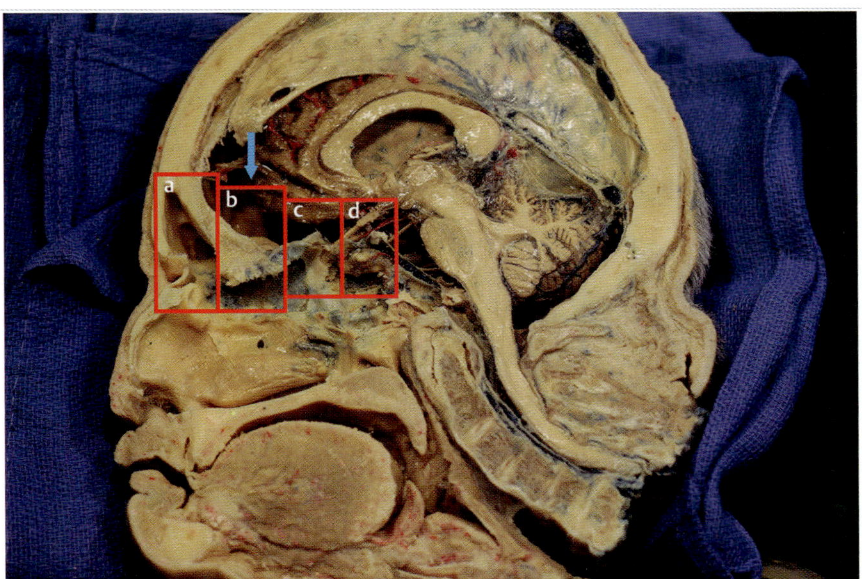

Fig. 17.1 Illustration of the skull base in sagittal view, divided into different areas of the endoscopic approach. **(a)** Transfrontal; **(b)** transcribriform (*blue arrow*); **(c)** transplanal and transtuberculum; **(d)** transellar.

aspect as it determines the feasibility of this approach and allows better-directed care from the initial stages. Focus on symptoms like nasal obstruction, changes in personality, headaches, anosmia, or recurrent CSF rhinorrhea. Assess overall health and surgical candidacy.

- **Imaging studies**[1,2,7]:
  - **High-resolution computed tomography (CT) scan**:
    - It is used to visualize bony anatomy, check for skull base defects and tumor calcification, and evaluate the integrity of the cribriform plate.
  - **MRI with and without contrast with skull base protocol:** The imaging modality offers superior soft tissue resolution and can be used to delineate tumor boundaries, evaluate vascular involvement, and detect potential perineural or intracranial spread.
  - **CT angiography:**
    - It helps identify vascular encasement/displacement. It is beneficial for cases where there are larger tumors or many complex anatomical variations.
- **Nasal endoscopy:** This examination, performed by the ear, nose, and throat (ENT) physician, allows for direct visualization of the lesion (if intranasal), nasal septum, and turbinates. It can be used to assess mucosal involvement by lesion and planning surgical approaches.
- **Functional tests:**
  - **Olfactory testing:** Evaluate preexisting smell function to counsel on postoperative anosmia risks.
  - **Neuropsychological testing:** Useful for comprehensive evaluation of frontal lobe dysfunction in those patients with significant mass effect/edema in the frontal lobes.
- **Laboratory workup**:
  - **Coagulation profile**:
    - Need to check for a bleeding disorder to prepare for surgical risk/rule in candidacy for surgery.
  - **CSF leak studies:** Beta-2 transferrin testing confirms CSF presence in nasal discharge.
- **Multidisciplinary evaluation**[8,9]: Neurosurgery, otolaryngology, ophthalmology, and radiology will join forces to ensure that all stages of patient care (preoperative, surgical planning, procedure, postoperative care, and follow-up) are optimal.
- At our institution, any patient undergoing scheduled skull base surgery is evaluated by the center for preoperative medicine, where a thorough evaluation is performed to minimize complication risks. Additional testing is tailored on an as-needed basis.

17.2 Indications and Contraindications

17.2.1 Indications

- Tumors involving the anterior skull base (specifically the cribriform plate), such as esthesioneuroblastomas, sinonasal carcinomas, or meningiomas.[4]
- CSF leaks localized to the cribriform plate.
- Skull base defects due to trauma or previous surgery.[1] Fractures of the anterior skull base may require surgical correction to repair dural tears, restore structure, and prevent CSF leaks.
- Inflammatory or infectious conditions refractory to medical treatment such as fungal sinusitis that may necessitate surgical debridement and reconstruction.

17.2.2 Contraindications

- Extensive vascular involvement or encasement of major vessels such as the anterior cerebral vasculature.
- Significant medical comorbidities precluding general anesthesia.
- Inadequate endoscopic visualization or expertise.

Note: Most contraindications are relative and must be evaluated on a case-by-case basis, along with the expertise of the operating team available.

17.3 Informed Consent

Informed consent should address the following:

- Purpose of the surgery and expected outcomes.
- Risks including CSF leaks, anosmia, intracranial infections, and hemorrhage.
- Possibility of neurological deficits, stroke, or vision loss.
- Recovery expectations and the potential need for further interventions.

17.4 Instruments

- High-definition endoscope (0-, 30-, 45-, and 70-degree scopes).
- Image guidance system.
- Drills with endonasal attachment.
- Standard paranasal sinus endoscopic tray.
- Ultrasonic aspirator; consider using a more aggressive tip in highly calcified tumors.
- Long suctions (Frazier for drilling and Fukushima for tumor resection and microsurgical technique).
- Microdebrider.
- Needle tip Bovie.
- Endonasal bipolar cautery (Storz, Endopen).
- Skull base repair materials: autologous tissue grafts (e.g., fascia lata) and synthetic materials (e.g., DuraMatrix).
- Hemostatic agents.

17.5 Patient Preparation

- **Patient counseling:** Explain the possibility of postoperative anosmia, temporary nasal congestion, CSF leak, need for lumbar drain in the postoperative period, and the need for follow-up care. Ensure patients understand the recovery timeline and restrictions.
- **Anesthesia preparation:**
  - Patients undergo general anesthesia with oral endotracheal intubation. The tube is taped toward the left side of the patient as the surgical team stands to the patient's right side.
  - Patients at risk of adrenal insufficiency, particularly those with chronic steroid use or hypothalamic–pituitary involvement, receive stress dose corticosteroids (e.g., hydrocortisone) to prevent perioperative adrenal crisis.
  - In case of neuromonitoring (cranial nerve/brainstem), short-acting muscle relaxants are used during induction to allow for neuromuscular recovery to conduct intraoperative monitoring. Anesthetic agents are carefully selected to ensure they do not interfere with neuromonitoring signals (e.g., total intravenous anesthesia with propofol and remifentanil).
  - Emergency drugs, such as vasopressors and anticonvulsants, should be readily available to address potential complications like sudden hypotension, seizure activity, or significant blood loss.
  - Ensure a backup plan for airway management in case of difficulty during extubation, especially in prolonged cases where airway swelling might occur.
- **Foley catheter placement and monitoring:** A Foley catheter is essential for accurate monitoring of fluid intake and output.
- **Blood loss communication and coagulation management:** Maintaining clear communication regarding estimated blood loss is crucial, especially as some tumors can result in significant hemorrhage and potentially lead to disseminated intravascular coagulation (DIC). In such cases, immediate action is required. If concerns arise from the surgical or anesthesia team, a coagulation panel should be ordered without delay, and any abnormal results must be promptly addressed and corrected.
- **Equipment preparation:** Verify the availability of all necessary instruments, including navigation systems and surgical trays, to avoid intraoperative delays.[3,8,9]
- **Infection control:** Address existing sinonasal infections with culture-directed antibiotics and ensure resolution before surgery.[7]

Note: In these cases, the abdomen and thigh are prepped in case a fat graft and/or fascia lata is needed for reconstruction.

17.6 Patient Positioning

- Upon arrival to the operating room, the patient must be safely transferred onto the operating table. Thereafter, general anesthesia is administered.
- After anesthesia has had its desired effect, the patient starts off in a supine position and the head of the bed is elevated by 15 to 20 degrees[1,2] by utilizing the back-up function in the operating table.
- Elevation allows venous draining and reduces intraoperative bleeding. The patient's head just needs to be secured using a Mayfield head holder.[10] The head is gently placed on extension to facilitate access to the anterior part of the skull base.
- The head is also gently rotated toward the right side (operator side) with small lateral flexion to

the left. All these moves facilitate the surgeons' more natural and comfortable access to the instruments through the nostrils.
- **Image guidance:** Co-registration is done with anatomical landmarks; surface refinement might be needed to increase accuracy.[3] Reassess the positioning for comfort, stability, and access to the nasal cavity and anterior skull base after sterilization and draping.

17.7 Technique

- The nasal cavity is prepared by inserting nasal pledges soaked in a vasoconstrictive agent (e.g., oxymetazoline or epinephrine).[1] Wait for 5 to 10 minutes before moving forward to allow the vasoconstrictor to take effect.
- We then prep the nose, nostrils, and the upper lip with ophthalmic Betadine (diluted Betadine). We also prep and drape the periumbilical area and the thigh.
- ENT will perform tailored ethmoidectomy, ranging up to full anterior and posterior ethmoidectomies to clear ethmoid air cells and provide access to the skull base. This approach will likely require a Draf III procedure (► Fig. 17.2), especially if the tumor extends to the frontal sinus' posterior table.
- Reconstruction techniques should be planned prior to surgery as pointed out by Gardner and Snyderman.[11] For instance, a nasal septal flap might not be ideal in some scenarios owing to tumor involvement. Autografts/allografts are possible options to augment the primary flap to achieve complete coverage. An extracranial pericranial flap is an option if other choices are unfeasible.
- The skull base is identified by removing the bony partitions of the ethmoids with precaution. If a sphenoidotomy is required, access the sphenoid sinus by removing its anterior wall. This step can be used to look for posterior extension of a lesion into the planum sphenoidale.
- Identification, dissection, and ligation of the posterior and anterior ethmoidal arteries are performed. Avoid ligating these arteries near the periorbital to avoid retraction and potential orbital hematoma.
- Exposure of the cribriform plate is done by utilizing blunt dissection tools to elevate the mucosa covering it. It is important to preserve as much of the mucosa as possible to later reconstruct the skull base. The neurosurgeon will use a high-speed diamond burr and drill through the thin bone of the cribriform plate while taking special care to preserve neurovascular structures. A stepwise approach involved:
  - After coagulating and ligating the ethmoidal arteries, anterior osteotomies must be made right behind the posterior wall of the frontal sinus, with extension to the crista galli, allowing for separation of anterior cranial plates from the dura. The planum sphenoidale and tuberculum sella can be removed separately.
  - Lateral extension of bone removal can be conducted to the midorbit if the lamina papyracea has been removed, allowing for visualization of all dura that may be involved in the lesion.
  - Coagulate the dura and tumor (if indicated) to achieve hemostasis prior to exposure and tumor devascularization.
  - Dissect and remove the crista galli in the end, usually after dissecting the dura.
- The dura mater must be exposed carefully avoiding unnecessary tears and perforations. Make the dural incision and expose the tumor—if that is the indication of the surgery. The approach of dura exposure is dependent on the type of tumor and its exact location. Tumor debulking and resecting is performed using microsurgical instruments under direct endoscopic visualization.
- Ensure clear margins are obtained while simultaneously avoiding critical structures such as the optic nerves or frontal lobes. Examine the surgical margins of the dura using histology to confirm complete resection.
- After this is achieved, it is time to begin reconstruction of the skull base to help prevent CSF leaks and any other defects that can arise from improper reconstruction.
- At our institution, for cases with intradural extension, we usually start with an inlay layer of a collagen matrix graft such as DuraMatrix. Ensure the patient's head is extended adequately to allow gravity to hold each layer in its place. This is followed by an onlay layer of the fascia lata, followed by the vascularized nasoseptal flap. This is reinforced in the edges with small pieces of Surgicel.

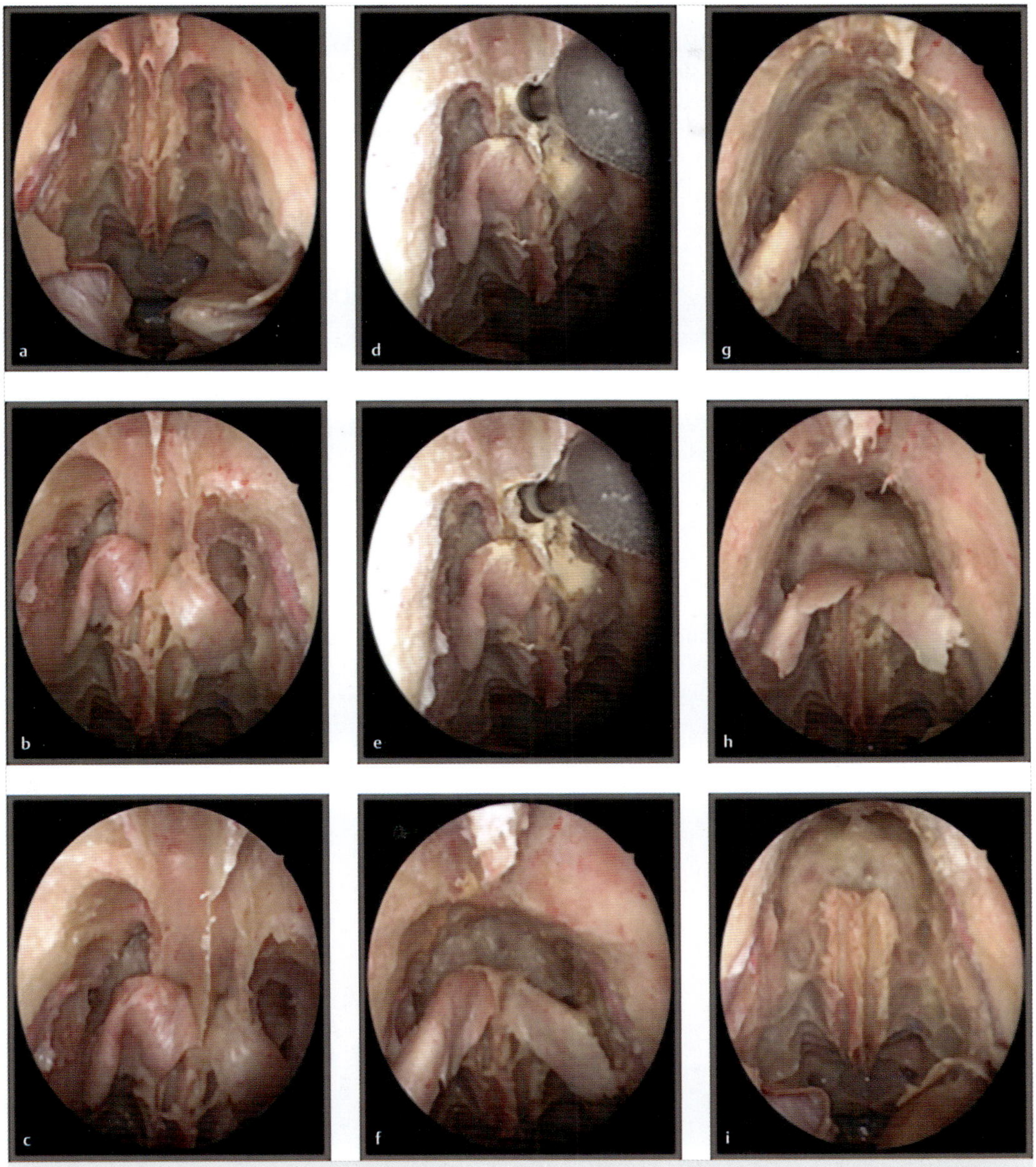

Fig. 17.2 Endoscopic view of a Draf III as a step for a transcribriform approach. **(a)** View of the cribriform plate and frontal recess. **(b)** Bilateral identification of the first olfactory fiber. **(c)** View after partial drilling of the frontal sinus floor. **(d)** Drilling of the bony junction between the two frontal sinuses. **(e)** Visualization of the left frontal sinus. **(f)** View after communicating both frontal sinuses. **(g)** Further drilling of the anterior table of the frontal sinus. **(h, i)** Final aspect after a complete drill out of the frontal sinuses. (Reproduced from Dassi CS, Demarco FR, Mangussi-Gomes J, et al. The frontal sinus and frontal recess: anatomical, radiological and surgical concepts. Int Arch Otorhinolaryngol 2020;24(3): e364–e375.)

- The bulk of the flap is also covered with small cut pieces of Gelfoam followed by Merocel packing. It is important that the flap is in contact with the lateral nasal wall or sinus to prevent contraction from occurring. Bleeding is controlled throughout by using hemostatic agents such as absorbable paddies/sponges, and bipolar cautery technique.
- Ensure the field is fully dry before closing the procedure and pack the nose. The integrity of the repair must be inspected along with testing for adequate ventilation in the nasal cavity.

17.7.1 Relevant Anatomy

Refer to ▶ Fig. 17.3 and ▶ Fig. 17.4 to observe the relationship between the cribriform plate and surrounding structures.

17.8 Postoperative Care

- Monitor for CSF leakage, infection, and nasal obstruction.
- Initiate saline nasal sprays to maintain mucosal health and decrease crusting.
- Prophylactic antibiotics and, if needed, anticonvulsants.
- Postoperative CT of the head helps assess the amount of pneumocephalus and rule out intracranial hemorrhage.
- Lumbar drain is usually kept for 3 days; we drain 5 to 10 mL/h pending on the amount of pneumocephalus.

17.9 Complications

- CSF leaks and associated meningitis.
- Loss of olfactory function (anosmia).
- Intracranial hemorrhage or ischemia.
- Orbital complications such as vision loss or extraocular movement deficits.
- Sinonasal complications, including adhesions and infections.

17.10 Management Pearls

- Preoperative imaging is critical for surgical planning and navigation.
- A multilayer skull base reconstruction with a vascularized nasoseptal flap decreases

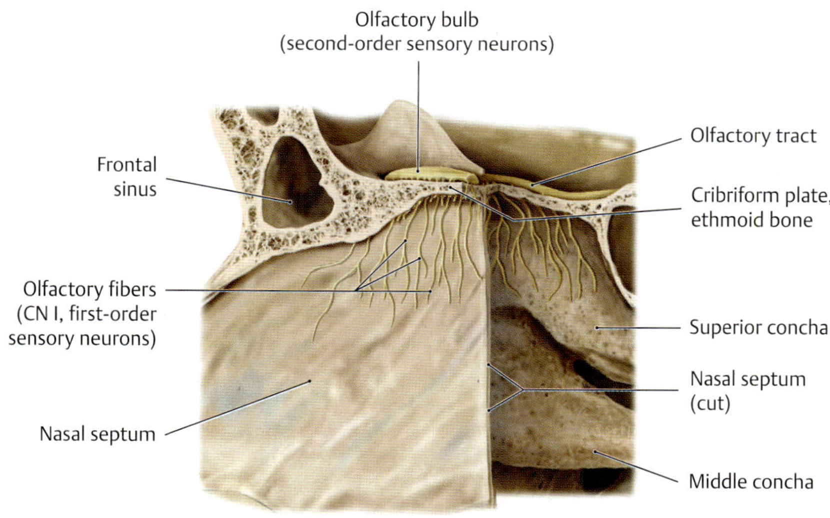

Fig. 17.3 Fiber bundles in the olfactory mucosa pass from the nasal cavity through the cribriform plate of the ethmoid bone into the anterior cranial fossa, where they synapse in the olfactory bulb. (Reproduced from Schuenke M, Schulte E, Schumacher U. THIEME Atlas of Anatomy. Head, Neck and Neuroanatomy. Illustrations by Voll M and Wesker K. Fourth Edition. © Thieme 2025.)

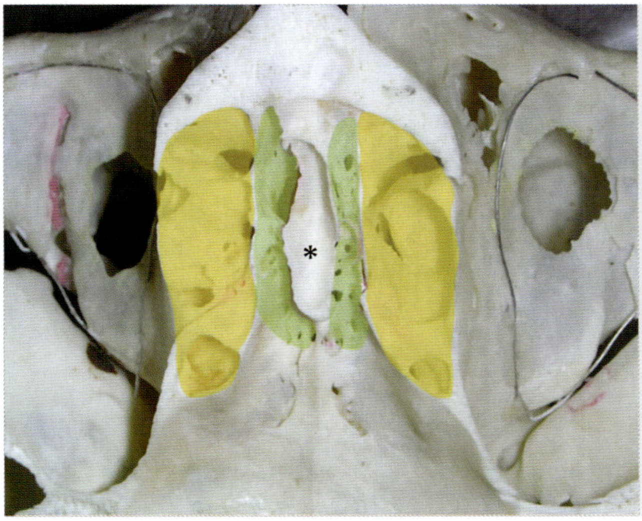

Fig. 17.4 Image of a dry skull showing the relationship between the ethmoidal roof (*yellow area*) and cribriform plate (*green area*). The crista galli (pneumatized in this case; *black asterisk*) separates the two cribriform plates. (Reproduced from Lenzi R, Vinciguerra A, Maccari A, Pipolo C. In: Felisati G, Chiapasco M, ed. Sinonasal Complications of Dental Disease and Treatment: Prevention–Diagnosis–Management. 1st Edition. © 2015 Thieme Publishers, Stuttgart.)

postoperative CSF leaks in combination with a lumbar drain. However, make sure the nasal septum does not have tumor involvement.
- Use of intraoperative fluorescence or endoscopic Doppler can enhance safety.
- Employ a multidisciplinary team for comprehensive care, including neurosurgery and otolaryngology.

17.11 Emerging Technologies

- Advanced intraoperative navigation systems with augmented reality.
- Fluorescent imaging for real-time identification of critical structures.
- Biodegradable and bioengineered materials for skull base repair.
- Robotic-assisted endoscopy for improved precision and ergonomics.

References

[1] Radulesco T, Penicaud M, Dessi P, Michel J. Endoscopic surgery for sinonasal tumors: the transcribriform approach. J Stomatol Oral Maxillofac Surg. 2017; 118(4):248–250

[2] Kassam AB et al. Endoscopic endonasal skull base surgery: analysis of complications in the authors' initial 800 patients. J Neurosurg. 2011; 114(6):1544–1568

[3] Kassam AB, Gardner P, Snyderman C, Carrau R, Mintz A. Expanded endonasal approach: fully endoscopic, completely transnasal approach to the middle third of the clivus, petrous bone, middle cranial fossa, and infratemporal fossa. Neurosurg Focus. 2005; 19(1):E6

[4] Cavallo LM, Messina A, Cappabianca P, et al. Endoscopic endonasal surgery of the midline skull base: anatomical study and clinical considerations. Neurosurg Focus. 2005; 19(1):E2

[5] Stamm AC, Pignatari SS, Vellutini E. Transnasal endoscopic surgical approaches to the clivus. Otolaryngol Clin North Am. 2006; 39(3):639–656, xi

[6] Vellutini Ede A, Balsalobre L, Hermann DR, Stamm AC. The endoscopic endonasal approach for extradural and intradural clivus lesions. World Neurosurg. 2014; 82(6 Suppl): S106–S115

[7] Wang EW, et al. ICAR: endoscopic skull-base surgery. Int Forum Allergy Rhinol. 2019; 9(S3):S145–S365

[8] Liu JK, Christiano LD, Patel SK, Tubbs RS, Eloy JA, et al. Surgical nuances for removal of olfactory groove meningiomas using the endoscopic endonasal transcribriform approach. Neurosurg Focus. 2011; 30(5):E3

[9] Lee JM, Ransom E, Lee JY, Palmer JN, Chiu AG. Endoscopic anterior skull base surgery: intraoperative considerations of the crista galli. Skull Base. 2011; 21(2):83–86

[10] Perneczky A, Fries G. Endoscope-assisted brain surgery: part 1–evolution, basic concept, and current technique. Neurosurgery. 1998; 42(2):219–224; discussion 224–225

[11] Gardner PA, Snyderman CH. Endonasal transcribriform approach to the anterior cranial fossa. In: Gardner PA, Snyderman CH, eds. Master Techniques in Otolaryngology–Head and Neck Surgery: Skull Base Surgery. 1st ed. Philadelphia, PA: Lippincott Williams & Wilkins; 2014

18 Transclival

A. Karim Ahmed, Wataru Ishida, Nicholas R. Rowan, and Debraj Mukherjee

18.1 Background

- Lesions of the clivus may be classified as malignant or benign neoplasms, and nontumoral lesions.
- Common malignant neoplasms encountered in the clivus include chordoma, metastasis, multiple myeloma/plasmacytoma, lymphoma, and osteosarcoma.
- In contrast, paraclival malignancies, which may involve the clivus by spatial extension, include nasopharyngeal carcinoma, traditionally arising from the fossa of Rosenmüller (posterolateral pharyngeal recess), and chondrosarcoma from the petroclival synchondrosis.
- Similarly, benign neoplasms may involve the clivus directly, such as osteoblastoma, or include the clivus by extension. Benign lesions extending into the clivus include pituitary macroadenoma, meningioma, and chondroblastoma. Nontumoral lesions of the clivus include ecchordosis physaliphora (benign notochordal remnant similar to the malignant counterpart chordoma), fibrous dysplasia, and other nontumoral lesions involving the clivus by extension, including dermoid/epidermoid cyst, arachnoid cyst, neuroenteric cyst, and mucocele.[1,2,3,4,5]
- The endoscopic endonasal transclival approach is used mainly for ventral extradural lesions involving the clivus. In general, the clivus may be approached via the anterior, anterolateral, or posterolateral approach.
- Variants to the anterior transclival approach include the transsphenoidal (upper clivus), transoral, transcervical, transantral, bilateral Le Fort I maxillotomy, transbasal, transpalatal, and Caldwell–Luc approach.[6,7]
- Laterally, once the pterygopalatine ganglion is unroofed and lateralized, a transpterygoid approach can be useful to increase the lateral working angle and access to the infratemporal fossa/paraclival region, which may be necessary for some very extensive clival lesions.[8,9]
- The advent of the endoscopic endonasal transclival approach has drastically improved the feasibility of accessing clival lesions, particularly those extradural and in the midline, while minimizing the morbidity associated with traditional open approaches.
- Lesions of the clivus most commonly include chordoma, chondrosarcoma, metastasis, plasmacytoma, lymphoma, and noncancerous lesions.
- This chapter will outline the relevant anatomy, classification by clival location, associated risk factors, and technical nuances of the endoscopic endonasal approach.

18.2 Indications and Contraindications

- The anterior endoscopic endonasal transclival approach is primarily used for extradural ventral pathologies of the clivus or those paraclival (off-midline) lesions without significant lateral extent beyond critical neurovascular structures, such as the internal carotid artery (ICA). In such cases, an endoscopic endonasal transclival approach may be supplemented with an open anterolateral (i.e., anterior petrosectomy) or posterolateral (i.e., far lateral) approach.[10,11,12,13,14,15,16]
- Relative contraindications to this approach include lesions extending lateral to the oculomotor nerves in the upper clivus, lateral to the abducens nerves or petroclival fissure in the middle clivus, and lateral to the lower cranial nerves (CN) or vertebral arteries in the lower clivus. The endoscopic transclival approach may extend down to the odontoid tip depending on the nasal axial line; however, intradural lesions below the limits of the clivus represent a particularly challenging reconstructive entity with higher rates of postoperative cerebrospinal fluid (CSF) leak.[17,18,19,20]

18.3 Informed Consent

- Following standard procedure, informed consent is obtained for all patients undergoing surgery.
- In addition to the rare and serious adverse events (i.e., death, stroke, coma, paralysis, bleeding, infection), informed consent for the

anterior transclival procedure is outlined by anatomy-specific pathology.
- Although substantially lower risk than that of the transoral approach, dysphagia related to pharyngeal muscle mobilization should be described in the endoscopic endonasal transclival approach.
- Cranial nerve dysfunction is included in the informed consent for upper clival (CNs III, IV, V), middle clival (CNs VI, VII, VIII), or lower clival pathologies (CNs IX, X, XI, XII).
- Patients are also counseled about vascular injuries, including internal jugular and internal carotid injuries—notably, the parapharyngeal ICA lies in closest proximity to the Rosenmüller fossa. Informed consent should also include reconstructive adjuncts such as synthetic grafts, autologous fat/fascia, and a pedicled nasal septal flap with the risk of potential CSF leak.

18.4 Instruments

- Frameless stereotactic neuronavigation and rigid endoscopy (Karl Storz Endoscopy, Tuttlingen, Germany) are mainstays for endoscopic endonasal procedures.
- Neuronavigation should be registered to both computed tomography (CT) and magnetic resonance imaging (MRI) to aid in identifying bony landmarks, adjacent critical structures, and extent of lesion resection. Frameless guidance may be facilitated by both a specified neuronavigation wand device or navigation-registered instruments (i.e., drill, suction tip).
- Endoscopes should be low profile, typically 18 cm in length and 4 mm in diameter, to prevent crowding of the surgical field. Angled tip instruments and angled endoscopes may be required to visualize and access narrow spaces not in direct trajectory.
- An array of endoscopic surgical instruments are required, including but not limited to monopolar and bipolar cautery, Cottle and other elevators, high-speed drills, up- and downgoing Kerrison punches, micro-Doppler, sickle knife, curettes, backbiting forceps, thrombin matrix solution (Floseal, Baxter, Deerfield, IL), cotton pledgets, and endoscopic forceps.[21,22,23]

18.5 Patient Preparation

- Lesions of the clivus should be evaluated with high-resolution MRI with thin cuts through the skull base and thin-cut CT scan with possible CT angiogram (CTA) or diagnostic cerebral angiogram depending on vascular involvement of the lesion.
- Constructive interference steady-state (CISS) sequences on MRI is particularly helpful to identify the cisternal segments for CNs adjacent to the clivus. Systemic staging via positron emission tomography (PET)/CT is warranted in cases of known or suspected primary or metastatic malignancy.
- Lesions of unknown malignancy or significance should be evaluated by biopsy as this has further implications for surgical management and future treatments, though lesions thought to be chordoma or chondrosarcoma should have attempted gross total resection upfront of technically feasible.[3,24,25,26,27,28,29]
- An appropriate operating table capable of rotating and reverse Trendelenburg positioning, to promote venous drainage and reduce intraoperative blood loss, is of paramount importance.
- If a neural integrity monitor (NIM) for laryngeal muscle electromyogram (EMG; CN X) is desired, this is attached to the endotracheal tube prior to intubation.
- By convention, and for most right-handed surgeons, the endotracheal tube is secured to the left lower lip of the patient, an orogastric tube is inserted to decompress the stomach, and the patient is turned away from the anesthesia setup.
- Intraoperative neuromonitoring, including somatosensory evoked potentials (SSEPs) and free-running electroencephalography (EEG), are mainstays of skull base surgery.
- Additional monitoring, such as EMG of the trapezius muscle (CN XI), tongue (CN XII), or brainstem auditory evoked response (BAER; CNs VII and VIII) occurs on a location-specific basis.[21,30,31,32]
- Such neurophysiologic monitoring is an important adjunct to a detailed understanding of the patient's pathology, imaging, anatomy, and adjacent neurovascular structures.

18.6 Patient Positioning

- The following case involves a 65-year-old woman who initially presented with syncopal episodes. She was evaluated by a neurologist who ordered imaging that incidentally demonstrated a clival mass with nasopharyngeal extension, without any other associated neurologic symptoms. The patient underwent a biopsy with an outside otolaryngologist, and pathology was consistent with a conventional type chordoma. She was then referred to our center for further management (▶ Fig. 18.1 and ▶ Fig. 18.2).
- The patient was placed supine with the head tilted, translated laterally toward the primary surgeon, elevated for venous return, and in slight extension (note the amount of head extension varies with craniocaudal location of pathology, with increased extension for upper clivus/sellar lesions).
- Following standard prep and registration, epinephrine-soaked pledgets were placed in the nasal cavity.

18.7 Technique

- Operative video demonstrating this technique can be found in **Video 18.1**.
- The endonasal approach proceeded with outfracturing of the inferior and middle turbinates bilaterally.
- A Cottle elevator identified and elevated the submucoperichondrial and periosteal plane.
- A posterior septectomy was performed; in cases of significant septal deviation, a formal septoplasty may be necessary.
- Monopolar cautery was used from the choana down to approximately 2 cm anteriorly on the nasal septum and a posterior septal window was created with the mucosa elevated.
- One should maintain caution when elevating the mucosa from the rostrum as to not violate the posterior septal artery should a nasoseptal flap be required. A high-speed drill was used to resect the residual septum and vomer.
- The prior biopsy site in the nasopharynx was identified. Using monopolar cautery, and a series of blunt and sharp dissection techniques, an approximately 2-cm-wide by 1.5-cm-tall swath of mucosa and underlying mucoperiosteum was resected from the superior aspect of the nasopharynx surrounding the prior biopsy site and corresponding with the mid-clivus; this tissue was sent for permanent pathology.
- Next, the eustachian tube was held out laterally on either side and an inverted U-shaped flap

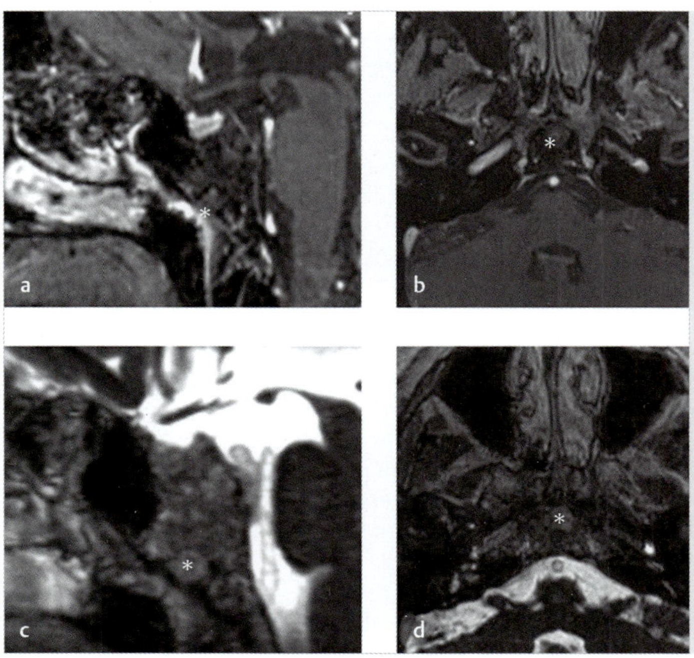

Fig. 18.1 Preoperative MRI of anterior clival chordoma. **(a)** Midsagittal T1 postcontrast MRI. **(b)** Axial T1 postcontrast MRI. **(c)** Midsagittal high-resolution T2 constructive interference steady state (CISS). **(d)** Axial T2 CISS. The *asterisk symbol* (*) denotes tumor of the clivus.

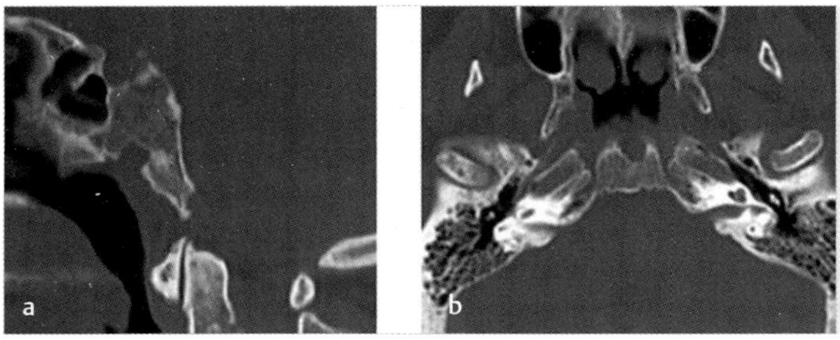

Fig. 18.2 Preoperative CT of lytic clival chordoma. **(a)** Midsagittal CT showing lytic lesion of the anterior clivus. **(b)** Axial CT.

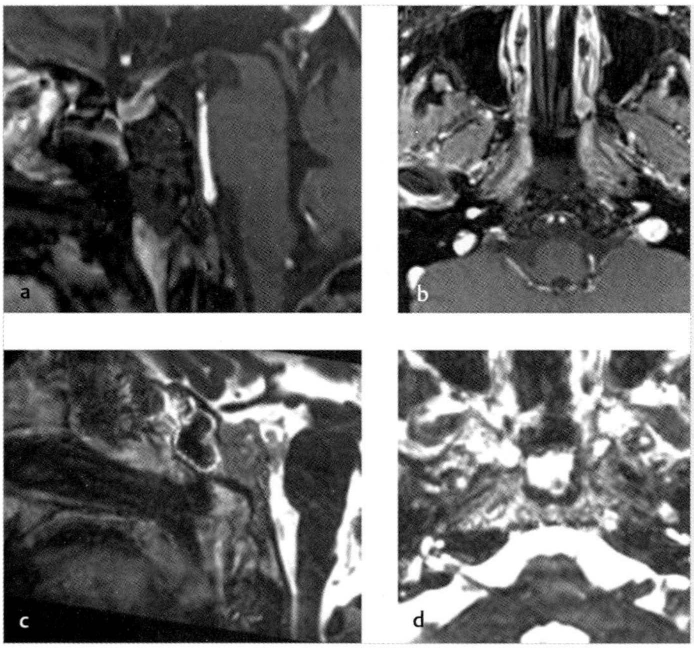

Fig. 18.3 Postoperative MRI of anterior clival chordoma with gross total resection. **(a)** Midsagittal T1 postcontrast MRI. **(b)** Axial T1 postcontrast MRI. **(c)** Midsagittal high-resolution T2 constructive interference steady state (CISS). **(d)** Axial T2 CISS.

was created to reflect down all the residual mucosa of the nasopharynx. This mucosa was skeletonized off the bone. Using meticulous sharp and blunt dissection techniques, the tumor was subsequently resected. A piece of this lesion was sent for frozen pathology, which was consistent with chordoma.

- At the posterior aspect of the tumor, there was no connection with any critical structures. The venous plexus may bleed significantly, but can be controlled with injectable thrombin solution (Floseal, Baxter) and cotton pledgets. In the present case, any bleeding in the cancellous bone of the clivus was controlled with the same materials.
- Following gross total resection of the tumor, the surgical cavity was thoroughly irrigated. Image guidance was used to confirm a broad dissection cavity and gross total resection had been achieved. The inverted-U flap was rotated up to cover the exposed bone, with invaded soft tissue removed. There was some exposed bone of the mid-clivus that was intentionally left uncovered given concerns of aspiration of any packing that was placed in the nasopharynx. Bilateral Doyle splints were placed in the nares and sutured in place.
- The patient recovered well with no CSF leak and no postoperative deficits. Postoperative imaging confirmed gross total resection (► Fig. 18.3). She completed 42 fractions of image-guided intensity-modulated radiotherapy (IMRT) for a total dose of 68.88 Gy 3 months after surgery with no residual tumor

on her most recent MRI at 7 months postoperatively.

- Owing to multileaf collimators and image guidance, IMRT utilizes equivalent total dose of photons, as opposed to classic adjuvant proton therapy in chordoma, with favorable steep dose fall-off minimizing radiation to adjacent critical structures with comparable survival and local control rates to that of proton therapy.[33]

18.8 Postoperative Care

- The postoperative care following an endoscopic endonasal transclival approach in the perioperative period first involves careful observation for unintended neurologic or vascular complication and postoperative routine imaging. Further postoperative management may be specific to the location in the clivus. For instance, lesions involving the upper clivus/sella require careful observation of endocrine status and sodium regulation.[14,34]
- Attention should be paid to the potential for postoperative CSF leak, especially in cases with intraoperative high-flow CSF leaks. Although adjunctive measures such as bedrest, ICP-lowering medications such as acetazolamide, or lumbar drainage may be used in the setting of a postoperative leak, reoperation with skull base reconstruction may be required for persistent CSF leak.
- Adjuvant chemoradiation, systemic imaging, and surveillance imaging may also be warranted depending on lesion pathology.[35,36,37,38]

18.9 Complications

- Of the possible complications inherent to the endoscopic endonasal transclival approach, the most severe and rare comprise unintended vascular injury to the carotid, basilar, or vertebral arteries, for which intraoperative micro-Doppler and meticulous operative technique are essential.
- CN injury, particularly CN VI, may also be encountered and further emphasizing the importance of a detailed three-dimensional understanding of the anatomy, patient imaging, stereotactic navigation, and intraoperative neuromonitoring.
- More common complications include CSF leak, retropharyngeal abscess, surgical site infection, and sodium dysregulation particularly in pathologies involving the upper clivus and sella.[13,39]
- Risks related to the transclival approach may be stratified based on anatomic-specific approach—to the upper, middle, or lower clivus.
- Emerging from the interpedicular cistern, the oculomotor nerves and subjacent posterior communicating arteries limit the lateral exposure of the upper clivus and must be carefully identified to prevent neurovascular compromise. Limited by the sellar floor and pituitary gland, this access often requires pituitary transposition, which may be accomplished in three ways: extradural, interdural, and intradural.
- The extradural approach is safest in minimizing arterial (inferior hypophyseal artery) or venous outflow disruption to the pituitary. The interdural approach identifies a plane between meningeal and periosteal layers, which communicate with the cavernous sinus and preserve the venous outflow of the meningeal layer. This approach requires coagulation of the inferior hypophyseal arteries, but the gland may still be adequately perfused by the superior hypophyseal arteries. Finally, intradural transposition has the highest rate of pituitary and venous outflow disruption, requiring the gland to be detached from the meningeal layer.[13,14,39,40,41,42]

18.10 Management Pearls

- The clivus is formed by the synostosis of the basisphenoid and basiocciput, of the sphenoid and occipital bones, respectively. Derived from the synonymous Latin clivus ("slope"), it is a wedge-shaped bone at the center of the skull base and occipitocervical junction, bounded by the petroclival fissures laterally, dorsum sella superiorly, and foramen magnum inferiorly.
- Cranial to caudal, the clivus may be divided into three regions—upper (sellar), middle (sphenoidal), and lower (nasopharyngeal) clivus. From the endonasal view, the dural portion of the abducens nerves divides the upper and middle clivus, and the dural meatus of the glossopharyngeal nerve divides the middle and

lower clivus.[40,43] The laterally situated dural portion of the abducens nerve forms the fibrous Dorello canal for the passage of the nerve, which passes *under* Gruber's (petrosphenoidal) ligament and *above* the petrolingual ligament.

- The pharyngobasilar fascia, an extension of the superior constrictor muscles, extends from soft palate to the base of the skull, investing the anterior muscular layer. The longus capitis and rectus capitis anterior attach to the superior and inferior clival lines, respectively, lateral to the pharyngeal tubercle.
- The pharyngeal tubercle demarcates the posterior pharynx, and serves as the attachment point for the pharyngeal and anterior longitudinal ligament. The supracondylar groove in the lower clivus is the site of attachment for the atlanto-occipital membrane, useful for localizing the hypoglossal canal—located inferomedial to the jugular foramen.
- Inferior to the glossopharyngeal nerve, the lower clivus is laterally bounded by the sigmoid sinus and the jugular bulb. In the nasopharyngeal approach, the paraclival ICA comes in closest proximity to the fossa of Rosenmüller.[24,25,39,44,45]
- The upper clivus (sellar) is inferolaterally limited by the dural entry of the abducens nerve and cranially by the dorsum sella. A superior transclival approach may provide access to the interpedicular cistern, basilar apex, midbrain, floor of the third ventricle (tuber cinereum), trochlear nerve, tentorial incisura, and mamillary bodies.
- The middle (sphenoid) clivus allows access to the cisternal abducens nerve, prepontine cistern, ventral pons, and anteroinferior cerebellar arteries (AICAs). The paraclival ICA and petroclival fissure laterally limit the middle clivus. It is important to note that the vidian nerve, within the pterygoid wedge, tracks back to the lacerum segment of the ICA, along its lateral aspect, which may be visualized in the transpterygoid approach by following the vidian canal posteriorly.[24,25]
- The lower (nasopharyngeal) clivus may be accessed once the nasopharyngeal fascia, longus capitis, and rectus capitis muscles are dissected. At the caudal extent, one is able to visualize the anterior craniocervical junction, associated ligaments (atlanto-occipital membrane, apical ligament, cruciate ligament, and tectorial membrane), foramen magnum, atlanto-occipital joint, anterior arch of the atlas, and tip of the odontoid.
- Disruption of these ligamentous structures may contribute to craniocervical instability. Drilling of the jugular tubercle laterally exposes the cisternal segments of CNs IX to XI and the ventral occipital condyle. Notably the medial occipital condyle, approximately 5 mm inferior to the hypoglossal canal, may be carefully drilled to expose the intradural entry point of the vertebral artery at the first dentate ligament.
- In the posterolateral nasopharynx, the eustachian tube can be laterally mobilized or transected to expose the inferior petroclival fissure, parapharyngeal space, and parapharyngeal ICA. Owing to the close proximity of the parapharyngeal ICA, this maneuver should be done with great care, with the assistance of image guidance and micro-Doppler. For additional lateral exposure, the pterygoid process can be removed, following the supracondylar groove laterally and opening the poststyloid compartment to expose the parapharyngeal ICA, jugular foramen, hypoglossal canal, and associated CNs IX to XII.[42,44,45,46]

References

[1] Neelakantan A, Rana AK. Benign and malignant diseases of the clivus. Clin Radiol. 2014; 69(12):1295–1303
[2] Jozsa F, Das JM. Metastatic lesions of the clivus: a systematic review. World Neurosurg. 2022; 158:190–204
[3] Nardi C, Maraghelli D, Pietragalla M, et al. A practical overview of CT and MRI features of developmental, inflammatory, and neoplastic lesions of the sphenoid body and clivus. Neuroradiology. 2022; 64(8):1483–1509
[4] Gagliardi F, Spina A, Boari N, Narayanan A, Mortini P. Solitary lesions of the clivus: what else besides chordomas? An extensive clinical outlook on rare pathologies. Acta Neurochir (Wien). 2015; 157(4):597–605, discussion 605
[5] Chan JYW, Wong STS, Wei WI. Surgical salvage of recurrent T3 nasopharyngeal carcinoma: Prognostic significance of clivus, maxillary, temporal and sphenoid bone invasion. Oral Oncol. 2019; 91:85–91
[6] Agosti E, Saraceno G, Qiu J, et al. Quantitative anatomical comparison of transnasal and transcranial approaches to the clivus. Acta Neurochir (Wien). 2020; 162(3):649–660
[7] Rabadán A, Conesa H. Transmaxillary-transnasal approach to the anterior clivus: a microsurgical anatomical model. Neurosurgery. 1992; 30(4):473–481, discussion 482
[8] Asmaro K, Rock J, Craig J. Expanded endonasal approach for resection of extradural infratemporal fossa trigeminal schwannoma: 2-dimensional operative video. Oper Neurosurg (Hagerstown). 2020; 19(4):E396–E397

[9] Mehta GU, Raza SM. Endoscopic endonasal transpterygoid approach to petrous pathologies: technique, limitations and alternative approaches. J Neurosurg Sci. 2018; 62(3): 339–346

[10] Er A, Bozdag M. Anatomical location of the vertebrobasilar junction: computed tomography morphometrics for planning endoscopic transsphenoidal transclival approaches. Folia Morphol (Warsz). 2020; 79(3):445–449

[11] Sato D, Hasegawa H, Shin M, Kondo K, Saito N. Combined endoscopic endonasal transtubercular and transclival approaches for large neurenteric cyst in posterior cranial fossa: a case report and literature review. Surg Neurol Int. 2021; 12:554

[12] Revuelta Barbero JM, Subramaniam S, Noiphithak R, et al. The eustachian tube as a landmark for early identification of the abducens nerve during endonasal transclival approaches. Oper Neurosurg (Hagerstown). 2019; 16(6):743–749

[13] Little RE, Taylor RJ, Miller JD, et al. Endoscopic endonasal transclival approaches: case series and outcomes for different clival regions. J Neurol Surg B Skull Base. 2014; 75 (4):247–254

[14] Belotti F, Tengattini F, Mattavelli D, et al. Transclival approaches for intradural pathologies: historical overview and present scenario. Neurosurg Rev. 2021; 44(1):279–287

[15] Doglietto F, Ferrari M, Mattavelli D, et al. Transnasal endoscopic and lateral approaches to the clivus: a quantitative anatomic study. World Neurosurg. 2018; 113:e659–e671

[16] Kshettry VR, Thorp BD, Shriver MF, et al. Endoscopic approaches to the craniovertebral junction. Otolaryngol Clin North Am. 2016; 49(1):213–226

[17] Kobets A, Ammar A, Dowling K, Cohen A, Goodrich J. The limits of endoscopic endonasal approaches in young children: a review. Childs Nerv Syst. 2020; 36(2):263–271

[18] Bossi Todeschini A, Montaser AS, Hardesty DA, Carrau RL, Prevedello DM. The limits of the endoscopic endonasal transclival approach for posterior fossa tumors. J Neurosurg Sci. 2018; 62(3):322–331

[19] Essayed WI, Singh H, Lapadula G, Almodovar-Mercado GJ, Anand VK, Schwartz TH. Endoscopic endonasal approach to the ventral brainstem: anatomical feasibility and surgical limitations. J Neurosurg. 2017; 127(5):1139–1146

[20] Hussaini AS, Clark CM, DeKlotz TR. Perioperative considerations in endoscopic skull base surgery. Curr Otorhinolaryngol Rep. 2020; 8(2):129–135

[21] Shkarubo AN, Koval KV, Chernov IV, Andreev DN, Panteleyev AA. Endoscopic endonasal transclival approach to tumors of the clivus and anterior region of the posterior cranial fossa (results of surgical treatment of 136 patients). World Neurosurg. 2019; 121:e246–e261

[22] Solari D, Villa A, De Angelis M, Esposito F, Cavallo LM, Cappabianca P. Anatomy and surgery of the endoscopic endonasal approach to the skull base. Transl Med UniSa. 2012; 2:36–46

[23] Liu JK, Patel J, Goldstein IM, Eloy JA. Endoscopic endonasal transclival transodontoid approach for ventral decompression of the craniovertebral junction: operative technique and nuances. Neurosurg Focus. 2015; 38(4):E17

[24] Murjani B, Bhosale R, Ramaswami E, Kadam S, Ramchandani A. Anatomical variations of clivus: a descriptive anatomical study. Surg Radiol Anat. 2021; 43(6):945–951

[25] Hofmann E, Prescher A. The clivus: anatomy, normal variants and imaging pathology. Clin Neuroradiol. 2012; 22(2):123–139

[26] Folbe AJ, Svider PF, Liu JK, Eloy JA. Endoscopic resection of clival malignancies. Otolaryngol Clin North Am. 2017; 50(2): 315–329

[27] Mark IT, Van Gompel JJ, Inwards CY, Ball MK, Morris JM, Carr CM. MRI enhancement patterns in 28 cases of clival chordomas. J Clin Neurosci. 2022; 99:117–122

[28] Yuh SJ, Woulfe J, Corsten MJ, Carrau RL, Prevedello DM, Kassam AB. Diagnostic imaging dilemma of a clival lesion and its clinical management implications. J Neurol Surg B Skull Base. 2014; 75(3):177–182

[29] Olson JT, Wenger DE, Rose PS, Petersen IA, Broski SM. Chordoma: ^{18}F-FDG PET/CT and MRI imaging features. Skeletal Radiol. 2021; 50(8):1657–1666

[30] Elangovan C, Singh SP, Gardner P, et al. Intraoperative neurophysiological monitoring during endoscopic endonasal surgery for pediatric skull base tumors. J Neurosurg Pediatr. 2016; 17(2):147–155

[31] Thirumala PD, Kassasm AB, Habeych M, et al. Somatosensory evoked potential monitoring during endoscopic endonasal approach to skull base surgery: analysis of observed changes. Neurosurgery. 2011; 69(1) Suppl Operative:ons64–ons76, discussion ons76

[32] Jean WC, Felbaum DR, Anaizi A, DeKlotz TR. Endoscopic endonasal approach for transclival resection of a petroclival meningioma: a technical note. Cureus. 2016; 8(6):e641

[33] Sahgal A, Chan MW, Atenafu EG, et al. Image-guided, intensity-modulated radiation therapy (IG-IMRT) for skull base chordoma and chondrosarcoma: preliminary outcomes. Neuro-oncol. 2015; 17(6):889–894

[34] Wong AK, Raviv J, Wong RH. Sellar trough technique for endoscopic endonasal transclival repair. Surg Neurol Int. 2020; 11:99

[35] Marchioni D, Musumeci A, Fabbris C, De Rossi S, Soloperto D. Endoscopic transnasal surgery of clival lesions: our experience. Eur Arch Otorhinolaryngol. 2018; 275(5): 1149–1156

[36] Mangussi-Gomes J, Beer-Furlan A, Balsalobre L, Vellutini EA, Stamm AC. Endoscopic endonasal management of skull base chordomas: surgical technique, nuances, and pitfalls. Otolaryngol Clin North Am. 2016; 49(1):167–182

[37] Raza SM, Gidley PW, Kupferman ME, Hanna EY, Su SY, DeMonte F. Site-specific considerations in the surgical management of skull base chondrosarcomas. Oper Neurosurg (Hagerstown). 2018; 14(6):611–619

[38] Sen C, Triana AI, Berglind N, Godbold J, Shrivastava RK. Clival chordomas: clinical management, results, and complications in 71 patients. J Neurosurg. 2010; 113(5):1059–1071

[39] Hardesty DA, Montaser A, Kreatsoulas D, et al. Complications after 1002 endoscopic endonasal approach procedures at a single center: lessons learned, 2010–2018. J Neurosurg. 2021; 136(2):393–404

[40] Funaki T, Matsushima T, Peris-Celda M, Valentine RJ, Joo W, Rhoton AL, Jr. Focal transnasal approach to the upper, middle, and lower clivus. Neurosurgery. 2013; 73(2) Suppl Operative: ons155–ons190, discussion ons190–ons191

[41] Altafulla JJ, Rai R, Shrager S, et al. Transclival venous circulation: anatomic study. World Neurosurg. 2019; 121: e136–e139

[42] Labib MA, Belykh E, Cavallo C, et al. The endoscopic endonasal eustachian tube anterolateral mobilization strategy: minimizing the cost of the extreme-medial approach. J Neurosurg. 2020; 134 (3):831–842
[43] Fernandez-Miranda JC, Morera VA, Snyderman CH, Gardner P. Endoscopic endonasal transclival approach to the jugular tubercle. Neurosurgery. 2012; 71(1) Suppl Operative:146–158, discussion 158–159
[44] Rai R, Iwanaga J, Shokouhi G, et al. A comprehensive review of the clivus: anatomy, embryology, variants, pathology, and surgical approaches. Childs Nerv Syst. 2018; 34(8):1451–1458
[45] Patel CR, Fernandez-Miranda JC, Wang WH, Wang EW. Skull base anatomy. Otolaryngol Clin North Am. 2016; 49(1):9–20
[46] Mintelis A, Sameshima T, Bulsara KR, Gray L, Friedman AH, Fukushima T. Jugular tubercle: morphometric analysis and surgical significance. J Neurosurg. 2006; 105(5):753–757

19 Transodontoid

Zachary A. Warren, Vijay A. Patel, Christopher R. Roxbury, and Sean P. Polster

19.1 Background

- Odontoidectomy is performed to allow for decompression of the craniovertebral junction (CVJ) for pathological conditions that result in symptomatic cervicomedullary compression. This region is subject to a myriad of conditions, including congenital (e.g., Chiari malformation, basilar invagination), degenerative (e.g., odontoid pannus), infectious, inflammatory (e.g., rheumatoid arthritis), neoplastic, and traumatic conditions.
- Surgical intervention for decompression and/or fixation is recommended in symptomatic and/or unstable cases.[1]
- Owing to its proximity to vital neurological structures, injury to this region may present with neck pain, myelopathy, sensorimotor deficits, lower cranial neuropathies, and/or dysphagia.
- While the transoral route has historically been the standard approach for odontoidectomy, the endoscopic transnasal approach is a minimally invasive alternative, and should be especially considered in pathology superior to the palatine line. The palatine line is evaluated on sagittal imaging by drawing a line along the plane of the hard palate toward the CVJ.

19.2 Indications and Contraindications

- The endonasal corridor has been explored by de Almeida et al to delineate access afforded from an anterior transnasal approach; the nasopalatine line connects the most inferior point of the nasal bone to the most posterior point of the hard palate in the midsagittal plane. The intersection of this line at the vertebral column delineates the inferior extent of surgical dissection, with a mean angle of 27.1 degrees.[2] Additional access can be granted through combined supplementary approaches.

19.3 Informed Consent

- It is obtained through a thorough discussion with the patient, covering the risks, benefits, and available alternatives to the proposed procedure. Additionally, the expected functional outcomes following posterior cervical fusion are reviewed, including potential effects on neck range of motion and overall postoperative recovery.

19.4 Instruments

- The endoscopic endonasal approach (EEA) begins by fixing the patient's head in a neutral position using a Mayfield skull clamp.
- Pre- and postpositioning somatosensory evoked potentials are used for intraoperative neuromonitoring to monitor cortical responses and global perfusion as well as motor evoked potentials to monitor the descending (anterior) motor pathway.

19.5 Patient Preparation

- The integrity of the CVJ must be assessed through radiographic studies, namely, computed tomography (CT) and magnetic resonance imaging (MRI). CVJ stability is also evaluated clinically with a detailed neurological examination as well as with flexion–extension plain films (only to be considered in the nonobtunded patient where instability is not certain; ▶ Fig. 19.1).
- Diagnosis requires the integration of history, physical examination, and radiographic studies before embarking on a treatment plan. Otolaryngology consultation may be necessary to perform flexible laryngoscopy for assessment of lower cranial neuropathies.
- Surgery is performed under general anesthesia. After the patient has been safely intubated, the bed is turned 90 or 180 degrees, depending on the operating room configuration. Gram-negative and gram-positive coverage for surgical prophylaxis is typically achieved with perioperative ceftriaxone.

19.6 Patient Positioning

- The patient is placed supine and secured with Mayfield pins. The table is turned in line with the projection screens in the operating room.

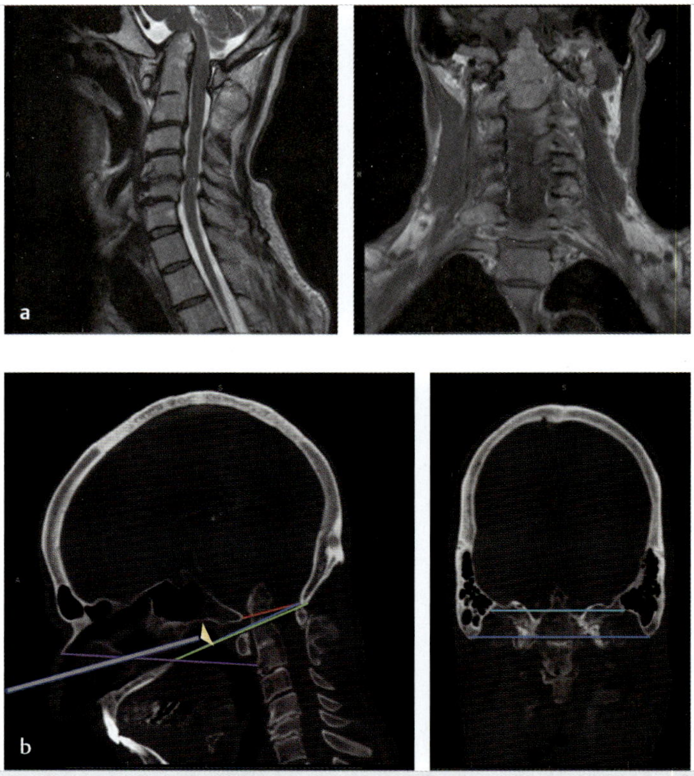

Fig. 19.1 Radiographic parameters/lines. **(a)** Sagittal and coronal T2-weighted MRI example case. **(b)** Radiographic parameters for surgical evaluation with silver endoscope in place with flexibility of soft tissue for viewing angles (view of ▶ Fig. 19.2, ▶ Fig. 19.3, and ▶ Fig. 19.4). Sagittal view: McRae's line (*red*): Connects the basion and opisthion. The tip of the odontoid process normally projects below this line; therefore, basilar invagination is diagnosed when the tip crosses this line. Chamberlain's line (*blue*): Connects the posterior border of the hard palate and opisthion. The tip of the odontoid process projects normally not more than 3 mm above this line. McGregor's line (*green*): Connects the posterior edge of the hard palate to the most caudal point of the occipital curve. The tip of the odontoid process projects normally not more than 5 mm above this line. Nasopalatine line for EEA access (*purple*): Connects the most inferior point of the nasal bone to the most posterior point of the hard palate in the midsagittal plane to define the inferior access extent. Coronal view: Digastric line (*teal*): The tip of the odontoid process is normally located 11 to 21 mm below this line. Bimastoid line (*blue*): The tip of odontoid process projects normally not more than 10 mm above this line.

- For right-handed surgeons working from the right side of the patient's head, a large shoulder bump is placed under the patient's left shoulder to facilitate turning the patient toward the surgeons without rotating the head.
- Padding is placed underneath the left shoulder and arm to prevent positioning-related neuropathy.
- The head is kept in a relatively neutral position to prevent malalignment of the craniocervical junction.

19.7 Technique

- First described by Kassam et al in 2005, transnasal odontoidectomy offers an alternative to traditional transoral approaches, which were historically morbid. The endonasal corridor spares critical anatomical structures involved with swallowing and phonation.[1]
- Nasal access is obtained by bilateral inferior turbinate lateralization to maximize exposure. A posterior one-third septectomy is performed with monopolar electrocautery. Exposure

remains below the level of posterior septal arteries to preserve a nasoseptal flap pedicle in the event of an intraoperative cerebrospinal fluid (CSF) leak.
- The exposed bony septum is resected to allow for bilateral access. Electrocautery is used to create vertical incisions for the rhinopharyngeal (RP) flap, and care is taken to stay medial to the eustachian tube to minimize iatrogenic parapharyngeal carotid injury.
- An incision carried laterally along the inferior surface of the sphenoid sinus floor with electrocautery leads to the design of an inferiorly based U-shaped flap (▶ Fig. 19.2).
- Once elevated, the RP flap is gently tucked beneath the soft palate to allow for unimpeded access to the CVJ (C1 and C2).
- Using a high-speed drill, the anterior arch of C1 is resected. Further drilling starting from the apex inferiorly, the dens is carefully cored out and removed in a superior to inferior fashion.
- Tectorial membrane visualization marks as the posterior aspect of resection once the odontoid is removed (▶ Fig. 19.3).
- Staged intraoperative repositioning may also be considered in settings of significant neural compression.[3]
- Stereotactic navigation, intraoperative CT, or Omnipaque fluoroscopy may be used to confirm adequate decompression.
- The RP flap is retrieved from the oropharynx and draped over the odontoidectomy defect. Fibrin glue is used to adhere the flap to its native anatomical position (▶ Fig. 19.4).

19.8 Postoperative Care

- At the end of the case, a nasogastric tube is placed under direct endoscopic guidance to avoid surgical site disruption. Septal Doyle splints are secured with a 3-0 nylon suture to maintain nasal integrity and minimize synechiae formation.

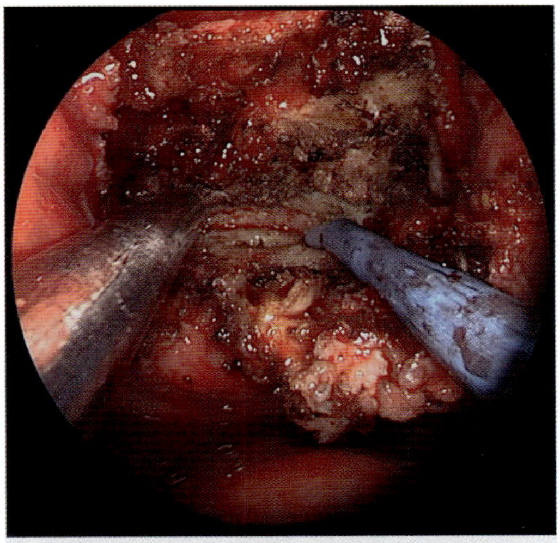

Fig. 19.2 Rhinopharyngeal flap elevation.

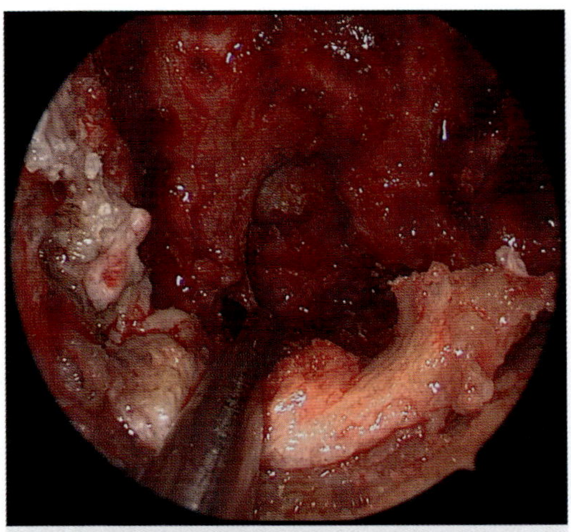

Fig. 19.3 Odontoidectomy defect.

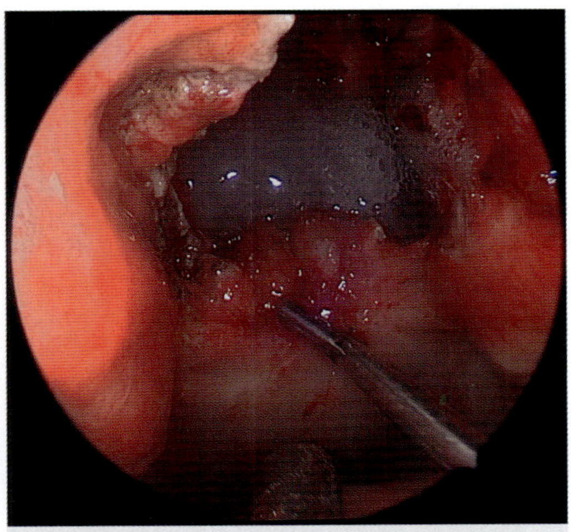

Fig. 19.4 Rhinopharyngeal flap inset.

- Typically, a staged atlantoaxial or occipitocervical stabilization is performed either the same day or a few days following EEA.
- A cervical collar is placed around the patient's neck until internal fixation is completed.

19.9 Complications

- In a comprehensive retrospective series of 34 patients who underwent an EEA for symptomatic odontoid pathology,[4] following surgery, all patients experienced stable or improved symptoms with successful decompression. Most complications were transient (86%), and dysphagia was significantly more common in patients who underwent occipitocervical fixation ($p = 0.02$). Significant complications included intraoperative CSF leak ($n = 1$), reoperation ($n = 2$), and infection ($n = 1$). The 90-day perioperative mortality rate was 2.9%.
- In a systematic review, Fang et al reported 85 patients who underwent transnasal odontoidectomy, with a mean age of 47.9 ± 24.8 years.[5] The most common indication was basilar invagination ($n = 41$, 48.2%), followed by odontoid pannus ($n = 20$, 23.5%). Postoperative complications following transnasal odontoidectomy included respiratory failure ($n = 6$, 7.1%) and velopharyngeal insufficiency ($n = 4$, 4.71%). Intraoperative complications included CSF leak ($n = 15$); three patients developed a postoperative CSF leak requiring reoperation for repair using abdominal fat graft and fibrin glue.
- An additional systematic review by Shriver et al comparing transoral versus transnasal odontoidectomy complications found no statistically significant difference between approaches, except tracheostomy, which was higher following transoral odontoidectomy (10.8 vs. 3.4%).[6]

19.10 Management Pearls

- *Anatomy*:
  - The odontoid process, or dens, is the superior projection of the axis, the second vertebrae. It is part of the CVJ, which is defined as the junction of the cranium and the cervical spine. It is comprised of two joints, the atlanto-occipital and atlantoaxial joints. The primary function of the atlanto-occipital joint is flexion and extension, whereas the atlantoaxial joint allows rotation and lateral flexion. The CVJ houses the spinal cord, vertebral arteries, and lower cranial nerves. The biomechanics of the CVJ are unique at each vertebra and segment; disruption can be devastating neurologically.[7]
- *Ligaments*:
  - **Alar ligaments:** These are paired ligaments that originate from each side of the dens and attach to the medial occipital condyles bilaterally. Slightly wider at their attachment, they have a V-shaped appearance. It serves to limit lateral movement at the atlanto-occipital joint.
  - **Transverse ligament:** This is the strongest and most crucial ligament of the CVJ in regard to stability. It runs horizontally, originating from the medial tubercles on either aspect of the axis, and firmly affixes the odontoid process to the axis, preventing posterior migration.
  - **Tectorial membrane:** This is a broad structure that covers the odontoid process and ligaments continuous with the posterior longitudinal ligament. The tectorial membrane spreads out as it extends superiorly to its attachment at the basilar groove of the occipital bone.
  - **Apical ligament:** It extends from the tip of the odontoid process to the basion and the anterior and midline aspect of the foramen magnum. It is a minor contributor to CVJ stability and is often vestigial.[8]
  - **Anterior atlanto-occipital membrane:** This is a thin membrane that connects the anterior atlas to the anterior rim of the foramen magnum. It forms the anterior wall of the supraodontoid space.

References

[1] Kassam AB, Snyderman C, Gardner P, Carrau R, Spiro R. The expanded endonasal approach: a fully endoscopic transnasal approach and resection of the odontoid process: technical case report. Neurosurgery. 2005; 57(1) Suppl:E213–, discussion E213

[2] de Almeida JR, Zanation AM, Snyderman CH, et al. Defining the nasopalatine line: the limit for endonasal surgery of the spine. Laryngoscope. 2009; 119(2):239–244
[3] Algattas HN, Okonkwo DO, Snyderman C, Gardner PA, Wang EW, Zenonos GA. Staged repositioning in endoscopic endonasal odontoidectomy maximizes decompression while allowing preservation of the C1 anterior arch: a technical note. World Neurosurg. 2021; 151:118–123
[4] Zwagerman NT, Tormenti MJ, Tempel ZJ, et al. Endoscopic endonasal resection of the odontoid process: clinical outcomes in 34 adults. J Neurosurg. 2018; 128(3):923–931
[5] Fang CH, Friedman R, Schild SD, et al. Purely endoscopic endonasal surgery of the craniovertebral junction: a systematic review. Int Forum Allergy Rhinol. 2015; 5(8): 754–760
[6] Shriver MF, Kshettry VR, Sindwani R, Woodard T, Benzel EC, Recinos PF. Transoral and transnasal odontoidectomy complications: a systematic review and meta-analysis. Clin Neurol Neurosurg. 2016; 148:121–129
[7] Offiah CE, Day E. The craniocervical junction: embryology, anatomy, biomechanics and imaging in blunt trauma. Insights Imaging. 2017; 8(1):29–47
[8] Liu YT, Yang TC, Jung SM, Lee CC. Probable pathogenesis, diagnosis, and management of untreated arteriovenous malformation with cyst formation: case report and literature review. Acta Neurol Belg. 2018; 118(4):603–605

Part II

Endovascular Techniques

II

20 Transfemoral Approach for Catheter-Based Cerebral Angiography

Andre Monteiro, Ryan C. Turner, Mehdi Bouslama, and Elad I. Levy

20.1 Background

- The transfemoral approach for catheter-based cerebral angiography is a core technical skill in the armamentarium of any dual-trained neurosurgeon, interventional neurologist, or interventional neuroradiologist.
- The approach involves the use of the groin region as the puncture site to catheterize the femoral artery and navigate appropriate catheter systems through the aorta and aortic arch to reach the carotid and vertebral arteries.
- Transfemoral cerebral angiography serves as a minimally invasive vascular imaging technique for diagnostic and therapeutic management of cerebrovascular diseases.
- The two main approaches for modern catheter-based cerebral angiography are transfemoral and transradial access.[1,2,3] Other less commonly used access sites include the brachial artery and the carotid artery.[4]
- The field of interventional cardiology migrated toward a radial-first approach decades ago due to less operative pain, early ambulation, and lower risk of life-threatening groin hematomas than the femoral approach.[2,3,5]
- Nevertheless, transfemoral access was still the favored approach in the field of neurointervention, only recently being challenged by the radial-first paradigm shift.[3] Reasons for this practice are that, contrary to coronary artery catheterization, in which the radial artery route provides a straight path to the target vessels, the cervical and intracranial vasculature require overcoming the acute aortic arch angles and vessel tortuosity encountered when accessed from the transradial anatomical route.[1]
- Conversely, transfemoral access provides a direct and less complex route to the vasculature typically targeted during neurointervention. Therefore, the transfemoral approach remained the most practiced for neurointervention, despite longer patient immobilization and higher risk of groin hematoma.[1,3]
- Nevertheless, the technology for femoral access-site closure devices and sheaths has improved over the years, making hematomas with serious consequences a rare event.[5,6]

20.2 Indications and Contraindications

- The transfemoral approach for catheter-based cerebral angiography is regarded as the "gold standard" for imaging of the cervical and cerebral vasculature to evaluate the presence of cerebrovascular diseases, such as carotid stenosis or dissection; cervical and intracranial aneurysms; arteriovenous fistulas and malformations; intracranial arterial dissection, stenosis, or occlusion; venous thrombosis; dural venous sinus stenosis (e.g., in idiopathic intracranial hypertension); and venous malformations (e.g., vein of Galen malformations).
- This approach is also indicated as a minimally invasive procedure for treatment of the aforementioned cerebrovascular diseases. In comparison to other access sites, the transfemoral approach is especially indicated when challenging aortic arch angulation (e.g., type III aortic arches), subclavian stenosis or occlusion, and radial, brachial, or subclavian artery anatomical anomalies are present.
- The transfemoral approach for catheter-based cerebral angiography provides a straightforward path to the cervical and intracranial vasculature in most patients. Nevertheless, bearing in mind all of the patient's anatomical and pathological conditions is key to avoiding unnecessary risks, and a few additional features must be taken into consideration prior to choosing this approach.
- In patients with a previous history of groin dissection, hematoma, or stenting, this approach should be avoided if possible. For treatment of patients who are receiving triple antithrombotic therapy (i.e., dual antiplatelets plus anticoagulant agents), the transfemoral approach may carry higher risk of serious

hematoma and other access sites should be considered if possible.[7,8]
- In purely diagnostic (e.g., not therapeutic) procedures in patients with an uncomplicated anatomical transradial route, that approach may also be preferred over the transfemoral approach, but this largely depends on the operator preferences and the patients' previous experiences with angiograms.[5]

20.3 Instruments

- Personnel required for performing a transfemoral catheter-based cerebral angiogram:
  - Neurosurgeon, neurologist, or radiologist with endovascular training.
  - Trained angiosuite nurses and technologists.
  - Radiology technicians.
- Mandatory materials (▶ Fig. 20.1):
  - Sterile prep stick.
  - Angiography drape.
  - Micropuncture kit containing an 18- to 22-gauge needle, a 0.035-in microwire, and a dilator.
  - InQwire J-wire (Merit Vascular).
  - Femoral sheath, ranging from 4 to 9 Fr.
  - Sterile gauze.
  - Heparinized saline with pressurized bag (for sheath flush).
  - Radiopaque iodine-based contrast medium (e.g., iopamidol injection).
  - 10-mL syringes.
  - 5 mL of local anesthetic agent (e.g., 2% lidocaine).
  - Hemostat.
- Nonmandatory materials include the following:
  - Ultrasound device with probe cover and gel.
  - Nitrex microwire (Medtronic).
  - InQwire Diagnostic Guide Wire (Merit Vascular).
  - Skin marker.
  - Closure devices (e.g., Angio-Seal, Terumo Interventional; Mynx, Cordis Johnson and Johnson; Vasc Band, Teleflex).

20.4 Patient Positioning

- Supine with legs flexed.

20.5 Technique

- The step-by-step process to perform the transfemoral approach for cerebral angiograms is as follows:
  1. Sterile preparation and draping of both groins.
  2. *Identification of anatomical bony landmarks:* A common site used for skin puncture when cannulating the femoral artery is the midpoint between the anterosuperior iliac spine and pubic tubercle (2–3 cm below the midpoint of the inguinal ligament).
  3. Palpation of the above-mentioned groin region with two fingers to identify the pulsation and course of the femoral artery.

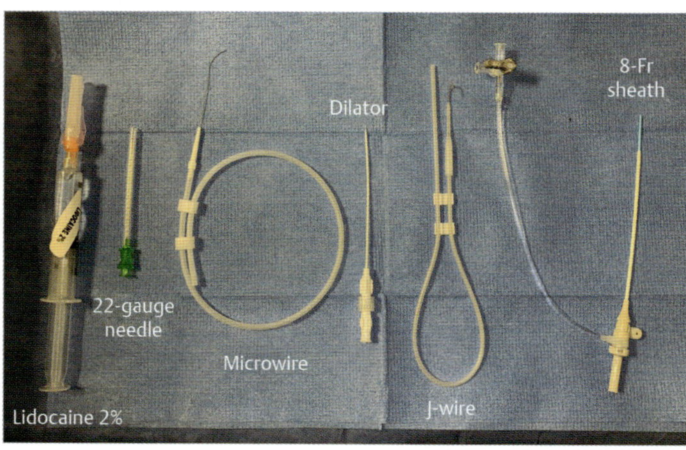

Fig. 20.1 Equipment required to perform a transfemoral approach for catheter-based cerebral angiography.

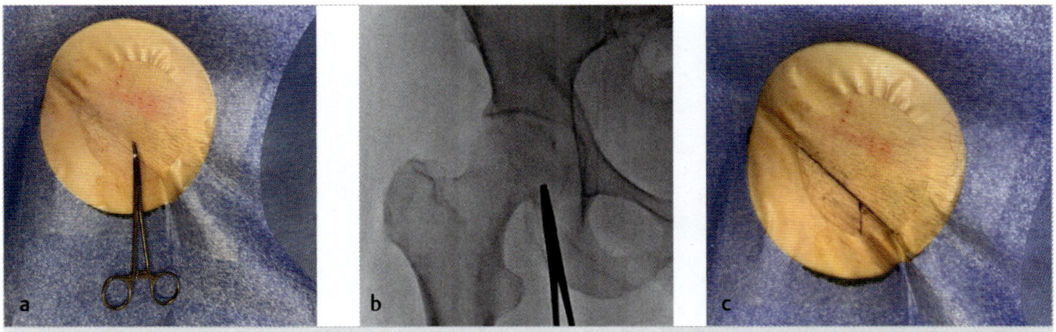

Fig. 20.2 (a) Hemostat placed at the point where the femoral artery is palpated. (b) Fluoroscopic image confirming hemostat placement over the femoral head. (c) Horizontal line to denote the femoral head with a medially directed vertical line to indicate the palpated course of the femoral artery.

4. Placement of the tip of the hemostat at the palpated point (▶ Fig. 20.2a).
5. Acquisition of an anteroposterior fluoroscopic view to confirm the location of the hemostat over the lower portion of the femoral head (▶ Fig. 20.2b).
6. Use the skin marker to mark (draw) a horizontal line denoting the femoral head with a medially directed vertical line to indicate the palpated course of the femoral artery (▶ Fig. 20.2c).
7. Injection of local anesthetic agent:
   a) Based on operator preference, the skin can be infiltrated with 6 to 10 mL of local anesthetic along the course of the needle path or with 2 to 3 mL to create a skin wheal.
   b) Less local anesthetic may provide easier palpation of the vessel, however with increased patient discomfort (which is rarely an issue).
   c) More local anesthetic may make palpation of the vessel difficult, which in turn can affect vessel localization. Ultrasound imaging can be used to better locate the vessel.
8. With two fingers, one above and one below the horizontal line, palpation of the artery is repeated for confirmation of its location. The micropuncture needle (22 gauge) is inserted at a 45-degree angle until the return of arterial blood is achieved (▶ Fig. 20.3a).
   a) *Certain visual cues are useful in this step:* While advancing the needle and approaching the artery, the needle itself may pulse in conjunction with the pulsatile flow, indicating the proper trajectory.
   b) If the needle is in the correct location based on tactile feedback (i.e., feeling of "punch" through the arterial wall) but no blood return is seen, consider the possibility that the vessel is heavily calcified and the needle tip became occluded. In this case, switching to the use of a larger caliber needle (18 gauge) usually results in a successful puncture.
9. Once needle access is achieved, the left hand is used to stabilize the needle while being careful to not move it. The right hand is used to thread the microwire through the needle for approximately half of its length (▶ Fig. 20.3b, c).
10. The needle is then backed out of the artery over the microwire while being careful to not dislodge or remove the microwire (▶ Fig. 20.3d).
11. The dilator is inserted over the microwire (▶ Fig. 20.3e).
12. The dilator's inner sheath and the microwire are removed (▶ Fig. 20.4a–c).
13. An InQwire J-wire is inserted through the dilator into the artery for approximately half of its length (▶ Fig. 20.4d).
   a) Alternatives to the InQwire J-wire include the Nitrex wire (soft tip, longer length), InQwire wire (straight tip, longer length),

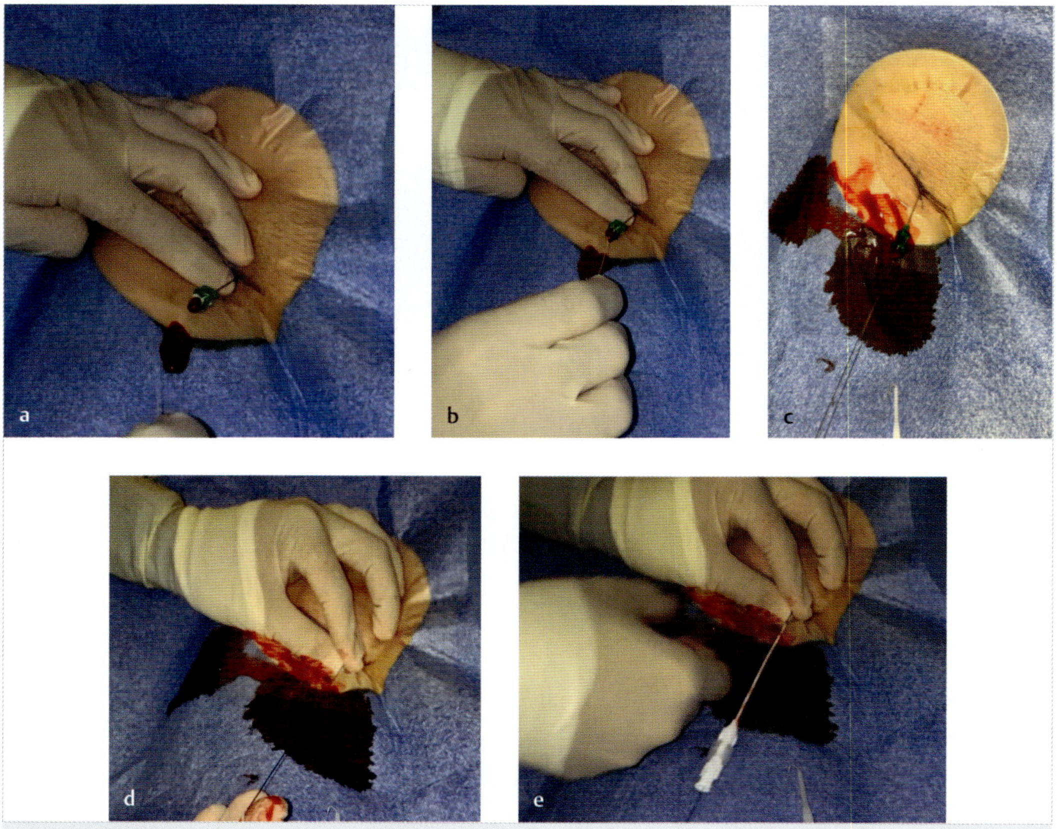

Fig. 20.3 **(a)** A 22-gauge needle inserted at a 45-degree angle with blood return obtained. **(b)** The left hand stabilizing the needle, while the right hand inserts the 0.035-in microwire. **(c)** The microwire is inserted up to half of its length. **(d)** The needle is removed while maintaining the microwire in place. **(e)** The dilator is inserted over the microwire.

and the Torq wire (Merit). Usually the choice of the 0.035-in wire depends on the operator's preference.

14. The dilator is removed (▶ Fig. 20.4e).
15. The desired sheath is inserted over the selected J-wire (▶ Fig. 20.4e).
16. The sheath's inner dilator and the selected J-wire are removed.
17. Back bleeding from the sheath is allowed (▶ Fig. 20.5).
18. The femoral sheath is flushed with the pressurized heparinized saline.
19. At this point, femoral access has been obtained. Further steps would involve the maintenance of femoral access or short-term subsequent intervention, manual compression, and the use of closure devices.

20.6 Complications

- Despite the optimized technique for the transfemoral approach for cerebral angiography described in this chapter, procedure-related complications may arise, mostly depending on where along the femoral artery the puncture is done:
  - High puncture:
    - Increased likelihood of retroperitoneal hematoma.
  - Low puncture:
    - Increased likelihood of catheterizing a smaller branch arising from the femoral artery, which can result in occlusion of the smaller vessel.
- If catheterization of a smaller branch is recognized prior to the use of the dilator, the

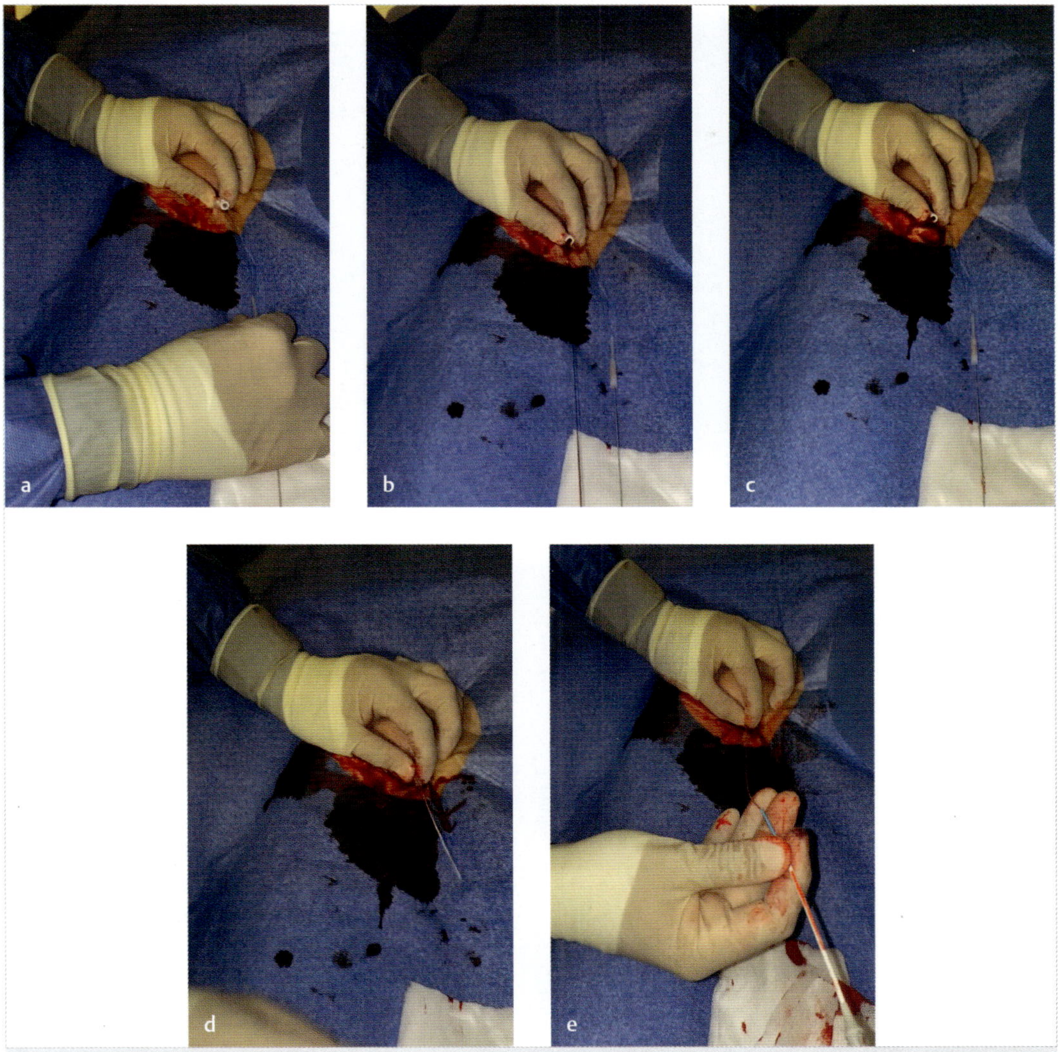

Fig. 20.4 **(a)** Dilator in place with microwire. **(b)** Inner sheath of the dilator removed with the microwire still in place. **(c)** Both the microwire and the inner sheath of the dilator removed. **(d)** InQwire J-wire (Merit Vascular) inserted into the dilator. **(e)** Dilator removed; InQwire J-wire left in place and an 8-Fr sheath being inserted.

procedure should be stopped to correct the access.

- If catheterization of a smaller branch is identified only at the end of the procedure, manual compression of the puncture site should be performed because an intravascular closure devices can cause occlusion of the branch in this situation.
  - Increased risk of iatrogenic arteriovenous fistula.
  - Increased risk of iatrogenic pseudoaneurysm.
- *Additional challenges*:
  - If blood return is not obtained even after switching to a larger caliber needle, consider the use of ultrasound imaging guidance. If no pulsatility is observed with the use of ultrasound, consider switching the access site (e.g., to the contralateral femoral artery or the radial artery).

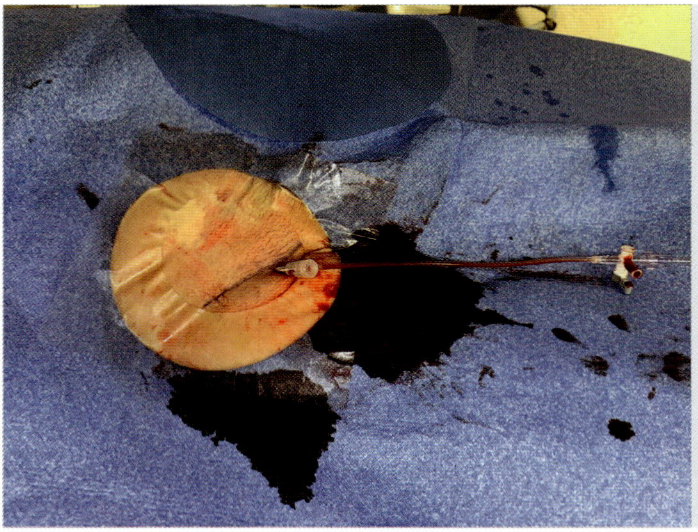

Fig. 20.5 An 8-Fr femoral sheath successfully placed.

- ∘ If venous blood return is observed, the needle can be left as a landmark to indicate the puncture site, after which a more lateral puncture should be attempted.
- ∘ If resistance is encountered when advancing the microwire:
  - Stop advancing the microwire.
  - Obtain fluoroscopic imaging to confirm the microwire trajectory and avoid further complications. Coiling of the tip of the microwire can be an indication of extravascular location. If the microwire is seen to be partially within the vessel, gentle manipulation to steer it or switching to the Nitrex can be done. Using further force to pull the microwire can result in dissection.
  - Of note, if the needle and microwire need to be removed after unsuccessful attempts to correct the puncture site, the removal of both in one motion is preferred. If resistance is felt when attempting to remove the microwire alone, no further pulling should be done to avoid shearing of the device and accidentally leaving it in the patient.

20.7 Management Pearls

- Anatomical landmarks, tactile feedback to elicit the femoral artery pulse, and fluoroscopy must be used in combination to ensure safe femoral access. In addition, the use of ultrasound is highly recommended in cases of challenging access to avoid further complications.
- Although femoral access consists of relatively simple steps, it is important to become familiar with the variety of tools available for this procedure. Being able to switch to different tools, such as the Nitrex (Medtronic) and InQwire (Merit Vascular) wires, and use them efficiently when needed are key to the prevention of hematomas, dissections, and branch occlusions.
- To prevent postprocedural complications, attention during closure is as important as obtaining access.
- In modern neurosurgery, the cerebrovascular surgeon should be proficient in a wide range of both open and endovascular techniques.
- Currently, dual training (i.e., open and endovascular surgery) for cerebrovascular surgeons is extremely important to provide patients with the best options and consider their preferences and concerns when offering treatment.
- Therefore, the ability to perform procedures such as the transfemoral approach for catheter-based cerebral angiography is a fundamental technique for modern neurosurgeons to achieve a successful and safe practice.

References

[1] Levy EI, Boulos AS, Fessler RD, et al. Transradial cerebral angiography: an alternative route. Neurosurgery. 2002; 51(2):335–340, discussion 340–342

[2] Tso MK, Rajah GB, Dossani RH, et al. Learning curves for transradial access versus transfemoral access in diagnostic cerebral angiography: a case series. J Neurointerv Surg. 2022; 14(2):174–178

[3] Siddiqui AH, Waqas M, Neumaier J, et al. Radial first or patient first: a case series and meta-analysis of transradial versus transfemoral access for acute ischemic stroke intervention. J Neurointerv Surg. 2021; 13(8):687–692

[4] Mokin M, Snyder KV, Levy EI, Hopkins LN, Siddiqui AH. Direct carotid artery puncture access for endovascular treatment of acute ischemic stroke: technical aspects, advantages, and limitations. J Neurointerv Surg. 2015; 7(2): 108–113

[5] Monteiro A, Cappuzzo JM, Aguirre AO, et al. Transradial versus transfemoral approach for neuroendovascular procedures: a survey of patient preferences and perspectives. World Neurosurg. 2022; 163:e623–e627

[6] Shah VA, Martin CO, Hawkins AM, Holloway WE, Junna S, Akhtar N. Groin complications in endovascular mechanical thrombectomy for acute ischemic stroke: a 10-year single center experience. J Neurointerv Surg. 2016; 8(6): 568–570

[7] Oneissi M, Sweid A, Tjoumakaris S, et al. Access-site complications in transfemoral neuroendovascular procedures: a systematic review of incidence rates and management strategies. Oper Neurosurg (Hagerstown). 2020; 19(4): 353–363

[8] Siddiqui AH, Monteiro A, Hanel RA, et al. Triple therapy versus dual-antiplatelet therapy for dolichoectatic vertebrobasilar fusiform aneurysms treated with flow diverters. J Neurointerv Surg. 2023; 15(7):655–663

21 Radial Access

Brandon M. Fox, Joshua S Catapano, and Andrew F. Ducruet

21.1 Background

- Radial access has become an increasingly popular alternative to femoral access for neuroendovascular procedures because of the well-established superior safety of this approach and the success of early adopters who have applied this approach to neurovascular angiography and interventions. This chapter provides a technical overview of the transradial approach, from setup to closure, and highlights procedural steps that are key to the successful application of this approach to neuroendovascular practice, including access, catheter navigation and reformation, and hemostasis. It provides a high-level overview of fundamental radial access technique that is tailored to trainees, early-career neurointerventionalists developing their transradial skillset, and established physicians transitioning to a radial-first practice.
- The transradial approach has emerged as a viable alternative to the transfemoral approach for many diagnostic and neurointerventional procedures.
- The rationale for this evolution in practice has been largely derived from multiple large interventional cardiology trials that have demonstrated a decreased rate of complications and all-cause mortality, among other benefits.[1,2,3]
- These benefits are largely derived from the superficial anatomical location of the radial artery, which facilitates both ease of access and reliable hemostasis.

21.2 Indications and Contraindications

- The majority of neurointerventions can be accomplished safely and effectively via the transradial approach.

21.3 Patient Positioning

- The patient is positioned supine with the right arm fully adducted by their side and the elbow extended.
- The forearm is supinated, and the wrist is extended over a towel roll to bring the radial artery closer to the skin surface.
- Tape secures this position along the palmar aspect of the hand.
- This positioning places the access point at a craniocaudal location similar to that in the transfemoral approach.
- Thus, the remainder of room setup is grossly unchanged for radial access, including placement of monitors and controls as well as the optimal location for the interventionalist and assistants.
- The lateral distal wrist is prepped and draped wide enough to allow some flexibility in the location of the access point.
- There are two other key features specific to patient positioning for radial access:
  - First, the sphygmomanometer cuff is placed on the proximal left arm to allow a left vertebral arteriogram to be accomplished using a left subclavian injection if left vertebral catheterization is not successful.
  - Second, a pulse oximeter is placed on the right hand to monitor right hand perfusion continuously.

21.4 Technique

- The superficial anatomical location and readily palpable pulse of the radial artery make it tempting to access the artery without ultrasound guidance.
- However, before attempting access, ultrasound should be used to characterize the radial artery as it approaches the wrist and select an optimal access point (**Video 21.1**).
- The ultrasound probe is then held in a fixed position at the desired access site, and the subcutaneous and periarterial tissue overlying the radial artery is infiltrated with lidocaine.
- Under continuous ultrasound visualization, the radial artery is punctured using a 21-gauge needle via the single-wall technique, and access is confirmed with the return of arterial flow from the access needle.

- A 0.021-inch guidewire is then introduced via the access needle, with care taken not to advance through resistance.
- Gentle pressure is applied over the access site while the access needle is removed over the guidewire.
- Placement of the radial introducer sheath is accomplished over the guidewire with smooth, continuous force, and the guidewire is then removed.
- Next, a vasodilatory cocktail of verapamil 2.5 mg, 1 mL of 2% preservative-free lidocaine, 5,000 U of heparin, and 0.1 µg of nitroglycerin is diluted with blood from the introducer sheath and then slowly injected.
- A radial arteriogram is routinely obtained at this point to assess for anatomical variants and radial vasospasm.
- Of note, vasodilatory cocktail administration can be repeated if delayed radial artery spasm develops.
- Other strategies to address radial artery spasm include application of a warm compress over the access site, compression of the ipsilateral ulnar artery, and increased depth of sedation.

21.4.1 Catheter Navigation and Reformation

- For diagnostic procedures, a hydrophilic Simmons-2 catheter over a 0.035-inch Glidewire is introduced into the radial artery via the sheath.
- If radial and brachial artery anatomy are found to be favorable on the initial arteriogram, with no significant tortuosity or loops, then the wire and catheter can be slowly advanced together under live fluoroscopy into the proximal brachial artery while monitoring the advancing wire for sudden direction changes or increased resistance that could indicate inadvertent entry into a smaller arterial branch.
- Once the wire and catheter have been successfully navigated to the proximal brachial artery, live fluoroscopy can be used to navigate to the subclavian artery and, from there, to the aorta while avoiding its major branches.
- If radial or brachial tortuosity or loops are identified, then a roadmap can be used to assist with navigation. Complete arterial loops can be challenging to navigate, even with optimal visualization, and can lead to radial access failure.
- Our experience is that the optimal method of forming the selective catheter is across the aortic arch, without reflecting the guidewire off the aortic valve. To accomplish this, the guidewire is first navigated into the descending aorta.
- Next, the catheter is advanced until its secondary curve is near the peak of the arch. The wire is then retracted while rotating and applying forward pressure to the catheter. This maneuver will cause the secondary curve to reduce, with herniation of the formed catheter into the ascending aorta (▶ Fig. 21.1).
- There are two common alternative strategies for catheter formation:
  - The first is to create a 180-degree turn in the guidewire by reflecting it off the aortic valve and then form the catheter by advancing its secondary curve over this turn in the wire.
  - The second strategy is to navigate the catheter into the common carotid artery, with its secondary curve near the artery's origin, and then rotate and slowly advance the catheter until its secondary curve reduces and it herniates into the aorta.
- Once the catheter is formed, diagnostic cerebral angiography typically proceeds in the left to right order.

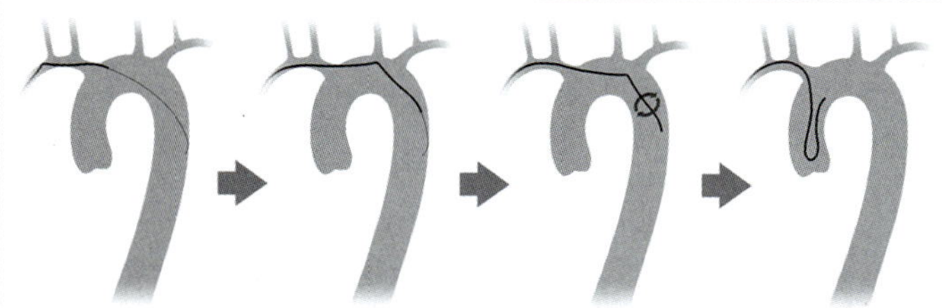

Fig. 21.1 Reformatting the Simmons-2 catheter. (Used with permission from Barrow Neurological Institute, Phoenix, Arizona.)

21.4.2 Hemostasis

- An inflatable radial artery band is used to achieve patent hemostasis, with the goal of applying the minimum necessary pressure for the minimum amount of time to minimize the risk of radial artery occlusion.
- To achieve this, the radial band is fully inflated over the access site, the sheath is removed, the band is slowly deflated until bleeding occurs, and then 2 mL of air is used to reinflate the band and stop the bleeding.
- This level of inflation is maintained for 30 minutes for diagnostic procedures and for up to 2 hours for interventional procedures under dual antiplatelet therapy and anticoagulation, after which the band is slowly deflated in a stepwise manner, with reinflation should bleeding recur.

21.5 Complications

- Ultrasound should be used routinely for radial access due to the high risk of access failure and other complications, including radial artery occlusion, that are associated with multiple failed access attempts.
- Complete arterial loops can be challenging to navigate, even with optimal visualization, and can lead to radial access failure. When a complete loop is encountered, a microcatheter system with a 0.014- to 0.024-inch microwire can be used to navigate the loop, which will frequently lead to loop reduction once the wire is passed distally.
- A small-caliber radial artery and/or high radial bifurcations can also present a challenge to radial access due to the increased risk of radial artery spasm. In such cases, a longer sheath can be used, and careful procedure planning is critical for minimization of system exchanges.

21.6 Management Pearls

- There is a well-established initial learning curve when transitioning to radial access for interventionalists accustomed to cerebrovascular access via the transfemoral approach.[4,5]
- Hands-on training with experienced neurointerventionalists and persistence are both key to safe and effective adoption of this method. Smaller radial artery caliber, anatomical variation, and difficulty of contralateral access are challenges specific to radial access.

21.7 Disclosures

- Andrew F. Ducruet is a consultant for Medtronic, Penumbra, Cerenovus, Koswire, Balt, Stryker, and Oculus, and has ownership interest in Aneuvas.

Acknowledgments

- We thank the staff of Neuroscience Publications at Barrow Neurological Institute for assistance with manuscript and video preparation.

References

[1] Jolly SS, Yusuf S, Cairns J, et al. RIVAL trial group. Radial versus femoral access for coronary angiography and intervention in patients with acute coronary syndromes (RIVAL): a randomised, parallel group, multicentre trial. Lancet. 2011; 377(9775):1409–1420

[2] Romagnoli E, Biondi-Zoccai G, Sciahbasi A, et al. Radial versus femoral randomized investigation in ST-segment elevation acute coronary syndrome: the RIFLE-STEACS (Radial Versus Femoral Randomized Investigation in ST-Elevation Acute Coronary Syndrome) study. J Am Coll Cardiol. 2012; 60(24): 2481–2489

[3] Catapano JS, Ducruet AF, Nguyen CL, et al. Propensity-adjusted comparative analysis of radial versus femoral access for neurointerventional treatments. Neurosurgery. 2021; 88(6):E505–E509

[4] Zussman BM, Tonetti DA, Stone J, et al. A prospective study of the transradial approach for diagnostic cerebral arteriography. J Neurointerv Surg. 2019; 11(10):1045–1049

[5] Catapano JS, Fredrickson VL, Fujii T, et al. Complications of femoral versus radial access in neuroendovascular procedures with propensity adjustment. J Neurointerv Surg. 2020; 12(6): 611–615

22 Direct Carotid Artery Puncture

Kunal P. Raygor, Ammad A. Baig, Wasiq Khawar, Mehdi Bouslama, Ryan C. Turner, Rosalind Lai, and Jason Davies

22.1 Background

- Direct carotid artery puncture allows for expedited access to the common carotid artery (CCA) and facilitates catheterization of the intracranial vasculature.
- Any endovascular therapy conventionally initiated by femoral or radial artery access is feasible via a carotid puncture.
- Two primary techniques exist for direct carotid artery puncture for intracranial endovascular therapy: percutaneous and surgical cutdown (open).
- In practice, patients with extreme vessel tortuosity in the aortic arch or carotid takeoff often cannot receive treatment at an acceptable speed and risk profile due to difficulty accessing the carotid artery through the femoral or radial approach.
- Rapid access is particularly critical for patients suffering from acute ischemic stroke (AIS), intracranial hemorrhage, or other illnesses requiring immediate intervention.[1]
- Carotid puncture has been shown to be a valuable alternative for mechanical thrombectomy and carotid artery stenting (CAS)[1,2]; it has also been used for access to perform intracranial aneurysm embolization procedures in patients with severe vessel tortuosity when other access methods are ineffective.[3,4]

22.2 Indications and Contraindications

- Anatomical variations linked to technically difficult carotid access have been discussed at length in the literature, typically in connection with CAS and AIS cases.[2,4]
- Carotid artery puncture is a reasonable and feasible option when interventionalists fail to gain access through the transfemoral or transradial route. Elderly patients with severe atherosclerotic disease, including disease that causes severe femoral artery stenosis or occlusion, as well as inaccessibility of the CCA through the radial route due to severe vasospasm are some of the more common indications for direct carotid puncture.
- Severe arch calcifications should also be considered during treatment planning as a direct carotid puncture may avoid complications due to arch emboli. Other common indications for both percutaneous carotid puncture and direct surgical carotid cutdown technique include anatomical variations of the aortic arch such as bovine arch, type II and particularly type III aortic arches; CCA and internal carotid artery tortuosity, significant angulation or loops, and ostial stenosis at the carotid takeoff are other carotid-specific indications.
- Intra-arterial therapy for AIS is an emergent indication because time is of importance in these cases, and failure to obtain access elsewhere leaves no other option. At most facilities, suspected stroke patients undergo head and neck computed tomography angiography (CTA) as part of the CT stroke protocol. When several of the aforementioned anatomical variants are visible on CTA, direct carotid artery puncture should be considered for endovascular access. In terms of disease indications, endovascular intra-arterial therapy for anterior circulation large vessel occlusion strokes including mechanical thrombectomy with a stent retriever and/or aspiration catheter is most commonly reported.[2,5,6]
- Intracranial aneurysm coil embolization is the second most commonly reported[4,7] disease process for which direct carotid puncture is indicated for access. Direct carotid access is also reported[8,9] for CAS.
- Caution should be exercised in performing carotid puncture on patients in whom intravenous thrombolysis with tenecteplase (TNK) or tissue plasminogen activator (tPA) was administered in the context of an AIS.
- In the case of percutaneous access, thrombolytics may increase the risk of neck hematoma as well as rapid airway compromise.
- In the case of surgical cutdown, thrombolytics significantly increase the risk of soft tissue bleeding.

- The cutdown approach may also be inappropriate in the acute setting due to the increased time to puncture compared to the percutaneous approach.[2]

22.3 Instruments

- Percutaneous access:
  - Ultrasound.
  - Sterile ultrasound probe cover.
  - Micropuncture kit (21-gauge needle, 0.018-inch microwire, 5-Fr dilator).
  - 6-Fr sheath.
  - 0.035-inch angled Glidewire (Terumo Corp, Tokyo, Japan).
  - Lidocaine 1%.
- Surgical cutdown:
  - Standard surgical instruments.
  - Monopolar and bipolar cautery.
  - Vessel loops.
  - 5–0 or 6–0 Prolene suture on a tapered needle.
  - Micropuncture kit (21-gauge needle, 0.018-inch microwire, 5-Fr dilator).
  - 6-Fr sheath.
  - 0.035-in angled Glidewire.

22.4 Patient Preparation

- The most common indication for carotid puncture is anatomical variations, with either significant tortuosity or extreme angulation of the parent vessels.
- These features are usually assessed by angiographic imaging, including CTA, digital subtraction angiography (DSA), or magnetic resonance angiography. At many centers, patients suspected of having an AIS undergo a CT stroke study (consisting of noncontrast CT, CTA, and CT perfusion) that captures the vasculature from the aortic arch to the vertex, according to the treatment protocol.
- Unfortunately, the extent of vessel tortuosity is often not appreciated until the patient is on the angiography table undergoing attempted femoral or radial artery access. For instance, patients receiving DSA during an evaluation for carotid artery stenosis may be found to have highly variant aortic arch anatomy that is not amenable to femoral or radial artery access.[1,2,4]
- Decisions regarding the induction of general anesthesia (GA) and endotracheal intubation require consideration of individual patient comorbidities and tolerability.
- Although the airway is completely controlled with GA, the induction risks transient hypotension that can be deleterious in patients with reduced cardiopulmonary reserve.
- Conversely, the utilization of monitored anesthesia care (MAC) or moderate (conscious) sedation with fentanyl and midazolam (for example) combined with a local anesthetic requires a cooperative patient without preexisting cardiac or pulmonary comorbidities.
- Patients with comorbid chronic obstructive pulmonary disease or obstructive sleep apnea will be at higher risk of hypoventilation and associated carbon dioxide retention, which can even further worsen pulmonary pressures and lead to more severe cardiopulmonary instability. Of course, in well-chosen patients and with an experienced proceduralist, MAC or moderate sedation can be used safely and has been shown to be as effective and safe as GA in transfemoral flow diversion of intracranial aneurysms.[10]
- No significant differences in stroke, myocardial infarction, and death were found in the general anesthesia versus local anesthesia for carotid surgery (GALA) trial[11]; however, a recent review by the American College of Surgeons National Surgical Quality Improvement Program (ACS NSQIP) demonstrated shorter hospital stays and operative durations and lower odds of pulmonary complications in patients who received MAC than those who received GA.[12]

22.5 Patient Positioning

- With both percutaneous and open techniques, the patient's head is rotated 10 to 15 degrees contralaterally, and the neck is extended using a rolled towel or sheet between the scapulae.

22.6 Technique

- As mentioned, percutaneous and surgical cutdown (open) are the primary techniques for direct carotid puncture. One report demonstrated no statistically significant difference in clinical outcomes between patients undergoing percutaneous versus open surgical access.[13]

- Either conscious sedation or GA can be utilized for both techniques.
- The neck is then prepared in the usual sterile fashion, and a local anesthetic (lidocaine 1% without epinephrine) is injected along a line that traced the medial border of the sternocleidomastoid (SCM) muscle. For percutaneous access, the carotid artery is palpated using the second and third fingers and visualized using ultrasound guidance. Ultrasound imaging can ensure that the puncture site is below the carotid bifurcation to avoid inadvertently catheterizing the external or internal carotid artery.
- Puncture of the carotid artery between the sternal and clavicular heads of the SCM muscle helps prevent the formation of a neck hematoma due to avulsion of muscular arteries and veins.
- The ideal carotid puncture site is 2 to 3 cm above the superior edge of the clavicle.
- Under ultrasound guidance, the micropuncture needle is inserted into the skin about 1 cm above the clavicle at a 45- to 60-degree angle to avoid deflection of the access instruments by the clavicle.
- After slight resistance and blood, pulsation waves are transmitted through the needle, and the needle is advanced through the arterial wall until brisk backflow through the needle is encountered.
- This single-wall puncture is critical to avoid hematoma formation.
- A soft 0.018-inch microwire is then advanced under fluoroscopic visualization into the external carotid artery, after which a 5-Fr dilator is advanced over the microwire.
- The guidewire is removed, and cervical angiography is performed so that a 0.035-inch angled Glidewire can be advanced under roadmap guidance.
- The dilator is then removed, and an appropriately sized sheath is advanced over the Glidewire. The intervention then proceeds as per the interventionalist's preferences.
- Of note, given the proximity of the sheath within the carotid artery, it is often preferable to avoid a traditional guide catheter, proceeding through the sheath with the intermediate catheter directly. This allows the interventionalist to downsize the sheath and minimize closure risks. After completion of the intervention, the arteriotomy is closed through manual compression after sheath removal or via the use of a percutaneous closure device.
- Although manual compression for 20 to 30 minutes is a well-established method for arteriotomy closure with low risk of hematoma formation, it is not without risk as the force of the compression could significantly reduce cerebral perfusion or could even precipitate the occlusion of a newly placed carotid stent.
- Percutaneous closure devices such as the Angio-Seal (Terumo Medical, Somerset, NJ) may also be considered, although their use in the carotid artery is currently off-label and risks embolization should the device not deploy properly.
- Multiple studies have shown the safety and efficacy of Angio-Seal closure in the carotid artery[2,3,4,14,15]; however, other devices, including the Mynx (Cordis, Miami Lakes, FL)[1] and StarClose (Abbott Vascular, Abbott Park, IL),[2] have been associated with neck hematomas.
- For surgical cutdown access, the head and neck are positioned and prepared in the same fashion as for percutaneous access.
- A single dose of cefazolin is administered systemically immediately prior to skin incision.
- A transverse skin incision is made between the sternal and clavicular heads of the SCM. Alternatively, a longitudinal incision can be made along the medial border of the SCM.
- The platysma is divided and subplatysmal flaps are made to facilitate exposure.
- The avascular plane is followed deep until the carotid sheath is identified and opened. The internal jugular vein is mobilized laterally, and any small traversing veins are ligated and cut.
- For incisions 2 to 3 cm superior to the clavicle, the omohyoid muscle may be encountered en route to the carotid sheath.
- Division of the omohyoid can be done safely and with no clinically significant morbidity.
- The CCA is then circumferentially isolated both proximal and distal to the planned puncture site and umbilical tape or vessel loops are applied for vascular control.
- The open approach to the CCA allows direct visualization of the artery so that a 5–0 or 6–0 monofilament suture can be applied in a purse-string fashion at the planned puncture site.

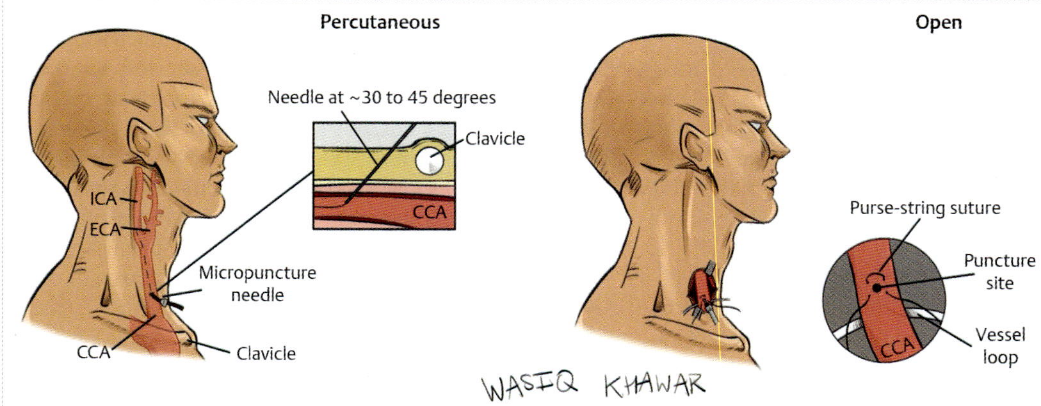

Fig. 22.1 Schematic illustration of the percutaneous access technique. Micropuncture needle access site and angle of entry **(left)**. Surgical cutdown (open) access utilizing a purse-string suture at the puncture site **(right)**. CCA, common carotid artery; ECA, external carotid artery; ICA, internal carotid artery.

- The carotid artery is then accessed using a micropuncture needle, microwire, and dilator, similar to the percutaneous technique. After completion of the desired intervention, closure of the arteriotomy is performed by tying the preloaded purse-string suture.
- After hemostasis is achieved, the platysma and skin are closed in layers.
- Relevant anatomy is provided in ▶ Fig. 22.1.

22.7 Postoperative Care

- Patients should be monitored in the intensive care unit postoperatively with hourly neurologic checks and with neck circumference checks.
- The neck circumference should be measured immediately upon arrival in the unit and should be monitored frequently to avoid overlooking a growing neck hematoma.
- In addition, CTA can be obtained to search for active extravasation to confirm an arterial source of a neck hematoma; however, the index of suspicion should be very low for an arterial source, and definitive management should be pursued as soon as possible.

22.8 Complications

- Two primary complications can arise as a result of direct carotid artery access for endovascular intervention.
  - First, as with any arterial access, advancement of microwires and dilators can lead to vessel dissection and intraluminal thrombus. Care must be taken to utilize roadmap guidance whenever possible during access to avoid this.
  - Second, neck hematomas as a result of insufficient manual compression or failed percutaneous device closure can be deadly because the hematoma can compress the airway. If a neck hematoma is observed, emergent intubation is indicated. If a neck hematoma is observed after a surgical cutdown, the incision should be opened emergently and proper hemostasis must be obtained prior to reclosing the incision.

22.9 Management Pearls

- Anatomical variations linked to technically difficult carotid access and aortic arch anomalies can sometimes complicate intracranial interventions.
- Direct carotid artery puncture expedites access to the CCA and facilitates catheterization of the intracranial target vessel.
- Two primary techniques exist for direct carotid artery puncture for intracranial endovascular therapy: percutaneous and surgical cutdown (open).
- Mechanical thrombectomy, CAS, and coil embolization of intracranial aneurysms are

among the interventions that can be performed using direct carotid access.
- Vessel dissection, intraluminal thrombus, and hematoma formation, as well as air embolism, are some of the complications that can occur following direct carotid access.
- Air embolism is a unique risk of carotid access compared to peripheral access, and care must be taken to ensure that no air bubbles are included in the contrast material or heparinized saline solution infused during the procedure.
- In addition, the risk of neck hematoma is increased in patients who require dual antiplatelet therapy or systemic heparin therapy with therapeutic activated clotting times or in patients in whom large-bore catheters (8 Fr) are used. Extra care must be taken to avoid neck hematomas in these patients.

Acknowledgments

- The authors thank Paul H. Dressel BFA for formatting the illustration and Carrie Owens MSILS and Debra J. Zimmer for editorial assistance.

References

[1] Jadhav AP, Ribo M, Grandhi R, et al. Transcervical access in acute ischemic stroke. J Neurointerv Surg. 2014; 6(9): 652–657
[2] Mokin M, Snyder KV, Levy EI, Hopkins LN, Siddiqui AH. Direct carotid artery puncture access for endovascular treatment of acute ischemic stroke: technical aspects, advantages, and limitations. J Neurointerv Surg. 2015; 7(2): 108–113
[3] Blanc R, Mounayer C, Piotin M, Sadik JC, Spelle L, Moret J. Hemostatic closure device after carotid puncture for stent and coil placement in an intracranial aneurysm: technical note. AJNR Am J Neuroradiol. 2002; 23(6):978–981
[4] Nii K, Kazekawa K, Onizuka M, et al. Direct carotid puncture for the endovascular treatment of anterior circulation aneurysms. AJNR Am J Neuroradiol. 2006; 27(7):1502–1504
[5] Colombo E, Rinaldo L, Lanzino G. Direct carotid puncture in acute ischaemic stroke intervention. Stroke Vasc Neurol. 2020; 5(1):71–79
[6] Roche A, Griffin E, Looby S, et al. Direct carotid puncture for endovascular thrombectomy in acute ischemic stroke. J Neurointerv Surg. 2019; 11(7):647–652
[7] Maruyama F, Ishibashi T, Kato N, et al. Direct carotid exposure approach in the treatment of anterior circulation unruptured intracranial aneurysms for elderly patients. Interv Neuroradiol. 2021; 27(4):503–510
[8] Texakalidis P, Giannopoulos S, Kokkinidis DG, et al. Direct transcervical access vs the transfemoral approach for carotid artery stenting: a systematic review and meta-analysis. J Endovasc Ther. 2019; 26(2):219–227
[9] Guimaraens L, Theron J, Casasco A, Cuellar H. Carotid artery stenting by direct percutaneous puncture. J Vasc Surg. 2011; 54(1):249–251
[10] Griessenauer CJ, Shallwani H, Adeeb N, et al. Conscious sedation versus general anesthesia for the treatment of cerebral aneurysms with flow diversion: a matched cohort study. World Neurosurg. 2017; 102:1–5
[11] Lewis SC, Warlow CP, Bodenham AR, et al. GALA Trial Collaborative Group. General anaesthesia versus local anaesthesia for carotid surgery (GALA): a multicentre, randomised controlled trial. Lancet. 2008; 372(9656):2132–2142
[12] Burton BN, Finneran Iv JJ, Harris KK, et al. Association of primary anesthesia type with postoperative adverse events after transcarotid artery revascularization. J Cardiothorac Vasc Anesth. 2020; 34(1):136–142
[13] Dorfer C, Standhardt H, Gruber A, Ferraz-Leite H, Knosp E, Bavinzski G. Direct percutaneous puncture approach versus surgical cutdown technique for intracranial neuroendovascular procedures: technical aspects. World Neurosurg. 2012; 77(1): 192–200
[14] Blanc R, Piotin M, Mounayer C, Spelle L, Moret J. Direct cervical arterial access for intracranial endovascular treatment. Neuroradiology. 2006; 48(12):925–929
[15] Kim HY, Choo SW, Roh HG, et al. Efficacy of femoral vascular closure devices in patients treated with anticoagulant, abciximab or thrombolytics during percutaneous endovascular procedures. Korean J Radiol. 2006; 7(1):35–40

23 Transcarotid Artery Revascularization

Nanthiya Sujijantarat, Joseph P. Antonios, Andrew B. Koo, Daniela Renedo, Ryan M. Hebert, and Charles C. Matouk

23.1 Background

- Carotid stenosis is responsible for 16% of ischemic strokes and is prevalent in patients with high cardiovascular risk.[1] Etiologies of carotid stenosis include carotid atherosclerosis, carotid web, carotid dissection, and secondary vasculopathy, with carotid atherosclerosis being the most common etiology. In a population of patients with carotid stenosis, carotid revascularization has been shown to be efficacious in reducing the long-term risk of stroke.[2,3,4] In the most current clinical practice guidelines, the European Society for Vascular Surgery (ESVS) and Society for Vascular Surgery (SVS) recommend carotid revascularization in symptomatic patients with 50 to 99% stenosis.[5] In asymptomatic patients with life expectancy greater than 5 years, carotid intervention is recommended when the stenosis is 60 to 99%.
- Transcarotid artery revascularization (TCAR) is a minimally invasive hybrid approach to carotid revascularization. In the TCAR procedure, carotid stenting is performed via a transcarotid approach rather than a traditional transfemoral approach, using flow reversal as a neuroprotection strategy.
- Similar to transfemoral carotid artery stenting (TF-CAS), TCAR achieves the goal of carotid revascularization by means of endovascular carotid balloon angioplasty and stenting.
- However, in the TCAR procedure, vascular access sheath is established in the common carotid artery (CCA) rather than the femoral artery.
- The main advantages of transcarotid access are the ability to bypass a difficult arch or tortuous vessel anatomy and a stable base construct that can allow for a safe delivery of an endovascular device.
- The use of a dedicated transcarotid system requires that the CCA be sufficiently exposed.
- The small open exposure allows the sheath entry site to be closed primarily with sutures, thus reducing the risks of access site complications associated with unreliable closure technique, which can be catastrophic in the neck region especially in the context of dual antiplatelet therapy use. Since crossing the carotid lesion with a wire is associated with potential embolic risks but is a necessary step for balloon angioplasty and stenting, TF-CAS typically starts with the deployment of a distal protection device to capture any emboli dislodged during this process.
- However, this protection strategy requires that the carotid lesion be crossed unprotected at least once for the deployment of the distal embolic protection device. This step and the recapturing of distal projection device are believed to be the most dangerous steps in terms of embolic risks during TF-CAS.
- In the TCAR procedure, the neuroprotection strategy involves the establishment of extracorporeal shunt via flow reversal from the CCA to the femoral vein, rather than the physical deployment of a distal embolic protection device.
- Thus, the carotid lesion is never crossed unprotected, and the balloon angioplasty and stenting procedure is done completely under flow reversal neuroprotection.
- TCAR has a lower perioperative stroke risks compared to TF-CAS,[6] and comparable perioperative stroke risks compared to carotid endarterectomy (CEA),[7] but is associated with shorter procedural time and shorter cross-clamp time compared to CEA.[8]
- TCAR was previously approved for patients with carotid stenosis needing revascularization who were deemed to be at a high risk of complications during CEA.
- In April 2022, the Food and Drug Administration (FDA) expanded the TCAR indication to include patients with a normal risk of complications.[9]
- Several trials investigating the utility of TCAR have been performed:
  - *Safety and Efficacy Study for Reverse Flow Used During Carotid Artery Stenting Procedure*[10]:
    - The ROADSTER trial is a single-arm, prospective, multi-institutional clinical trial evaluating the use of ENROUTE Transcarotid Neuroprotection System (NPS) in patients who were considered high risk for CEA. These high-risk criteria include contralateral carotid

occlusion, tandem stenosis, high cervical stenosis, restenosis after CEA, hostile neck, bilateral carotid stenosis, as well as physiologic factors such as advanced age (> 75 years), greater than two-vessel coronary artery disease (CAD), angina, advanced heart failure, recent myocardial infarction (MI; 3 days to 6 weeks prior to procedure), chronic obstructive pulmonary disease (COPD), chronic renal insufficiency, and contralateral cranial nerve injury. Patients with asymptomatic stenosis ≥ 70% and symptomatic stenosis ≥ 50% were included. Symptomatic patients were defined as symptoms within preceding 180 days. The primary end point was a composite of all strokes, deaths, and MI at 30 days.
  - A total of 105 patients were included in the study. Technical success was reported in 99% of the cases. At 30 days postprocedure, the primary end point was achieved in 3.5% of patients. Stroke rates were reported to be 1.4%. MI occurred in 0.7% of the patients, with an overall mortality of 1.4%. Of note, 26% of the patients in the cohort were symptomatic, while 75% were asymptomatic.
- **Reverse to Procedure**[11,12]:
  - The ROADSTER-2 trial is an open-label, single-arm, postapproval registry for TCAR patients who were considered to be high risk for CEA by the above criteria. The primary end point was procedural success, defined as technical success and absence of stroke, MI, or death within 30 days. In total, 632 patients were enrolled in the study. Within the 30-day time frame, the primary end point was achieved in 96.5% of the patients. The stroke rates were reported to be 1.9%. MI occurred in 0.9%, while death occurred in 0.4% of the patients.[11]
  - At an extended time period between 30 and 365 days, the outcomes were available in 155 patients.[12] In this long-term follow-up, there was no MI or stroke. In all, 2.6% patients died from non-neurological causes. A technical success rate of 98.7% was achieved. Twenty-three percent patients were symptomatic.
- *ROADSTER-3*[13]:
  - The ROADSTER-3 trial is ongoing at the time of writing; it is an open-label, single-arm, multicenter postapproval study. Unlike ROADSTER-1 and ROADSTER-2, ROADSTER-3 enrolls patients who are determined to be standard risk for CEA. The study will enroll 400 patients and is estimated to complete in May 2025.

23.2 Indications and Contraindications

- Several landmark trials have been published on the indications for carotid revascularization for symptomatic[2,3,4] and asymptomatic[14,15] patients.
- The current guidelines recommend carotid intervention in symptomatic patients with 50 to 99% stenosis and in asymptomatic patients with 60 to 99% stenosis if life expectancy is greater than 5 years.[5]
- Our institution's practice for symptomatic patients follows this guideline. However, the decision to perform carotid revascularization for asymptomatic carotid stenosis is typically made on a case-by-case basis.
- Generally, intervention for asymptomatic patients is reserved for cases with progressive stenosis, contralateral carotid occlusion, or other factors that put them at a higher-than-average stroke risk. Because all three modalities of carotid revascularization (CEA, TCAR, TF-CAS) are offered at our institution, the decision between the three modalities depends on patient-specific factors such as vascular anatomy, plaque anatomy, existing comorbidities, and any potential contraindications to dual antiplatelet therapy use.
- TCAR is typically offered for patients with surgical carotid stenosis who have (1) sufficient collateral circulation for flow reversal, defined as the presence of ipsilateral posterior communicating artery (PComA) or anterior communicating artery (AComA); (2) favorable plaque morphology for carotid stenting, specifically no heavily calcified plaque; (3) no contraindication to stenting, specifically no contraindication to dual antiplatelet therapy use; and (4) sufficient "landing zone" for CCA sheath, with at least a 5-cm distance between the CCA at the level of the clavicle and the carotid bifurcation.

- Because TCAR is a carotid stenting procedure, it is contraindicated in patients with any contraindications to stenting. These include the inability to tolerate antiplatelet therapy or lesions unamenable to stenting.
- TCAR is also contraindicated in patients with severe local changes from prior surgery or radiation that reach the threshold of precluding safe neck dissection for vascular access.

23.3 Patient Preparation

- Computed tomography angiography (CTA) of the head and neck for evaluation of the landing zone, plaque morphology, degree of stenosis, and circle of Willis.
- Carotid ultrasound for quantifying the degree of stenosis by flow measurements.
- Magnetic resonance imaging (MRI) of the brain to quantify stroke burden in patients who are symptomatic.
- General anesthesia (GA) or monitored anesthesia care (MAC) with a local block can be used.
  - If GA is chosen, endotracheal intubation is recommended over laryngeal mask airway.[16] Neuromonitoring baselines in the form of somatosensory evoked potential (SSEP) and electroencephalogram (EEG) should be established.
  - At our institution, motor evoked potential (MEP) is not performed.
- With reference to the personnel, in addition to the primary operator, necessary personnel include standard operating room (OR) team (a surgical scrub technologist and a circulator nurse), anesthesia team, interventional radiology (IR) technologist(s), and a neuromonitoring personnel.
  - Necessary equipment are as follows:
    - C-arm X-ray or a single plane X-ray.
    - IR table:
      - ENROUTE Transcarotid NPS (Silk Road Medical, Sunnyvale, CA).
        - Currently, there is no approved substitute for the device.
      - ENROUTE Transcarotid Stent System (Silk Road Medical, Sunnyvale, CA).
        - Any approved carotid stent may be used as a substitute. However, the carotid stents currently on the market are made with the length suitable for TF-CAS, which is typically longer and may be technically more challenging to deploy in the transcarotid system.
      - Carotid balloon of choice:
        - Any monorail balloon of choice may be used.
      - A 4-Fr micropuncture kit for establishment of venous access.
      - A 0.035-inch Bentson wire or a 0.035-inch wire of choice for establishment of venous access.
      - Iodinated contrast agent.
      - Knife.
      - Hemostat.
      - Balloon insufflator.
      - Local anesthetic of choice (for establishment of venous access, especially if performed under MAC anesthesia).
    - Standard OR instruments for CEA are used. These include a carotid clamp, vessel loop, hemostatic matrix, and a 5–0 or 6–0 Prolene for closure of the carotid puncture site.
- The balloon and stent should be prepared prior to the start of the procedure according to the instructions provided on the package.
- All TCAR equipment should be flushed and assembled.

23.3.1 Venous Access

- Using a standard micropuncture technique, an 8-Fr venous sheath is inserted over a 0.035-inch wire into the right femoral vein.
- We routinely use the right side for convenience. The venous sheath is then secured to the skin using a 2–0 or 3–0 Silk suture.

23.3.2 Transcarotid Exposure

- Prior to draping, a triangular depression between the sternal and clavicular heads of the sternocleidomastoid (SCM) muscle is palpated.
- An ultrasound can be used to localize the point at which the CCA is most superficial proximally in that triangle, as well as the point at which CCA bifurcates. The distance between these two points is measured to ensure there is enough landing zone for the sheath (~5 cm).
- A transverse incision about 4 to 5 cm long is planned over the superior border of the clavicle straddling the borders of the two heads of the SCM muscle.

- After infiltration with local anesthetics with epinephrine, the skin and platysma are cut sharply with a no. 10 blade.
- Then, an avascular plane is developed below the soft tissues and divided. A 4 × 4 inch sponge can be used to massage the tissues to increase their conspicuity at this point.
- The surgical plane between the two heads of the SCM is developed using primarily blunt dissection.
- The internal jugular vein (IJV) is identified and skeletonized at the medial border.
- The small crossing veins may be observed and should be divided as needed to safely retract the IJV laterally.
- These veins can avulse and produce bleeding if not dealt with upfront.
- The CCA and sometimes the vagus nerve can be visualized once the IJV is retracted laterally (▶ Fig. 23.1).
- A short segment of the CCA should be mobilized circumferentially and secured with a double-looped umbilical tape (▶ Fig. 23.2).

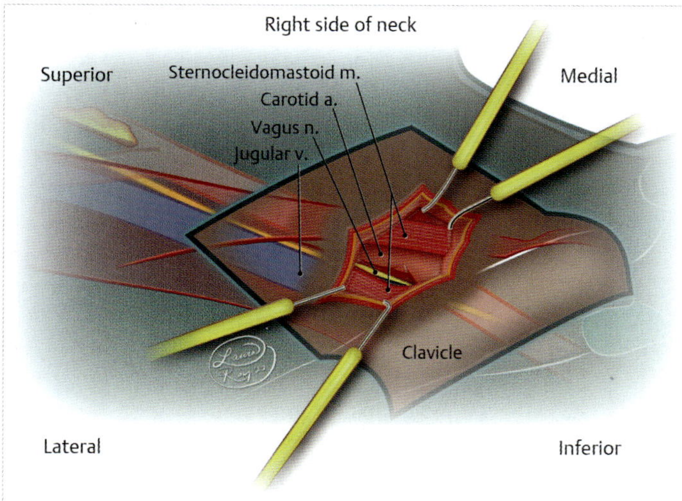

Fig. 23.1 Overview of the typical anatomy encountered during the initial part of the neck dissection. a., artery; m., muscle; n., nerve; v., vein.

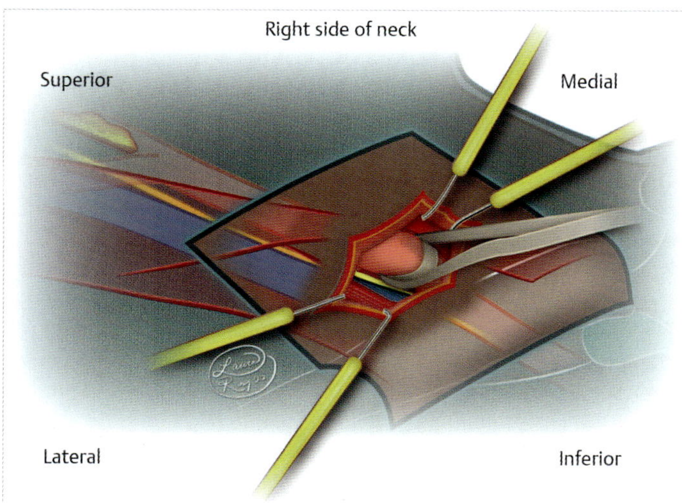

Fig. 23.2 Isolation of the common carotid artery is achieved with the use of the umbilical tape.

- An umbilical tape is preferred over a standard vessel loop to secure the CCA, as the increased friction with the vessel wall facilitates manipulation during the next steps of the procedure.

23.3.3 Insertion of the Transcarotid Sheath

- Once the CCA is secured loosely with the umbilical tape, the patient is heparinized with an activated clotting time (ACT) goal of greater than 250 sec.
- A "U-stitch" is placed at the site of planned micropuncture with a 5–0 or a 6–0 Prolene double-barreled stitch.
- A 21-gauge micropuncture needle is slowly advanced through the anterior wall of the CCA to the black marker on the needle, using a bimanual technique while placing counter tension on the CCA.
- Arterial back-bleeding should be demonstrated. An 0.018-inch microguidewire is inserted 3 cm into the CCA (a point marked on the needle included in the kit), and a 4-Fr microsheath is advanced 3 cm inside the vessel.
- The inner dilator and microguidewire are removed.
- Brisk back-bleeding should be confirmed again.
- Control angiographic runs are performed at this point to confirm proper positioning and to rule out vessel dissection or injury.
- Under a roadmap guidance, an 0.035-inch ENROUTETM J-wire is navigated to the distal CCA, proximal to the lesion ("stop short technique"), and the arterial sheath is inserted.
- Alternatively, the J-wire can be positioned through the microsheath in the external carotid artery (ECA) if more purchase is required for safe sheath insertion and the lesion does not involve the CCA.
- The sheath is secured to the surrounding drapes at three points using 2–0 silk stitches.
- The side ports are purged of air, and a control run is performed to rule out dissection and confirm proper positioning. ▶ Fig. 23.3a demonstrates a typical position of the transcarotid sheath.
- If the CCA is located deep in the surgical field, an alternative tunneling technique without foot plate can be used in place of the standard technique to achieve a shallower angle of approach for the sheath.
- In this approach, a small nick incision is made over the chest wall and a snap instrument used to create a subcutaneous tunnel under the clavicle into the surgical field.
- DeBakey forceps are placed in the tunnel and the micropuncture needle is guided between the arms of the DeBakey forceps to the planned CCA puncture site.
- This technique ensures that the micropuncture needle does not create a new channel through the skin and subcutaneous tissues.
- When utilizing this technique, the foot plate of the arterial sheath is removed and discarded. ▶ Fig. 23.3b demonstrates the insertion of the

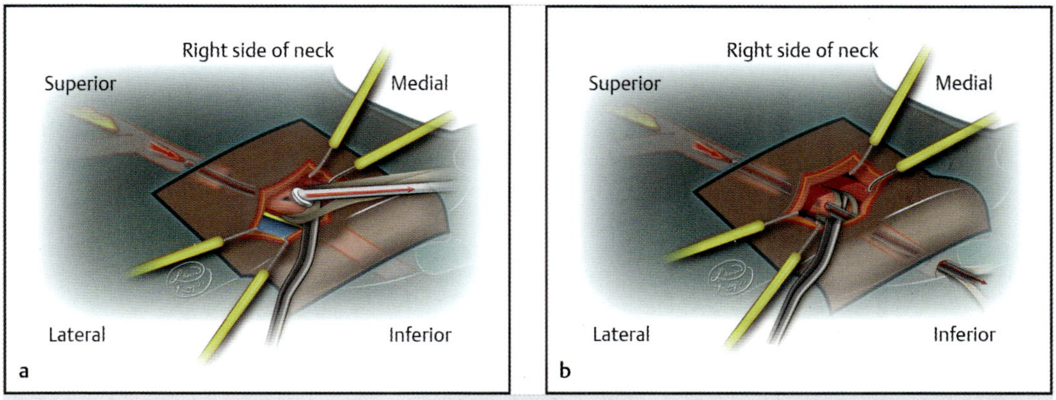

Fig. 23.3 Insertion of the transcarotid arterial sheath using **(a)** the standard technique with foot plate and **(b)** the tunneling technique.

transcarotid sheath using the tunneling technique.

23.3.4 Flow Reversal

- Once the flow line and controller are connected to the arterial and venous sheaths, an extracorporeal arteriovenous shunt is established (▶ Fig. 23.4).
- The high-flow setting is generally used. The venous sheath is flushed with heparinized saline to confirm rapid blood flow through the circuit.
- At this point, passive flow reversal is established.
- A TCAR timeout is performed to ensure blood pressure is maintained over 160 mm Hg systolic and the heart rate is greater than 70 bpm. All endovascular devices should be prepped and ready on the table.
- Using one hand to hold slight tension on the umbilical tape, the CCA is then clamped just proximal to the arterial sheath.
- This step establishes active flow reversal. With one hand on the STOP button of the controller, a gentle angiographic run is performed.
- When the contrast bolus reaches the petrous segment, release the STOP button, but continue with fluoroscopy.
- A flow reversal is confirmed when contrast bolus is seen flowing retrogradely in the cervical ICA after the STOP button is released.
- If this is not achieved, it is possible that flow reversal may not be sufficient, and a deployment of distal embolic protection device should be considered before proceeding with the next step.

23.3.5 Carotid Balloon Angioplasty and Stenting

- A standard carotid balloon angioplasty and stenting procedure is performed.
- The flow line and controller should be left connected for a few minutes after completing the procedure to clear any remaining debris.
- The carotid clamp can then be removed to restore passive flow reversal.

23.3.6 Closing

- Prior to disconnecting, the arterial flow line stopcock should be turned off to the patient.
- The arterial flow line is then disconnected from the arterial sheath. Blood that remains in the flow line and controller can be auto-transfused back to the femoral vein.
- The transcarotid sheath is removed, and the previously placed U-stitch is tied.
- The puncture site is then inspected and a rescue 6–0 Prolene stitch used as necessary. Meticulous hemostasis should be ensured in the surgical site.
- We typically administer IV protamine after a test dose to reduce the risk of surgical site hematoma and groin hematoma.
- A standard closure in layers is then performed.

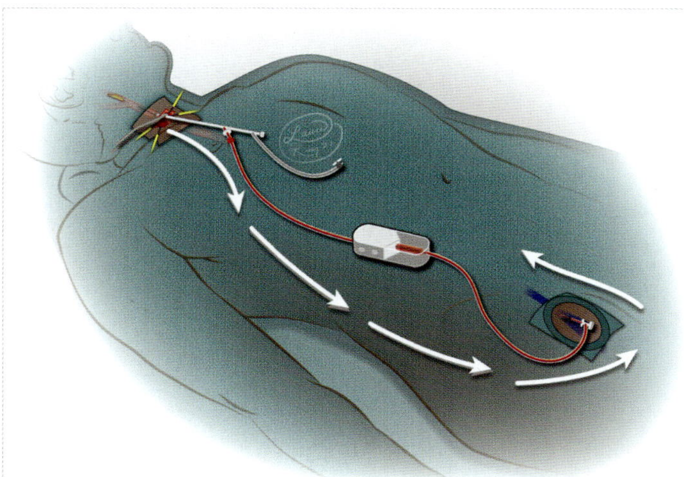

Fig. 23.4 Overview of the right transcarotid artery revascularization (TCAR) procedure is pictured here, with the carotid sheath connected to the flow line, controller, and the right femoral vein.

23.4 Patient Positioning

- The patient is positioned supine on the angiogram table.

23.5 Technique

- The following anatomical factors should be evaluated if a TCAR procedure is being considered:
  - Circle of Willis (CoW):
    - Because the neuroprotection strategy for TCAR involves flow reversal, the CoW should be evaluated for collateral circulation to ensure sufficient flow reversal. Although the absolute requirement is not well established, we typically look for the presence of ipsilateral PComA or AComA.
  - Landing zone:
    - A landing zone of approximately 5 cm is recommended for a safe sheath insertion. This is a length from the puncture site to the carotid lesion, and can be measured with an ultrasound when the incision is planned. Occasionally, if the lesion only involves ICA and not CCA, more wire purchase can be obtained by navigating the wire into the ECA.
  - Lesion morphology:
    - As previously discussed, a lesion should be amenable to stenting if TCAR is being considered. Notably, a concentric, heavily calcified lesion is typically not suitable, although this is not an absolute contraindication.

23.5.1 Setting Up

- At our institution, TCAR is performed in a hybrid neurovascular operating room with biplane. If this is unavailable, a single plane or a C-arm can be utilized.
- The TCAR procedure can be performed under GA or MAC, as mentioned previously. GA is helpful when the technique is first adopted.
- The endotracheal tube (ETT) should be positioned contralateral to the surgical field.
- The preinduction blood pressure should be noted.
- During timeout, the following should be mentioned:
  - *Blood pressure:* In general, blood pressure should be maintained at about the patient's preinduction baseline.
  - *Zoll pad:* A Zoll pad may be placed prior to starting the procedure due to the risk of asystole during balloon angioplasty.
  - Medications:
    - *Dual antiplatelet therapy:* Verify that the patient has been sufficiently loaded with dual antiplatelet therapy prior to the procedure.
    - *Perioperative antibiotics:* Give weight-appropriate antibiotics with skin flora coverage prior to incision unless there is any contraindication.
    - *Heparin:* Give weight-appropriate heparin IV bolus prior to placing the carotid stitch.
    - *Glycopyrrolate:* It may be considered prior to carotid balloon angioplasty, depending on the patient's baseline heart rate.
    - *Protamine:* It may be considered at the end of the procedure to reduce the risk of access site complications.
- If GA is used, neuromonitoring baseline is established after intubation.
- A small bolster is placed under the patient's shoulders to extend the neck, and the head is turned contralaterally.
- The positions of the CCA and the carotid bifurcation are marked under ultrasound guidance.
- The ipsilateral neck, upper chest, and groin are prepped in a standard sterile fashion.
- We routinely use the right femoral venous puncture. All equipment is prepped and flushed prior to the start of the procedure. ▶ Fig. 23.4 details an overview of the procedure when all equipment is in place. **Video 23.1** details procedural implementation.

23.6 Postoperative Care

23.6.1 Immediate Postoperative Period and In-Hospital Course

- Postoperatively, TCAR patients undergo close monitoring of vital signs, surgical site, and neurological exam. Care should be taken not to allow precipitous hypotension or vital sign changes that may sometimes be associated with recent balloon angioplasty and stretching of the carotid baroreceptors. Currently, the blood pressure guideline for the poststenting period remains a topic of debate. In general, if there are no neurologic changes or neuromonitoring changes during the procedure, we maintain the systolic BP between 100 and 160 mm Hg to avoid precipitous hypotension as well as hyperperfusion injury. The decision for BP management postprocedure should be tailored to the patient's preoperative baseline and intraprocedural course. In the immediate postoperative period, the patient is typically maintained flat with the right leg straight for 1 to 2 hours due to venous femoral puncture in the context of heparin load and antiplatelet use. Thereafter, the head of the bed may be mobilized slowly. The patient then undergoes a bedside nursing swallow evaluation and is allowed to eat. A dual antiplatelet regimen is maintained. A postoperative carotid ultrasound can be considered to establish a new baseline if this is desired by the proceduralist. At our institution, we do not routinely obtain postprocedure carotid ultrasound as it is often difficult to interpret in the context of recent local tissue manipulation. The in-hospital course then follows a routine course for any carotid revascularization. The patient is maintained on dual antiplatelet regimen and is discharged when he or she meets discharge criteria.

23.6.2 Outpatient Follow-up

- Because we typically close the wound with absorbable sutures, the first follow-up is typically at 1 month with a carotid ultrasound. If desired or if the patient is deemed high risk, a 2-week follow-up can be considered for routine clinical check.

23.7 Complications

23.7.1 Complications during Execution

- *Steep angle of approach, precluding safe sheath insertion:* After exposure, if the angle of approach is too steep and is felt to preclude safe sheath insertion, the tunneling technique may be used instead. This technique is detailed above.
- *Insufficient landing zone for a safe sheath insertion:* The CTA of the neck should be studied prior to selecting the TCAR procedure to ensure sufficient landing zone for the arterial sheath (~5 cm). If the lesion only involves the ICA but not the CCA, the J-wire can be guided into the ECA to increase wire purchase prior to the arterial sheath insertion. Occasionally, additional CCA length can be gained by placing a higher bump underneath the patient's shoulders. Care should be taken not to overextend the head.
- Loss of neuromonitoring signals:
  - Loss of neuromonitoring signals should be dealt with in a protocolized fashion, similar to other neurosurgical procedures.
    - Ensure all neuromonitoring needles are in proper positions.
    - Examine any use of anesthetic agents that may affect signals.
    - Blood pressure should be noted and augmented if appropriate.
    - If the signal loss occurs after carotid clamping, release the carotid clamp. The CTA of the head and neck should be studied prior to the procedure to ensure sufficient collateral circulation to tolerate cross-clamping.
    - Perform angiographic runs to rule out intracranial occlusion.
  - Insufficient active flow reversal:
    - If the angiographic run demonstrates insufficient flow reversal, deployment of distal embolic protection device can be considered prior to proceeding to the next steps.
  - Flow reversal intolerance:
    - Intolerance of flow reversal occurs in about 1 to 2% of patients.[8] Definition of intolerance includes changes in neuromonitoring signals or hemodynamic instability.
  - In MAC or local anesthesia, intolerance also includes altered level of consciousness, change in neurologic examination, as well as reported symptoms of shortness of breath and dizziness, among others.
  - In one study, intolerance of flow reversal occurred in 8 out of 297 patients who underwent TCAR under MAC/local anesthetics.[8] Four of these patients were able to complete the case by changing flow reversal from high to low, and one had to be converted

to GA. The authors found no association between flow reversal and tandem stenoses, prior stroke, hostile neck, or prior procedure. However, there was a trend toward significance with COPD and contralateral carotid occlusion.
  - If there is evidence of flow reversal intolerance, the following actions should be considered:
    - Changing flow reversal setting from high to low.
    - Conversion to GA if the case is done under local anesthesia/MAC.
    - Blood pressure elevation for hypotensive patients or if intraprocedural BP is much lower than the preoperative baseline BP.
    - Increase oxygenation.
    - Complete the procedure in an expedient fashion.
  - If the above methods do not reverse the evidence of flow reversal intolerance, the procedure should be aborted.
  - Asystole during balloon angioplasty.
    - Asystole or extreme bradycardia can occur not uncommonly during balloon angioplasty due to stretching of the carotid baroreceptors. This reaction is typically short-lived and resolves when the balloon is deflated. Pretreatment with atropine is typically used at our institution. A Zoll pad may also be placed prior to the start of the procedure. During bradycardia or asystole, it is important to remind the anesthesiologist not to overreact as the episode will typically self-resolve.

23.7.2 Complications after Execution

- Postoperative neck hematoma:
  - At our institution, the patient is typically reversed with protamine prior to closing to reduce the incidence of postoperative hematoma. Because the TCAR incision is just above the clavicle and much more inferior in the neck compared to the incision for CEA, local hematoma from TCAR causing respiratory compromise or swallowing issues is relatively rare. When respiratory or swallowing symptoms occur, they are most commonly associated with intubation or manipulation of the vagus nerve, rather than a local hematoma. Nevertheless, if the postoperative hematoma becomes symptomatic, it should be evacuated promptly.
- Cranial nerve injury:
  - In a multi-institutional study, TCAR is associated with a lower risk of cranial nerve injury compared to CEA (0.3 vs. 3.8%, $p = 0.01$).[7] Cranial nerve injury specifically refers to vagus nerve injury due to its course in relation to CCA. In this study, vagus nerve injury resulting in hoarseness was reported in 1 out of 103 TCAR cases. This resolved within 6 months without intervention.
  - In our experience, hoarseness that resolves within 1 to 2 days following the procedure is typically attributable to irritation from the ETT and requires no intervention. A short course of steroids can be considered if difficulty swallowing is concomitantly reported. If hoarseness persists, a direct laryngoscopy can be considered to diagnose an underlying vagus nerve injury. Other complaints may include voice change or difficulty swallowing. Our institutional experience is similar to what is reported in that all cases resolved within 6 months without intervention.
- Worsened neurological status or postoperative stroke:
  - The stroke rates following TCAR are similar to CEA at 30 days (1.0 vs. 1.1%) and 12 months (2.8 vs. 3.0%) postoperatively.[7] All strokes in the TCAR group that occurred within 30 days were in symptomatic patients. In symptomatic patients, neurological deficits following an otherwise uncomplicated procedure may manifest in a recrudescence of prior stroke symptoms. These cases can typically be managed by blood pressure augmentation, although evidence for exact blood pressure guideline in these circumstances is lacking. In practice, we typically augment systolic blood pressure by 10 to 20% from the baseline at which recrudescence of prior symptoms occurs. An MRI of the brain without contrast should be performed to rule out new infarcts.

References

[1] Petty GW, Brown RD, Jr, Whisnant JP, Sicks JD, O'Fallon WM, Wiebers DO. Ischemic stroke subtypes: a population-based study of incidence and risk factors. Stroke. 1999; 30(12): 2513–2516

[2] Clinical alert: benefit of carotid endarterectomy for patients with high-grade stenosis of the internal carotid artery. National Institute of Neurological Disorders and Stroke Stroke and Trauma Division. North American Symptomatic Carotid Endarterectomy Trial (NASCET) investigators. Stroke. 1991; 22(6):816–817

[3] Mayberg MR, Wilson SE, Yatsu F, et al. Carotid endarterectomy and prevention of cerebral ischemia in symptomatic carotid stenosis. Veterans Affairs Cooperative Studies Program 309 Trialist Group. JAMA. 1991; 266(23):3289–3294

[4] Rothwell PM, Eliasziw M, Gutnikov SA, et al. Carotid Endarterectomy Trialists' Collaboration. Analysis of pooled data from the randomised controlled trials of endarterectomy for symptomatic carotid stenosis. Lancet. 2003; 361(9352):107–116

[5] Naylor AR, Ricco JB, de Borst GJ, et al. Esvs Guidelines Committee. Esvs Guideline Reviewers. Editor's Choice: Management of atherosclerotic carotid and vertebral artery disease—2017 Clinical Practice Guidelines of the European Society for Vascular Surgery (ESVS). Eur J Vasc Endovasc Surg. 2018; 55(1):3–81

[6] Malas MB, Dakour-Aridi H, Wang GJ, et al. Transcarotid artery revascularization versus transfemoral carotid artery stenting in the Society for Vascular Surgery Vascular Quality Initiative. J Vasc Surg. 2019; 69(1):92–103.e2

[7] Kashyap VS, King AH, Foteh MI, et al. A multi-institutional analysis of transcarotid artery revascularization compared to carotid endarterectomy. J Vasc Surg. 2019; 70(1):123–129

[8] Teter K, Rockman C, Lamparello P, et al. Risk factors for and intraoperative management of intolerance to flow reversal in TCAR. Ann Vasc Surg. 2022; 79:41–45

[9] FDA. ENROUTE Transcarotid Stent System – P140026/S016. FDA. 2023. Accessed April 23, 2025 at: https://www.fda.gov/medical-devices/recently-approved-devices/enroute-transcarotid-stent-system-p140026s016

[10] Kwolek CJ, Jaff MR, Leal JI, et al. Results of the ROADSTER multicenter trial of transcarotid stenting with dynamic flow reversal. J Vasc Surg. 2015; 62(5):1227–1234

[11] Kashyap VS, Schneider PA, Foteh M, et al. ROADSTER 2 Investigators*. Early Outcomes in the ROADSTER 2 study of transcarotid artery revascularization in patients with significant carotid artery disease. Stroke. 2020; 51(9):2620–2629

[12] Kashyap VS, So KL, Schneider PA, et al. One-year outcomes after transcarotid artery revascularization (TCAR) in the ROADSTER 2 trial. J Vasc Surg. 2022; 76(2):466–473.e1

[13] National Library of Medicine. Post-approval Study of Transcarotid Artery Revascularization in Standard Risk Patients With Significant Carotid Artery Disease. ClinicalTrials.gov. 2023. Accessed April 23, 2025 at: https://clinicaltrials.gov/ct2/show/NCT05365490

[14] Endarterectomy for asymptomatic carotid artery stenosis. Executive Committee for the Asymptomatic Carotid Atherosclerosis Study. JAMA. 1995; 273(18):1421–1428

[15] Halliday AW, Thomas D, Mansfield A, Steering Committee. The Asymptomatic Carotid Surgery Trial (ACST). Rationale and design. Eur J Vasc Surg. 1994; 8(6):703–710

[16] Wang SK, Motaganahalli RL. Anesthetic considerations in transcarotid artery revascularization. Semin Vasc Surg. 2020; 33(1–2):10–15

Part III

Peripheral Nerve Surgery

III

24 Supraclavicular Brachial Plexus Exposure

Kitty Y. Wu, Robert J. Spinner, and Alexander Shin

24.1 Background

- The supraclavicular brachial plexus includes the intradural roots, spinal nerves, and trunks, While the retroclavicular space includes the divisions. The subclavian artery and vein are positioned near the plexus and the first rib. The subclavian artery is found within the interscalene triangle (between the anterior and middle scalene muscles), while the vein is anterior to the anterior scalene muscle. The exposure of the supraclavicular brachial plexus is challenging even in the best situations. This becomes even more difficult when the anatomy is altered by anatomical variations or postinjury scarring.
- High-speed injuries such as motorcycle or motor vehicle accidents are associated with supraclavicular brachial plexus injuries. In contrast, lower-velocity injuries, commonly from falls, result in infraclavicular injuries and are often associated with shoulder fractures or dislocation.
- Upper plexus or pan-plexus injuries are the most common injury patterns and can lead to postganglionic (neuromas-in-continuity or ruptures outside the spinal canal) injuries and preganglionic (within the spinal canal) avulsions.
- Entrapments tend to affect the lower plexal elements, particularly the C8–T1 roots and the lower trunk, at the level of the scalene muscles. This can be associated with bony abnormalities, such as a cervical rib or elongated C7 transverse process.

24.2 Indications and Contraindications

- Exposure to the supraclavicular brachial plexus is performed for the treatment of patients with peripheral nerve injuries, tumors, and entrapments.
- This may be done either alone or in conjunction with distal exposures of the brachial plexus (retroclavicular, infraclavicular, axillary, and arm regions).
- Patients who are demonstrating spontaneous clinical recovery should be managed expectantly without surgical intervention.
- The rare patient who is medically unable to tolerate general anesthesia or adhere to postoperative instructions or therapy protocols would be contraindicated for surgery.

24.3 Instruments

- Intraoperative handheld nerve stimulator.
- Vessel loops.
- Microsurgical instruments if nerve reconstruction is necessary.

24.4 Patient Preparation

- Comprehensive clinical examination.
- Clavicle, shoulder, or other upper extremity radiographs in cases of associated orthopaedic injuries.
- Chest X-ray to rule out diaphragmatic elevation.
- Computed tomography (CT)/magnetic resonance (MR) angiography in cases of suspected vascular injury.
- CT myelogram or high-resolution brachial plexus/cervical MRI.
- Nerve conduction and needle electromyography studies.

24.5 Patient Positioning

- The patient is positioned supine with the neck rotated to the contralateral side. A bump is placed between the scapulae to protract the shoulder, and the head is gently extended.
- A modified beach chair position further allows for improved exposure. The endotracheal tube is secured facing the contralateral side.

24.6 Technique

- Total inhaled IV anesthesia is utilized, with the addition of intraoperative neurophysiology including motor or somatosensory evoked potentials to aid in decision-making.

- Once intraoperative testing is complete, patients are placed under a general anesthetic.
- Paralytics are avoided to allow for intraoperative nerve stimulation of viable nerves when present.
- The neck, chest, and entire limb (and often both legs in anticipation of autologous nerve graft harvest) are prepped and draped (**Video 24.1**).
- A transverse incision 2 to 3 cm above the clavicle along a Langer's line, crossing the sternocleidomastoid toward the trapezius muscles, is made (▶ Fig. 24.1).
  - If desired or required, an oblique incision following the posterior aspect of the sternocleidomastoid from the mid-neck to the medial clavicle can be incorporated with the transverse incision.
  - The oblique or zigzag incisions provide greater exposure but are less cosmetic and often unnecessary.
- The transverse incision is centered on the external jugular vein, which is often visible. Wide subplatysmal flaps are raised cranially and caudally.

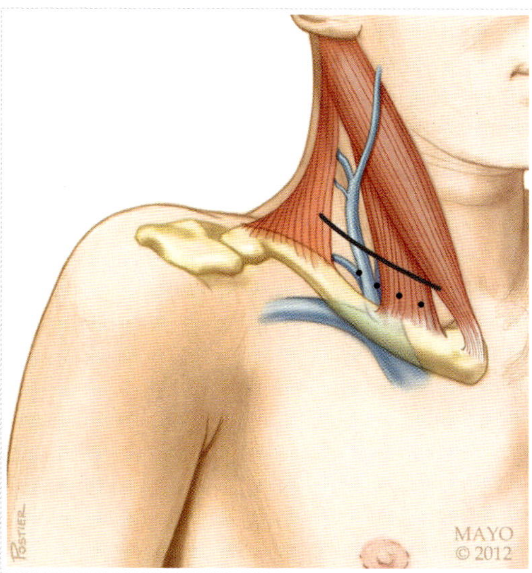

Fig. 24.1 Incision planning. For the majority of brachial plexus explorations and reconstructions, we utilize a transverse incision two to three fingerbreadths above the clavicle crossing the sternocleidomastoid toward the trapezius (*solid line*). For thoracic outlet decompression, we use a shorter incision one to two fingerbreadths above the clavicle (*dotted line*). (Used with permission of Mayo Foundation for Medical Education and Research, all rights reserved.)

- The external jugular vein and cervical plexus nerves are dissected free and protected (▶ Fig. 24.2). The dissection is perpendicular following the cleidal head of the sternocleidomastoid either medial or lateral to the external jugular vein (the vein can also be ligated if necessary) toward the clavicle. The retroclavicular space is exposed.
- The cleidal head of the sternomastoid can be taken down from the clavicle with electrocautery to facilitate medial exposure.
- The omohyoid is identified, and its tendinous bowtie is located. Laterally, it is dissected deep to the clavicle toward the suprascapular ligament. After being mobilized, the omohyoid is divided and tagged with sutures to facilitate retraction and exposure of the retroclavicular space (▶ Fig. 24.3). The fat pad is dissected and mobilized laterally. Some fat can be included in the retractors, which can be readjusted to protect the internal jugular vein.
- The brachial plexus is identified. The upper trunk near its trifurcation is an excellent landmark.
- Just cephalad to the clavicle, the suprascapular nerve (laterally) and the posterior and anterior divisions of the upper trunk can be identified. The mnemonic "S.P.A." can be used to identify the structures from lateral to medial: suprascapular nerve, posterior division, and anterior division of the upper trunk.

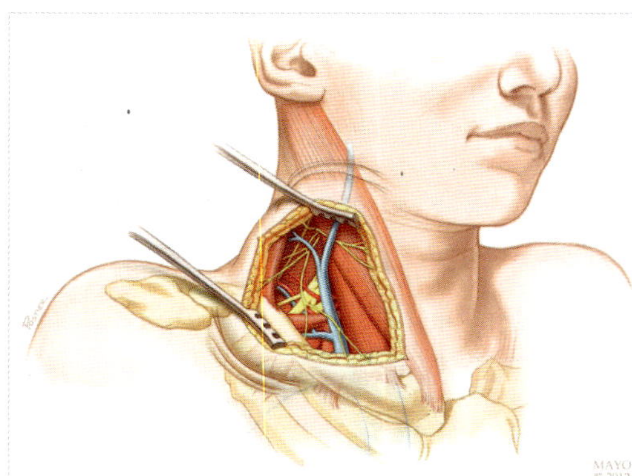

Fig. 24.2 Subplatysmal dissection. After raising subplatysmal flaps superiorly and inferiorly, the external jugular vein and cervical plexus are exposed. (Used with permission of Mayo Foundation for Medical Education and Research, all rights reserved.)

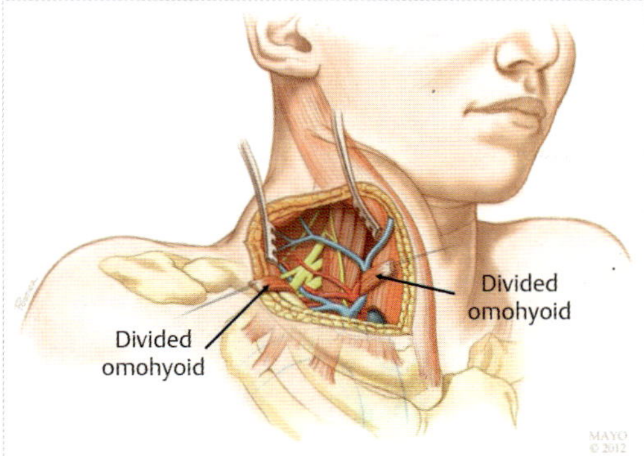

Fig. 24.3 Division of the omohyoid. The omohyoid is dissected medially beyond its tendinous bowtie and laterally toward the suprascapular ligament. It is then divided and tagged with sutures to be used for gentle retraction. (Used with permission of Mayo Foundation for Medical Education and Research, all rights reserved.)

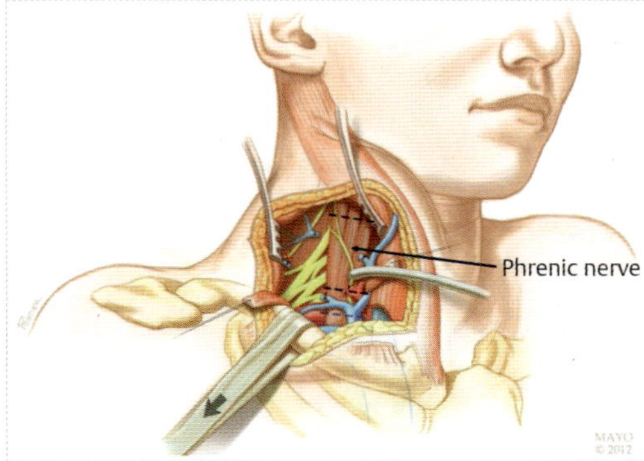

Fig. 24.4 Exposure of the brachial plexus. The phrenic nerve (*arrow*), and its contribution from C5, is identified coursing over the anterior scalene muscle. A portion of the anterior scalene can be resected (*dotted lines*) to allow for proximal exposure. (Used with permission of Mayo Foundation for Medical Education and Research, all rights reserved.)

- Vessel loops placed around each of these nerves can help retract them safely.
- Mobilization of the suprascapular nerve and the divisions is facilitated by dissection deep to the clavicle. The subclavius muscle and crossing suprascapular vessels are divided.
- The clavicle is mobilized by subperiosteal dissection and retracted with an umbilical tape, if necessary.
- The suprascapular nerve is dissected toward the suprascapular ligament (it can be dissected from an infraclavicular or posterior approach as well).
- The long thoracic nerve is seen lateral to the middle scalene. It lies deep to the suprascapular nerve, which in turn lies deep to the omohyoid muscle.
- Proximal dissection with identification of the phrenic nerve and its contribution from C5 (phrenic nerve is innervated by C3, C4, C5) is the next step (▶ Fig. 24.4).
- The phrenic nerve passes obliquely from laterally superiorly to medially inferiorly (as does the small subclavius nerve, which arises from the upper trunk). This is distinct from other nerves run the opposite trajectory.
- Stimulation of the phrenic nerve with a handheld nerve stimulator should result in hemidiaphragmatic contraction if uninjured. Care should be taken when dissecting the anterior scalene as an accessory phrenic nerve is often present.
- The upper trunk is traced to the C5 and C6 nerves. The C5–T1 spinal nerves can be identified. C5 is the most superficial and each of these spinal nerves in sequence is slightly deeper. These nerves can be traced proximally to their respective foramina.
- A portion of anterior scalene can be divided or resected to allow proximal exposure (▶ Fig. 24.4). The dorsal scapular nerve (supplying rhomboid and levator scapulae muscles) may be seen proximally, arising from C5.
- The middle trunk/C7 is then identified lateral to the anterior scalene.
- Exposure of the lower trunk is not routinely performed for adult posttraumatic cases, as the results of reconstruction of these nerves has historically been poor.
- For thoracic outlet syndrome and select tumor cases, exposure of the lower trunk and the C8 and T1 spinal nerves may be necessary.
- When the C8–T1 nerves are exposed, the subclavian artery is identified and mobilized deep to the anterior scalene as necessary, and then protected in a red vessel loop (▶ Fig. 24.5). The thyrocervical trunk is ligated if necessary.

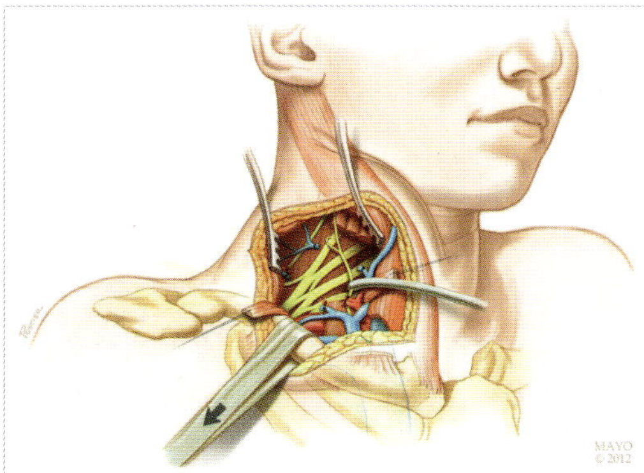

Fig. 24.5 Exposure of the C8–T1 nerve roots. The subclavian artery is mobilized deep to the anterior scalene to aid in exposure of the C8–T1 nerve roots. Care must be taken to avoid injury to the pleura, lymphatics, and thoracic duct (in the left neck) (*Black arrow* indicates direction of retraction). (Used with permission of Mayo Foundation for Medical Education and Research, all rights reserved.)

- The location of the phrenic nerve must be considered with medial dissection. The vertebral artery may also be seen medially.
- When identifying the C8 and T1 roots, care must be taken to avoid injury to the apical lung, lymphatics, and thoracic duct (in the left neck).
- For thoracic outlet decompression, variant bony anatomy such as a cervical rib or elongated transverse process are addressed.
  - Fibers of the middle scalene are divided if they are causing tethering or compression.
  - The first rib may also be removed as needed.
- The spinal accessory nerve(SAN), which is a cranial nerve and not part of the brachial plexus per se, is commonly used as a nerve transfer in brachial plexus reconstructions. It is most easily found just medial to the medial edge of the fascia overlying the anterior edge of the trapezius.
- The SAN is traced as distally as possible (to facilitate reach to recipient nerve) while preserving the proximal branch to the trapezius.
- Superficial supraclavicular nerves may be seen in this location, but they will not produce robust trapezius muscle contraction when stimulated.
- The spinal accessory nerve can also be identified more cranially, in the posterior triangle of the neck, approximately 1.5 cm superior to the great auricular nerve as it passes through or deep to the sternocleidomastoid muscle.
- For distal dissection, one must follow the spinal accessory nerve through vascular lymphoid tissue, which should be controlled with bipolar cautery.

24.7 Postoperative Care

- Postoperative care is dictated by the subsequent nerve repair methods that are employed based on the results of intraoperative exploration. Often, patients are placed in a shoulder immobilizer to allow for soft tissue rest and protection of the nerve grafts or repairs for 3 weeks. Patients are then able to start gentle range of motion while waiting for reinnervation. Directed physical therapy may also be helpful to assist with relearning when motor recovery starts.

24.8 Complications

- Vascular injury to the external jugular vein and subclavian and axillary arteries/veins.
- Lymphatic injury and lymphocele (especially with left-sided supraclavicular dissection).
- Iatrogenic phrenic nerve injury.
- Pneumothorax.

24.9 Management Pearls

- In cases of dense scar or nerve ruptures, a few tricks may be helpful (▶ Fig. 24.6).
- We prefer dissection lateral to the anterior scalene muscle as described. Dissection medial to the phrenic nerve can be done to identify C5, and the C5 nerve stump can be transposed anterior to the phrenic nerve.[1]
- Dissection of the long thoracic nerve (C5–C7) from its identification lateral to the medial scalene can also be done proximally to identify the undersurface of the C6 spinal nerve, in cases of rupture.
- A handheld Doppler ultrasound can be used intraoperatively to map the subclavian artery in severely scarred fields.

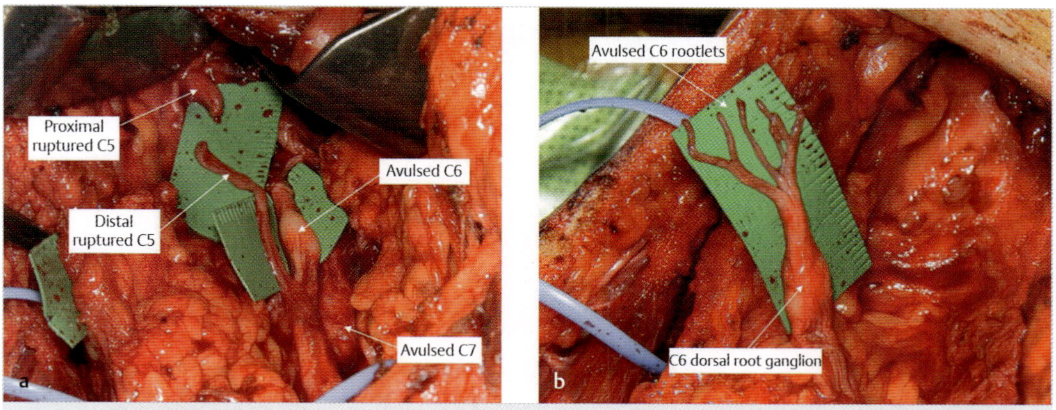

Fig. 24.6 Illustrative case. A 20-year-old man sustained a traumatic left pan-brachial plexus injury following a motor vehicle accident. Supraclavicular exploration demonstrated **(a)** avulsion of the phrenic nerve, postganglionic rupture of the C5, and **(b)** preganglionic avulsion of C6 and C7 with visualization of the C6 rootlets and dorsal root ganglion (B). Proximal = left/superior; distal = right/inferior.

- Clavicular osteotomy is rarely used in traumatic brachial plexus injuries but may be necessary in cases of malignant peripheral nerve sheath tumors in this region.

Reference

[1] Hinchcliff KM, Bishop AT, Shin AY, Spinner RJ. Relocating the C5 nerve stump in C5 nerve grafting to prevent iatrogenic phrenic nerve injury. Acta Neurochir (Wien). 2021; 163(3):829–834

25 Infraclavicular Brachial Plexus Exposure

Kitty Y. Wu, Robert J. Spinner, and Alexander Shin

25.1 Background

- Understanding the surgical exposure to the infraclavicular brachial plexus is important for the management of peripheral nerve injuries and tumors. This can be performed independently or in conjunction with exposure of the brachial plexus in the supraclavicular fossa, the retroclavicular region, or the axilla and proximal arm.
- With ruptured or avulsed supraclavicular injuries, retracted distal targets may be easier to be identified in the infraclavicular region. Additionally, identifying nerves in an unscarred, undistorted area can in turn facilitate accurate target identification.
- The infraclavicular brachial plexus encompasses the divisions, cords, and terminal branches of the brachial plexus and the axillary artery.
- Usually, the exposure of the infraclavicular brachial plexus is fairly straightforward and quick; however, in the cases where there is scarring from previous surgery or injury, this can become quite challenging.

25.2 Indications and Contraindications

- The infraclavicular brachial plexus may need to be exposed in cases of patients with obstetric, traumatic, or iatrogenic brachial plexus injuries that are not demonstrating adequate spontaneous recovery to allow for functional recovery.
- Similarly, patients with malignant or benign peripheral nerve or soft tissue tumors in this anatomical region may need a similar exposure to ensure the infraclavicular brachial plexus is identified and protected during tumor resection.
- Patients who are demonstrating spontaneous clinical recovery should be managed expectantly without surgical intervention.
- Patients who are medically unable to tolerate general anesthesia or unable to adhere to postoperative instructions or therapy protocols are contraindicated from undergoing this procedure.

25.3 Instruments

- Intraoperative handheld nerve stimulator.
- Vessel loops.
- Microsurgical instruments if nerve reconstruction is necessary.

25.4 Patient Preparation

- Comprehensive clinical examination.
- Clavicle, shoulder, or other upper extremity radiographs in cases of associated orthopedic injuries.
- Chest X-ray for rule out diaphragmatic elevation.
- Computed tomography (CT) or magnetic resonance (MR) angiography in cases of suspected vascular injury.
- CT myelogram or brachial plexus/cervical MRI for assessment of root avulsions.
- Nerve conduction and needle electromyography studies.

25.5 Patient Positioning

- Typically, the patient is positioned supine, and the neck, chest, and the entire limb are prepped and draped in the usual sterile fashion.

25.6 Technique

- Total inhaled IV anesthesia should be used if this is being performed in conjunction with a supraclavicular brachial plexus exploration with the use of motor or somatosensory evoked potentials to aid in intraoperative decision making; otherwise, patients are placed under a general anesthesia (**Video 25.1**).
- An oblique deltopectoral incision is performed from the clavicle to a point anterior to the axilla, centered upon or slightly medial to the coracoid process.
  - The incision can be made on its own or incorporated into a longer incision crossing the clavicle for a combined exposure of the supraclavicular plexus (as a T or zigzag) or one extending into the arm (▸ Fig. 25.1).

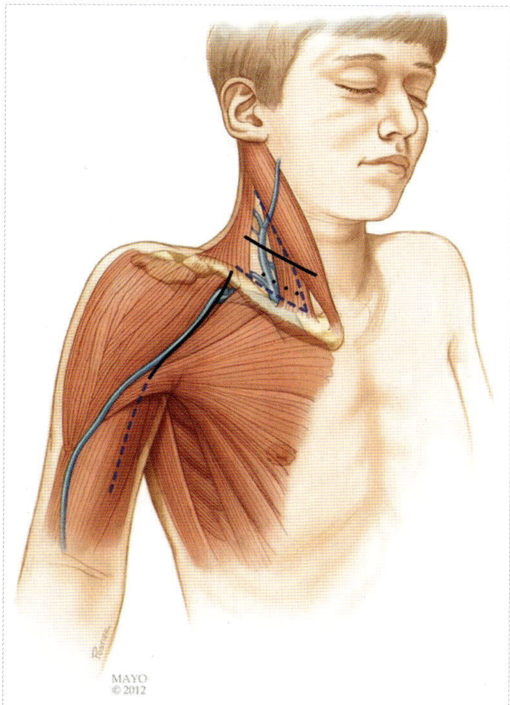

Fig. 25.1 Incision planning. A deltopectoral incision is marked out overlying the cephalic vein (*solid black line*). This can be incorporated into a separate or a longer incision for combined exposure of the supraclavicular plexus (*dashed lines*). (Used with permission of Mayo Foundation for Medical Education and Research, all rights reserved.)

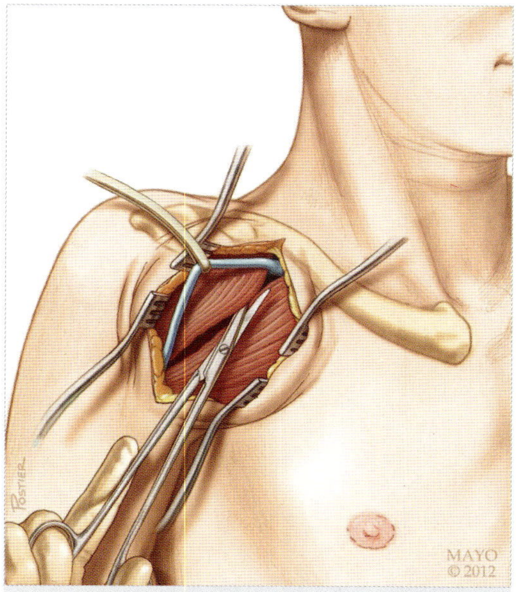

Fig. 25.2 Deltopectoral dissection. The cephalic vein is identified and retracted laterally to allow for dissection between the deltoid and pectoralis major. (Used with permission of Mayo Foundation for Medical Education and Research, all rights reserved.)

- The deltopectoral interval is then deepened and the cephalic vein is identified. The cephalic vein is mobilized laterally (our preference) or medially, and the interval between the deltoid (laterally) and the pectoralis major (medially) is developed (▶ Fig. 25.2).
- The pectoralis minor is seen arising from the ribs and inserting into the coracoid process.
- The conjoined tendon (comprised the coracobrachialis more medially and the short head of the biceps laterally) attaches into the coracoid more caudally.
- The pectoralis minor is defined and mobilized and a finger is passed beneath it (▶ Fig. 25.3).
- Stay sutures are placed in the pectoralis minor and it is released at its tendinous insertion while protecting the brachial plexus beneath.
- Deeper retractors are placed to reflect the pectoralis minor muscle.
    - Care is taken to avoid placement of the teeth of the retractor laterally deep to the coracoid.
    - The fat pad over the neurovascular elements is swept away with a wet sponge and retracted.
- The infraclavicular brachial plexus can now be exposed and starts with sequentially exposing parts of and then identification of the entire "M" of the more superficial aspect of the infraclavicular brachial plexus (▶ Fig. 25.4).

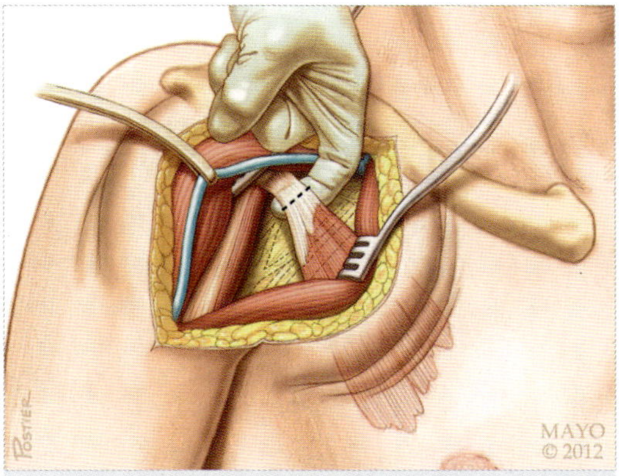

Fig. 25.3 Mobilization of pectoralis minor. The pectoralis minor tendon is seen inserting onto the coracoid. Stay sutures can be placed and then the pectoralis minor tendon released at its tendinous insertion (*dotted line*) while protecting the brachial plexus underneath. (Used with permission of Mayo Foundation for Medical Education and Research, all rights reserved.)

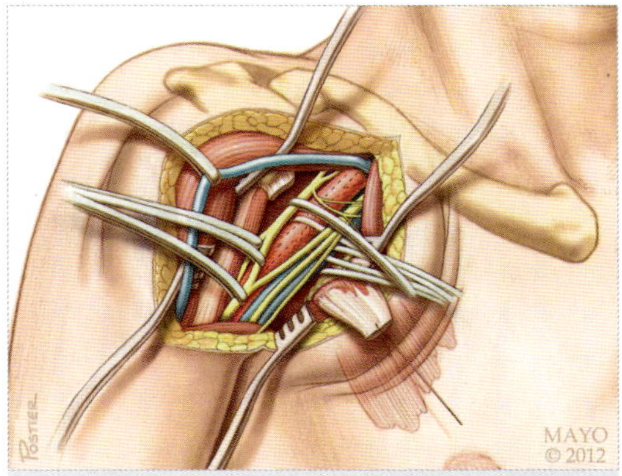

Fig. 25.4 Exposure of medial and lateral cord. The infraclavicular plexus can then be exposed including the medial and lateral cords, so named given their relationship to the axillary artery. (Used with permission of Mayo Foundation for Medical Education and Research, all rights reserved.)

- The lateral cord is first encountered. Medially to it, the axillary artery can be palpated and protected.
  - We use (colored) vessel loops (blue for nerves and red for vessels) for easy identification of these structures and to provide gentle retraction.
- The lateral cord is traced distally to identify its lateral cord contribution to the median nerve and the musculocutaneous nerve (present in about 90% of cases in this location but arising more distally in the arm in 10% of cases).
- A handheld nerve stimulator is used to confirm the anatomy (if possible) and gauge the extent of the pathology; more sophisticated intraoperative neurophysiology can be used after the pathology has been fully displayed.
- The median nerve is then identified, which lies just anterior to the axillary artery.
- The medial cord and the ulnar nerve may be identified as necessary. The upper portion of the pectoralis major insertion may be released as needed to help with better exposure distally.
- For exposure of the posterior cord and its branches (axillary and radial nerves), identification of the axillary artery is imperative.
- The posterior cord is superoposterior to the axillary artery proximally and lateral more distally. The plane of dissection is lateral to the lateral cord (▶ Fig. 25.5).
- The axillary nerve is smaller and lateral compared to the radial nerve.
  - Proximal branches to the triceps often originate from the radial nerve but may also be seen branching off the axillary or ulnar nerves.
  - The axillary nerve can be traced into the quadrilateral space.
  - During the deep exposure of the axillary nerve, the more superficial branches to the musculocutaneous (and coracobrachialis) nerves, which may be out of the field, need to be protected.
- A separate posterior approach may be necessary for reconstruction of the axillary nerve, and if needed preoperatively, placing a bump under the shoulder helps to facilitates the posterior approach.
- For exposure in the retroclavicular space, the clavicle should be exposed. Retraction superiorly

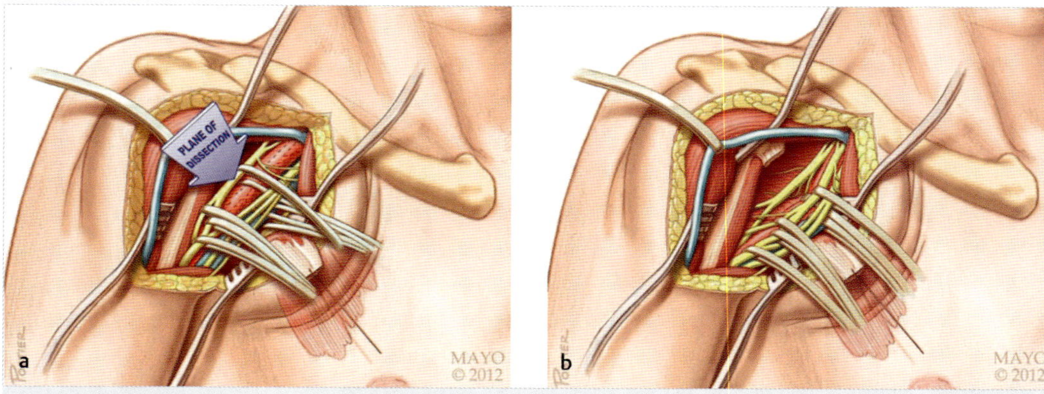

Fig. 25.5 Exposure of the posterior cord. **(a)** The posterior cord is identified by dissection in a plane lateral to the lateral cord. **(b)** The other elements of the brachial plexus are retracted medially to allow for exposure of the posterior cord. The axillary nerve is smaller and lateral to the radial nerve. (Used with permission of Mayo Foundation for Medical Education and Research, all rights reserved.)

(or inferiorly) often opens the retroclavicular space sufficiently.

- The subclavius fascia and muscle are divided, and the cords can be traced proximally.
- The ansa pectoralis (arising from divisions) is noted.
- By the medial pectoral nerve, the thoracoacromial trunk (used as a recipient artery for free functioning muscle transfer) is identified and protected. Other nerves and branches, including the suprascapular nerve, can be dissected as necessary.
- The suprascapular nerve can be identified passing obliquely toward the suprascapular ligament at the level of the coracoid. We have only used clavicular osteotomy in cases of malignant peripheral nerve sheath tumors in this region, as clavicular osteotomy is not necessary for the majority of traumatic brachial plexus reconstruction.
- If the clavicle needs to be osteotomized, a preplaced low contour clavicle plate should be applied prior to osteotomy to facilitate anatomical repair.

25.7 Postoperative Care

- Postoperative care is dictated by the subsequent nerve repair methods that are employed based on the results of intraoperative exploration.
- Often, patients are placed in a shoulder immobilizer to allow for soft tissue rest and protection of the nerve grafts or repairs for 3 weeks.
- Patients are them able to start gentle range of motion while waiting for reinnervation.
- Physical therapy may be indicated when muscle recovery is noted as part of the relearning process.

25.8 Complications

- Vascular injury to the subclavian, brachial, or axillary vessels or hematoma.

25.9 Management Pearls

- In cases of a dense scar, a few tricks may be helpful.
- Finding the cephalic vein and the deltopectoral interval may be done more readily near clavicle in the deltopectoral triangle.
- The clavicle can be further exposed by detaching some of the clavicular head of the pectoralis major fibers.
  - A muscle splitting approach through the pectoralis major can be done. Taking down the entire pectoralis major insertion or the conjoined tendon origin may allow for a safer dissection, especially in cases of prior vascular surgery and bypass grafting.

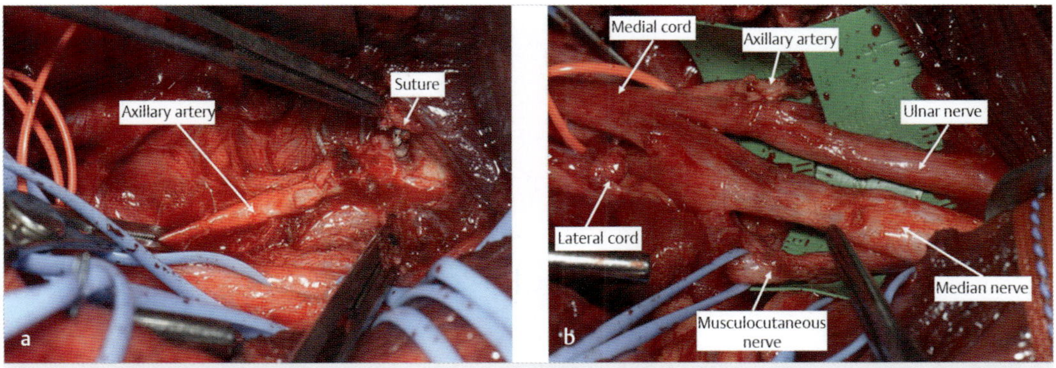

Fig. 25.6 Illustrative case. A 21-year-old woman with an iatrogenic infraclavicular brachial plexus and axillary artery injury following left shoulder dislocation and subscapularis tendon reconstruction with capsular tightening. **(a)** Suture material is seen ligating the axillary artery and elements of the infraclavicular brachial plexus. **(b)** There was dense scarring and nonconducting neuromas-in-continuity of all terminal branches (probe). Reconstruction was performed with autologous cable grafting over a 7-cm segment in the lateral and medial cord contributions to the median nerve, in addition to the median, musculocutaneous, axillary, radial, and ulnar nerves and interposition saphenous vein grafting of the axillary artery. Proximal = left; distal = right.

  - The pectoralis major muscle or conjoined tendon should be tagged and repaired at the end of the case with nonabsorbable sutures.
- An intraoperative Doppler can be used to map the course of the artery or vascular graft (▶ Fig. 25.6).
- While some surgeons use a transaxillary approach for thoracic outlet surgery, we tend to use it only for small superficial tumors in the axilla. While this is a well-hidden and a cosmetic incision, it provides limited exposure that is not amenable to most reconstructive cases.

26 Ulnar Nerve Compression at the Elbow

Brynn Alison Hathaway, Rachael M. Payne, Benjamin Harris Timmins, and Susan E. Mackinnon

26.1 Background

- The ulnar nerve arises from the medial cord of the brachial plexus, running posteromedial to the brachial artery in the upper medial arm.
- It then pierces the medial intermuscular septum and travels between this and the medial head of the triceps.[1] The arcade of Struthers is formed by a confluence of the brachial fascia (BF), internal brachial ligament (IBL), and medial intermuscular septum (MIS) approximately 8 cm proximal to the medial epicondyle.[2]
- In our opinion, the presence of the IBL below the ulnar nerve is the prerequisite component necessary to make the "arcade of Struthers" clinically significant.
- As the nerve travels distally toward the elbow, it passes into the fibro-osseous cubital tunnel posterior to the medial epicondyle and medial to the olecranon.[1] An anomalous anconeus epitrochlearis is estimated to be present in 3 to 34% of the population and can cause compression at the elbow.[3]
- After passing through the cubital tunnel, the nerve travels deep into the forearm between the two heads of the flexor carpi ulnaris (FCU) muscle. The fascia between the FCU heads, also known as Osbourne's ligament,[4] is a compression site.
- A distal MIS is the frequent site of compression if the nerve is transposed and we excise this septum to prevent that problem.
- As the nerve traverses between the FCU and the flexor digitorum profundus (FDP) muscles in the forearm, it runs medial to the ulnar artery and gives off motor branches to the FCU and ring and small finger FDP.
- The topography of the ulnar nerve at the elbow from medial to lateral is the FCU, FDP, sensation, and intrinsic muscles.
- The dorsal cutaneous branch exits the ulnar nerve proper in this region roughly 9 cm proximal to the wrist crease.[1]
- The distal ulnar nerve and its associated pathologies are described in another chapter.
- The cubital tunnel is the most common site of ulnar nerve compression and is the second most common compression neuropathy overall.[1,4]
- Common causes of compression at the elbow include prolonged elbow flexion,[5] posttraumatic or postsurgical scarring, and nerve subluxation.[6]
- Less common etiologies include congenital variations such as cubitus valgus, anomalous musculature such as anconeus epitrochlearis, low and prominent medial triceps muscle, or abnormally thick Osborne's fascia.[1]
- Compression at this level typically manifests clinically as numbness in the small and ulnar ring fingers with weakness of the intrinsic muscles of the hand.[7]

26.2 Indications and Contraindications

- Patients with mild cubital tunnel syndrome are treated conservatively with activity modifications, nerve glide exercises, and nocturnal splinting.
- Importantly, patients with classic cubital tunnel syndrome and normal electrodiagnostic studies frequently have weak middle trapezius muscles resulting in increased tension on the lower trunk and ulnar nerve and improve with physical therapy.
- Patients with recalcitrant symptoms, severe disease on nerve conduction studies (NCS), atrophy, or motor weakness should be considered for surgical intervention.
- Contraindications to surgical intervention include poor surgical candidates, those with cervical radiculopathy, thoracic outlet syndrome, or systemic motor/sensory neuropathy.

26.3 Instruments

- Relevant equipment includes a standard hand table, sterile tourniquet, microbipolar electrocautery, Mackinnon tenotomy scissors (Fischer-USA), standard hand surgery tray, pain pump, and suction drain.

26.4 Patient Preparation

- Diagnosis of the severity of cubital tunnel syndrome is based on a combination of factors.
- Symptoms include paresthesia and numbness in the small and ring fingers, aching in the medial aspect of the proximal forearm worsened with repeated elbow flexion, hand weakness, decreased grip strength, clumsiness, and lack of dexterity.
- Examination findings consistent with cubital tunnel syndrome can be identified by inspection, palpation, sensory and motor evaluation, and provocative maneuvers. On inspection, hypothenar wasting and intrinsic atrophy may be noted.
- Nerve subluxation or "perching" can be found by palpating for abnormal movement of the nerve out of the ulnar groove and onto the medial epicondyle during elbow flexion. A positive Tinel sign at the cubital tunnel may also be present.[4]
- Sensation can be measured by static or dynamic two-point discrimination, the Ten Test, or Semmes–Weinstein monofilament tests.[8] The senior author utilizes these tests as well as a standardized pain questionnaire completed at initial evaluation and subsequent postoperative visits to monitor progress (▶ Fig. 26.1).
- Motor weakness can be confirmed with a positive Froment test, Wartenberg sign, or ulnar clawing[9] (see Fig. 30.1 and Fig. 30.2 in Chapter 30).
- Provocative maneuvers such as cubital tunnel compression test and elbow flexion tests have good sensitivity and specificity.[10] The senior author also advocates using the Scratch Collapse Test (SCT) given its high accuracy in detecting compression location.[11,12]

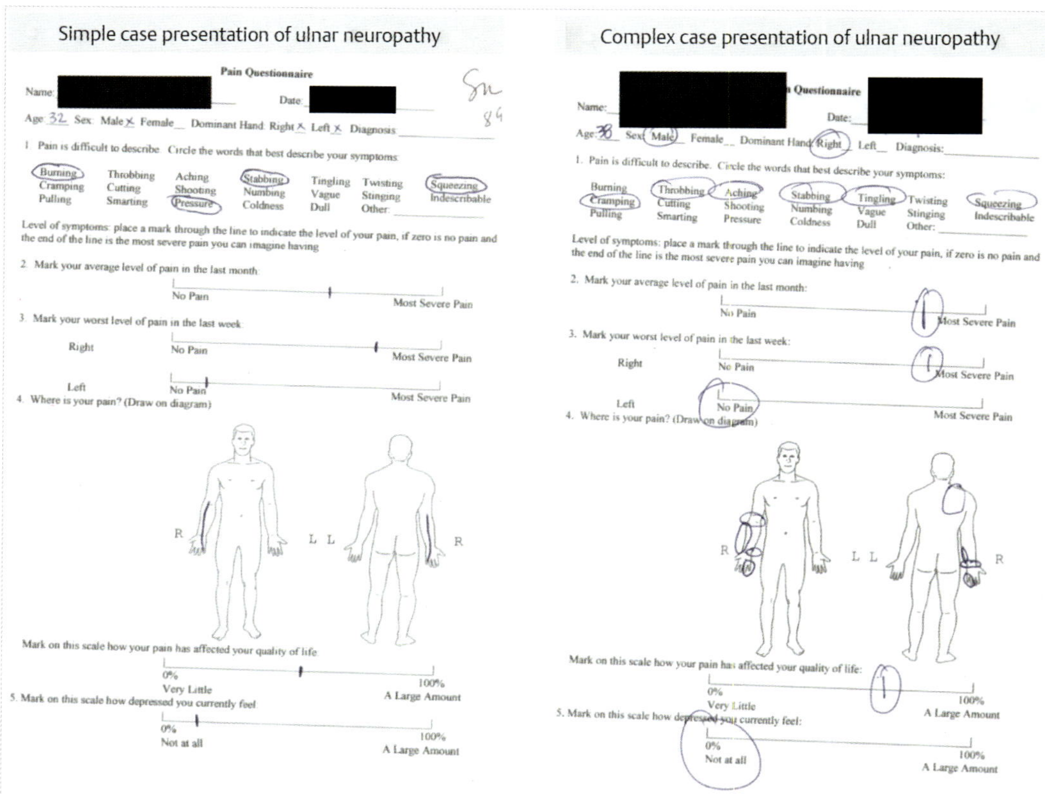

Fig. 26.1 Pain evaluation questionnaire examples for ulnar neuropathy. The questionnaire provides an illustrative view of the patient's perception and description of their pain, and quantifies severity and the effect on their quality of life. The senior author has each patient complete this evaluation at the initial visit and postintervention visits. (Reproduced from Davidge KM, Boyd KU. Ulnar Nerve Entrapment and Injury. In: Mackinnon S, ed. Nerve Surgery. 1st Edition. New York: Thieme; 2015.)

- The SCT can also be used to establish the hierarchy of cubital tunnel, Guyon's canal, arcade of Struthers, and any associated parascapular muscle imbalance.
- NCS and electromyographic (EMG) studies are useful adjuncts to evaluate the level of compression, degree of axonal injury versus demyelination, and progression of ulnar neuropathy. Studies have shown these to be 80 to 96% sensitive for ulnar nerve entrapment at the elbow.[13]
- Understanding the degree of axonal injury and need for (compound muscle action potential [CMAP]) and receptivity to (fibrillations, positive sharp waves [PSWs]) distal muscle target reinnervation is critical in determining if additional procedures such as anterior interosseous nerve (AIN) supercharge end-to-side transfers or adductor digiti minimi (ADM) nerve end-to-side turbocharging are indicated (reduced CMAP) or will be successful (presence of fibrillations, PSWs).[14,15]
- The procedure is performed under general anesthesia.
- We recommend neither pre- nor postoperative brachial plexus blocks be used due to risk of injury to the plexus.
- Intraoperatively, a pain catheter is placed under direct vision and connected to a continuous local anesthetic delivery pump (On-Q or similar pump) until its removal on postoperative day (POD) 2 or 3.

26.5 Patient Positioning

- The patient is positioned supine with their arm on the hand table under a sterile tourniquet.

26.6 Technique

- The medial epicondyle and a point 3.5 cm distal (noting the likely location of a medial antebrachial cutaneous [MABC] nerve branch) are marked for reference.
- The incision is marked along the course of the ulnar nerve posterior to the medial epicondyle (▶ Fig. 26.2).

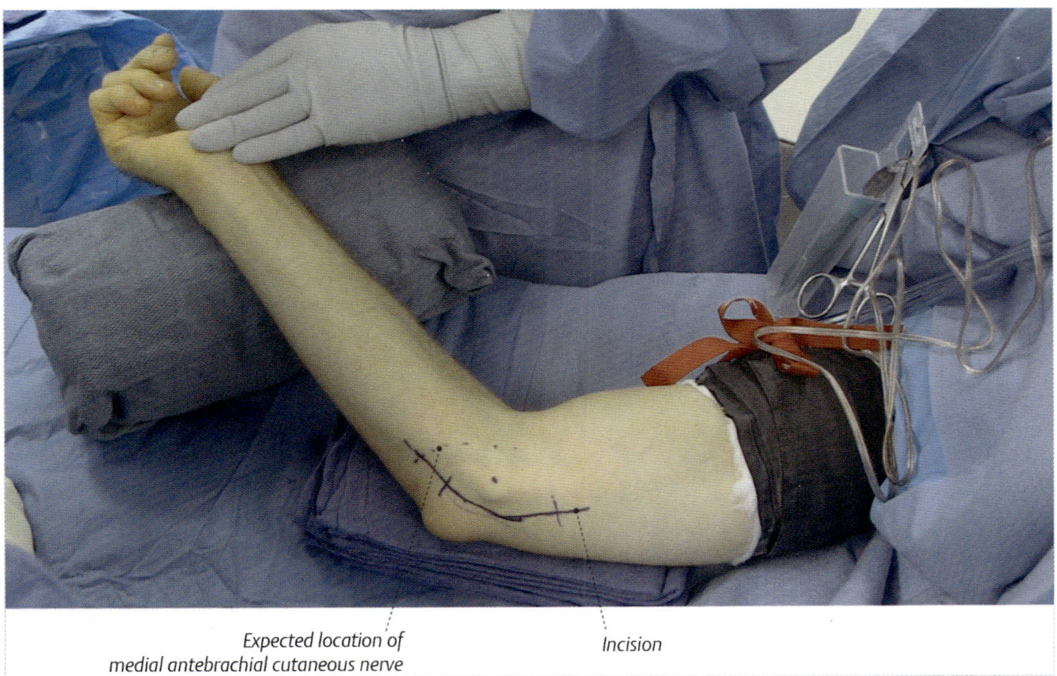

Fig. 26.2 Positioning of the arm and high location of the sterile tourniquet. The skin incision is marked along the course of the ulnar nerve posterior to the medial epicondyle. A mark is placed along this incision 3.5 cm distal to the medial epicondyle corresponding to the likely location of the MABC nerve branch or branches. (Reproduced from Davidge KM, Boyd KU. Ulnar Nerve Entrapment and Injury. In: Mackinnon S, ed. Nerve Surgery. 1st Edition. New York: Thieme; 2015.)

- The skin is incised and blunt dissection is used to identify and protect cutaneous branches superficial to the muscular fascia (▶ Fig. 26.3).
- Proximal to the medial epicondyle, the septum of the medial triceps is palpated to locate the ulnar nerve along its posterior border (▶ Fig. 26.4).
- Using Mackinnon tenotomy scissors, the ulnar nerve is followed distally, and Osbourne's band is opened. The fascia overlying the FCU muscle is incised and its two heads bluntly separated.
- Dissecting on the superficial surface of the nerve, the deep fascia of the FCU can safely be divided. Release of the deep FCU fascia is continued until there is no longer compression of the nerve (▶ Fig. 26.5).
- Returning to the proximal dissection, the septum of the medial triceps is transversely dissected and excised while avoiding injury to deep veins anteriorly.
- The senior author advocates for routine submuscular transposition of the nerve. Skin and soft tissue flaps are raised medially to expose the flexor-pronator fascia, which are then incised to create step-lengthening flaps. A distally based proximal flap can be elevated off the muscle with traction alone, while a proximally based distal flap is elevated sharply.

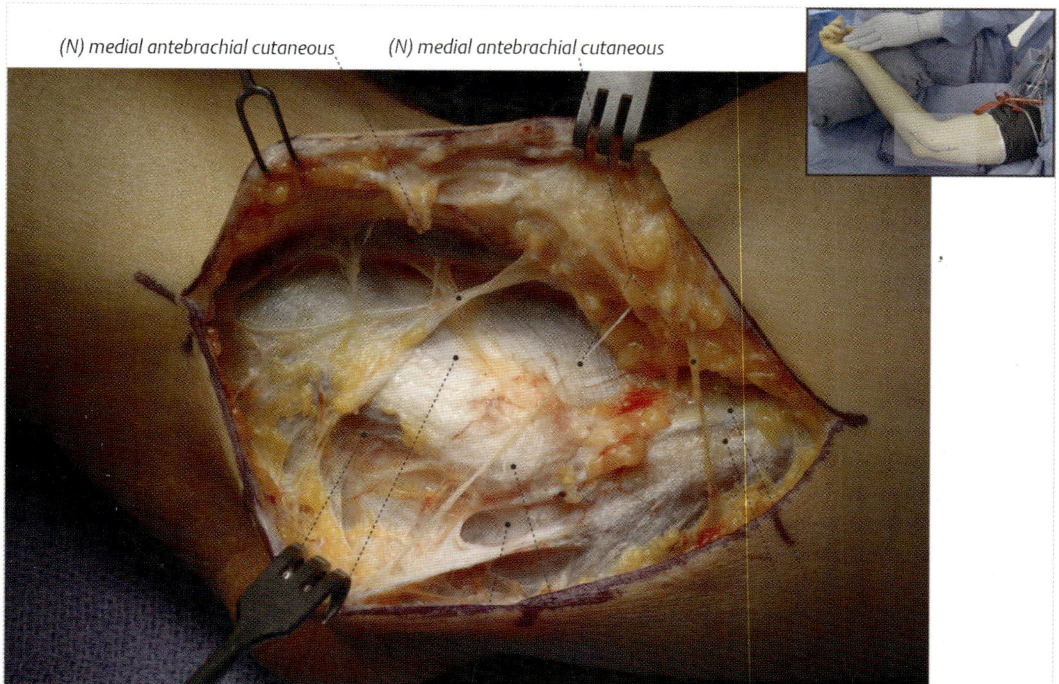

Fig. 26.3 Dissection to the level of the muscular fascia showing branches of the MABC nerve. The main branch can reliably be found 3.5 cm distal to the medial epicondyle. It is important to preserve these branches to decrease the likelihood of a painful post-operative neuroma. (Reproduced from Davidge KM, Boyd KU. Ulnar Nerve Entrapment and Injury. In: Mackinnon S, ed. Nerve Surgery. 1st Edition. New York: Thieme; 2015.)

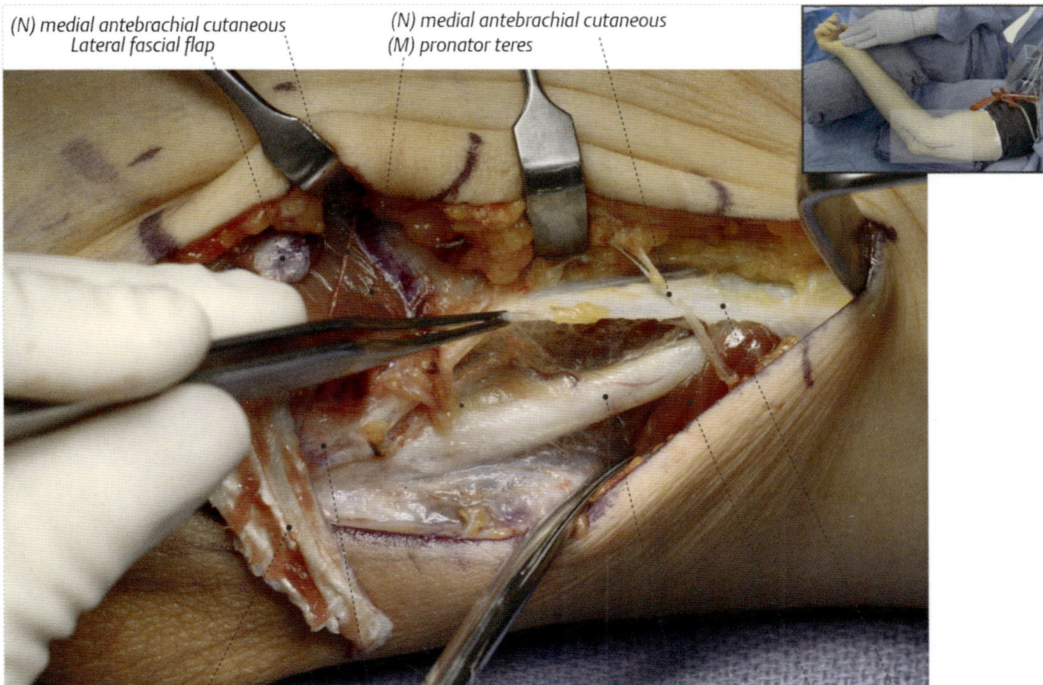

Fig. 26.4 Identification and dissection of the medial intermuscular septum prior to resection. Failure to resect this septum often leads to a pressure point causing compression of the ulnar nerve after transposition. (Reproduced from Davidge KM, Boyd KU. Ulnar Nerve Entrapment and Injury. In: Mackinnon S, ed. Nerve Surgery. 1st Edition. New York: Thieme; 2015.)

- Within the muscle, distal septi between the FCU and flexor-pronator group are excised to prevent additional compression after nerve transposition (▶ Fig. 26.6).
- Proximally, the flexor-pronator complex is released to the level of the brachialis.
- Distally, limited 1-inch flexor-pronator slide is then completed to allow for nerve transposition in a submuscular position. Only after this dissection is complete is the ulnar nerve mobilized and transposed to its new anterior position.
- A neurolysis of the FCU from the ulnar nerve motor branch proximally allows transposition without placing tension on the nerve (▶ Fig. 26.7).
- After transposition, the ulnar nerve's course is inspected to ensure no new points of compression have been created.
- The nerve is then secured in place by closing the step-lengthening flaps very loosely, allowing enough room for at least two fingerbreadths within the sling.
- After the tourniquet is released, palpate proximally to check for an IBL that runs below the nerve in an oblique course and will create a functional arcade of Struthers with the associated MIS and the BF. Prior to final skin

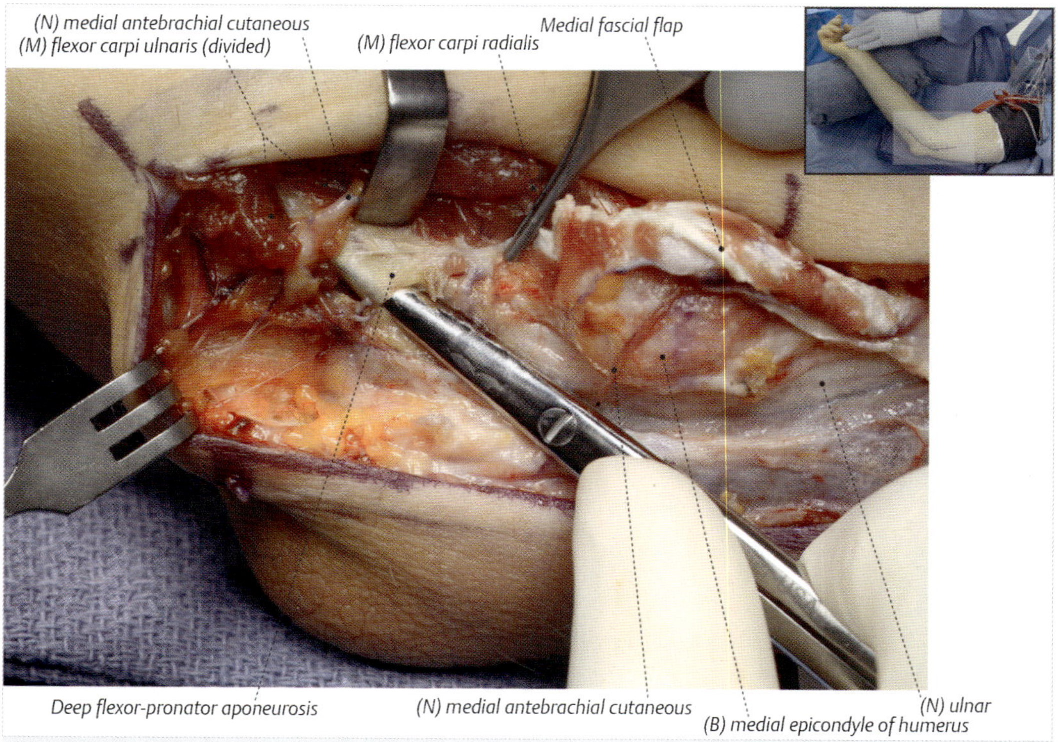

Fig. 26.5 Decompression of the ulnar nerve through Osbourne's band, FCU fascia, and deep fascial of FCU. After dissection it is important to check that there are no further kink points along the course of the nerve once the nerve has been transposed. (Reproduced from Davidge KM, Boyd KU. Ulnar Nerve Entrapment and Injury. In: Mackinnon S, ed. Nerve Surgery. 1st Edition. New York: Thieme; 2015.)

closure, a small surgical drain and pain catheter are placed. See accompanying **Video 26.1**.

26.7 Postoperative Care

- In the senior author's practice, patients are placed in a long arm splint with 45 degrees of elbow flexion and forearm pronation immediately postoperatively. The splint, drain, and pain catheter are removed on POD 2 or 3 and patients are seen by a certified hand therapist. Gentle movement is encouraged to prevent scar tissue from tethering the nerve. The patient may begin strengthening at 1 month postoperatively and is released from all restrictions at 2 months. During postoperative visits, repeat pain questionnaires are collected to evaluate for monitoring recovery and symptom resolution.

26.8 Complications

- General complications include infection, hematoma, bursa, or seroma. Specific complications include nerve injury including MABC, distal kinking with transposition or

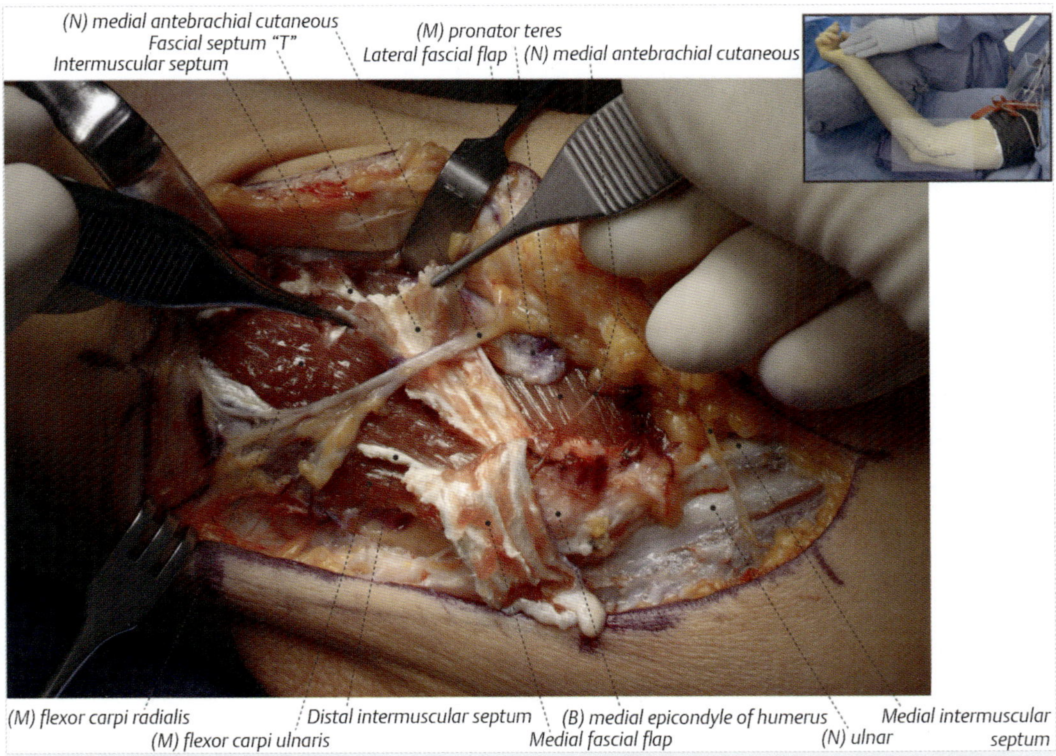

Fig. 26.6 Identification for resection of the "T" intermuscular septum within the flexor-pronator mass. This septum must be resected to avoid creation of new pressure points causing compression of the transposed ulnar nerve. (Reproduced from Davidge KM, Boyd KU. Ulnar Nerve Entrapment and Injury. In: Mackinnon S, ed. Nerve Surgery. 1st Edition. New York: Thieme; 2015.)

release, incomplete decompression and/or persistent or recurrent symptoms.
- Special risks include iatrogenic injury to the MABC nerve.

26.9 Management Pearls

- Ulnar compression neuropathy at the elbow is one of the most common compressive neuropathies of the upper extremity.[1]
- Large meta-analyses have not shown superiority of simple decompression versus transposition in the treatment of cubital tunnel syndrome.[16,17]
- Patient factors, such as etiology, severity, location, and presence of nerve subluxation, and surgeon preference influence the choice of surgical technique.
- Martin-Gruber anastomoses are motor connections between the median and ulnar nerves distal to the medial epicondyle. These anomalous connections have been shown in 15 to 40% of patients undergoing NCS.[1]
- In the senior author's practice, anterior transposition of the ulnar nerve to the submuscular position with flexor pronator slide is routinely performed.

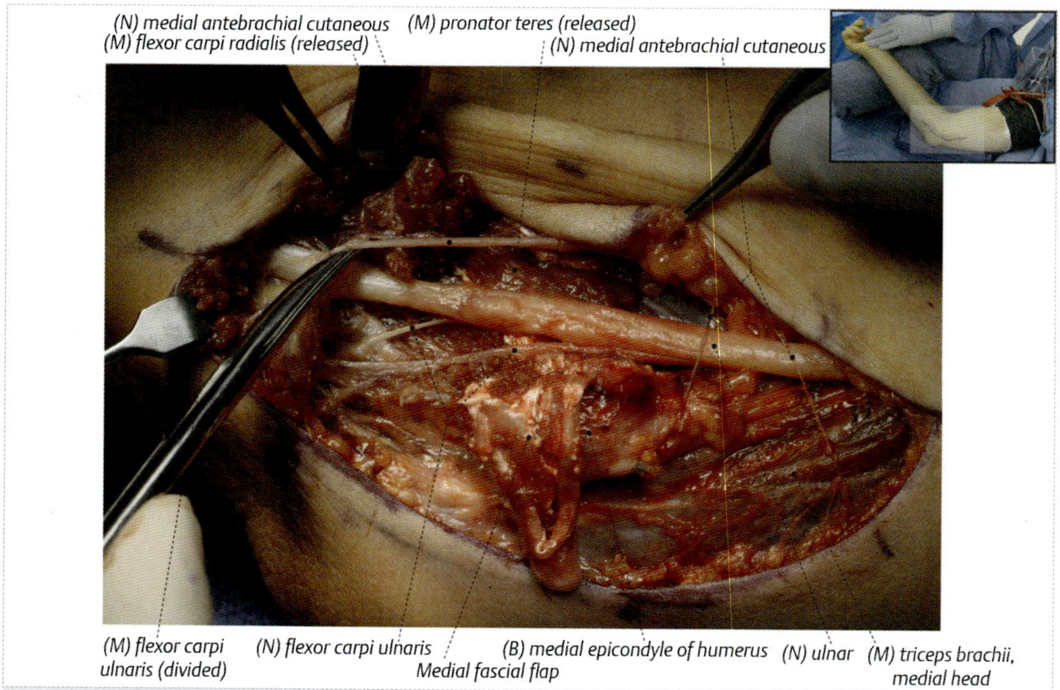

Fig. 26.7 After resection and preparation of for sub muscular transposition the ulnar nerve is mobilized and moved into its transposed position. Neurolysis of the FCU motor branch may be required to allow transposition. The course of the ulnar nerve is rechecked for any points of compression or kinking. (Reproduced from Davidge KM, Boyd KU. Ulnar Nerve Entrapment and Injury. In: Mackinnon S, ed. Nerve Surgery. 1st Edition. New York: Thieme; 2015.)

References

[1] Davidge KM, Boyd KU. Ulnar Nerve Entrapment and Injury. In: Mackinnon SE, ed. Nerve Surgery. 1st ed. New York, NY: Thieme; 2015:251–288

[2] Bezuhly M, O'Brien J, Lalonde D. Nerve entrapment syndromes. In: Neligan P, ed. Plastic Surgery. Vol. 6. Hand and Upper Limb. 3rd ed. London: Elsevier; 2013:503–515

[3] Maslow JI, Johnson DJ, Block JJ, Lee DH, Desai MJ. Prevalence and clinical manifestations of the anconeus epitrochlearis and cubital tunnel syndrome. Hand (N Y). 2020; 15(1):69–74

[4] Patterson JMM, Novak CB, Mackinnon SE. Compression neuropathies. In: Green's Operative Hand Surgery. 8th ed. Philadelphia, PA: Elsevier; 2022:1085–1126

[5] Apfelberg DB, Larson SJ. Dynamic anatomy of the ulnar nerve at the elbow. Plast Reconstr Surg. 1973; 51(1):76–81

[6] Novak CB, Mehdian H, von Schroeder HP. Laxity of the ulnar nerve during elbow flexion and extension. J Hand Surg Am. 2012; 37(6):1163–1167

[7] Becker RE, Manna B. Anatomy, Shoulder and Upper Limb, Ulnar Nerve. Treasure Island, FL: StatPearls Publishing; 2022

[8] Dy CJ, Mackinnon SE. Ulnar neuropathy: evaluation and management. Curr Rev Musculoskelet Med. 2016; 9(2):178–184

[9] Bertelli JA, Tavares KE. Little finger abduction and adduction testing in ulnar nerve lesions. Hand Surg Rehabil. 2018; 37(6):368–371

[10] Novak CB, Lee GW, Mackinnon SE, Lay L. Provocative testing for cubital tunnel syndrome. J Hand Surg Am. 1994; 19(5):817–820

[11] Cheng CJ, Mackinnon-Patterson B, Beck JL, Mackinnon SE. Scratch Collapse Test for evaluation of carpal and cubital tunnel syndrome. J Hand Surg Am. 2008; 33(9):1518–1524

[12] Brown JM, Mokhtee D, Evangelista MS, Mackinnon SE. Scratch Collapse Test localizes Osborne's band as the point of maximal nerve compression in cubital tunnel syndrome. Hand (N Y). 2010; 5(2):141–147

[13] Todnem K, Michler RP, Wader TE, Engstrøm M, Sand T. The impact of extended electrodiagnostic studies in ulnar neuropathy at the elbow. BMC Neurol. 2009; 9:52

[14] Dengler J, Dolen U, Patterson JMM, et al. Supercharge end-to-side anterior interosseous-to-ulnar motor nerve transfer restores intrinsic function in cubital tunnel syndrome. Plast Reconstr Surg. 2020; 146(4):808–818

[15] Davidge KM, Yee A, Moore AM, Mackinnon SE. The supercharge end-to-side anterior interosseous-to-ulnar motor nerve transfer for restoring intrinsic function: clinical experience. Plast Reconstr Surg. 2015; 136(3):344e–352e

[16] Chung KC. Treatment of ulnar nerve compression at the elbow. J Hand Surg Am. 2008; 33(9):1625–1627

[17] Macadam SA, Gandhi R, Bezuhly M, Lefaivre KA. Simple decompression versus anterior subcutaneous and submuscular transposition of the ulnar nerve for cubital tunnel syndrome: a meta-analysis. J Hand Surg Am. 2008; 33(8):1314.e1–1314.e12

27 Median Nerve Decompression at the Proximal Forearm for Pronator and Anterior Interosseous Nerve Syndromes

Oliver Mrowczynski, Sonia S. Majid, Neel Patel, Elias Rizk, and Kimberly Harbaugh

27.1 Background

- The median nerve is lateral to the brachial artery with which it travels in the medial arm. As the nerve approaches the medial elbow, it courses anteriorly below the bicipital aponeurosis and above the brachialis and the brachial artery and passes between the superficial and deep heads of the pronator teres.
- After passing through the pronator teres, the median nerve reaches the deep portion of the flexor digitorum superficialis (FDS), running between the FDS and flexor digitorum profundus (FDP).
- Five to 8 cm from the medial epicondyle and in the region of the FDS arch, the median nerve gives off the anterior interosseous nerve (AIN) on the posterior and radial side.[1]
- The AIN continues to travel in the deep compartment of the arm between the FDP medially and the flexor pollicis longus (FPL) laterally and innervates the FPL, the radial half of the FDP, and the pronator quadratus.
- Pronator syndrome (PS) results from compression or irritation of the median nerve at the elbow region. The inciting cause is typically a dense tendon of the pronator teres or fibrous edge of the FDS. The nerve can also be compressed by the bicipital aponeurosis. Anatomical variants including a supracondylar process with Struthers' ligament or anomalous muscles are less frequent causes.[2,3] Patients have aching in the forearm especially with pronation, numbness in the median distribution including the palm, and variable degrees of weakness in finger flexion.
- PS is generally caused by irritation/compression by tendons in the pronator muscle or the fibrous edge of the FDS with anatomical variants being much less common.
- AIN syndrome results in a pure motor palsy of the FPL, FDP to the index and to a variable degree the middle finger (FDP), and the pronator quadratus without cutaneous sensory symptoms. AIN syndrome occurs most commonly due to Parsonage–Turner syndrome (PTS) but may result from entrapment by fibrous tendon/muscle bands as with PS.[2,3] It can also occur due to compression from trauma, following supracondylar fracture, or due to mass lesions in the area, or arterial thrombus.[4] Examination reveals preservation of sensation but weakness most notably in flexion of the tips of the thumb and the index finger resulting in an inability to produce an "OK sign."
- Typically, AIN palsy patients are observed for a minimum of 3 to 6 months for nerve improvement before considering surgical decompression.

27.2 Indications and Contraindications

- In patients whose evaluation and workup are consistent with PS and who fail conservative therapy with anti-inflammatories, rest, and physical therapy, surgery may be offered.
- For AIN patients, a period of at least 3 to 6 months is usually recommended as most of these are due to PTS and should improve spontaneously. This is particularly important in patients who have a classic presentation with sudden onset of severe pain followed by weakness.
- Contraindications to surgical intervention are a clear diagnosis of PTS with no signs of physical nerve compression, or symptoms/signs of alternative diagnoses such as carpal tunnel syndrome or cervical radiculopathy.

27.3 Instruments

- We use a nerve stimulator and intraoperative neuromonitoring to delineate the median nerve, AIN, and the branches.

27.4 Patient Preparation

- A thorough history and physical examination are critical for initial localization of the median nerve symptoms to the forearm.

- We do not routinely obtain X-rays unless palpation suggests the presence of a supracondylar process.
- Electrodiagnostic studies (EDX) are usually obtained and may be normal in patients with PS but are typically positive in AIN patients. Looking for voluntary motor units is important in AIN patients as their presence suggests continuity and recovery.
- EDX can also exclude other pathologies such as carpal tunnel syndrome and cervical radiculopathy.
- Imaging is usually carried out. We prefer magnetic resonance imaging (MRI) as it allows for detection of denervation myositis, mass lesions, and assessment for compressive bands/ muscles.
  - In our experience, it is less operator dependent than ultrasound, but some find high-definition ultrasound to be very useful.

27.5 Patient Positioning

- Patients are positioned with the arm on an arm board.

27.6 Technique

- We utilize general anesthesia with a laryngeal mask airway and avoid paralytics to allow for nerve stimulation at the time of surgery.
- A 6-cm incision at the proximal forearm is made along the lateral border of the pronator teres muscle.
  - For patients with PS, the incision can be extended proximally if needed in a lazy S fashion, making sure that the incision does not cross the cubital crease perpendicularly.
- The fascia is opened, and a plane is developed between the pronator teres and brachioradialis muscles to identify the median nerve and brachial artery.
- The median nerve is released proximally and then distally as it passes through the pronator teres and under the FDS. Care is taken to avoid injury to the motor branches of the median nerve in this step.
- It is important to look for and release any dense bands of the pronator teres.
- The AIN is identified and released in PS and AIN syndrome and is typically found on the posterolateral side of the median nerve approximately 5 cm from the medial epicondyle and at approximately the midpoint of the pronator teres muscle.[1]
- Once fully decompressed, hemostasis is assured, the wound is irrigated and closed with interrupted absorbable sutures in the deep dermal layer and a running subcuticular stitch in the skin.
- Paper tapes are placed over the incision and a dry gauze is wrapped loosely around the elbow region (**Video 27.1**).

27.7 Postoperative Care

- Splints are not used, but patients may use a sling for comfort if needed.
- Patients are instructed to avoid lifting for 2 weeks and to return to the clinic in 2 to 4 weeks for wound check and functional examination.
- Occupational hand therapy is ordered for selected patients with persistent motor deficits.

27.8 Complications

- In addition to wound complications and infection, injury to the median nerve motor branches that arise in the proximal forearm region can occur if care is not taken at initial exposure and median nerve dissection.
- The initial branch of the AIN, which innervates the FPL, arises 1 to 6 cm from the AIN origin and can be injured if not identified and avoided.
- Injury to the lateral antebrachial cutaneous branch of the musculocutaneous nerve located lateral to the biceps muscle tendon is also possible and may lead to a painful neuroma.
- Finally, injury to the brachial artery and/or its branches may occur.

27.9 Management Pearls

- Liberal use of nerve stimulation and meticulous dissection are important to avoid injury to median nerve motor branches and associated vasculature.
- Parsonage–Turner syndrome should be strongly considered in the differential diagnosis in these patients, with expectant management in those showing improvement.

References

[1] Tubbs RS, Custis JW, Salter EG, Wellons JC, III, Blount JP, Oakes WJ. Quantitation of and superficial surgical landmarks for the anterior interosseous nerve. J Neurosurg. 2006; 104(5): 787–791

[2] Johnson RK, Spinner M, Shrewsbury MM. Median nerve entrapment syndrome in the proximal forearm. J Hand Surg Am. 1979; 4(1):48–51

[3] Koo JT, Szabo RM. Compression neuropathies of the median nerve. J Am Soc Surg Hand. 2004; 4:156–175

[4] Eversmann W. Operative Hand Surgery. 3rd ed. New York, NY: Churchill Livingstone; 1993

28 Posterior Interosseous Nerve Entrapment and Decompression

Sonia S. Majid, Oliver Mrowczynski, Neel Patel, Elias Rizk, and Kimberly Harbaugh

28.1 Background

- The posterior interosseus nerve (PIN) is a branch of the radial nerve (RN) at the region of the proximal forearm.
- The RN travels in the distal arm between the brachioradialis (BR) and brachialis/biceps muscles.
- In the proximal forearm, it branches into deep and superficial RNs and gives off several motor branches. The deep RN passes under the leading edge of the supinator muscle (the arcade of Frohse) where it can be compressed. In this location, the nerve can be referred to as the PIN although others reserve that term for the nerve after it exits the supinator in the dorsal forearm.
- Other areas of compression include the fascia of the extensor carpi radialis brevis (ECRB) and the vascular leash of the recurrent radial vessels although this is debated.[1,2]
- Compression of the PIN can result in clinical weakness or functional loss of finger/thumb extension and lack of ulnar wrist extension.
- Because the BR and extensor carpi radialis longus (ERCL) and ECRB are innervated proximal to the site of compression, wrist extension is preserved but with radial deviation.
- Pain in the proximal dorsal forearm and/or with pressure over the PIN at the radial head is common.
- When examining finger extension, it is important to have the patient attempt to extend the fingers with the palm on a flat surface. The hand intrinsic action on the volar hood in the digits produces extension at the interphalangeal joints and should not be mistaken for residual or return of the PIN function.
- The PIN does not have cutaneous representation, so sensory loss would indicate an upstream RN compression or cervical radiculopathy.
- Conservative treatment includes anti-inflammatory agents, ice, rest, and occupational therapy.

28.2 Indications and Contraindications

- Surgery is reserved for patients with PIN compression that does not improve with conservative measures for at least 3 months.

28.3 Instruments

- Disposable nerve stimulator or formal neuromonitoring is usually used to assess the PIN and other motor branches. Intraoperative ultrasound may be used for localization.

28.4 Patient Preparation

- Electrodiagnostic studies are helpful to exclude upstream RN compression, cervical radiculopathy, and Parsonage–Turner syndrome. They can also assess for spontaneous PIN recovery.
- Magnetic resonance imaging may be obtained in some cases to assess for masses, denervation myositis, and PIN compression and/or inflammation. Inflammation of the extensor origin suggesting lateral epicondylitis (tennis elbow) can also be assessed.
- High-definition ultrasound is used in some centers.

28.5 Patient Positioning

- The patient is positioned supine with the arm abducted on the arm board.

28.6 Technique

- We typically use general anesthesia with a laryngeal mask airway. Paralytics are avoided to allow for intraoperative nerve stimulation.
- We typically use the technique described by Hall et al[3] with dissection at the lateral border of BR, but dissection along the medial BR border may also be used.[1]

- An incision is made through the skin along the junction between the BR and wrist extensors.
- The deep fascia is opened and the plane between the BR and ECRL is developed.
- The superficial RN is identified and tracked proximally.
- Intermittent stimulation during the case is carried out to identify motor branches and the deep RN.
- The bifurcation of the deep and superficial RN is identified. This is usually within 1 to 1.5 inches from the antecubital crease.[1,2]
- The deep RN/PIN arises from the posterior side of the RN and is decompressed as it passes under the leading fibrous edge of the supinator (arcade of Frohse) to travel between the muscle's superficial and deep heads.
- At the distal edge of the supinator, the branches of the PIN come off at right angles and can be injured if care is not taken during this part of the dissection.
- Once release is completed, the wound is irrigated and closed with absorbable sutures and paper tapes.
- A gauze dressing is applied, and an elastic wrap is used selectively. We do not use a drain, splint, or sling (**Video 28.1**).

28.7 Postoperative Care

- Patients are instructed to avoid heavy lifting for 2 weeks and to return for follow-up in 3 to 4 weeks.

28.8 Complications

- In addition to routine risks, injury to the recurrent radial vessels, motor branches of the RN, or PIN is possible.
- Injury to the lateral or posterior antebrachial cutaneous nerves in the region of the incision is also possible.

28.9 Management Pearls

- Meticulous dissection and nerve stimulation are important to avoid injury to motor and vascular branches at the site of PIN compression.
- Acute PIN palsy associated with pain is likely due to a brachial neuritis (Parsonage–Turner syndrome) and should be monitored for 3 to 6 months for spontaneous recovery prior to surgery.

References

[1] Kim DH, Murovic JA, Kim YY, Kline DG. Surgical treatment and outcomes in 45 cases of posterior interosseous nerve entrapments and injuries. J Neurosurg. 2006; 104(5): 766–777

[2] Rinker B, Effron CR, Beasley RW. Proximal radial compression neuropathy. Ann Plast Surg. 2004; 52(2):174–180, discussion 181–183

[3] Hall HC, MacKinnon SE, Gilbert RW. An approach to the posterior interosseous nerve. Plast Reconstr Surg. 1984; 74(3): 435–437

29 Median Nerve Decompression at the Wrist for Carpal Tunnel Syndrome

Neel Patel, Oliver Mrowczynski, Sonia S. Majid, Elias Rizk, Kimberly Harbaugh

29.1 Background

- Carpal tunnel syndrome (CTS) is the most common upper extremity peripheral nerve entrapment, and carpal tunnel release (CTR) is the most common hand surgery performed in United States.[1]
- The median nerve (MN) supplies motor fibers to most of the thenar muscles and the lumbricals to the index and middle fingers. It transmits sensory input from the thumb, index, middle, and radial half of the ring fingers.
- Common symptoms include aching pain at the wrist that radiates proximally and paresthesia of the median digits. Symptoms are typically worse at night and with activities such as driving and using the phone. Dropping objects is another frequent complaint. Motor weakness described as clumsiness may be noted later in the disease course, at which point the digits are usually described as numb.
- Repetitive motions may increase the risk of CTS.
- Other risk factors include hypothyroidism, pregnancy, diabetes, inflammatory and rheumatic diseases, and trauma.[2]

29.2 Indications and Contraindications

- In patients with a clear history, examination, and electrophysiology studies consistent with CTS and severe pain or denervation on electromyogram (EMG), surgery is offered early. In patients with mild or moderate CTS, we often recommend a short period of conservative treatment, which includes wrist splints, rest, and nonsteroidal anti-inflammatory agents. Steroid injections may also be considered but are not standard in our practice.[3,4]
- After initial course of conservative treatment, additional treatments are not likely to improve CTS as noted in one review where greater than 50% of patients who received additional conservative treatment still progressed to surgery.[5]
- Contraindications to surgical intervention are a clear diagnosis of proximal pathology or a reversible cause such as uncontrolled diabetes, pregnancy, gout, etc. In elderly patients with severe CTS (complete thenar atrophy, numbness but no pain), surgery is unlikely to be helpful. In those with pain, the pain typically improves but the sensory and motor function may not.

29.3 Instruments

- Standard surgical tools are utilized.

29.4 Patient Preparation

- Clinical history and examination are the primary methods of diagnosis of CTS.
- A Tinel response with percussion and pain with compression of the MN at the wrist, increased paresthesia with wrist flexion/extension, deficits in median sensation, and/or atrophy of the thenar muscles are consistent with the diagnosis of CTS.
- Adjunct testing includes electrodiagnostic studies (EDX) and/or imaging. We prefer EDX as they give a baseline function of the nerve, detect ongoing denervation, and can assess other conditions such as cervical radiculopathy or peripheral neuropathy.[6]
- The nerve latencies often improve but do not necessarily return to normal following CTR.
- In diabetic patients in particular, peripheral neuropathy may proceed despite successful CTR.
- Postoperative EDX that improve significantly but remain in the abnormal range may then be misinterpreted as recurrent or persistent CTS.
- Baseline EDX preoperatively helps prevent unnecessary reoperation in those cases.
- We utilize ultrasound and magnetic resonance imaging (MRI) studies selectively in patients with atypical presentation.
- In addition, MRI studies are usually obtained in patients with recurrent symptoms in whom reoperation is being considered.

29.5 Patient Positioning

- Patients are positioned with the hand on an arm board.
- No tourniquet is used, and we do not routinely give preoperative antibiotics.

29.6 Technique

- We utilize local anesthesia with/without mild sedation and avoid paralytics. We avoid nerve blocks and tourniquets.
- Surgical management of CTS includes endoscopic or open release.
- Both approaches are equally effective.[7] We prefer the open technique as it does not require tourniquet use and can be done with local alone or with minimal intravenous anesthesia.
- Local anesthetic is infiltrated along the incision line.
- A 2- to 3-cm skin incision is made in the palm starting at the distal wrist crease in line with the web space between the third and fourth digits.
- A small Weitlaner retractor is placed. Points of bleeding in the subcutaneous tissues are cauterized with a pair of bipolar forceps.
- The midportion of the transverse carpal ligament is divided with the scalpel.
- The distal and proximal portions of the transverse carpal ligament are then divided under direct vision with a tenotomy scissor.
- It is helpful to have the wrist in a neutral or slightly flexed position and elevate the subcutaneous tissues away from the ligament with a handheld retractor. This allows the MN to fall away from the ligament.
- The distal release extends to the distal fat pad. We extend the proximal release subcutaneously to include the distal forearm fascia.
- The wound is then irrigated, and hemostasis is assured.
- The wound is closed with a single inverted absorbable stitch in the deep dermis and a running nonabsorbable monofilament suture in the skin.
- The incision is covered with bacitracin ointment, iodine gauze, and a folded gauze.
- Opened 4 × 4 gauze pads are placed between the fingers and the hand is then wrapped with gauze and an elastic wrap overlying. We do not use a splint (**Video 29.1**).

29.7 Postoperative Care

- We recommend ice and elevation for 24 hours and acetaminophen with codeine for pain. Patients are instructed to keep the dressing intact for 5 days. They are also instructed to avoid pulling activities with the wrist flexed to avoid bowstringing of the flexor tendons.
- Patients return for wound check and suture removal at 10 to 14 days postoperatively.
- Occupational hand therapy is reserved for rare patients with wound sensitivity, hypertrophic scar, or persistent sensorimotor deficits.

29.8 Complications

- Complications include infection, wound dehiscence, weakness, numbness, incisional pain, and pain at the wrist or basal joint of thumb.

29.9 Management Pearls

- Although a simple and rewarding procedure, CTR demands meticulous attention to detail since the complications of wound infection, pain, and nerve injury in the hand of the patient can lead to significant loss of function and quality of life.
- The MN may take an angular approach to the carpal tunnel.[8] A persistent median artery may accompany the MN and should be spared during CTR.
- Redo-CTR has increased risk of nerve injury or pain syndrome due to scar formation. We extend the incision above the wrist in reoperation cases to identify the nerve in the unscarred region.

References

[1] Einhorn N, Leddy JP. Pitfalls of endoscopic carpal tunnel release. Orthop Clin North Am. 1996; 27(2):373–380

[2] Padua L, Cuccagna C, Giovannini S, et al. Carpal tunnel syndrome: updated evidence and new questions. Lancet Neurol. 2023; 22(3):255–267

[3] Page MJ, Massy-Westropp N, O'Connor D, Pitt V. Splinting for carpal tunnel syndrome. Cochrane Database Syst Rev. 2012; 2012(7):CD010003

[4] Marshall S, Tardif G, Ashworth N. Local corticosteroid injection for carpal tunnel syndrome. Cochrane Database Syst Rev. 2007(2):CD001554

[5] Baker NA, Livengood HM. Symptom severity and conservative treatment for carpal tunnel syndrome in association with eventual carpal tunnel release. J Hand Surg Am. 2014; 39(9): 1792–1798
[6] Jablecki CK, Andary MT, So YT, Wilkins DE, Williams FH, AAEM Quality Assurance Committee. Literature review of the usefulness of nerve conduction studies and electromyography for the evaluation of patients with carpal tunnel syndrome. Muscle Nerve. 1993; 16(12):1392–1414
[7] Michelotti BM, Vakharia KT, Romanowsky D, Hauck RMA. A prospective, randomized trial comparing open and endoscopic carpal tunnel release within the same patient. Hand (N Y). 2020; 15(3):322–326
[8] Payne R, Nasralah Z, Sieg E, Rizk EB, Glantz M, Harbaugh K. The angular course of the median nerve in the distal forearm and its anatomical importance in preventing nerve injury in a modern era of carpal tunnel release. J Neurosurg. 2017; 126(3):979–984

30 Guyon's Canal Decompression

Rachael M. Payne, Ruby L. Taylor, Benjamin Harris Timmins, and Susan E. Mackinnon

30.1 Background

- Ulnar nerve compression at the wrist, specifically Guyon's canal, is the second most common site of ulnar nerve compression.[1] At this distal location, the ulnar nerve bifurcates into superficial sensory and deep motor branches, providing sensation to the small finger and ulnar half of the ring finger as well as innervation of the ulnar-mediated intrinsic hand muscles (hypothenar muscles [abductor digit minimi, flexor digiti minimi brevis, opponens digiti minimi], interosseous muscles, third and fourth lumbricals, adductor pollicis, and the deep head of flexor pollicis brevis). Thus, classic symptoms associated with Guyon's canal syndrome include pain, numbness, and tingling involving the small and ring finger, and weakness with fine motor tasks including clumsiness and lack of dexterity.
- In the senior author's practice, the deep motor branch of the ulnar nerve is always decompressed during Guyon's canal release; however, this operative step can be challenging due to the inability to visualize this nerve branch until after release of the hypothenar musculature is performed. It is also imperative to extend the skin incision proximal to the wrist crease in a Brunner fashion to decompress the distal antebrachial fascia, which is the most compressive structure.

30.2 Indications and Contraindications

- Conservative management with activity modification, neutral wrist splinting, and anti-inflammatory medications can be attempted but is generally ineffective long term.[2,3] One exception to this is compression caused by repetitive trauma, which can respond favorably to activity modification.[4] Surgical treatment is usually recommended, especially with severe or persistent symptoms.

30.3 Instruments

- Relevant equipment items include a hand table, tourniquet, microbipolar electrocautery, and standard surgical instruments for hand surgery (no. 15 blade, double hook retractors, Fischer Mackinnon tenotomy scissors [no conflict of interest], Senn retractors, Weitlaner retractor, and Adson forceps with teeth).

30.4 Patient Preparation

- History and physical examination are key elements in diagnosis.
- Our pain questionnaire supplements history-taking and provides valuable details regarding pain character, intensity, location, and its impact on patient.[1,5]
- On examination, thorough motor and sensory testing should be compared to the contralateral unaffected extremity.[6]
- Motor evaluation begins with visual inspection for atrophy of the first dorsal interossei muscle dorsally and hypothenar eminence volarly.[1]
- Intrinsic muscle strength can be evaluated by measuring pinch strength and having the patient abduct their index and small fingers against resistance.
- We use a "teeter totter" test to measure abductor digit minimi strength by having the patient push the tips of the small fingers strongly against each other to see which is stronger.
- We also test strength of resisted abduction of small fingers with the elbow extended and flexed to evaluate for ulnar Sunderland zero ischemic changes at the elbow versus Guyon's canal.
- Intrinsic muscle weakness can result in specific examination findings.
- For example, clawing of the ring and small fingers (Duchenne's sign) can be observed due to unopposed action of the long extensors at the metacarpophalangeal joints and long flexors at the interphalangeal joints, while an abducted position of the small finger (Wartenberg's sign)

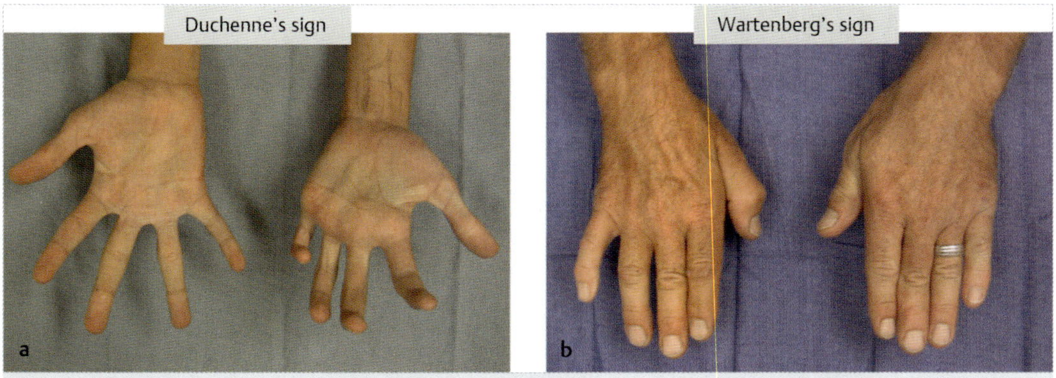

Fig. 30.1 Clawing and Wartenberg's sign. **(a)** Intrinsic muscle weakness can manifest as clawing (Duchenne's sign) of the ring and little fingers due to an unopposed action of the long extensors at the metacarpophalangeal joints and long flexors at the interphalangeal joints. **(b)** Wartenberg's sign is the abducted posture of the little finger due to unopposed action of the extensor digiti minimi. (Reproduced from Davidge KM, Boyd KU. Ulnar nerve entrapment and injury. In: Mackinnon S, ed. Nerve Surgery. 1st Edition. New York: Thieme; 2015.)

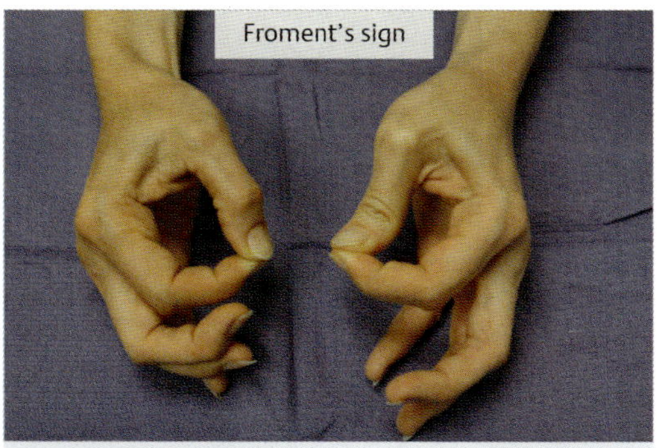

Fig. 30.2 Right hand Froment's sign. A way to evaluate weakness of the first dorsal interosseous and thumb adductor muscles is to have the patient pinch. A positive Froment's sign is the overt flexion of the thumb interphalangeal joint associated with this weakness. Having the patient hold a piece of paper during pinch, then having the examiner pull the paper away, will help elicit this sign. (Reproduced from Davidge KM, Boyd KU. Ulnar nerve entrapment and injury. In: Mackinnon S, ed. Nerve Surgery. 1st Edition. New York: Thieme; 2015.)

can result from unopposed extensor digiti minimi (▶ Fig. 30.1).

- A positive Froment's sign occurs when the patient's thumb flexes as the examiner pulls a piece of paper away from being grasped in the first web space (▶ Fig. 30.2).
- This is due to dorsal interosseous and thumb adductor weakness, which results in compensatory flexor pollicis longus activation during pinch. In contrast to ulnar nerve compression at the elbow, compression at Guyon's canal spares flexor carpi ulnaris and flexor digitorum profundus to the small and ring fingers.
- Therefore, ulnar wrist flexion and flexion of the distal interphalangeal joints of the small and ring fingers against resistance are preserved.
- Sensation can be most readily assessed with the Ten Test,[7] but static and moving two-point discrimination as well as Semmes–Weinstein monofilament testing are helpful adjuncts.
- Evaluating sensation of the dorsal cutaneous branch of the ulnar nerve is useful in differentiating ulnar nerve compression at the elbow (dorsal-ulnar hand sensation reduced) from Guyon's canal (dorsal-ulnar hand sensation spared), while compression at either site can lead to diminished sensation at the small finger and ulnar half of the ring finger (▶ Fig. 30.3).
- Ulnar sensory loss is distinguished from radial and median nerve territories by assessing sensation with the Ten Test at the dorsal-ulnar hand versus the dorsal first web space (superficial radial nerve) and at the small finger pulp versus the index finger pulp (median nerve).

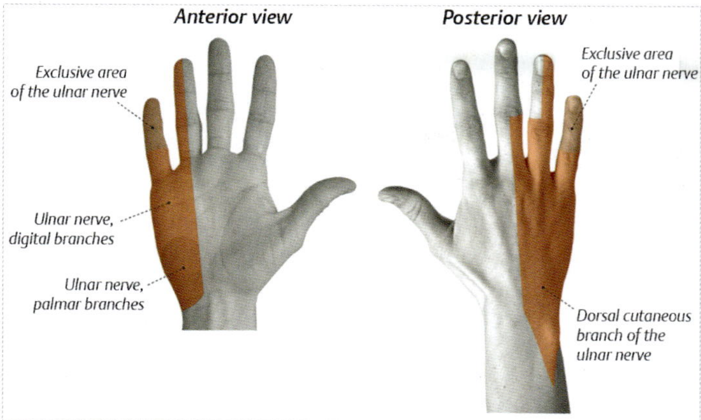

Fig. 30.3 Ulnar nerve sensory innervation. The ulnar nerve innervates the ulnar aspect of the anterior/posterior hand. The exclusive area of the ulnar nerve to test for sensation is located on the distal aspect of the little finger. (Reproduced from Davidge KM, Boyd KU. Ulnar nerve entrapment and injury. In: Mackinnon S, ed. Nerve Surgery. 1st Edition. New York: Thieme; 2015.)

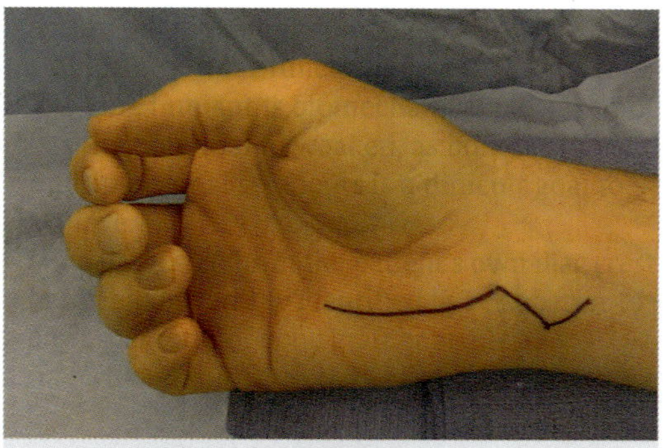

Fig. 30.4 Steps in the surgical decompression of the ulnar nerve at the level of the Guyon canal. Incision for the Guyon canal. Incision is made ulnar to the thenar crease and taken proximally across the wrist in a Brunner fashion. (Reproduced from Davidge KM, Boyd KU. Ulnar nerve entrapment and injury. In: Mackinnon S, ed. Nerve Surgery. 1st Edition. New York: Thieme; 2015.)

- Finally, percussion over the hypothenar eminence typically results in a positive Tinel's sign when there is nerve compression in Guyon's canal.
- The Scratch Collapse Test (SCT) with ethyl chloride hierarchy may demonstrate two entrapment points (distal forearm vs. deep motor site).[8] Nerve conduction and electromyographic (EMG) studies can aid in diagnosis when it is not clear, help localize the site(s) of compression, or exclude brachial plexus neuropathy, C8–T1 radiculopathy, or a systemic motor neuropathy.[9,10]

30.5 Patient Positioning

- The patient is placed in supine position with the affected arm abducted and the wrist slightly extended.

30.6 Technique

- Guyon's canal decompression is accomplished using torniquet control and loupe magnification.
- First, an incision is made approximately 6 mm ulnar to the thenar crease, extending proximal to the wrist crease as a modified Brunner incision.
- The palmaris brevis muscle is divided with microbipolar electrocautery.
- When present, the small cutaneous branch from the ulnar nerve located near the distal aspect of the dissection is protected.
- Next, thick antebrachial fascia proximal to the wrist crease is released sharply with tenotomy scissors.
- The ulnar neurovascular bundle is then swept ulnarly and protected under a retractor.
- The hook of the hamate and leading edge of the hypothenar muscle are identified.
- The deep motor branch enters at the leading edge of the hypothenar muscle but is under the muscle and therefore not visualized, so extreme care is taken as tenotomy scissors are used to divide the tendinous leading edge of the hypothenar muscle along the hook of the hamate.
- The deep motor branch is visualized and decompressed once this is performed

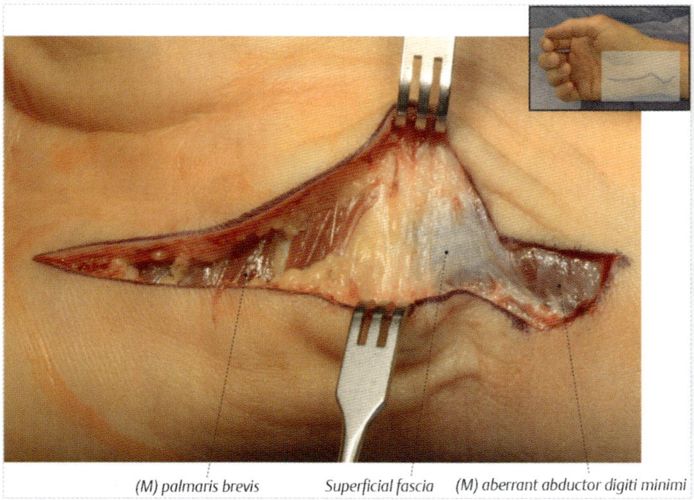

Fig. 30.5 Initial exposure for the Guyon canal. Upon initial exposure, the palmaris brevis is identified. In some cases, a crossing cutaneous palmar branch of the ulnar nerve is identified and protected in the distal third of the incision. (Reproduced from Davidge KM, Boyd KU. Ulnar nerve entrapment and injury. In: Mackinnon S, ed. Nerve Surgery. 1st Edition. New York: Thieme; 2015.)

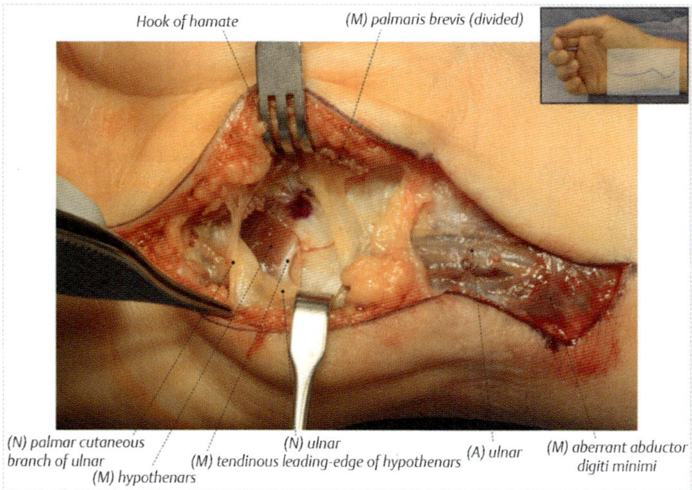

Fig. 30.6 Identification of the hypothenar muscles for orientation. By sweeping the ulnar nerve and vessels medially, the hypothenar muscles are identified medial to the marked hook of the hamate (*purple*). The deep motor branch of the ulnar nerve courses deep to this muscle. The palmar cutaneous branch of the ulnar nerve is identified and protected through this exposure. (Reproduced from Davidge KM, Boyd KU. Ulnar nerve entrapment and injury. In: Mackinnon S, ed. Nerve Surgery. 1st Edition. New York: Thieme; 2015.)

(▶ Fig. 30.4, ▶ Fig. 30.5, ▶ Fig. 30.6, ▶ Fig. 30.7, ▶ Fig. 30.8, and ▶ Fig. 30.9).

30.7 Postoperative Care

- A well-padded dressing is applied and removed on postoperative day 2 to 3. At this time, the patient is provided an over-the-counter wrist neutral splint to wear at night and during the day as needed. Gentle motion of the fingers and wrist is encouraged, but strengthening is restricted for 4 weeks. Hand therapy is initiated at the first postoperative visit and is continued for 2 months. Sutures are removed at approximately 2 weeks.

30.8 Complications

- Complications are rare but include infection, delayed wound healing, nerve injury, and/or poor scarring.

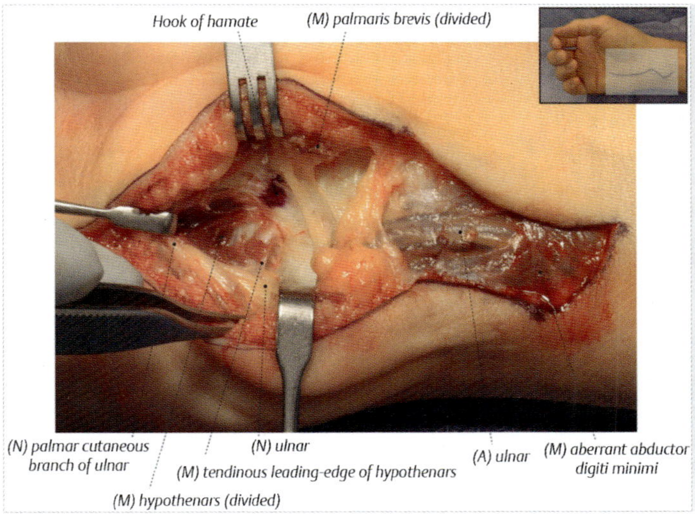

Fig. 30.7 Identification of the tendinous leading edge of the hypothenar muscles. The tendinous leading edge of the hypothenar muscles can compress the deep motor branch of the ulnar nerve. This tendon was exposed by partially dividing the muscular tissue superficial to the tendon. The deep motor branch cannot be visualized until this tendon structure is divided. (Reproduced from Davidge KM, Boyd KU. Ulnar nerve entrapment and injury. In: Mackinnon S, ed. Nerve Surgery. 1st Edition. New York: Thieme; 2015.)

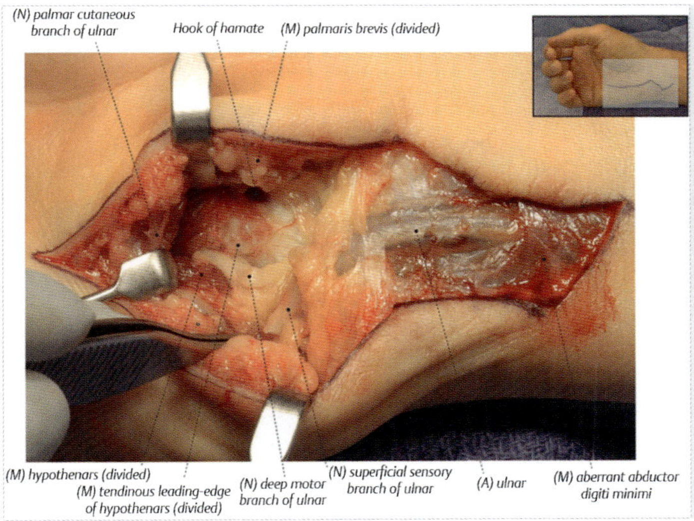

Fig. 30.8 Decompression of the deep motor branch of the ulnar nerve. The deep motor branch of the ulnar nerve is decompressed by dividing the tendinous leading edge of the hypothenar muscles. (Reproduced from Davidge KM, Boyd KU. Ulnar nerve entrapment and injury. In: Mackinnon S, ed. Nerve Surgery. 1st Edition. New York: Thieme; 2015.)

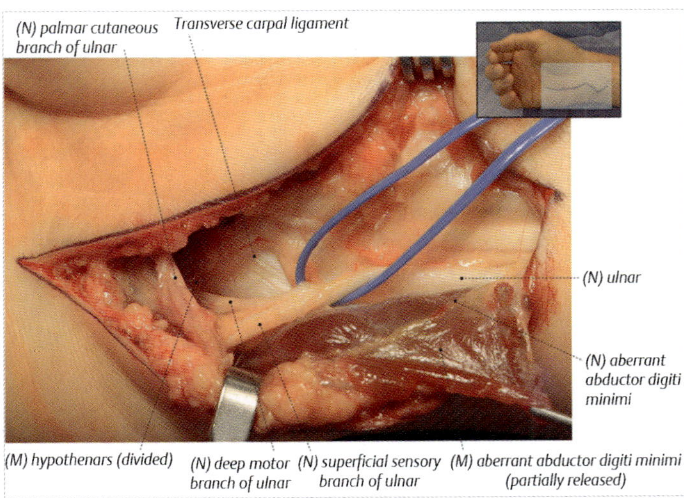

Fig. 30.9 Decompression of the ulnar nerve through the Guyon canal. The ulnar nerve is decompressed through the Guyon canal, and any antebrachial fascia is released. In this case, an aberrant abductor digiti minimi muscle was identified and divided. (Reproduced from Davidge KM, Boyd KU. Ulnar nerve entrapment and injury. In: Mackinnon S, ed. Nerve Surgery. 1st Edition. New York: Thieme; 2015.)

30.9 Management Pearls

- Specific release of the deep motor branch of the ulnar nerve is challenging due to the inability to visualize this nerve branch until after release of the hypothenar musculature is performed. Therefore, one must approach this step with caution and complete understanding of anatomical landmarks to avoid nerve injury.

References

[1] Mackinnon SE Nerve Surgery. New York, NY: Thieme; 2015

[2] Brzović Z. Neuralni kompresivni sindromi na rukama [Nerve compression syndromes of the arm]. Acta Med Iugosl. 1989; 43(5):373–395

[3] Lee JH, Lee JK, Park JS, et al. Characteristics of surgically treated Guyon canal syndrome: a multicenter retrospective study. J Plast Reconstr Aesthet Surg. 2022; 75(9):3269–3278

[4] Almeida V, de Carvalho M. Lesion of the deep palmar branch of the ulnar nerve: causes and clinical outcome. Neurophysiol Clin. 2010; 40(3):159–164

[5] Poppler LH, Mackinnon SE. The role of the peripheral nerve surgeon in the treatment of pain. Neurotherapeutics. 2019; 16(1):9–25

[6] Kenney RJ, Hammert WC. Physical examination of the hand. J Hand Surg Am. 2014; 39(11):2324–2334, quiz 2334

[7] Strauch B, Lang A, Ferder M, Keyes-Ford M, Freeman K, Newstein D. The Ten Test. Plast Reconstr Surg. 1997; 99(4):1074–1078

[8] Davidge KM, Gontre G, Tang D, et al. The "hierarchical" Scratch Collapse Test for identifying multilevel ulnar nerve compression. Hand (N Y). 2015; 10(3):388–395

[9] Dimberg EL. Electrodiagnostic evaluation of ulnar neuropathy and other upper extremity mononeuropathies. Neurol Clin. 2012; 30(2):479–503

[10] Pearce C, Feinberg J, Wolfe SW. Ulnar neuropathy at the wrist. HSS J. 2009; 5(2):180–183, quiz 184–185

31 Tarsal Tunnel Syndrome

Andrew S. Jack and Line Jacques

31.1 Background

- Tarsal tunnel syndrome (TTS) is an entrapment syndrome due to compression of the tibial nerve (TN) as it courses through the fibro-osseus tarsal tunnel (roofed by the flexor retinaculum) at the medial aspect of the foot between the medial malleolus and calcaneal tuberosity.
- Although rare and often a diagnostic challenge, TTS is an important consideration in patients presenting with foot pain as surgical treatment via decompression (much like carpal tunnel release for its analogous upper extremity entrapment carpal tunnel syndrome) in appropriately selected patients can yield excellent long-term results. That being said, akin to many other chronic pain syndromes, reported outcomes within the literature vary greatly due to the previously mentioned diagnostic challenges that TTS poses and difficulty in patient selection that this then brings.
- The sciatic nerve has nerve root contributions originating from L4–S2. It is comprised of a medial (tibial) and lateral (common peroneal) division.
- The medial or TN component is formed by the anterior divisions of the lumbosacral plexus contributions from the L4–S2 nerve roots, whereas the lateral or common peroneal component is formed by the posterior divisions of the lumbosacral plexus contributions from the L4–S2 nerve roots.[1,2,3]
- After exiting from the pelvis through the greater sciatic notch, the sciatic nerve divides in the posterior thigh a variable distance from the popliteal fossa into these respective nerves.
- The tibial division of the sciatic nerve innervates the majority of the hamstring muscles (semitendinosus, semimembranosus, and long head of the biceps femoris) as it passes them in the posterior thigh. The exception to the latter is the short head of the biceps femoris (supplied by the common peroneal nerve division).
- The medial component of the sciatic (TN) then continues inferiorly through the middle of the popliteal fossa, coursing deep to the two heads of the gastrocnemius muscle. It then passes under the fibrous/tendinous arch of the soleus muscle (soleal sling) in the proximal portion of leg where it then continues distally with the popliteal artery and vein.
- As the TN dives deep to the soleus muscle and passes the tendinous origin of the soleal sling, it can become compressed resulting in an entrapment syndrome known as soleal sling syndrome.
- During its course distally, the TN supplies motor innervation to the gastrocnemius muscle, the soleus muscle, and plantaris muscle in the proximal leg. Furthermore, it will also give off geniculate branches to the knee capsule, lateral collateral ligaments, and cruciate ligaments of the knee in proximity to the popliteal fossa, in addition to a cutaneous branch (the medial contributing branch to the sural nerve) that joins the sural communicating branch off the common peroneal nerve to form the sural nerve proper (supplies cutaneous innervation to the inferolateral portion of the lower leg and outermost portion of the foot).
- Once deep to the soleus, the TN continues posterior to the tibia, between the flexor digitorum longus (medially) and the flexor hallucis longus (laterally), both of which it supplies (in addition to the tibialis posterior muscle). Once at the foot, it passes between the medial malleolus and the Achilles tendon, through a structure known as the tarsal tunnel.
- The tarsal tunnel is covered superiorly (roof) by the flexor retinaculum, which attaches to the medial malleolus and calcaneal tuberosity.[1,2,3] In analogous fashion to the carpal tunnel being a site of entrapment for the median nerve in the upper extremity, the tarsal tunnel with its overlying flexor retinaculum can also serve as a site of entrapment for the TN in the lower extremity.
- As will be discussed in subsequent sections of this chapter, in brief, any condition or pathology decreasing the amount of space for the TN within the tarsal tunnel or preventing it from gliding normally within it can potentially cause TTS (whether the etiology be intrinsic or extrinsic to the nerve itself).

- In proximity to or even within this tunnel, the TN then divides into the medial plantar, lateral plantar, and calcaneal nerves (supplying cutaneous innervation to the medial, lateral, and calcaneal portion of the plantar foot surface, respectively).
- Motor innervation to the foot intrinsic muscles also arises from the medial (abductor hallucis, flexor digitorum brevis, and flexor hallucis brevis) and lateral (adductor hallucis, flexor digitorum minimi, abductor digiti minimi, and interossei) plantar nerves.
- TTS is a relatively rare condition and often underdiagnosed. Owing to its rarity, ongoing controversy pertaining to its etiology (e.g., in patients with diabetes), and low electrodiagnostic sensitivity, the incidence of TTS is largely unknown.[4,5,6]
- TTS can present at any age, but is slightly more common in females. Furthermore, due to varying electrodiagnostic criteria, patients presenting with TTS require a detailed history and clinical examination to establish the diagnosis (as it is considered a clinical diagnosis).
- That being said, many etiologies can cause TTS.
- Space-occupying lesions proximally (as shown in ▶ Fig. 31.1 and ▶ Fig. 31.2) such as peripheral nerve sheath tumors (schwannoma, neurofibroma), lipoma, ganglion cyst, venous varicosities, and accessory muscles can all result in signs and symptoms of TTS.
- In the distal aspect of the tarsal tunnel, traction neuritis associated with plantar fasciitis, fascial or ligamentous thickening, and posterior tibial tendon dysfunction, among others, can all also result in TTS.[4,5,6,7,8]
- Typically, patients will then complain of pain at the medial aspect of the ankle and the plantar foot (medial or lateral plantar nerve distribution). In keeping with other entrapment neuropathies, the pain is commonly worse at night, aggravated with activity and improved with rest. This may consist of sharp, burning, or electrical/lancinating-like pain that is intermittent or constant (depending on severity and etiology). Moreover, patients may also complain of sensory symptoms such as numbness and/or tingling; however, weakness is rarer. Pressure at the tunnel (exacerbating nerve

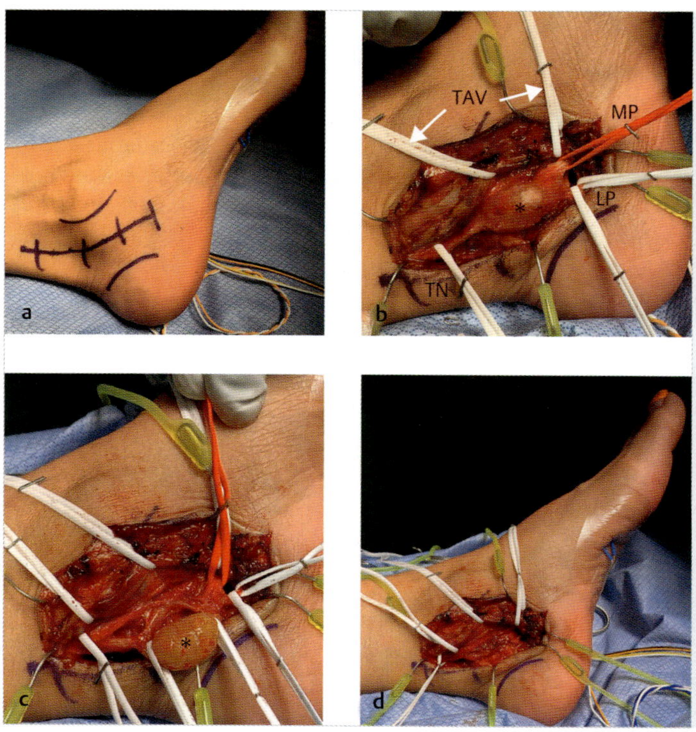

Fig. 31.1 Magnetic resonance neurogram depicting a tibial nerve schwannoma resulting in tarsal tunnel syndrome. **(a)** Coronal T2-weighted fat-suppressed sequence. **(b)** Sagittal T2-weighted fat-suppressed sequence. **(c)** Axial T1-weighted fat-suppressed sequence with gadolinium. **(d)** Sagittal T1-weighted fat-suppressed sequence with gadolinium.

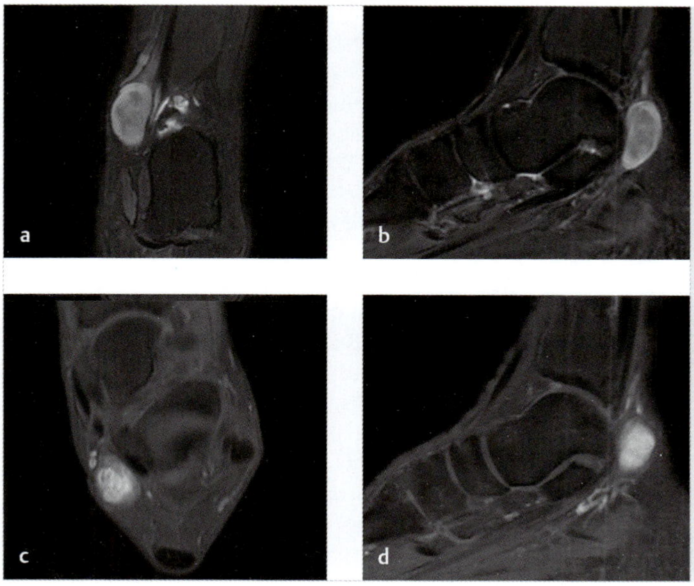

Fig. 31.2 **(a)** Intraoperative photographs from a left tibial nerve neurolysis and tarsal tunnel decompression for schwannoma resection showing supine positioning and incision marked. Throughout the dissection, **(b)** vasculature and nerve branches are isolated with vessel loops and externally neurolyzed to then allow **(c)** internal tibial neurolysis and tumor resection, **(d)** after which the epineurium is reapproximated with 8–0 Prolene suture. LP, lateral plantar nerve; MP, medial plantar nerve; TAV, tibial artery and vein; TN, tibial nerve; *asterisk* = tibial nerve schwannoma.

compression), dorsiflexion and/or eversion, and Tinel's provocation may all reproduce the symptoms.

31.2 Indications and Contraindications

- Failure of conservative therapy for TTS or progression of symptoms necessitates surgery.
- Poor operative candidates or noncompressive causes of TTS may preclude patients from surgery.

31.3 Patient Preparation

- Nerve conduction studies (NCS) and electromyography (EMG) should be performed to help confirm the diagnosis. NCS may show increased motor latency over the abductor hallucis and abductor digiti minimi (> 5.8 milliseconds), decreased sensory nerve conduction (< 41 milliseconds), and reduced amplitude of evoked response.
- However, as mentioned, electrodiagnostic studies need to be interpreted cautiously and be considered in a clinical context as they can also be fraught with diagnostic inaccuracy and decreased sensitivity. For example, previous studies have shown EMG of the intrinsic foot musculature to have a false-positive rate of 10 to 43%.[4,6,8]
- In keeping with other rare entrapment neuropathies, radiological imaging is integral to the diagnostic workup of a patient. Plain X-rays of the ankle can help detect osteophytes, malunions, deformities, accessory bones, and previous trauma at the ankle.[4]
- Moreover, ultrasound (US) is a cost-effective and reliable investigational tool, and US of the contralateral tarsal tunnel is an easy way of obtaining a control comparator. It can detect occupying mass lesions or fusiform TN thickening, as well as loss of the TN fascicular pattern.
- US also affords the ability to investigate whether or not there is a dynamic component by visualizing in real time what happens to the TN with particular ankle movements (which can also then be correlated to what the patient experiences clinically).
- Although US can be very helpful in the diagnosis of TTS, magnetic resonance imaging (MRI)/ magnetic resonance neurography (MRN) is considered the gold standard in accurately characterizing the anatomy of the TN, retinaculum, mass lesions, and pertinent surrounding anatomy.[4]
- MRN (as seen in ▶ Fig. 31.1) can provide information about the neurovascular bundle as it passes into the tarsal tunnel, focal or diffuse enlargement of the TN, fascicular hyperintensity

or disruption, neuroma formation, in addition to end-target muscle denervation (fatty infiltration and atrophy) in the distribution of the nerve.
- Finally, the authors also advocate that MRN be used in cases of failed peripheral nerve surgery in which patients often have a complex clinical and electrodiagnostic presentation with persistent or recurrent symptomatology.
- MRN is an invaluable diagnostic tool, and can also serve as an important prognostic tool, as well as help with preoperative planning and postoperative follow-up.

31.4 Patient Positioning

- Under general anesthetic, the patient is positioned supine on the hospital operating room table. All appropriate pressure points are padded and the patient's lower extremity undergoing decompression is positioned such that the thigh is flexed, leg extended and externally rotated using a surgical bump, pillows, padding, and tape to help with this (▶ Fig. 31.2a).

31.5 Technique

- Although several different decompression approaches to the TN at the tarsal tunnel have been previously described with each having their own respective advantages and disadvantages, herein described is the authors' preferred method including a stepwise depiction of the surgical anatomy.
- The patient's lower extremity from the knee down is washed appropriately following anesthesia and positioning. A marking pen is used to mark a proposed incision midway between the medial malleolus and the Achilles tendon/calcaneal tuberosity extending proximally toward the medial leg and distally toward the instep across the flexor retinaculum (▶ Fig. 31.2a).
- The extremity from the knee distal with the surgical site is sterilized using preparation solution and draped in the usual sterile fashion. Sterile electrodes are then placed into the tibialis anterior, abductor hallucis, and abductor digiti minimized, and sensory electrodes are placed into the plantar aspect of the foot for neurophysiological and electrodiagnostic monitoring/testing.
- A no. 15 scalpel blade is used to incise the skin and carry the incision down through the dermis to the subcutaneous tissue.
- A combination of blunt and sharp dissection is used to release the subcutaneous tissue and fascia using a combination of McCabe/Jake dissector, tenotomy scissors, and bipolar cautery.
- Flexible skin hooks (silastic ends) are then placed to maintain the exposure.
- Starting at the proximal end, dissection is carried down through the subcutaneous tissue and opened fascia. The extensor digitorum tendon is then palpated with the posterior tibial artery and vein(s) also being located through palpation ventral and medial in the exposure with the latter two then being isolated with a vessel loop for protection (▶ Fig. 31.2b).
- Attention is then turned just posterior and lateral to these where the TN is then found. The TN is then followed a bit more proximally and externally neurolyzed with a vessel loop being placed around it (▶ Fig. 31.2b).
- Bipolar stimulation is then used to confirm identification of the TN with an electrodiagnostic threshold being determined. The TN is followed distally, continuing the external neurolysis in the process until it begins to dive beneath the flexor retinaculum.
- Care must be taken to then protect the nerve (and posterior tibial artery/veins as these can entwine the TN) by separating the nerve from the flexor retinaculum above with a dissector (and the retinaculum then being released over top of the dissector or slowly with tenotomy scissors on top of the nerve).
- Dissection is continued toward the instep of the foot until the entirety of the tarsal tunnel is unroofed and flexor retinaculum incised. Typically, as the TN courses through the tarsal tunnel or near its distal end, it will trifurcate into its terminal branches (medial plantar, lateral plantar, and calcaneal branches).
- The authors will usually completely neurolyze these as well, clearing them of any septations or adhesions within the tarsal tunnel.
- Decompression is not typically carried any more distal than absolutely necessary (into the distal instep or plantar foot due to the difficulty with wound healing and pain that can then ensue).

- Once being satisfied with the TN decompression, the authors will then stimulate it proximally as well as its branches distally (in addition to having the neurophysiologist perform somatosensory and motor evoked potentials) to determine a threshold (and thus if there is any improvement postdecompression).
- The wound is then irrigated copiously with warm saline and any hemostasis required being obtained.
- The subcutaneous and dermal layers are closed using interrupted inverted 3-0 Vicryl sutures.
- Owing to the inherent difficulty of skin healing in this area (often thin skin with little subcutaneous tissue or fat, and area of high tension), the authors reapproximate the skin using interrupted vertical/horizontal mattress 3-0 Prolene sutures.
- Steri-Strips and gauze are then placed over top with an ankle wrap or tensor bandage also being placed.

31.6 Complications

- Wound complications.
- Damage to local vessels.

31.7 Management Pearls

- TTS should be managed according to the underlying etiology.
- For patients with reversible causes of TTS, those with pain only, or intermittent symptomatology, an initial trial of conservative/nonoperative management is often pursued. This includes activity modification, progressive mobilization, orthotic shoes, night splinting, physical therapy (potentially including taping, bracing, stretching, icing, massage), medications such as nonsteroidal anti-inflammatory medication, neuropathic and/or neuromodulatory pain medication (gabapentin, pregabalin, nortriptyline, amitriptyline, among others), and corticosteroid injection, among others.
- Surgical intervention for TTS is directed toward the removal of the causative mass or the decompression of the identified site causing symptoms. Owing to the wide range of clinical and diagnostic criteria that is often applied to TTS, not surprisingly a corresponding wide variation in outcomes has also been described in the literature.
- Patient selection, underlying etiology, timing of surgical intervention (with protracted symptomatology potentially increasing the likelihood of intraneural fibrosis and muscle wasting), surgical technique, and understanding of the involved anatomy all also play a crucial role in determining a patient's outcome. That being said, in the right circumstances, tarsal tunnel decompression has been shown to be safe and result in good to excellent results in 44 to 96% cases.[4,5,7,9,10,11,12]
- Much has been published about the role of tarsal tunnel decompression in the setting of diabetes (with/without electrodiagnostic evidence of entrapment); however, tarsal tunnel decompression for this indication remains controversial and is beyond the scope of this chapter.
- It is the authors' contention that one of the best indications for surgical intervention resulting in symptomatic relief is the presence of a space-occupying lesion (as shown in ▶ Fig. 31.1).

References

[1] Kim D, Husdon A, Kline D. Atlas of Peripheral Nerve Surgery. 2nd ed. Philadelphia, PA: Elsevier Saunders; 2013

[2] Kim D, Midha R, Murovic J, Spinner R. Kline and Hudon's Nerve Injuries: Operative Results for Major Nerve Injuries, Entrapments, and Tumors. 2nd ed. Philadelphia, PA: Elsevier Saunders; 2008

[3] Kline D, Husdon A, Kim D. Atlas of Peripheral Nerve Surgery. Philadelphia, PA: Saunders; 2001

[4] Ahmad M, Tsang K, Mackenney PJ, Adedapo AO. Tarsal tunnel syndrome: a literature review. Foot Ankle Surg. 2012; 18(3): 149–152

[5] Doneddu PE, Coraci D, Loreti C, Piccinini G, Padua L. Tarsal tunnel syndrome: still more opinions than evidence. Status of the art. Neurol Sci. 2017; 38(10):1735–1739

[6] McSweeney SC, Cichero M. Tarsal tunnel syndrome: a narrative literature review. Foot (Edinb). 2015; 25(4):244–250

[7] Gould JS. Recurrent tarsal tunnel syndrome. Foot Ankle Clin. 2014; 19(3):451–467

[8] Pomeroy G, Wilton J, Anthony S. Entrapment neuropathy about the foot and ankle: an update. J Am Acad Orthop Surg. 2015; 23(1):58–66

[9] Day FN, III, Naples JJ. Endoscopic tarsal tunnel release: update 96. J Foot Ankle Surg. 1996; 35(3):225–229

[10] Hendrix CL, Jolly GP, Garbalosa JC, Blume P, DosRemedios E. Entrapment neuropathy: the etiology of intractable chronic heel pain syndrome. J Foot Ankle Surg. 1998; 37(4):273–279

[11] Kaplan PE, Kernahan WT, Jr. Tarsal tunnel syndrome: an electrodiagnostic and surgical correlation. J Bone Joint Surg Am. 1981; 63(1):96–99

[12] Pfeiffer WH, Cracchiolo A, III. Clinical results after tarsal tunnel decompression. J Bone Joint Surg Am. 1994; 76(8): 1222–1230

32 Common Peroneal Decompression

Andrew S. Jack and Line Jacques

32.1 Background

- The sciatic nerve has nerve root contributions originating from L4–S2.
- It is comprised of a medial (tibial) and lateral (common peroneal) division.
- The medial or tibial nerve component is formed by the anterior divisions of the lumbosacral plexus contributions from the L4–S2 nerve roots, whereas the lateral or common peroneal component is formed by the posterior divisions of the lumbosacral plexus contributions from the L4–S2 nerve roots.[1,2,3]
- After exiting from the pelvis through the greater sciatic notch, the sciatic nerve divides in the posterior thigh a variable distance from the popliteal fossa into these respective nerves.
- The common peroneal nerve (CPN) then continues deep and medial to the biceps femoris muscle and tendon as it proceeds distally into the leg. It courses around the neck of the fibula where it is usually quite superficial (and susceptible to injury as a result) as it enters the leg from the popliteal fossa.[2]
- The CPN will give off articular branches to the knee and superior tibiofibular joint as it passes these joints, as well as a lateral cutaneous nerve of the calf, which supplies sensation to the superolateral part of the calf and a sural communicating branch (or lateral sural contribution branch, which joins the medial sural contribution branch from the tibial nerve to form the sural nerve proper).
- Once past the neck of the fibula, the CPN runs deep to the peroneus longus (which attaches to the head of the fibula and its upper lateral surface). The overlying fascia and sharp fibrous bands from the peroneus longus can also serve as a site of entrapment for the CPN as it continues distally into the leg.
- The CPN divides a variable distance from the popliteal fossa (though typically after crossing the neck of the fibula and passing beneath the peroneus longus) into two main branches—the deep and superficial peroneal nerves.
- The superficial peroneal nerve continues in the lateral leg compartment between the peroneus longus and brevis supplying sensory innervation to the anterolateral leg and dorsal aspect of the foot (with the exception of a small area in the first web space between digits 1 and 2), as well as motor innervation to the peroneus longus and brevis for foot eversion.
- After its bifurcation, the deep peroneal nerve pierces the peroneus longus muscle and courses under the extensor digitorum longus to run between the tibialis anterior and the extensor digitorum longus in the superior portion of the leg, and between the tibialis anterior and the extensor hallucis longus in the inferior leg.
- As it moves distally through the anterior leg compartment on the interosseus membrane, it travels adjacent to the anterior tibial artery to the dorsal foot.
  - Along this route, it supplies motor innervation to the tibialis anterior, extensor digitorum longus, extensor hallucis longus, extensor digitorum brevis, and peroneus tertius to enable ankle and toe dorsiflexion.
  - It also supplies cutaneous sensory innervation to a small area of skin in the first web space.
- Relative to upper extremity entrapments such as carpal tunnel syndrome and cubital tunnel syndrome, common peroneal entrapment is relatively rare. That being said, it is still the most common lower extremity nerve entrapment.[4,5,6]
- Few epidemiological studies exist detailing the incidence and prevalence of CPN palsy with varying methodologies being used and as a result a wide range being reported. A prevalence ranging between approximately 19 and 40/100,000 people (or 0.6–1.2% of all neuropathies) has been reported in some studies, with others reporting this to be as high as 15%.[5,7,8,9,10]
- Depending on the etiology of the CPN palsy, different risk factors exist. Moreover, different etiologies for CPN palsy will also portend a different epidemiological profile (e.g., traumatic CPN palsy will tend to affect more males than females at a younger age, in keeping with general trauma literature trends).
- With respect to entrapment of the CPN at the fibular neck, several risk factors have been detailed. As discussed above, the CPN courses

relatively superficially around the fibular neck where it is tethered, diving beneath the crural fascia of the peroneus longus. As a result, factors associated with CPN entrapment include thin body habitus (presumably resulting in decreased subcutaneous fat to protect the nerve) or precipitous weight loss such as after procedures aimed at reducing weight loss (such as gastric banding), consistent and/or constant sitting with legs crossed or other positioning that results in pressure/stretch on the CPN as it is tethered at the fibular neck (such as squatting—often referred to as "strawberry picker's knee"), as well as tobacco use and metabolic disorders (such as diabetes potentially resulting in a relative compromise of its perfusion or metabolic requirements).[2,10,11,12,13,14,15,16,17,18,19]

- CPN palsy can also be caused by tumors such as schwannomas and cysts such as intra- and extraneural cysts (as seen in ▶ Fig. 32.1),[20,21] iatrogenic injury from operative positioning (especially in a lithotomy position, lateral decubitus position, or with a hard popliteal fossa support),[2,22] and trauma,[23,24,25] among others.
- Any of the above etiologies resulting in CPN palsy will result in a constellation of signs and symptoms that typically includes foot drop (FD). This FD is a result of weakness to the tibialis anterior, extensor hallucis longus, and extensor digitorum longus (supplied by the deep peroneal nerve). FD in turn manifests as patients having to adopt an abnormal "high-stepping" gait to avoid tripping and falling resulting in further ankle injury.
- Owing to the CPN (specifically superficial peroneal nerve) also innervating the peroneus longus and brevis, in addition to the FD, patients will also typically present with an inversion deformity of the foot (due to unopposed action of the tibialis posterior muscle). This lack of eversion predisposes patients to traumatic ankle injury from forced inversion. Moreover, the FD may be either painless or painful. That being said, it is also possible that patients present with pure sensory symptoms such as decreased sensation and/or neuropathic pain radiating from the knee distally into the anterolateral leg and dorsal foot (superficial and deep peroneal nerve distributions as discussed above).

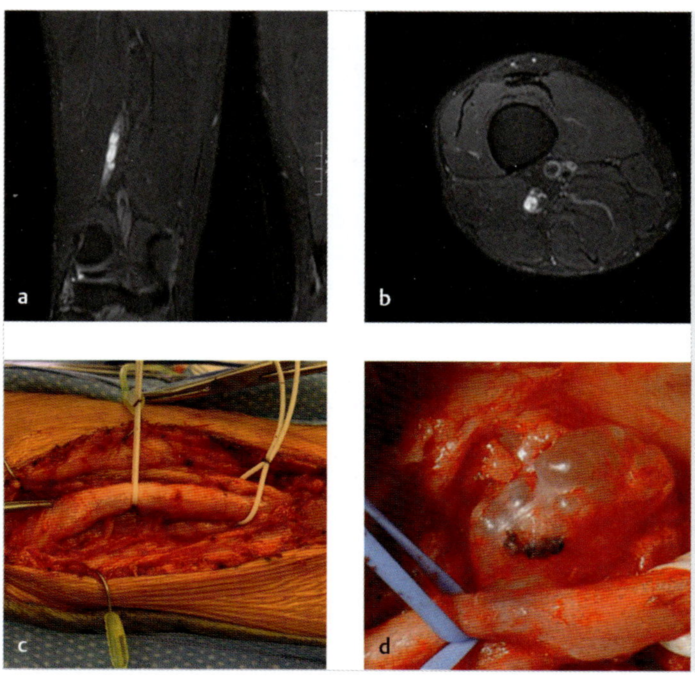

Fig. 32.1 **(a)** Coronal and **(b)** axial views of a magnetic resonance neurogram showing a right-sided intraneural ganglionic cysts of the common peroneal nerve (CPN) with **(c)** intraoperative photographs showing the corresponding patient's CPN (right-sided white vessel loop) and its bifurcation into superficial and deep (left-sided white vessel loop) peroneal nerves. **(d)** An intraoperative photograph of an extraneural ganglionic cyst compressing the right CPN from a different patient.

32.2 Indications and Contraindications

- Decompression can be performed when CPN lesions result in clinical symptoms such as FD; however, the decision to operate should be weighed after evaluating the patient's general operative risks and comorbidities.
- Any discussion with the patient regarding management also then requires a discussion about the natural history of CPN palsy that is going to be dictated by the etiology. Put simply, management will either be nonoperative (or conservative) including careful clinical (and potentially electrodiagnostic [ECx]/radiological) follow-up, physical therapy, and/or the use of foot orthoses or operative intervention.
- Studies detailing the outcome for conservative management of CPN palsy report "good outcomes" (typically defined as Medical Research Council [MRC] grade 4/5 or better) in 0 to 100% of cases. The substantially varied outcomes reported undoubtedly stems from the diverse etiologies for CPN palsy with many including CPN palsies attributable to entrapment, weight loss, idiopathic causes, postural and positioning factors, and compression from external orthosis, among others, all together.
- Generally speaking, for cases in which a reversible etiology is found such as a closed injury (from compression from a lower extremity cast or simple positioning), a trial on nonoperative management is sensible (needing to also take into account the duration and severity of symptomatology).
- However, in cases of CPN palsy due to irreversible causes or etiologies likely to progress (e.g., open traumatic or iatrogenic laceration, tumor resulting in significant deficits), upfront operative intervention is warranted. Good outcomes with conservative management were reported from studies examining the CPN from entrapment in only 25% of cases and from idiopathic causes in 0 to 60% of cases (again, the difficulty in determining the natural history of these cases being the heterogeneity of etiologies, low number of cases reported, and bias toward treatment).[5,26,27,28]
- Moreover, in a systematic review including meta-analysis comparing CPN outcomes stratified by etiology, a statistically significant difference was found favoring operative intervention compared to ankle-foot orthosis use ($p = 0.019$).[29] For idiopathic and entrapment-related cases (or those related to an irreversible or progressive cause as mentioned above) of CPN palsy, it is the authors' preference to discuss upfront surgical management with patients (again, taking into consideration the severity, duration, etc., of symptomatology).
- Outcomes after decompression and external ± internal neurolysis for CPN have been reported to be quite favorable in the literature with the majority of studies showing recovery to an MRC grade 4/5 or better in 80 to 100% of cases.[4,5,27,28,30,31,32,33,34,35,36,37,38,39]

32.3 Patient Preparation

- The localization of a lesion to the CPN at the fibular neck can usually be made on clinical grounds through careful history-taking and physical examination of their presenting symptomatology.
- This is then confirmed through ECx testing and/or imaging. The American Association of Neuromuscular and Electrodiagnostic Medicine (AANEM) published guidelines in 2005 regarding the utility of ECx; however, nerve conduction study guidelines were a level C recommendation based on class 3 evidence and insufficient data being available for delineating the role of electromyography (level U based on class 4 evidence).[5,40]
- Prior to any sort of operative intervention, it is the authors' practice to routinely perform imaging studies including ultrasound (US) and/or magnetic resonance imaging (MRI) including magnetic resonance neurography (MRN).
- Although somewhat controversial, this is the authors' preference for any entrapment or focal nerve pathology aside from a straightforward/classic presentation of carpal tunnel syndrome. This is because of the relatively higher incidence of finding other pathology to explain the patient's symptomatology (in the case of CPN entrapment, e.g., and as demonstrated in ▶ Fig. 32.1, the relative frequency of an associated intra- or extraneural ganglionic cyst that may then change management).[20,41]

- Compared to MRI, US has the added benefit of being able to visualize (and thus take into account dynamic changes) the CPN during lower extremity range of motion (e.g., to visualize whether the nerve is gliding appropriately).
- Typical CPN characteristics and measurements from US used to help diagnose (and prognosticate) include its cross-sectional area (expressed as a ratio compared to the contralateral CPN, more normal appearing proximal nerve, or as an absolute value at the level of maximal diameter in proximity to the fibular head and neck), as well as its echogenicity.
  - CPN cross-sectional area threshold values reported in the literature vary (depending on the particular study), but typically range from 8 to 12 mm^2 with resultant sensitivity and specificity varying from 47 to 91% and 53 to 100%, respectively.[5]
  - Several studies also report on the use of CPN hypoechogenicity as an early sign of intraneural edema.
- In contrast, MRI/MRN has the benefit of improved resolution and ability to visualize surrounding anatomy over US (such as visualizing intramuscular changes including edema, fatty infiltration, and fibrosis that may result from denervation). Studies evaluating the use of MRI/MRN for CPN palsy have found sensitivity and specificity ranging from 31 100% and 73 100%, respectively.[5]
- After confirming the clinical diagnosis through ECx, US, and/or MRI/MRN, a detailed discussion with the patient pertaining to the different management options ensues.

32.4 Patient Positioning

- Under general anesthetic, the patient is positioned prone on the operating room table on two large gel rolls (usually oriented parallel to the patient) with the arms resting next to them on arm boards and appropriately padded (▶ Fig. 32.2a).
- Next, the patient's lower extremity undergoing decompression is positioned such that it is maximally extended at the hip and knee, as well as externally rotated using pillows, surgical padding, and tape to help with this (▶ Fig. 32.2a).

32.5 Technique

- Although several different approaches to CPN surgical decompression have been previously described with each having their own respective advantages and disadvantages, herein described is the authors' preferred method including a stepwise depiction of the surgical anatomy:
- The authors place intraoperative neuromonitoring electrodes in the distribution of the ipsilateral superficial peroneal, deep peroneal, and tibial nerve distribution (typically the peroneus longus, tibialis anterior, and gastrocnemius muscle).
- Square-off drapes are then used to separate the surgical field for preparation from the mid-thigh to the mid-leg.
- A proposed skin incision is marked that parallels the course of the CPN starting medial to the biceps femoris tendon on the lateral aspect of the patient's posterior thigh and through the lateral aspect of the popliteal fossa, distally

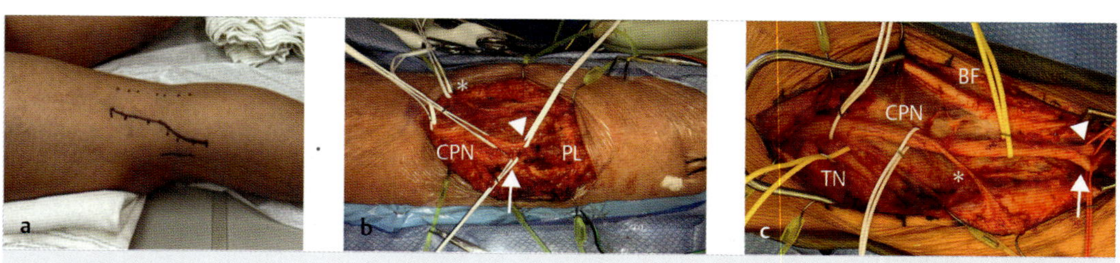

Fig. 32.2 **(a)** Intraoperative photographs from a left common peroneal decompression with prone positioning and incision marked. Throughout the dissection, individual nerve branches are isolated with vessel loops and externally neurolyzed (**b**: left CPN and **c**: right popliteal fossa, tibial, and CPN) to ensure all points of compression or tethering are released. BF, biceps femoris; CPN, common peroneal nerve; PL, peroneus longus; TN, tibial nerve; *arrow*: superficial peroneal nerve; *arrowhead*: deep peroneal nerve; *asterisk*: lateral sural communicating branch.

curving slightly anterolaterally around the neck of the fibula (▶ Fig. 32.2a).

- After the surgical field is sterilized with preparation solution, a no. 15 scalpel blade is used to incise the skin and carry the incision down through the dermis with bipolar cautery then being used from hemostasis.
- Skin hook retractors (silastic ends) are then used to maintain exposure and held in place with mosquito and/or Kelly clamps.
- A combination of blunt dissection using the McCabe or Jake dissector and Freer dissector is then used with bipolar cautery (as well as tenotomy scissors and bipolar cautery) to carry the exposure and incision down through the subcutaneous tissue to the fascia.
- Beginning at the rostral end of the exposure, the fascia lata is then opened and the CPN identified medial to the biceps femoris tendon (▶ Fig. 32.2c). The lateral communicating branch to the sural nerve off of the CPN is also typically identified, externally neurolyzed, and has a vessel loop placed around this to be mobilized out of the way to protect it (▶ Fig. 32.2b).
- The CPN is encircled with a vessel loop and externally neurolyzed. This parent nerve is then stimulated and electrophysiological threshold determined (as well as confirming this to be the CPN).
  - Typically, at higher stimulation parameters, there is spread to the tibial nerve with electrical stimulation signal being detected in electrodes placed in the gastrocnemius as well.
- The CPN is then followed distally performing an external neurolysis with the above-mentioned dissection techniques down toward the distal end of the exposure.
  - This is continued until just proximal to the fibular head and neck where there are usually tight fascial bands that are encountered with the peroneus longus fascia and fibular tunnel.
  - These are next released using a combination of bipolar cautery and tenotomy scissors.
- Another vessel loop is placed around the CPN just rostral to this and used to help retract it out of the way (in order to be able to undermine the fascia of the peroneus longus, which has then been identified—there are usually two layers of this).
- First, the superficial layer is released while protecting the branches of the CPN underneath.
- Once the superficial and deep fascial layers are released, the peroneus longus muscle can be seen (▶ Fig. 32.2b).
- As described above, the bifurcation of the CPN into its terminal superficial and deep peroneal nerves will occur at a variable distance from the popliteal fossa.
- Vessel loops are placed around each respective branch of the CPN and they are neurolyzed distally and proximally to ensure there are no further points of entrapment or tethering (▶ Fig. 32.2b, c).
- A large blunt dissector is next passed over top of the deep and superficial peroneal nerves down into the lateral and anterior compartments of the patient's leg over top of each nerve.
- The dissector should pass quite freely into each leg compartment paralleling the course of the superficial and deep peroneal nerves. The same maneuver at the rostral end of the exposure into the posterior aspect of the rostral thigh over top of the CPN is then performed to ensure that this is also completely free of entrapment or tethering.
- Finally, the CPN and its superficial and deep branches are stimulated one more time to determine their respective electrophysiological thresholds (which have often decreased after decompression).
- Of note, we will also have our neurophysiologist perform motor and sensory evoked potential signals before and after nerve release to determine any changes/improvements postdecompression.
- The wound is then copiously irrigated with a warm saline solution and any further hemostasis obtained.
- Vicryl 3–0 sutures are used to close the dermal layer in an interrupted inverted fashion and 3–0 Monocryl is used to reapproximate the skin and dermal layer over top of this in a running continuous fashion.
- Steri-Strips are then used to reapproximate the skin as well.

32.6 Complications

- Wound complications.
- Damage to local vessels.

32.7 Management Pearls

- CPN palsy should be treated according to the underlying etiology.
- For patients with reversible causes or those in which the natural history is expected to improve (such as a closed injury), an initial trial of conservative/nonoperative management is often pursued. This includes activity modification, physical therapy, medications such as nonsteroidal anti-inflammatory drugs, neuropathic and/or neuromodulatory pain medication (gabapentin, pregabalin, nortriptyline, amitriptyline, among others), among others.
- Surgical intervention for CPN palsy is directed toward the removal of the causative mass or decompression (and repair) of the identified site causing symptoms with external neurolysis ± internal neurolysis of the CPN.
- Outcomes after decompression and external ± internal neurolysis for CPN have been reported to be quite favorable in the literature, with the majority of studies showing recovery to an MRC grade 4/5 or better in 80 to 100% cases.

References

[1] Kim D, Husdon A, Kline D. Atlas of Peripheral Nerve Surgery. 2nd ed. Philadelphia, PA: Elsevier/Saunders; 2013

[2] Kim D, Midha R, Murovic J, Spinner R. Kline and Hudon's Nerve Injuries: Operative Results for Major Nerve Injuries, Entrapments, and Tumors. 2nd ed. Philadelphia, PA: Elsevier/Saunders; 2008

[3] Kline D, Husdon A, Kim D. Atlas of Peripheral Nerve Surgery. Philadelphia, PA: Saunders; 2001

[4] Broekx S, Weyns F. External neurolysis as a treatment for foot drop secondary to weight loss: a retrospective analysis of 200 cases. Acta Neurochir (Wien). 2018; 160(9):1847–1856

[5] Oosterbos C, Decramer T, Rummens S, et al. Evidence in peroneal nerve entrapment: a scoping review. Eur J Neurol. 2022; 29(2):665–679

[6] Poage C, Roth C, Scott B. Peroneal nerve palsy: evaluation and management. J Am Acad Orthop Surg. 2016; 24(1):1–10

[7] Cruz-Martinez A, Arpa J, Palau F. Peroneal neuropathy after weight loss. J Peripher Nerv Syst. 2000; 5(2):101–105

[8] Kandil MR, Darwish ES, Khedr EM, Sabry MM, Abdulah MA. A community-based epidemiological study of peripheral neuropathies in Assiut, Egypt. Neurol Res. 2012; 34(10):960–966

[9] Khedr EM, Fawi G, Allah Abbas MA, El-Fetoh NA, Zaki AF, Gamea A. Prevalence of common types of compression neuropathies in Qena Governorate/Egypt: a population-based survey. Neuroepidemiology. 2016; 46(4):253–260

[10] Shahar E, Landau E, Genizi J. Adolescence peroneal neuropathy associated with rapid marked weight reduction: case report and literature review. Eur J Paediatr Neurol. 2007; 11(1):50–54

[11] Elias WJ, Pouratian N, Oskouian RJ, Schirmer B, Burns T. Peroneal neuropathy following successful bariatric surgery. Case report and review of the literature. J Neurosurg. 2006; 105(4):631–635

[12] Farhad K, Traub R, Ruzhansky KM, Brannagan TH, III. Causes of neuropathy in patients referred as "idiopathic neuropathy.". Muscle Nerve. 2016; 53(6):856–861

[13] Lutte I, Rhys C, Hubert C, et al. Peroneal nerve palsy in anorexia nervosa. Acta Neurol Belg. 1997; 97(4):251–254

[14] Marciniak C. Fibular (peroneal) neuropathy: electrodiagnostic features and clinical correlates. Phys Med Rehabil Clin N Am. 2013; 24(1):121–137

[15] Meylaerts L, Cardinaels E, Vandevenne J, et al. Peroneal neuropathy after weight loss: a high-resolution ultrasonographic characterization of the common peroneal nerve. Skeletal Radiol. 2011; 40(12):1557–1562

[16] Åen O, Karaca FC, Türkçapar A. Neurological complication after laparoscopic sleeve gastrectomy: foot drop. Obes Surg. 2020; 30(3):957–960

[17] Weyns FJ, Beckers F, Vanormelingen L, Vandersteen M, Niville E. Foot drop as a complication of weight loss after bariatric surgery: is it preventable? Obes Surg. 2007; 17(9): 1209–1212

[18] Warner MA, Martin JT, Schroeder DR, Offord KP, Chute CG. Lower-extremity motor neuropathy associated with surgery performed on patients in a lithotomy position. Anesthesiology. 1994; 81(1):6–12

[19] Winfree CJ, Kline DG. Intraoperative positioning nerve injuries. Surg Neurol. 2005; 63(1):5–18, discussion 18

[20] Kokkalis ZT, Kalavrytinos D, Kokkineli S, et al. Intraneural ganglion cysts of the peroneal nerve. Eur J Orthop Surg Traumatol. 2021; 31(8):1639–1645

[21] Weyns F, Bringmans T, Vandevenne J, et al. Peripheral neuropathy caused by joint-related cysts: a review of 17 cases. Acta Neurochir (Wien). 2012; 154(10):1741–1753

[22] Garland H, Moorhouse D. Compressive lesions of the external popliteal (common peroneal) nerve. BMJ. 1952; 2(4799): 1373–1378

[23] Aprile I, Padua L, Padua R, et al. Peroneal mononeuropathy: predisposing factors, and clinical and neurophysiological relationships. Neurol Sci. 2000; 21(6):367–371

[24] Bowley MP, Doughty CT. Entrapment neuropathies of the lower extremity. Med Clin North Am. 2019; 103(2):371–382

[25] Pattyn R, Loder R, Mullis BH. Iatrogenic peroneal nerve palsy rates secondary to open reduction internal fixation for tibial plateau fractures using an intraoperative distractor. J Orthop Trauma. 2020; 34(7):359–362

[26] Berry H, Richardson PM. Common peroneal nerve palsy: a clinical and electrophysiological review. J Neurol Neurosurg Psychiatry. 1976; 39(12):1162–1171

[27] Kim DH, Kline DG. Management and results of peroneal nerve lesions. Neurosurgery. 1996; 39(2):312–319, discussion 319–320

[28] Tarabay B, Abdallah Y, Kobaiter-Maarrawi S, Yammine P, Maarrawi J. Outcome and prognosis of microsurgical decompression in idiopathic severe common fibular nerve entrapment: prospective clinical study. World Neurosurg. 2019; 126:e281–e287

[29] Klifto KM, Azoury SC, Gurno CF, Card EB, Levin LS, Kovach SJ. Treatment approach to isolated common peroneal nerve palsy by mechanism of injury: systematic review and meta-analysis of individual participants' data. J Plast Reconstr Aesthet Surg. 2022; 75(2):683–702

[30] Fares MY, Dimassi Z, Fares J, Musharrafieh U. Peroneal neuropathy and bariatric surgery: untying the knot. Int J Neurosci. 2020; 130(4):417–423
[31] George SC, Boyce DE. An evidence-based structured review to assess the results of common peroneal nerve repair. Plast Reconstr Surg. 2014; 134(2):302e–311e
[32] Maalla R, Youssef M, Ben Lassoued N, Sebai MA, Essadam H. Peroneal nerve entrapment at the fibular head: outcomes of neurolysis. Orthop Traumatol Surg Res. 2013; 99(6):719–722
[33] Yu JK, Yang JS, Kang SH, Cho YJ. Clinical characteristics of peroneal nerve palsy by posture. J Korean Neurosurg Soc. 2013; 53(5):269–273
[34] Vastamäki M. Decompression for peroneal nerve entrapment. Acta Orthop Scand. 1986; 57(6):551–554
[35] Terzis JK, Kostas I. Outcomes with microsurgery of common peroneal nerve lesions. J Plast Reconstr Aesthet Surg. 2020; 73(1):72–80
[36] Nirenberg MS. A simple test to assist with the diagnosis of common fibular nerve entrapment and predict outcomes of surgical decompression. Acta Neurochir (Wien). 2020; 162 (6):1439–1444
[37] Lale A, Kirkil C, Ozturk S, et al. The results of surgical decompression in the treatment of foot drop due to peroneal nerve entrapment after bariatric surgery. Surg Obes Relat Dis. 2020; 16(11):1684–1691
[38] Fabre T, Piton C, Andre D, Lasseur E, Durandeau A. Peroneal nerve entrapment. J Bone Joint Surg Am. 1998; 80(1):47–53
[39] Chow AL, Levidy MF, Luthringer M, Vasoya D, Ignatiuk A. Clinical outcomes after neurolysis for the treatment of peroneal nerve palsy: a systematic review and meta-analysis. Ann Plast Surg. 2021; 87(3):316–323
[40] Marciniak C, Armon C, Wilson J, Miller R. Practice parameter: utility of electrodiagnostic techniques in evaluating patients with suspected peroneal neuropathy: an evidence-based review. Muscle Nerve. 2005; 31(4):520–527
[41] Desy NM, Wang H, Elshiekh MA, et al. Intraneural ganglion cysts: a systematic review and reinterpretation of the world's literature. J Neurosurg. 2016; 125(3):615–630

Part IV

Spine Surgery

IV

33 Occipitocervical Fusion

Rohit Prem Kumar, Andrew Legarreta, Joseph Hudson, Hansen Deng, and D. Kojo Hamilton

33.1 Background

- Most pathologic events affecting the occipitocervical region are traumatic in origin. They can range from asymptomatic occipital condyle fracture to atlanto-occipital dislocation.
  - *Transverse ligament rupture:* This is classified into two categories by Dickman et al. Type 1 or intraligament tear is incapable of healing and requires C1–C2 fixation due to poor atlantoaxial stability. In type 2, the ligament is detached due to a bony avulsion fracture, and nonsurgical management is successful in 80% of cases with external orthosis. Fixation surgery can be considered for nonunion injuries after 3 to 4 months of immobilization.[1,2]
  - *Occipital condyle fracture:* It can routinely be managed with external cervical immobilization with follow-up in 6 weeks. In rare instances of disruption of the occiput–C1 joint, fusion should be utilized. Further classification is typically not warranted, regardless of the unilaterally of fracture.[3]
  - An isolated C1 fracture (Jefferson fracture) is based on the integrity of the transverse ligament. They are typically managed with external immobilization devices, but fusion can be considered in cases of transverse ligament disruption.[4]
- Additionally, large skull base tumors, rheumatologic disease, and infectious disease, among others, may require occipitocervical fusion to achieve the goals of surgical decompression and to maintain spinal stability.[5]
- Instability at the craniocervical junction can be vertical (cranial settling) or horizontal (atlantoaxial).[6]
- All adult patients with unstable lesions of the occipitocervical junction should be treated, as ligamentous injuries rarely heal by themselves.[1,7] Instrumentation is frequently required to achieve spinal stability.
  - Example: A 45-year-old man involved in a high-speed car accident presents with severe neck pain, limited neck movement, and mild neurological deficits in the upper extremities. Imaging reveals a displaced occipital condyle fracture on computed tomography (CT) and significant disruption of the alar and transverse ligaments on magnetic resonance imaging (MRI), indicating an unstable occipitocervical junction injury. Given the instability and ligamentous nature of the injury, surgical intervention with occipitocervical fusion is performed to achieve spinal stability and prevent further neurological damage.

33.2 Indications and Contraindications

- **Indications**:
  - Atlanto-occipital dislocation (▶ Fig. 33.1).[7,8]
  - Unstable C1 (Jefferson) fracture.[7,9]

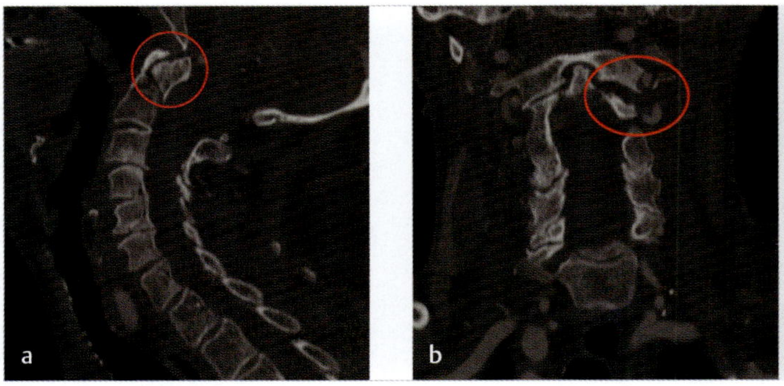

Fig. 33.1 CT image demonstrating a C1–C2 fracture (*red circles*) that required occiput to C3 fixation in **(a)** sagittal and **(b)** coronal views.

  - Basilar invagination requiring decompression (▶ Fig. 33.2).[6,9]
  - Atlantoaxial subluxation unsuitable for C1–C2 fixation.[7,9,10]
  - Cranial nerve deficit.[10]
  - Most commonly, cranial nerve XII is involved. Cranial nerves V, IX, X, and XI may also be affected.[11]
- **Contraindications**
  - Medical comorbidities placing the patient at high risk of intraoperative demise (other traumatic injuries, poor cardiopulmonary baseline, etc.)[7,9]
  - Previous posterior fossa decompression.[7,9]
  - Poor bone quality.[7,9]

33.3 Informed Consent

- Expected benefits:
  - Restoration of craniocervical stability.[5,6]
  - Neural decompression and pain relief.[5]
  - Preservation or improvement of neurologic function.[5]
- Potential complications:
  - Infection or poor wound healing.[12]
  - Bleeding or hematoma formation.[12]
  - Dural tear with CSF leak.[12]
  - Spinal cord, nerve root, or vertebral artery injury.[9]
  - Hardware malposition, loosening, or breakage.[13]
  - Nonunion (pseudarthrosis).[14]
  - Malalignment leading to pain, dysphagia, or motion loss.[15]
  - Airway complications (swelling, re-intubation).[16]
  - Anesthesia-related events (cardiopulmonary, thromboembolism).

33.4 Instruments

- Three-point fixation clamp (Mayfield).
- Wilson table with gel rolls.
- Fluoroscopy (C-arm).
- Occipital plating and rod system.
- High-speed and hand drills.

33.5 Patient Preparation

- **Preoperative diagnostics**:
  - *CT of the cervical spine without contrast (thin cut):* Carefully study the depth and angle of the C1 anterior tubercle, as this can vary significantly among patients. Measure the thickness of the suboccipital bone in preparation for screw placement. Evaluate for ponticulus posticus.
  - MRI of the cervical spine without contrast.
  - Consider CT angiography (CTA) of the neck to evaluate the location of vertebral arteries, as well as the carotid arteries, especially when C1 instrumentation is part of the planned construct.
  - *Full medical evaluation:* Patients with multiple medical comorbidities such as steroids, oral contraceptives, immunocompromise, and tobacco use can affect the fusion rate.
- **Anesthesia**:
  - General anesthesia.
  - Strict glideslope intubation with C-spine precautions.
  - Spinal cord injury patients may have significantly reduced vasomotor tone and require extensive fluid volume and vasopressors for hemodynamic stability.

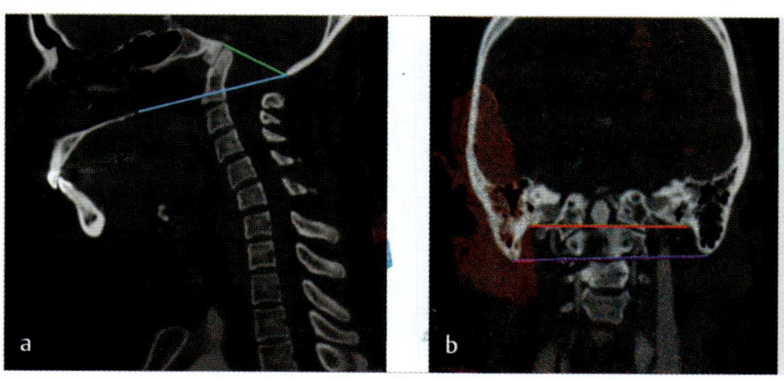

Fig. 33.2 CT image demonstrating a basilar invagination that required occiput to C4 fixation in **(a)** sagittal and **(b)** coronal views. The *lines* are the McRae (*green*), Chamberlain (*blue*), digastric (*red*), and bimastoid (*purple*) lines.

33.6 Patient Positioning

- Position the patient prone in three-point fixation.
- The eyes must be looking forward without lateral tilt.
- Confirm neutral alignment with fluoroscopy.

33.7 Technique

- A midline incision is made from the inion to the inferior aspect of the construct.
- A midline subperiosteal dissection is performed with care taken to stay in the avascular plane.
- Expose the foramen magnum and dorsal arches of the facet joints of the desired levels. Expose the occipital keel.
- Care should be taken to avoid violating interspinous ligaments during dissection.
- **Screw implantation:**
  - For occipitocervical arthrodesis to take place, a bony bridge must be established between the occiput and the upper cervical spine. Bone fusion requires two conditions: bone graft must be in continuity and motion must be minimized or eliminated.[3] It can be achieved with either bone alone or bone and instrumented fusion.[6]
  - *Occipital screws:* The thick surface of the occipital keel should be drilled prior to insertion of fixating bone screws. They should be tapped to full depth prior to insertion. Ideally, a bicortical purchase is achieved with screw placement. However, it is not necessary and may increase the risk of bleeding and spinal fluid leak. Four burr holes are made on the suboccipital bone paramedian.
  - *C1 lateral mass:* The technical difficulty of screw placement is due to the approach and entry point. The C2 nerve root and its associated venous plexus are closely associated with C1, and identifying the medial and lateral border of C1 is key, and requires meticulous hemostasis. The Lenke probe is used to identify the trajectory aiming toward the anterior tubercle on lateral fluoroscopy, then a tap is utilized. The entry point for the C1 lateral mass screw is the middle of the lateral mass. Typically, lag screws are used to facilitate rod placement.
  - Additional levels of cervical screw implants will be covered elsewhere in this book.
  - Appropriate decortication of the lamina should take place.
  - Bone grafting techniques depend on the surgical procedure and surgeon's preference. Options include autografts and allografts. Grafts can be cortical, cancellous, or mixed. Cortical bone is the strongest and should be used when strong structural support is required. Autografts are the gold standard and are associated with the highest rates of fusion. If neither autograft nor allograft is available, methyl methacrylate is an option. Autograft harvesting sites include the rib, iliac crest, skull, and fibula.
- Rod and plate screw systems are the most effective fusion techniques with varying options available (▶ Fig. 33.3).[5]

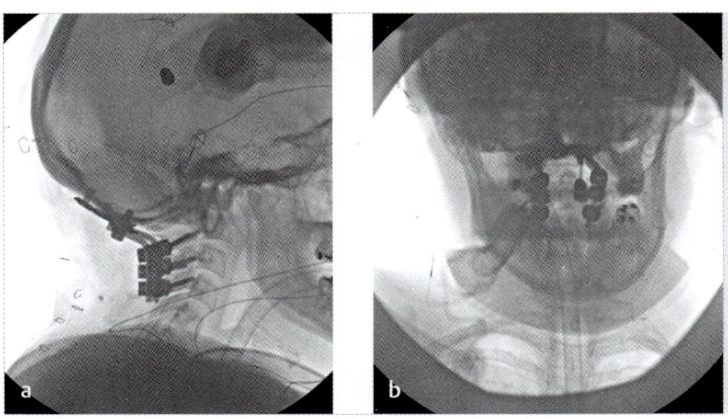

Fig. 33.3 Fluoroscopic image showing screw–rod constructs in **(a)** sagittal and **(b)** coronal views.

  - One option is a titanium rod contoured into a reverse "**U**" shape for appropriate craniocervical conformation.[6]
  - Another option is the inverted "**Y**" shape implant, which permits longer screws to prevent pullout.[9,13]
- **Relevant anatomy**:
  - The occipitocervical junction is the most mobile portion of the spine. It is integrated by three osseous structures: occiput, atlas, and axis. Membranes and ligaments protect the lower brainstem, cervical spinal cord, and vertebral arteries.
  - The major stabilizing components include the tectorial membrane, bilateral alar ligaments, and cruciate ligament.
  - A minor stabilization role is contributed by the anterior and posterior atlanto-occipital membranes and bony articulations.
  - The occipitoatlantoaxial joints have two synovial joints between the occipital condyles and the atlas.
  - The atlas (C1) is unique in that it contains no body. It consists of a ring with an anterior and posterior arch and two lateral masses. Its etymology is based on Greek mythology as a metaphor for Atlas supporting the entire world.
  - Disruption of the occipitocervical junction components can lead to permanent neurologic injury or death.
- **Variants and cross-reference**:
  - Other fixation strategies:
    - Suboccipital wiring.[9,17]
    - Suboccipital in-out buttons.[9,17]
    - Condylar screw fixation.[9,17]
  - Variant anatomy:
    - *Ponticulus posticus:* A bony prominence arising from the C1 posterior arch that partially or completely encircles the vertebral artery. It gives the false impression of a thick posterior arch able to accommodate C1 lateral mass screws.[18] It affects 8% of the population and can result in pinching of the vertebral artery.[7]
- **Video 33.1** provides additional expert tips and tricks for performing this technique.

33.8 Postoperative Care

- Care must be taken not to rush extubation and have a rebound of anesthesia medication. Difficult intubation, duration of surgery greater than 5 hours, and ≥ 6 vertebral levels of fusion are risk factors for postoperative airway complications (e.g., need to reintubate). These risk factors must be considered when determining the time and location of extubation.[16] Close postoperative monitoring is preeminent.
- Hard cervical collar for 6 to 12 weeks with radiographic follow-up is recommended. X-rays or CT scanning is sufficient.

33.9 Complications

- Penetration of the dura and cerebellum during occipital screw insertion.[12]
- Vertebral artery injury.
- Spinal cord injury.
- Spinal nerve root injury.
- Infection.[12]
- Malalignment leading to severely decreased range of motion, spinal stenosis,[15] pain, dysphagia, respiratory difficulties, and balance issues.
- **Special risk:** In cases of atlanto-occipital dislocation or fracture of C1, the C1 ring is often free-floating and unstable. A free-floating C1 ring is easily susceptible to rotational injury during screw insertion. This places the patient at high risk of injury to the vertebral arteries, neural elements, or both. The ring should be manually stabilized with a clamp to avoid these complications.[19] If this is not possible, this level should not be instrumented.

33.10 Management Pearls

- Determining the appropriate levels to end a fusion requires consideration of the patient's diagnosis, presentation, and radiographic findings.
- Committing a patient to occipitocervical fusion is potentially a highly morbid operation with an elevated risk of return to the operating room, and loss of 15 to 20 degrees of flexion/extension should be carefully discussed with the patient and family.[6,14,20]
- Although external fixation devices are critical in patients with craniocervical pathology, internal fixation is more effective, less costly, and less uncomfortable if immediate stabilization is required.[19]

33.11 Emerging Technologies

- 3D image-guided navigation and augmented reality overlays.[21]
- Robotic-assisted planning and screw placement.[21,22]
- Patient-specific 3D-printed plates and drill guides.[23]
- Percutaneous/endoscope-assisted approaches.[24]
- Advanced biologics (BMPs, stem cell scaffolds).[25,26]
- "Smart" drills/taps with breach detection feedback.[27,28]
- AI-driven surgical planning and risk stratification.[29]

References

[1] Kopparapu S, Mao G, Judy BF, Theodore N. Fifty years later: the "rule of Spence" is finally ready for retirement. J Neurosurg Spine. 2022; 37(2):149–156

[2] Dickman CA, Greene KA, Sonntag VKH. Injuries involving the transverse atlantal ligament: classification and treatment guidelines based upon experience with 39 injuries. Neurosurgery. 1996; 38(1):44–50

[3] Maserati MB, Stephens B, Zohny Z, et al. Occipital condyle fractures: clinical decision rule and surgical management. J Neurosurg Spine. 2009; 11(4):388–395

[4] Kim HS, Cloney MB, Koski TR, Smith ZA, Dahdaleh NS. Management of isolated atlas fractures: a retrospective study of 65 patients. World Neurosurg. 2018; 111:e316–e322

[5] Winegar CD, Lawrence JP, Friel BC, et al. A systematic review of occipital cervical fusion: techniques and outcomes. J Neurosurg Spine. 2010; 13(1):5–16

[6] Perin NI, Baldwin NG, Cooper PR. High cervical and occipitocervical plate, rod, wire, and bone techniques. In: Benzel's Spine Surgery Techniques, Complication Avoidance, and Management. 4th ed. Philadelphia, PA: Elsevier; 2017

[7] Lee DJ, Ahmadpour A, Ament JD, Goodarzi A, Panchal RR. When is occipitocervical fusion necessary for upper cervical injuries? Semin Spine Surg. 2017; 29(1):20–26

[8] Joaquim AF, Schroeder GD, Vaccaro AR. Traumatic atlanto-occipital dislocation-a comprehensive analysis of all case series found in the spinal trauma literature. Int J Spine Surg. 2021; 15(4):724–739

[9] Lu DC, Roeser AC, Mummaneni VP, Mummaneni PV. Nuances of occipitocervical fixation. Neurosurgery. 2010; 66(3) Suppl: 141–146

[10] Bhatia R, Desouza RM, Bull J, Casey ATH. Rigid occipitocervical fixation: indications, outcomes, and complications in the modern era. J Neurosurg Spine. 2013; 18(4):333–339

[11] Rogers MA, Crockard HA, Moskovich R, et al. Nystagmus and joint position sensation: their importance in posterior occipitocervical fusion in rheumatoid arthritis. Spine. 1994; 19(1):16–20

[12] Vender JR, Rekito AJ, Harrison SJ, McDonnell DE. The evolution of posterior cervical and occipitocervical fusion and instrumentation. Neurosurg Focus. 2004; 16(1):E9

[13] Hurlbert RJ, Crawford NR, Choi WG, Dickman CA. A biomechanical evaluation of occipitocervical instrumentation: screw compared with wire fixation. J Neurosurg. 1999; 90(1) Suppl:84–90

[14] Soriano-Baron H, Martinez-del-Campo E, Neal MT, Theodore N. Upper cervical and occipitocervical arthrodesis. In: Benzel's Spine Surgery Techniques, Complication Avoidance, and Management. 4th ed. Philadelphia, PA: Elsevier; 2017

[15] Phillips FM, Phillips CS, Wetzel FT, Gelinas C. Occipitocervical neutral position. Possible surgical implications. Spine. 1999; 24(8):775–778

[16] Sheshadri V, Moga R, Manninen P, et al. Airway adverse events following posterior occipito-cervical spinal fusion. J Clin Neurosci. 2017; 39:124–129

[17] Shasti M, Moshirfar A, Gum JL, Jazini E. Occipitocervical fusion: a review and current concepts. Semin Spine Surg. 2020; 32(1):100783

[18] Elliott RE, Tanweer O. The prevalence of the ponticulus posticus (arcuate foramen) and its importance in the Goel-Harms procedure: meta-analysis and review of the literature. World Neurosurg. 2014; 82(1–2):e335–e343

[19] Bisson EF, Guan J, Schmidt MH, Apfelbaum RI. Upper cervical screw fixation techniques. In: Benzel's Spine Surgery Techniques, Complication Avoidance, and Management. 4th ed. Philadelphia, PA: Elsevier; 2017

[20] Bhimani AD, Chiu RG, Esfahani DR, et al. C1-C2 fusion versus occipito-cervical fusion for high cervical fractures: a multi-institutional database analysis and review of the literature. World Neurosurg. 2018; 119:e459–e466

[21] Foley D, Hardacker P, McCarthy M. Emerging technologies within spine surgery. Life (Basel). 2023; 13(10):2028

[22] Vadalà G, De Salvatore S, Ambrosio L, Russo F, Papalia R, Denaro V. Robotic spine surgery and augmented reality systems: a state of the art. Neurospine. 2020; 17(1):88–100

[23] Tian X, Liu Y, Liu S, et al. Transforming spinal surgery with innovations in biologics and additive manufacturing. Mater Today Bio. 2025; 32:101853

[24] Huang CC, Fitts J, Huie D, Bhowmick DA, Abd-El-Barr MM. Evolution of cervical endoscopic spine surgery: current progress and future directions—a narrative review. J Clin Med. 2024; 13(7):2122

[25] Von Benecke JP, Tarsitano E, Zimmermann LA, Shakesheff KM, Walsh WR, Bae HW. A narrative review on recombinant human bone morphogenetic protein 2: where are we now? Cureus. 2024; 16(8):e67785

[26] Stephan SR, Kanim LE, Bae HW. Stem cells and spinal fusion. Int J Spine Surg. 2021; 15(s1) Suppl 1:94–103

[27] Ivanišević A, Boban Z, Jurić J, Vukojević K. Smart drill for a streamlined estimation of the drilling angle and channel length in orthopedic surgical procedures. Bioengineering (Basel). 2024; 11(6):630

[28] Massalimova A, Timmermans M, Cavalcanti N, et al. Automatic breach detection during spine pedicle drilling based on vibroacoustic sensing. Artif Intell Med. 2023; 144: 102641

[29] Yahanda AT, Joseph K, Bui T, et al. Current applications and future implications of artificial intelligence in spine surgery and research: a narrative review and commentary. Global Spine J. 2025; 15(2):1445–1454

34 Atlantoaxial Instability

Atul Goel, Krishna P. Nayak, and Abhidha Shah

34.1 Background

- The craniovertebral junction is a complex formation that supports the strongest and most mobile region of the spine.
- Some of the most critical neural and vascular structures transit this passage. The human spinal column has a **Y**-shaped configuration.
- The rostral "V" of the "Y," which is composed of the suboccipital bone, atlas, and axis vertebrae, constitutes the craniovertebral junction.
- The occipitoatlantal joint is the strongest joint, while the atlantoaxial joint is the most mobile joint of the spine. Mobility and stability are the hallmarks of the craniovertebral junction.
- The term *craniovertebral instability* can be synonymous with *atlantoaxial instability* because, whereas atlantoaxial instability is relatively common, occipitoatlantal instability is significantly infrequent and is rarely identified in cases with severe trauma and in children with "syndromic" affection.
- Atlantoaxial stabilization is a complex surgical procedure.
- The primary aims of surgery are to remove or denude the articular cartilage of the atlantoaxial articulation, introduce bone graft within the articular cavity, and subsequently perform metal fixation that will stabilize the region and permit bone fusion.
- The aim of the surgical procedure is to achieve solid arthrodesis of the atlantoaxial joint.
- Elimination of the source of power by sectioning the muscles and paralyzing the fulcrum of activity at the joints by denuding the articular cartilage and packing of bone grafts are critical surgical steps.
- The metal implant must be strong and capable of providing "zero" movement for a period of about 2 months and an opportunity for bone healing. Subsequently, the fused bone will be the primary source of stability.

34.2 Indications and Contraindications

- An abnormal increase in the atlantodental interval on dynamic lateral radiographs with the head in flexion and extension has been the criterion for diagnosing atlantoaxial instability. An increase in the atlantodental interval of more than 3 mm on flexion of the head is diagnostic of atlantoaxial instability.
- In children, an atlantodental interval of more than 5 mm is generally considered to indicate the presence of atlantoaxial instability.
- When the atlantodental interval reduces on extension, the atlantoaxial dislocation is "mobile" and "reducible" (▸ Fig. 34.1).[1,2]
- If the dislocation is reduced only partially on extension, the dislocation is called "partially reducible" atlantoaxial instability.
- If the dislocation does not reduce on extension, it is labeled as "fixed" or "irreducible" atlantoaxial instability (▸ Fig. 34.2).[3]

34.3 Instruments

- Gardner-Wells cervical traction.
- Osteotome.
- Electric drill/power drill.
- Two-hole titanium plate.
- Screws.

34.4 Patient Preparation

- Dynamic plain lateral radiographs, computed tomography (CT) scan, and magnetic resonance imaging (MRI) of the craniovertebral junction with the head in flexed and extended positions show the alteration in the atlantodental interval and confirm atlantoaxial instability in the anteroposterior and vertical perspectives.
- CT scan and MRI provide useful information regarding the nature of the primary and associated bone and soft tissue alterations.
- MRI and CT angiography show the relationship of the vertebral artery to the facets of C2 and C1. Such information can be crucial when lateral mass fixation techniques are employed.
- 3D CT scanning and 3D model reconstruction are emerging as useful imaging modalities. The 3D models can replicate the exact lifelike structure of the region.

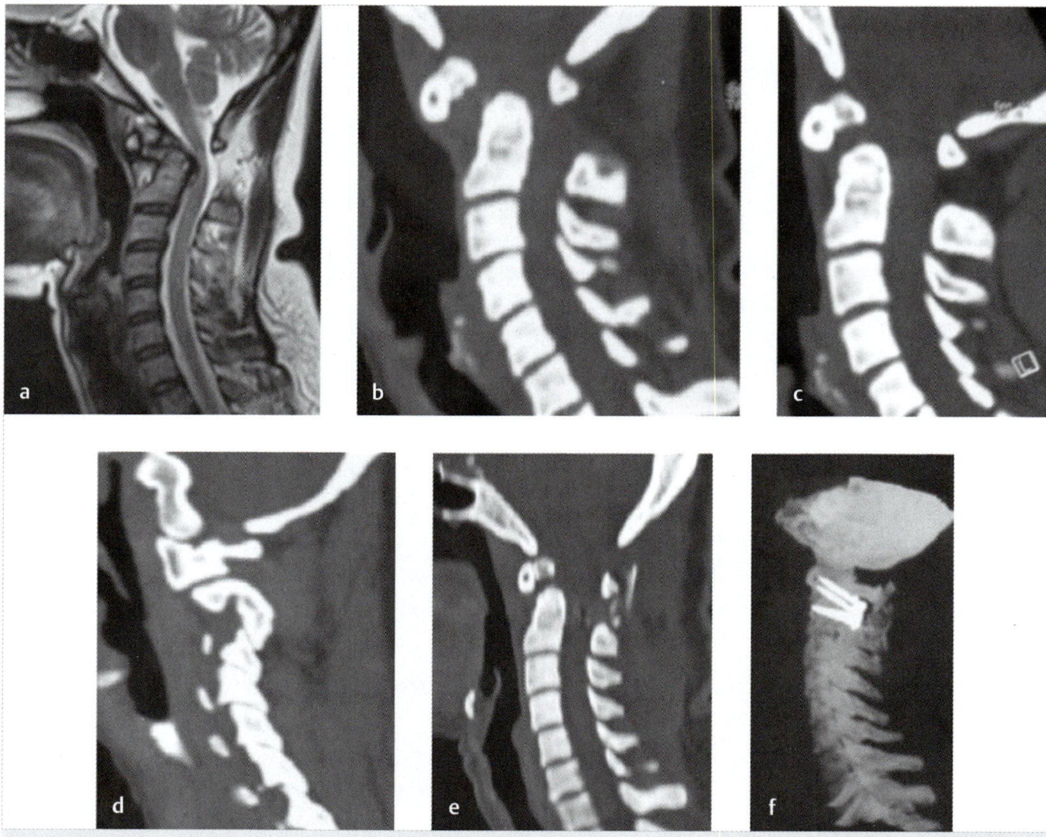

Fig. 34.1 Images showing mobile atlantoaxial dislocation. (a) T2-weighted magnetic resonance image showing os odontoideum, atlantoaxial dislocation, and cord compression. (b) Computed tomography (CT) scan with the head in flexion shows atlantoaxial dislocation. Os odontoideum can be seen. (c) CT scan with the head in extension showing reduction of the dislocation. (d) CT scan with the cut passing through the facets showing type 1 facetal instability. (e) Postoperative CT scan showing atlantoaxial fixation in reduced position. (f) Image showing the implants in the facets of the atlas and axis.

34.5 Patient Positioning

- After the induction of anesthesia, Gardner-Wells cervical traction is applied.
- The neck is held firmly, and the surgeon applies traction by holding the ring, and the patient is carefully turned prone. Traction should not be released during the entire surgical procedure to avoid any unwanted neck movements during anesthesia that paralyses the muscles.
- The head end of the operating table is elevated. The elevated head end of the table provides countertraction and reduces the venous congestion in the region of surgery. The elevated head position also allows a direct surgical vision to the operative field.
- The head is in a "floating" position, with the headrest being placed only for support.

34.6 Technique

- The techniques of fixation for atlantoaxial dislocation can be divided into *midline procedures* that involve the fixation of the arch of the atlas with the lamina of the axis and *lateral mass fixation procedures* that involve fixation of the facets of the atlas and the axis.

Goel and Laheri technique of lateral mass plate and screw fixation (▸ Fig. 34.3, ▸ Fig. 34.4, and ▸ Fig. 34.5 and Video 34.1)[1,2]:

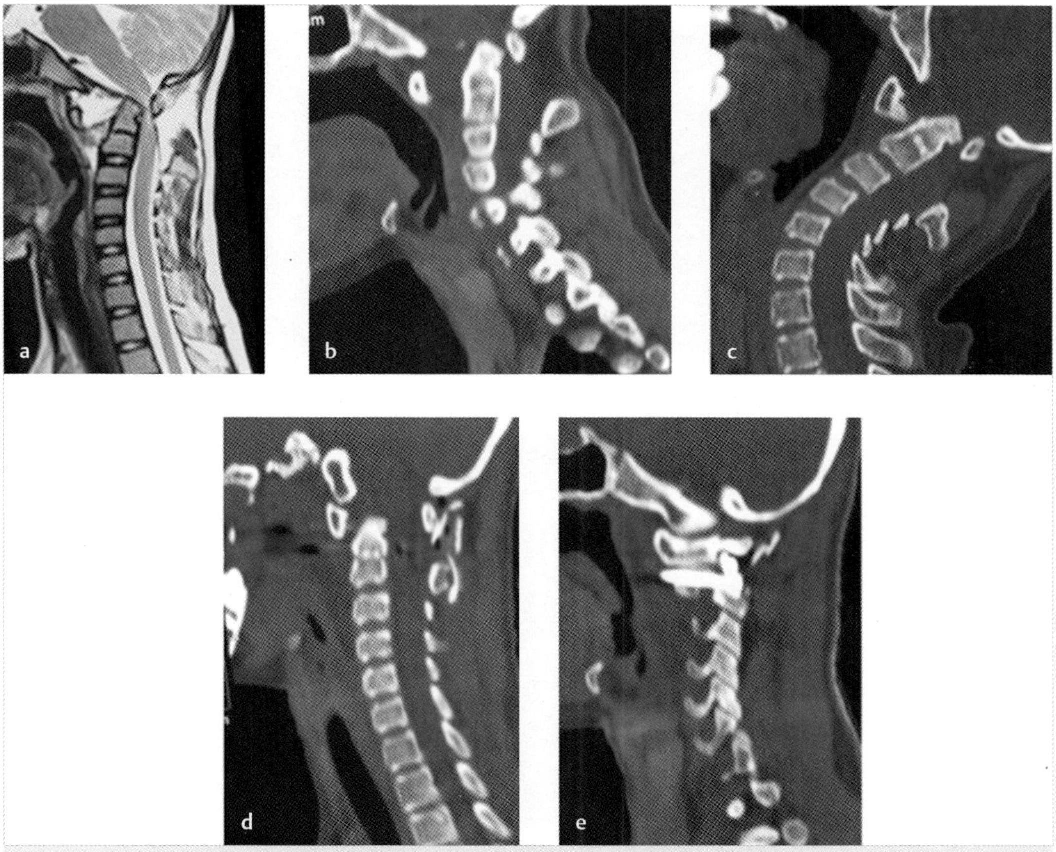

Fig. 34.2 Images showing “fixed” atlantoaxial dislocation. **(a)** T2-weighted magnetic resonance imaging (MRI) showing “irreducible” atlantoaxial dislocation and cord compression. **(b)** Computed tomography (CT) scan with the head in flexion showing severe atlantoaxial dislocation. **(c)** CT scan with the head in extension does not show any reduction in atlantoaxial dislocation. **(d)** Postoperative CT scan showing realignment of the craniovertebral junction and the atlantoaxial fusion. **(e)** Postoperative image through the facets showing lateral mass plate and screw fixation.

- *Surgical procedure*:
  - The large and stubby C2 spinous process forms the primary landmark during surgery.
  - A midline incision is made that extends from the suboccipital region to the neck and is approximately 4 cm above and below the C2 spinous process.
  - Subperiosteal dissection exposes the C2 spinous process and the lamina of the C2 vertebra.
  - Identification of the C2 pedicle then forms an important guiding landmark. The pedicle is then followed rostrally to expose the atlantoaxial articulation.
- *C2 ganglion*:
  - The C2 ganglion is located on the posterior face of the articulation and acts like a guard to the surgical gateway of the joint.[6] It can be elevated rostrally to widely expose the articular cavity.
  - In situations where the joint exposure is incomplete or less than satisfactory, sectioning of the C2 ganglion can be done safely.
- *Atlantoaxial joint*:
  - The atlantoaxial joint is widely exposed using the sharp edge of the osteotome introduced in the joint cavity and then turned in a screwing motion to denude articular cartilage and distract the joint.

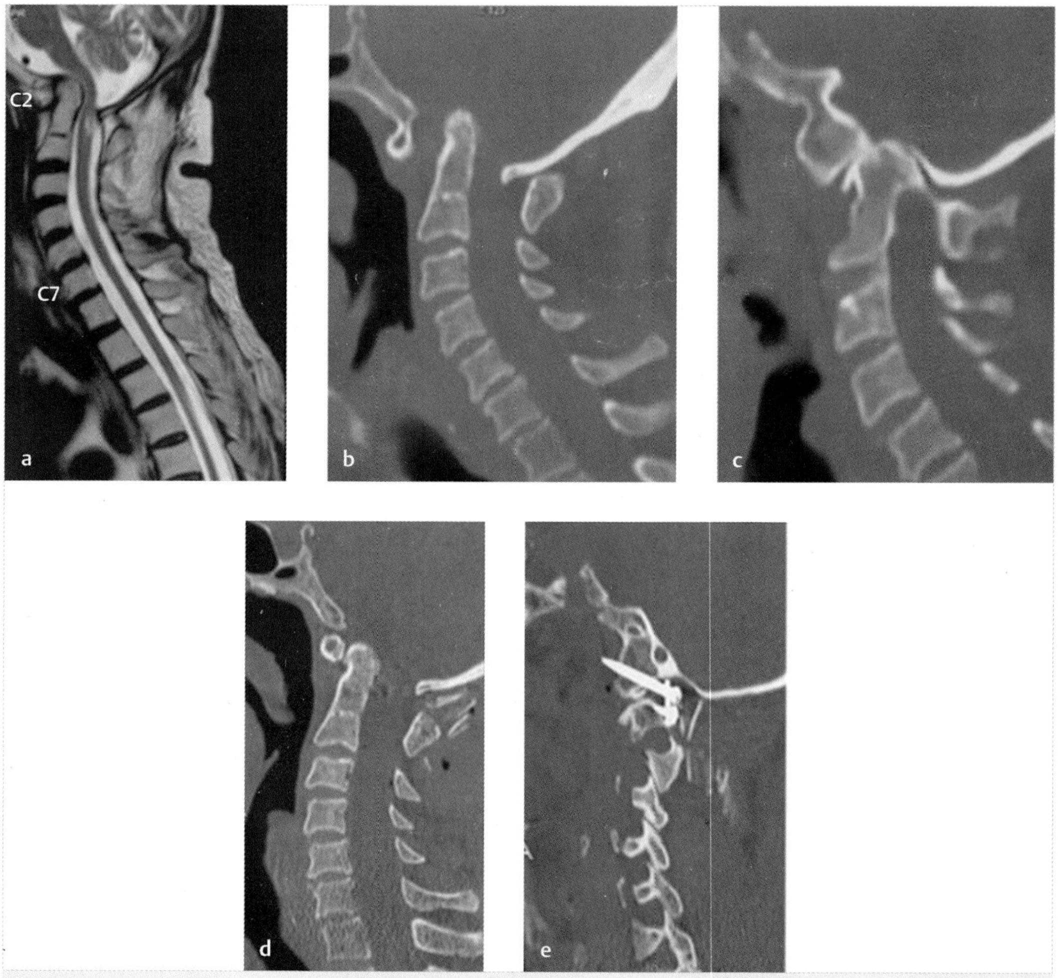

Fig. 34.3 Images of a patient with group A basilar invagination. **(a)** T2-weighted magnetic resonance imaging (MRI) showing severe indentation of the brainstem by the odontoid process. **(b)** Computed tomography (CT) scan with the head in flexion showing basilar invagination. **(c)** CT scan with the cut passing through the facets showing type 1 atlantoaxial dislocation. **(d)** Postoperative CT scan following distraction of the facets of the atlas and axis and subsequent instrumentation showing fixation with a reduction in basilar invagination and craniovertebral junction realignment. **(e)** Postoperative image with sagittal cut passing through the facets showing the metal construct.

  - The articular cartilage can also be denuded with the help of an electric drill.
  - Bone chips harvested from the iliac crest are then packed into the articular cavity.
- *Drilling*:
  - The lateral aspect of the lamina and a part of the pars of the axis are drilled to make the posterior surface of the lateral mass of the axis flat relative to the posterior surface of the facet of the atlas so that the metal plate can be placed snugly and parallel to the bone of the posterior surface of the facet of the atlas.
  - Drilling also helps reduce the length of the plate and place the screw more rostrally and almost directly into the pedicle–superior facet junction of the axis.
- *Screw implantation*:
  - Screws are implanted into the previously created guide holes made preferably with a power drill in the lateral mass of the atlas and

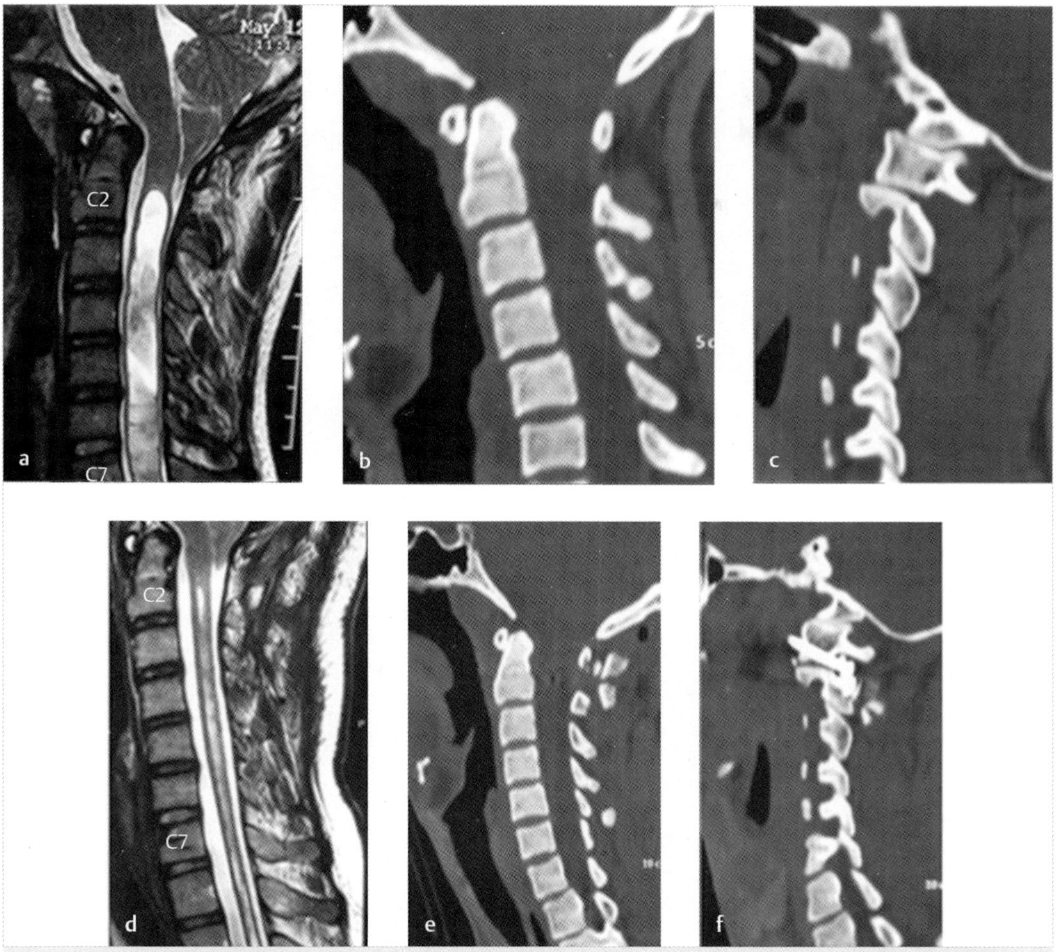

Fig. 34.4 Images of a patient with Chiari formation. **(a)** T1-weighted sagittal magnetic resonance imaging (MRI) showing Chiari formation and syringomyelia. **(b)** Computed tomography (CT) scan showing no craniovertebral junction bone anomaly. **(c)** CT scan with the cut passing through the facets showing type 2 facetal instability. **(d)** Postoperative T2-weighted MRI showing marked resolution of Chiari formation and syringomyelia. **(e)** Postoperative CT scan. **(f)** Postoperative CT image showing atlantoaxial fixation.

axis through a two-hole (~2 cm in length) metal (titanium) plate.

- First, a screw is placed into the facet of the atlas. The preferred site of screw insertion is at the center of the posterior surface of the facet of the atlas, 1 to 2 mm above the articular surface. The screw is directed at an angle of approximately 15 degrees medial to the sagittal plane and 15 to 30 degrees superior to the axial plane.
- Whenever necessary, careful drilling of the inferior surface of the lateral aspect of the posterior arch of the atlas in relation to its lateral mass can provide additional space for the placement of the plate and screw implantation.
- The articular surface of the facet of the atlas is a useful site for screw insertion. Such a site is more useful in children than in adult patients and in cases of basilar invagination.
- The pars interarticularis can be divided into nine compartments[7]; the superior and medial compartments can be preferentially used for screw implantation, as they are relatively safe for avoiding the vertebral artery.[7,8]

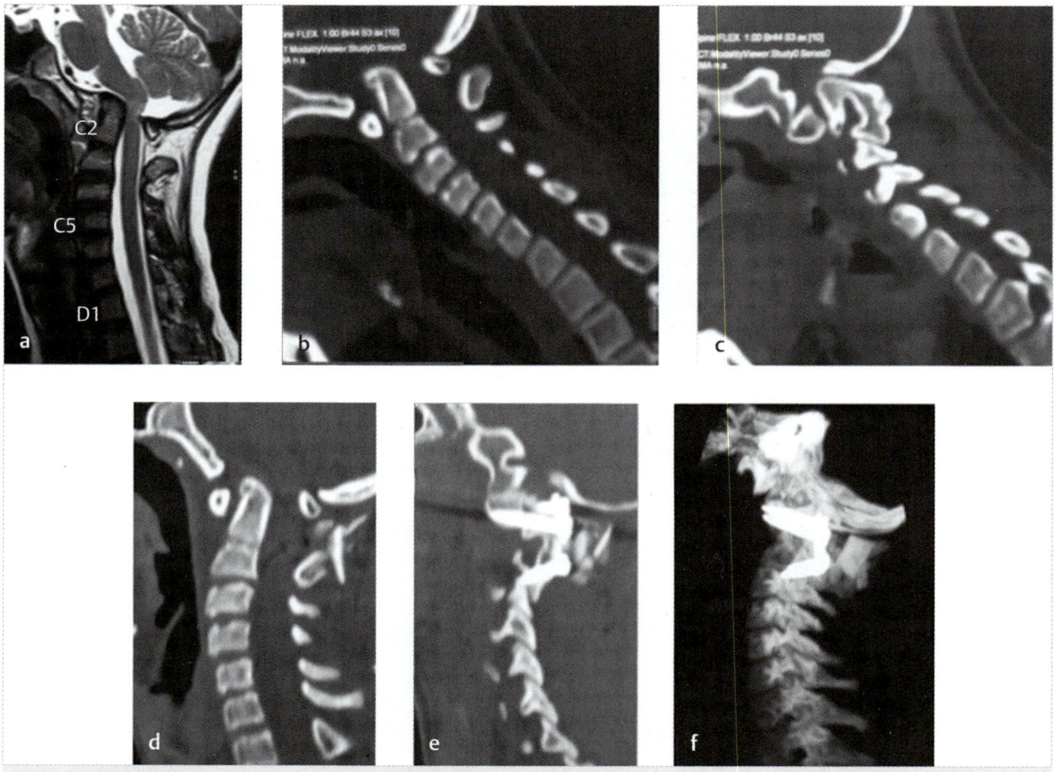

Fig. 34.5 Images of a patient with group A basilar invagination. **(a)** T2-weighted magnetic resonance imaging (MRI) showing severe indentation of the brainstem by the odontoid process. **(b)** Computed tomography (CT) scan with the head in flexion showing basilar invagination. **(c)** CT scan with the cut passing through the facets showing type 1 atlantoaxial dislocation. **(d)** Postoperative CT scan following distraction of the facets of the atlas and axis and subsequent instrumentation showing fixation with reduction in basilar invagination and craniovertebral junction realignment. **(e)** Postoperative image with the sagittal cut passing through the facets showing the metal construct and screw insertion in the inferior facet of C2. **(f)** Sagittal reconstructed image of a CT scan showing the implants.

- Neuronavigation can be of assistance in identifying the best and safest trajectory of the screw.
- The direction of screw implantation must be medial, superior, and toward the superior aspect of the body of the axis vertebra toward the midline.
- The medial surface of the pedicle of the axis is identified before screw implantation.
- The screw is directed approximately 25 degrees medial to the sagittal plane and 15 degrees superior to the axial plane. The angle of screw insertion varies depending on the local anatomy and the size of the bones.

• *Bone graft*:
  ◦ Large pieces of corticocancellous bone grafts from the iliac bone are then placed over the bone surface of the posterior elements of the atlas and axis.
  ◦ The muscles attached to the C2 spinous process are widely removed.
  ◦ The host bone is adequately prepared by removing all soft tissues and decortication of bone.

• After the wound is closed and the patient is turned supine, cervical traction is discontinued.

34.7 Postoperative Care

• The patients are mobilized as soon as possible and advised to wear a hard cervical collar for 3 months. Neck movements are strictly restricted during this time. After this period, normal life activities are permitted.

34.8 Complications

- It was observed that screw implantation in the superior facet of the C2 vertebra should be done under direct surgical vision after a wide and panoramic exposure. The medial surface of the C2 pedicle should be appropriately visualized prior to screw insertion. Neuronavigation is of great help in identifying the correct screw insertion site and direction. The screw insertion has to be sharply medial and directed toward the anterior tubercle of C1 for transarticular fixation and toward the vertebral body of C2 for interarticular fixation.
- A fixation procedure that involves only the atlantoaxial segment is biomechanically most stable. Inclusion of the occipital bone and the subaxial bone increases the length of the metal implant and unnecessarily stabilizes normal-functioning spinal segments. The long implant is biomechanically weak and has the potential to weaken, as bone fusion at multiple spinal segments is a difficult goal to achieve.
- Bone harvested from the patient's own iliac crest has been universally identified to be superior to any other form of bone graft or artificial material.[5]

34.9 Management Pearls

- Goel recently classified atlantoaxial dislocation based on the alignment of the facets observed on lateral profile imaging with the head in the neutral position (▶ Fig. 34.6)[4]:
  - Type 1 atlantoaxial facetal instability is when the facet of the atlas is dislocated anterior to the facet of the axis. Neural compression is a hallmark of type 1 atlantoaxial facetal dislocation, and the presenting symptoms are relatively acute.
  - Type 2 atlantoaxial facetal instability is when the facet of the atlas is dislocated posterior to the facet of the axis.
  - Type 3 atlantoaxial instability is when the facets of the atlas and axis are in alignment, and instability is diagnosed only based on a high degree of clinical suspicion and is confirmed by direct manual manipulation of bones during surgery.
  - As the atlantodental interval may not be altered and there may not be any dural or neural compression opposite the odontoid process, type 2 and 3 atlantoaxial facetal instability is sometimes labeled as "central" or "axial" atlantoaxial instability.[4] The presenting symptoms in both types 2 and 3 atlantoaxial

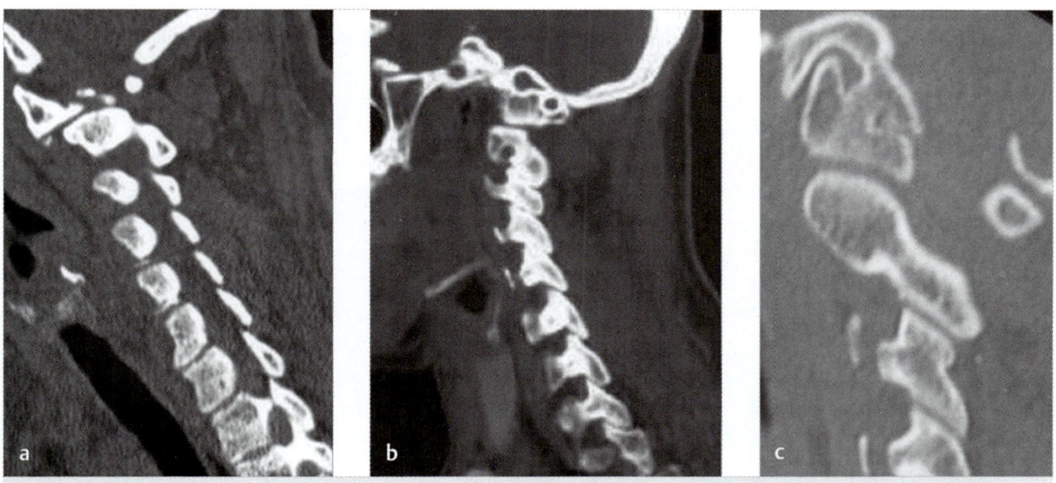

Fig. 34.6 Images showing Goel's classification of facetal instability. **(a)** Sagittal computed tomography (CT) image with the cut passing through the facets showing type 1 facetal instability. **(b)** Sagittal CT image showing type 2 facetal instability. **(c)** Sagittal CT image showing type 3 facetal instability.

facetal instability are usually chronic or long-standing.
  - In chronic and long-standing atlantoaxial dislocation, protective or reparative natural changes in the musculoskeletal and neural structures are prominent. Such changes include the complex of basilar invagination, Chiari formation, and syringomyelia.
- Anatomical peculiarities of the atlantoaxial region:
  - The craniovertebral junction is the most mobile and most stable region of the spine.
  - Both C1 and C2 are atypical bones.
  - C1 is in the form of a circle. The muscular attachment of C1 is essentially on the large transverse processes.
  - The C2 vertebra has a large spinous process. The majority of muscles acting at C2 are attached to the spinous process.
  - The facets of both C1 and C2 are larger than all other facets of the spine.
  - In terms of relative size, the transverse process of the atlas and the spinous process of the axis are the largest of the entire spine.
  - The facets of the atlas and axis are horizontally aligned and are placed one above the other in a brick-over-brick fashion. The cervical and dorsal spine facets are oblique in orientation, and the lumbar spine facets are more vertical in their alignment.
  - The vertebral artery is intimately related to the facet of C2.
  - The vertebral artery frequently makes a deep indentation into the inferior aspect of the facet of C2. The arterial indentation can sometimes be deep into the facet and is related to a "high" vertebral artery loop. Such a relationship of the artery with the facet of C2 makes screw implantation into the substance of the facet dangerous and identifies the need for precision.
  - The atlantodental joint in relationship with the odontoid process forms the axis of rotatory movements of the atlas over the axis.
  - The facets of the atlas and axis are the fulcrum or focus of all movements of the region.
- The exposure of the atlantoaxial joint can be difficult when the articulation is located rostrally, as in cases with basilar invagination. The exposure of the joint is relatively difficult in cases with assimilation of the atlas. The length of the clivus and degree of platybasia are other determinants of surgical difficulties in joint exposure.
- Actual vertebral artery exposure is unnecessary either lateral to the pars/pedicle of the axis or superior to the arch of the atlas.
- Lateral mass plate–rod and screw fixation technique can provide an opportunity to manipulate the facets of the atlas and axis independently by obtaining fixation points in their strongest elements. Such techniques are useful for realignment of the craniovertebral junction and are particularly useful in the treatment of basilar invagination and rotatory atlantoaxial dislocation.
- The screws used are 2.6 to 3 mm in diameter in adult patients and 2.6 to 2.8 mm in diameter in pediatric patients. Larger screws can be used, particularly when polyaxial screw–rod systems are used for fixation.
- The length of the required screw is calculated on the basis of the size of the lateral masses observed on the preoperative radiologic studies. The approximate lengths of the atlas screws are 26 to 30 mm in adults and 22 to 26 mm in children. The screws in the atlas and axis are almost similar in length.
- The lateral masses of the atlas and axis are firm and cortical in nature, and, although preferable, it is not mandatory that the screws engage both the posterior and anterior cortices. If the screw traverses beyond the anterior cortex, it will lie harmlessly in the displaced soft tissue.
- Alternative sites of C2 screw insertion:
  - In cases where the screw insertion in the superior facet of the C2 is not possible or has failed, the screw can be directed inferiorly and laterally and inserted into the inferior facet (▸ Fig. 34.5). The inferior facet is strong, and the vertebral artery is away from the course of the screw. Such screw insertion can be used as a salvage procedure.[9]
  - Goel first described the technique of insertion of screws into the large and stubby spinous process, lamina, and spinolaminar junction of the axis.[10] The technique of laminar screw insertion was further developed and popularized by Wright.[11] Considering the safety and biomechanical strength of screw implantation in the lamina, the technique is a popular choice.

- A "high-riding" vertebral artery is a frequent deterrent and poses difficulties in C2 screw insertion. It was observed that the bone cover over the vertebral artery was relatively thin and gentle, and careful drilling could expose the vertebral artery loop. Inferior and/or lateral mobilization of the loop permits direct screw insertion into the facet of the axis. The process of screw insertion is conducted with the vertebral artery under direct surgical vision. Such vertebral artery mobilization makes it possible to overcome the issues related to a high-riding vertebral artery.[12]

References

[1] Goel A, Laheri VK. Plate and screw fixation for atlanto-axial dislocation. Acta Neurochir (Wien). 1994; 129:47–53

[2] Goel A, Desai KI, Muzumdar DP. Atlantoaxial fixation using plate and screw method: a report of 160 treated patients. Neurosurgery. 2002; 51(6):1351–1356, discussion 1356–1357

[3] Goel A, Kulkarni AG, Sharma P. Reduction of fixed atlantoaxial dislocation in 24 cases: technical note. J Neurosurg Spine. 2005; 2(4):505–509

[4] Goel A. Goel's classification of atlantoaxial "facetal" dislocation. J Craniovertebr Junction Spine. 2014; 5(1): 3–8

[5] Goel A. Is "self-to-self" bone graft ideal for bone fusion after craniovertebral stabilization? World Neurosurg. 2012; 78(3–4):237–238

[6] Goel A. Cervical ganglion 2 (CG2) neurectomy: a window to the atlantoaxial joint. World Neurosurg. 2012; 78(1–2): 78–79

[7] Gupta S, Goel A. Quantitative anatomy of the lateral masses of the atlas and axis vertebrae. Neurol India. 2000; 48(2): 120–125

[8] Cacciola F, Phalke U, Goel A. Vertebral artery in relationship to C1-C2 vertebrae: an anatomical study. Neurol India. 2004; 52(2):178–184

[9] Goel A. Caudally directed inferior facetal and transfacetal screws for C1-C2 and C1-2-3 fixation. World Neurosurg. 2017; 100:236–243

[10] Goel A, Kulkarni AG. Screw implantation in spinous process for occipitoaxial fixation. J Clin Neurosci. 2004; 11(7): 735–737

[11] Wright NM. Posterior C2 fixation using bilateral, crossing C2 laminar screws: case series and technical note. J Spinal Disord Tech. 2004; 17(2):158–162

[12] Goel A, Rangnekar R, Shah A, Rai S, Vutha R. Mobilization of the vertebral artery: surgical option for C2 screw fixation in cases with "high riding" vertebral artery. Oper Neurosurg. 2020; 18(6):648–651

35 Instrumented Fixation of the Subaxial Cervical Spine

Mitch Paro, Maria Jose Cavagnaro, Matthew J. McPheeters, and Jeffrey P. Mullin

35.1 Background

- The subaxial cervical spine (SAC) is composed of vertebrae C3–C7 and the associated ligamentous and neurovascular structures. Fixation techniques use these bony structures as landmarks and fixation points for hardware placement. These include the pedicles, lateral masses (LM), facet joints (FJ), and laminae.
- Knowledge of the osseous anatomy and its relationships is critical for safe and accurate hardware placement with maximum biomechanical stability.[1,2]
- The pedicles connect the laminae with the vertebral bodies.[3] They are also the cranial and caudal limits of the neural foramina, which contain the exiting nerve roots.[4,5,6]
- The facets are the central weight-bearing and stabilizing elements of the SAC.
- The LM are bony prominences located between the superior articulating process (SAP) and the inferior articulating processes.
- The vertebral artery (VA) courses anterior to the LM of C7 and then ascends through the transverse foramina of C6–C1. To prevent injury, the course and morphology of the VA should be identified on preoperative imaging.[4]

35.2 Indications and Contraindications

- Different techniques of fixation exist, each with their own indications and contraindications:
  - LM screws (LMS):
    - Most widely used method of posterior fixation of the SAC.
    - Broad indications including degenerative conditions, instability from trauma, infection, and malignancy.[7]
  - Pedicle screws:
    - Cervical pedicle screws (CPS) provide a three-column fixation and, therefore, are associated with the highest biomechanical stability of any fixation method.
    - The indications for CPS are broad. However, LMS are still preferred by most surgeons due to familiarity and perceived safety. CPS may serve as a bailout option in cases of compromised LM. They may be preferable in deformity correction, occipitocervical fusion, or revision surgery.[4,8,9]
    - The major drawback of pedicle screws in the SAC is the technical difficulty of placement. The small pedicle diameter puts neurovascular structures at risk and pedicle trajectory requires a wide lateral angle of approach. A pedicle diameter of 4 mm is a generally accepted minimum value to accommodate CPS.[1,10,11]
  - Laminar screws (LS):
    - In the SAC, the laminae of C3–C6 are thin and LS are rarely used.[7] However, C7 has a more capacious lamina, and LS here are appropriate with a pullout strength similar to CPS.[12,13]
  - Transfacet screws (TFS):
    - Used at or caudal to C2–C3.[14]
    - At the cephalic levels, occipital bone protuberance can affect screw trajectory and TFS may not be feasible.
    - C6 and C7 have large facet angles, facilitating screw placement.[14,15]
  - Wiring:
    - Rarely used.
    - Alternative to screw-based methods when the latter are suboptimal or contraindicated.
    - Applicable to the pediatric population, where smaller anatomical dimensions make these patients poor candidates for screw-based fixation.[4]
    - Wire-based constructs also tend to have poor resistance to extension, lateral bending, and rotational forces.[4]

35.3 Patient Positioning

- Prone on a Jackson frame.

35.4 Technique

- LMS (*technique* [**Video 35.1**]):
  - *Magerl technique (most commonly used):* The screw entry point is localized 1 mm medial and 1 mm cranial to the LM midpoint. The

screw is advanced parallel to the FJ and 30 degrees laterally to avoid VA or nerve root injury (▶ Fig. 35.1 and ▶ Fig. 35.2).[4,16]

- *Roy-Camille technique:* The entry point is at the LM midpoint and the angulation is 10 degrees lateral. In the sagittal plane, the trajectory is perpendicular to the entry point.[4,17]
- Other techniques were described by Nazarian and Louis,[18] Anderson et al,[19] An et al,[20,21] and Joaquim et al,[4] and are comparable in safety and efficacy.
- The LM of C7 is often not substantial enough for a load-bearing screw. In these cases, a C7 pedicle screw and LS are excellent alternatives.
- If the cervical fusion construct includes the thoracic spine, then C7 screws can often be skipped.

- Pedicle screws (*technique* [**Video 35.1** and **Video 35.2**]):
  - The conventional technique uses an entry point 3 mm below the SAP with a medial trajectory of 45 degrees.[1]

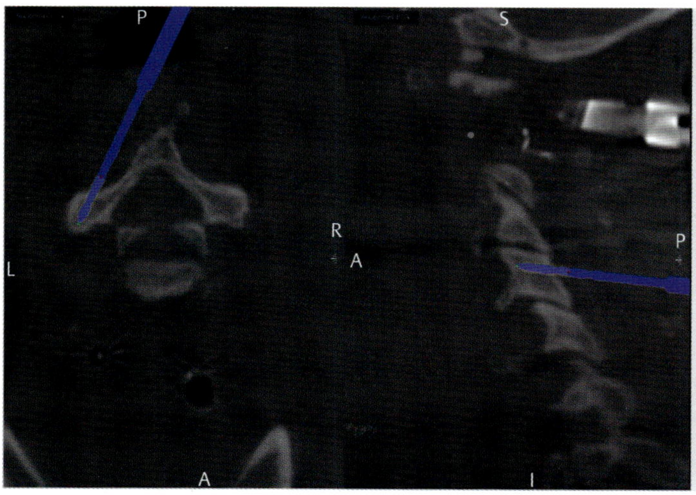

Fig. 35.1 CT neuronavigation image showing the C3 LMS trajectory.

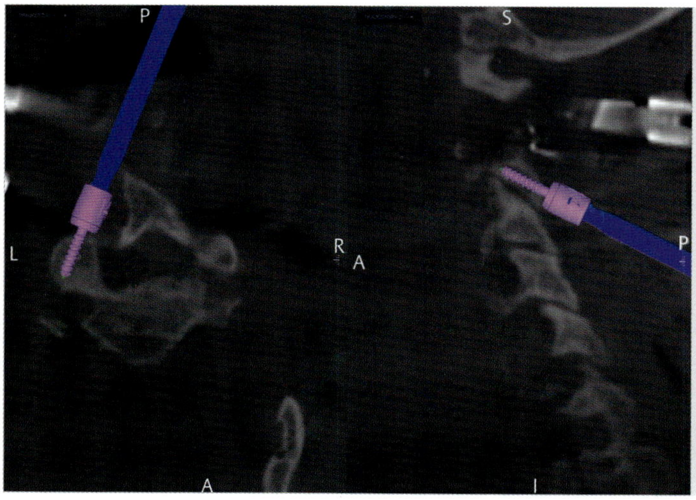

Fig. 35.2 CT neuronavigation image showing the C3 LMS pedicle screw placement.

- The sagittal inclination is slightly cephalad at C3 and C4 and parallel to the upper endplate at C5–C7 (▶ Fig. 35.3 and ▶ Fig. 35.4).[4]
- Variations on this technique have been described by Abumi et al[10] and Park et al.[11,22,23,24]

- LS:
  - The first pilot hole is made 4 mm caudal to the spinolaminar junction (SLJ).[4] Contralaterally, a second hole is made rostral to the SLJ. A tap is then performed toward the opposite lamina, using a ball-tipped probe to check for cortical violation. Screws are then passed from the SLJ to the lamina–LM junction bilaterally.
- TFS:
  - First described for SAC fixation by Roy-Camille et al.[4]
  - TFS have similar mechanical stability and superior pullout strength compared to LMS.[25,26]
  - *Takayasu technique:* The entry point bisects the caudal third of the LM.[14] The screw trajectory is 0 degrees in the coronal plane and 60 to 80 degrees inferior in the sagittal plane. Variations on this technique include the DelCanto,[27] Klekamp,[26] and Miyanji techniques.[25]
- Wiring:
  - For interspinous wiring, transverse drill holes are made at the base of two adjacent

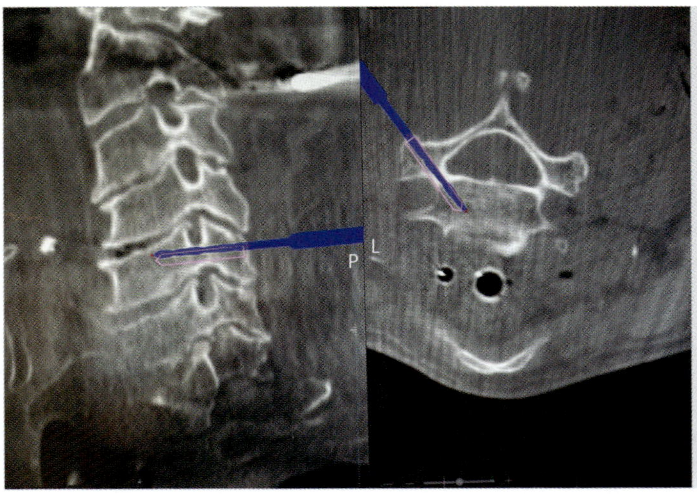

Fig. 35.3 CT neuronavigation image showing the C3 CPS trajectory.

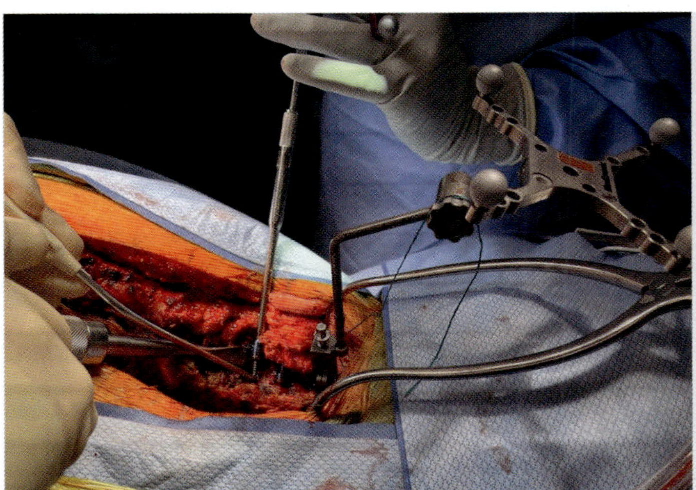

Fig. 35.4 Surgical picture showing the entry point and trajectory of CPS.

spinous processes (SP).[2] The cable is passed through the drill hole in the caudal SP, looped around the inferior edge of the SP, and passed again through the drill hole. It is then advanced through the drill hole in the cranial SP, looped around the superior edge of the SP, and passed again through the drill hole.

35.5 Complications

- LMS:
  - Anteromedial trajectory can lead to breach of the transverse or neural foramen.
  - An insufficient cranial trajectory can violate the FJ, leading to instability or pain.
- Pedicle screws:
  - Pedicle breach (PB).
    - Small breaches may not have any clinical consequence; there is no consensus regarding the dimensions of a safe zone.[28] PB rates of 6.7 to 27.9% have been reported, though not all were associated with complications or suboptimal outcomes.[29,30,31] A rate of 1.2% was reported with computed tomography (CT) based navigation.[32]
    - A lateral PB is more common than a medial breach. A lateral breach is more likely to cause VA injury while a medial breach is more likely to cause spinal cord injury.
    - A superior breach is more likely to injure the nerve root than an inferior breach.[31,33]
    - C3 CPS have the highest rate of PB, with decreasing rates at each subsequent level caudally.[34] Highly cortical pedicles may contribute to major breaches due to increased resistance during placement.[35]
    - Intraoperative CT navigation may reduce breach rates compared to fluoroscopy[35] or free-hand placement.[36]
  - A recent meta-analysis including 1,768 patients found higher rates of postoperative C5 palsy using CPS versus LMS. Otherwise, there were no significant differences in neural or vascular injury, revision rate, and hardware failure.[37,38]
  - Inadequate exposure can lead to screw malposition.[1,10,11] VA dominance and patient-specific VA anatomy can affect the safety of CPS.
- LS:
  - LS present a minimal risk of VA or nerve root injury.
  - However, cortical breech is possible. A relatively benign dorsal breach is more common than a ventral breach, which can injure the spinal cord.[7]
- TFS:
  - Takayasu et al reported a series of 81 TFS with no complications.[14,39]
  - Fracture of the inferior FJ is a risk of TFS placement, although proper entry and trajectory decrease the likelihood of this complication.[39]
- Wiring:
  - Complications are rare.
  - The most common complications are wire pullout, avulsion fractures, and hyperlordosis if there is excessive tension on the wire.[7]

35.6 Management Pearls

- In a cadaveric comparison of the Roy-Camille and Magerl techniques, Roy-Camille screws had a lower rate of nerve root injury but a higher rate of FJ violation.[40,41]
- Overall, LMS fixation has a low rate of major complications. A 2013 systematic review of 758 patients with LMS fixation showed a rate of nerve root injury of 3.9%, FJ violation of 0.6%, LM fracture of 1.9%, screw failure of less than 1.0%, and revision surgery of 2.3%. There were no VA or spinal cord injuries. A 2021 case series of 695 patients found a 7.3% rate of screw malpositioning and a 5.6% rate of LM fracture.[42]
- Some reports show that CPS have higher rates of fusion, better reduction, and earlier mobilization and rehabilitation compared to other methods.[8,9,43]
- To increase accuracy of pedicle screw placement, many surgeons use intraoperative fluoroscopy or perform a laminoforaminotomy prior to fixation.[44] The latter technique allows for direct visualization and palpation of the pedicle during screw placement. This technique may reduce the rate and severity of pedicle perforation compared to free-hand placement.[36]

35.7 Emerging Technologies

- **Navigation**:
  - Navigation systems utilize imaging obtained pre- or intraoperatively in conjunction with fiducialized surgical instruments to give the surgeon real-time, high-accuracy feedback on the accuracy of placement of spinal hardware, especially screws.
  - Intraoperative CT approaches for CPS placement have demonstrated high accuracy with no neurovascular complications.[31,45,46]
  - 3D-assisted CT navigation methods have higher safety and accuracy compared to fluoroscopy, with less radiation exposure to the surgical team and reduced operating room (OR) time.[11,28,37,47,48]
  - Stereotaxic errors may result from reference clamp movement during the procedure or high vertebral intersegmental mobility.[28,47] The force used during drilling, tapping, and screw placement may cause the array to shift and lose accuracy.[47] To avoid complications, the accuracy of the navigation should be periodically tested throughout the procedure by correlation with anatomical structures. If misalignment is noticed, another set of navigation images must be acquired.
- **3D template molds**:
  - 3D printing has been increasingly used in medical education and clinical practice, including in surgical fields.[49] In spine surgery, a recent application is the development of patient-specific, 3D-printed guides that direct screws along the pedicle trajectory with a high level of accuracy.[28,49] 3D templates can reduce OR time but mold design and printing can take up to several days.
- **Robotics**:
  - While some studies suggest that robotics increase the accuracy of CPS or LMS placement,[50,51,52,53,54] the experience of robot-assisted techniques for cervical instrumentation remains limited.[37,47,50]
  - Technical challenges include the acute angulation of screw trajectory, the mobility of the cervical spine, and the difficulty of digitally segmenting each level due to narrow disc spaces.[47,50]
  - Several surgical robotic systems are in clinical use; however, most are used for the lumbar and thoracic spine.[52]
  - In the United States, there are two systems available for cervical spine surgery: ExcelsiusGPS and Cirq Robotic Alignment Module.

References

[1] Jung YG, Jung SK, Lee BJ, et al. The subaxial cervical pedicle screw for cervical spine diseases: the review of technical developments and complication avoidance. Neurol Med Chir (Tokyo). 2020; 60(5):231–243

[2] Kim DH. Surgical Anatomy & Techniques to the Spine. Philadelphia, PA: Saunders; 2006

[3] Singh DK, Singh AK, Nayak S. Transfacetal screw fixation for subaxial cervical spine. Neurol India. 2022; 70(1):50–53

[4] Joaquim AF, Mudo ML, Tan LA, Riew KD. Posterior subaxial cervical spine screw fixation: a review of techniques. Global Spine J. 2018; 8(7):751–760

[5] Pech P, Daniels DL, Williams AL, Haughton VM. The cervical neural foramina: correlation of microtomy and CT anatomy. Radiology. 1985; 155(1):143–146

[6] Xu R, Kang A, Ebraheim NA, Yeasting RA. Anatomic relation between the cervical pedicle and the adjacent neural structures. Spine. 1999; 24(5):451–454

[7] Mikhail CM, Dowdell JE, III, Hecht AC. Posterior fusion for the subaxial cervical spine: a review of the major techniques. HSS J. 2020; 16(2):188–194

[8] Johnston TL, Karaikovic EE, Lautenschlager EP, Marcu D. Cervical pedicle screws vs. lateral mass screws: uniplanar fatigue analysis and residual pullout strengths. Spine J. 2006; 6(6):667–672

[9] Jones EL, Heller JG, Silcox DH, Hutton WC. Cervical pedicle screws versus lateral mass screws. Anatomic feasibility and biomechanical comparison. Spine. 1997; 22(9):977–982

[10] Abumi K, Kaneda K. Pedicle screw fixation for nontraumatic lesions of the cervical spine. Spine. 1997; 22(16):1853–1863

[11] Verma R, Krishan S, Haendlmayer K, Mohsen A. Functional outcome of computer-assisted spinal pedicle screw placement: a systematic review and meta-analysis of 23 studies including 5,992 pedicle screws. Eur Spine J. 2010; 19(3):370–375

[12] Ilgenfritz RM, Gandhi AA, Fredericks DC, Grosland NM, Smucker JD. Considerations for the use of C7 crossing laminar screws in subaxial and cervicothoracic instrumentation. Spine. 2013; 38(4):E199–E204

[13] Hong JT, Yi JS, Kim JT, Ji C, Ryu KS, Park CK. Clinical and radiologic outcome of laminar screw at C2 and C7 for posterior instrumentation–review of 25 cases and comparison of C2 and C7 intralaminar screw fixation. World Neurosurg. 2010; 73(2):112–118, discussion e15

[14] Takayasu M, Hara M, Yamauchi K, Yoshida M, Yoshida J. Transarticular screw fixation in the middle and lower cervical spine. Technical note. J Neurosurg. 2003; 99(1) Suppl:132–136

[15] Liu G, Ma W, Xu R, et al. Clinical application of combined fixation in the cervical spine using posterior transfacet screws and pedicle screws. J Clin Neurosci. 2013; 20(4):560–564

[16] Jeanneret B, Magerl F, Ward EH, Ward JC. Posterior stabilization of the cervical spine with hook plates. Spine. 1991; 16(3) Suppl:S56–S63

[17] Roy-Camille R, Salient G, Mazel C. Internal fixation of the unstable cervical spine by a posterior osteosynthesis with

plates and screws. In: Sherk HH, Dunn EJ, Eismont FJ, et al, eds. The Cervical Spine. 2nd ed. Philadelphia, PA: JB Lippincott; 1989:390–403
[18] Nazarian SM, Louis RP. Posterior internal fixation with screw plates in traumatic lesions of the cervical spine. Spine. 1991; 16(3) Suppl:S64–S71
[19] Anderson PA, Henley MB, Grady MS, Montesano PX, Winn HR. Posterior cervical arthrodesis with AO reconstruction plates and bone graft. Spine. 1991; 16(3) Suppl:S72–S79
[20] An HS, Coppes MA. Posterior cervical fixation for fracture and degenerative disc disease. Clin Orthop Relat Res. 1997; 335:101–111
[21] An HS, Gordin R, Renner K. Anatomic considerations for plate-screw fixation of the cervical spine. Spine. 1991; 16 (10) Suppl:S548–S551
[22] Park JH, Jeon SR, Roh SW, Kim JH, Rhim SC. The safety and accuracy of freehand pedicle screw placement in the subaxial cervical spine: a series of 45 consecutive patients. Spine. 2014; 39(4):280–285
[23] Lee S, Seo J, Lee MK, et al. Widening of the safe trajectory range during subaxial cervical pedicle screw placement: advantages of a curved pedicle probe and laterally located starting point without creating a funnel-shaped hole. J Neurosurg Spine. 2017; 27(2):150–157
[24] Jung YG, Lee S, Jeong SK, Kim M, Park JH. Subaxial cervical pedicle screw in traumatic spinal surgery. Korean J Neurotrauma. 2020; 16(1):18–27
[25] Miyanji F, Mahar A, Oka R, Newton P. Biomechanical differences between transfacet and lateral mass screw-rod constructs for multilevel posterior cervical spine stabilization. Spine. 2008; 33(23):E865–E869
[26] Klekamp JW, Ugbo JL, Heller JG, Hutton WC. Cervical transfacet versus lateral mass screws: a biomechanical comparison. J Spinal Disord. 2000; 13(6):515–518
[27] DalCanto RA, Lieberman I, Inceoglu S, Kayanja M, Ferrara L. Biomechanical comparison of transarticular facet screws to lateral mass plates in two-level instrumentations of the cervical spine. Spine. 2005; 30(8):897–902
[28] Mahmoud A, Shanmuganathan K, Rocos B, Sedra F, Montgomery A, Aftab S. Cervical spine pedicle screw accuracy in fluoroscopic, navigated and template guided systems: a systematic review. Tomography. 2021; 7(4):614–622
[29] Jo DJ, Seo EM, Kim KT, Kim SM, Lee SH. Cervical pedicle screw insertion using the technique with direct exposure of the pedicle by laminoforaminotomy. J Korean Neurosurg Soc. 2012; 52(5):459–465
[30] Yoshimoto H, Sato S, Hyakumachi T, Yanagibashi Y, Masuda T. Spinal reconstruction using a cervical pedicle screw system. Clin Orthop Relat Res. 2005(431):111–119
[31] Abumi K, Shono Y, Ito M, Taneichi H, Kotani Y, Kaneda K. Complications of pedicle screw fixation in reconstructive surgery of the cervical spine. Spine. 2000; 25(8):962–969
[32] Ito Y, Sugimoto Y, Tomioka M, Hasegawa Y, Nakago K, Yagata Y. Clinical accuracy of 3D fluoroscopy-assisted cervical pedicle screw insertion. J Neurosurg Spine. 2008; 9(5): 450–453
[33] Ghori A, Le HV, Makanji H, Cha T. Posterior fixation techniques in the subaxial cervical spine. Cureus. 2015; 7 (10):e338
[34] Yoshihara H, Passias PG, Errico TJ. Screw-related complications in the subaxial cervical spine with the use of lateral mass versus cervical pedicle screws: a systematic review. J Neurosurg Spine. 2013; 19(5):614–623
[35] Kotani Y, Abumi K, Ito M, Minami A. Improved accuracy of computer-assisted cervical pedicle screw insertion. J Neurosurg. 2003; 99(3) Suppl:257–263
[36] Miller RM, Ebraheim NA, Xu R, Yeasting RA. Anatomic consideration of transpedicular screw placement in the cervical spine. An analysis of two approaches. Spine. 1996; 21(20):2317–2322
[37] Soliman MAR, Khan S, Ruggiero N, et al. Complications associated with subaxial placement of pedicle screws versus lateral mass screws in the cervical spine: systematic review and meta-analysis comprising 1768 patients and 8636 screws. Neurosurg Rev. 2022; 45(3):1941–1950
[38] Yukawa Y, Kato F, Ito K, et al. Placement and complications of cervical pedicle screws in 144 cervical trauma patients using pedicle axis view techniques by fluoroscope. Eur Spine J. 2009; 18(9):1293–1299
[39] Liu GY, Xu RM, Ma WH, Ruan YP, Sun SH, Huang L. Anatomic comparison of transarticular screws with lateral mass screws in cervical vertebrae. Chin J Traumatol. 2007; 10(2):67–71
[40] Heller JG, Carlson GD, Abitbol JJ, Garfin SR. Anatomic comparison of the Roy-Camille and Magerl techniques for screw placement in the lower cervical spine. Spine. 1991; 16 (10) Suppl:S552–S557
[41] Stemper BD, Marawar SV, Yoganandan N, Shender BS, Rao RD. Quantitative anatomy of subaxial cervical lateral mass: an analysis of safe screw lengths for Roy-Camille and Magerl techniques. Spine. 2008; 33(8):893–897
[42] Al Barbarawi MM, Allouh MZ, Qudsieh SM, Barbarawi A. Cervical decompressive laminectomy and lateral mass screw-rod arthrodesis: surgical experience and analytical review of 4120 consecutive screws. Br J Neurosurg. 2021; 35(4):480–485
[43] Mao JZ, Agyei JO, Ghannam MM, et al. Navigation-guided subaxial cervical pedicle screws in revision spine surgery: 2-dimensional operative video. Oper Neurosurg (Hagerstown). 2021; 20(4):E312–E313
[44] Ludwig SC, Kramer DL, Balderston RA, Vaccaro AR, Foley KF, Albert TJ. Placement of pedicle screws in the human cadaveric cervical spine: comparative accuracy of three techniques. Spine. 2000; 25(13):1655–1667
[45] Arab A, Alkherayf F, Sachs A, Wai EK. Use of 3D navigation in subaxial cervical spine lateral mass screw insertion. J Neurol Surg Rep. 2018; 79(1):e1–e8
[46] Xu R, Haman SP, Ebraheim NA, Yeasting RA. The anatomic relation of lateral mass screws to the spinal nerves. A comparison of the Magerl, Anderson, and An techniques. Spine. 1999; 24(19):2057–2061
[47] Mao JZ, Soliman MAR, Karamian BA, et al. Anatomical and technical considerations of robot-assisted cervical pedicle screw placement: a cadaveric study. Global Spine J. 2023; 13 (7):1992–2000
[48] Shin BJ, James AR, Njoku IU, Härtl R. Pedicle screw navigation: a systematic review and meta-analysis of perforation risk for computer-navigated versus freehand insertion. J Neurosurg Spine. 2012; 17(2):113–122

[49] Shi J, Cavagnaro MJ, Xu S, Zhao M. The application of three-dimensional technologies in the improvement of orthopedic surgery training and medical education quality: a comparative bibliometrics analysis. Front Bioeng Biotechnol. 2022; 10: 852608

[50] Su XJ, Lv ZD, Chen Z, et al. Comparison of accuracy and clinical outcomes of robot-assisted versus fluoroscopy-guided pedicle screw placement in posterior cervical surgery. Global Spine J. 2022; 12(4):620–626

[51] Kostrzewski S, Duff JM, Baur C, Olszewski M. Robotic system for cervical spine surgery. Int J Med Robot. 2012; 8(2):184–190

[52] Lebl DR, Avrumova F, Abjornson C, Cammisa FP. Cervical spine navigation and enabled robotics: a new frontier in minimally invasive surgery. HSS J. 2021; 17(3):333–343

[53] Fan M, Liu Y, He D, et al. Improved accuracy of cervical spinal surgery with robot-assisted screw insertion: a prospective, randomized, controlled study. Spine. 2020; 45 (5):285–291

[54] Beyer RS, Nguyen A, Brown NJ, et al. Spinal robotics in cervical spine surgery: a systematic review with key concepts and technical considerations. J Neurosurg Spine. 2022; 38(1): 66–74

36 Posterolateral (Thoracolumbar)

Michael J. Strong, Krishna P. Nayak, and Jacob R. Joseph

36.1 Background

- Posterolateral spinal fusion is a surgical procedure used to treat various spinal pathologies resulting in spinal instability.
- This technique involves placing bone graft material between the dorsal bony surfaces, including the transverse processes, facet joints, and lamina of individual vertebrae to promote a single solid bony fusion.
- Instrumentation, typically in the form of a screw–rod construct, is placed to facilitate formation of the fusion mass.

36.2 Indications and Contraindications

- Patients presenting with spondylolisthesis or spinal deformity as a result of trauma or degenerative disc disease are commonly treated with posterolateral fusion.[1]
- In addition, patients who iatrogenically undergo destabilizing procedures such as osteotomies may require posterolateral fusion.
- Another indication is spinal instability that has not responded to conservative modalities including rest, physical therapy, interventional pain techniques, or oral medications.
- There are few contraindications to posterolateral fusion. Relative contraindications include spinal infections, osteoporosis, nicotine abuse, or poor medical status that may preclude safe recovery after surgery.

36.3 Instruments

- Pedicle screws.
- High-speed drill.
- Metal rods.
- Fluoroscopy.
- Intraoperative computed tomography (CT) system.
- Surgical navigation system (optional).

36.4 Patient Preparation

- In many cases, patients will have undergone magnetic resonance imaging of the spine, standing full-length scoliosis X-rays, and CT of the spine to help with surgical planning.[2]
- Most of these cases are performed under general anesthesia with an endotracheal breathing tube.
- Neurophysiologic monitoring, such as somatosensory evoked potentials, motor evoked potentials, and electromyogram (EMG), is used variably depending on the needs of the surgery and surgeon preference.

36.5 Patient Positioning

- Prone on the operating table.

36.6 Technique

- Posterolateral fusion involving pedicle screw fixation is typically used to augment other surgical techniques including decompression and interbody cage fusion. Steps for pedicle screw posterolateral fusion include the following:
  1. Exposure of the lamina, the facet joint complex including the inferior and superior articular processes, and the transverse process junction in a subperiosteal fashion without disrupting the facet joint capsule above and below the levels of spinal fusion.
  2. All of the soft tissue in between the vertebrae to be fused should be resected. This includes synovium in the facet joints, as well as ligamentous and muscular attachments to the lamina and the transverse processes.
  3. A high-speed drill is used to burr down the cortical bone of any lamina, inferior and superior articular processes, transverse processes, and synovium within the facet joint.
  4. Screws are placed within the pedicles of each vertebral segment being fused.
  5. Metal rods are placed connecting each screw.
  6. Bone graft material is laid out in the posterolateral portion of the spine as well as any exposed lamina. Bone graft material is also packed within the decorticated facet joint.

7. The muscles detached from the transverse processes are laid back over the bone graft, creating tension to hold the bone graft material in place.

36.7 Postoperative Care

- In order to promote healing of the bone into a single solid bony construct, patients are typically instructed to minimize bending, twisting, and lifting for a period of 6 to 12 weeks.
- Patients are also treated with physical therapy to enhance ideal body mechanics.
- An external bone stimulator or brace can be considered in certain circumstances.
- Routine interval imaging is performed to ensure that there are no signs of pseudoarthrosis or hardware failure.
- The typical time frame to establish solid fusion is 6 to 12 months.[3]

36.8 Complications

- Cerebrospinal fluid (CSF) leak.
- Injury to neural elements.
- Pseudoarthrosis.
- Need for additional surgery.

36.9 Management Pearls

- *Relevant anatomy:* Vertebral body, transverse process, superior and inferior articular processes, lamina, and pedicle.
- Arthrodesis of the facet joint will optimize the posterolateral fusion in addition to arthrodesis of the lamina and transverse processes.
- In order to promote posterolateral fusion, it is critical to remove all the soft tissue between the transverse processes, facets, and lamina in order for allow for adequate incorporation of the fusion mass into the vertebrae.
- Interbody fusions are a variant to posterolateral fusion. Posterolateral fusion is the classic method of spinal fusion and is extremely versatile. In many situations, both interbody fusion techniques and posterolateral fusion techniques are used simultaneously.

References

[1] Tajima N, Chosa E, Watanabe S. Posterolateral lumbar fusion. J Orthop Sci. 2004; 9(3):327–333
[2] Nouh MR. Spinal fusion-hardware construct: basic concepts and imaging review. World J Radiol. 2012; 4(5):193–207
[3] Burkus JK, Heim SE, Gornet MF, Zdeblick TA. Is INFUSE bone graft superior to autograft bone? An integrated analysis of clinical trials using the LT-CAGE lumbar tapered fusion device. J Spinal Disord Tech. 2003; 16(2):113–122

37 Transpedicular (Thoracolumbar)

Kaitlyn Melnick, Jonathan Munoz, and Daniel J. Hoh

37.1 Background

- The thoracic transpedicular approach is a dorsal approach to the ventral spine and has utility across numerous pathologies.
- It involves removal of the posterior elements including the pedicle in order to access the ventral epidural space, including the disc and/or vertebral body.
- This approach obviates the need for retraction of the thecal sac at the level of the spinal cord.
- This is a fundamental approach for all neurosurgeons.
- It was first described in 1978 by Patterson and Arbit.[1]
- There are four posterior or posterolateral approaches to the thoracic spine:
  - Dorsal midline:
    - This offers limited "blind" access to the ventral spine.
  - Transpedicular:
    - It provides access to the ventral epidural space, including most of the disc and vertebra, except for the posteromedial vertebral body wall.
  - Costotransversectomy:
    - It allows a greater corridor for accessing the complete disc space and vertebral body.
  - Lateral extracavitary:
    - It provides the widest operative corridor, but is a unilateral approach that has largely been replaced by the bilateral costotransversectomy for both maximal ventral access and exposure for placement of posterior instrumentation.
- Cadaveric anatomical studies have shown the extent of exposure of the ventral epidural spine for each technique at each thoracic level.[2]

37.2 Indications and Contraindications

- The thoracic transpedicular approach is commonly used for infection (discitis/osteomyelitis), trauma (disc herniation/fracture), or neoplasm.
- It is most frequently used for accessing the disc space in the setting of thoracic disc herniation or discitis.
- It can be used in select circumstances for ventral decompression in the setting of vertebral body fracture or neoplasm.

37.3 Patient Preparation

- The use of intraoperative monitoring may be indicated, and the anesthesia team should avoid muscle paralytics and volatile anesthetic. If there is concern for acute neurologic injury or potential risk of injury, mean arterial pressure (MAP) should be maintained above 85 mm Hg.
- Magnetic resonance imaging (MRI) is essential for assessing the location and extent of neural compression. Computed tomography (CT) provides bony detail. Standing X-rays demonstrate local, regional, and global alignment.
- Fluoroscopy is used to localize the level with special care in situations such as poorly visualized segments or transitional anatomy.
- Preincisional antibiotics should be administered but may be held in the setting of infection with the desire for effective culture.
- Intraoperative imaging (fluoroscopy, CT) is required for localization and for placement/confirmation of any instrumentation.

37.4 Patient Positioning

- The operation is performed with the patient in the prone position.

37.5 Technique

- A vertical midline incision over the relevant levels is made and the posterior spine is accessed using electrocautery dissection (see **Video 37.1**).

- If instrumentation is needed, placing it prior to decompression is preferred to avoid excessive passing of instruments over the exposed spinal cord, and immediate stabilization may be necessary if the spine is acutely unstable.
- The transpedicular approach is typically initiated with a conventional laminectomy. Next, the posterior elements are resected including the facets and transverse processes with a high-speed drill and/or rongeurs.
- The pedicles at the index level are skeletonized by drilling down the pedicle, leaving a cortical rim to protect the spinal cord and nerve roots (▶ Fig. 37.1).
- The pedicle cortical rim is then carefully removed with a small rongeur.
- A discectomy and/or partial vertebrectomy can then be performed with curettes or pituitary rongeurs through the absent pedicle (▶ Fig. 37.2).

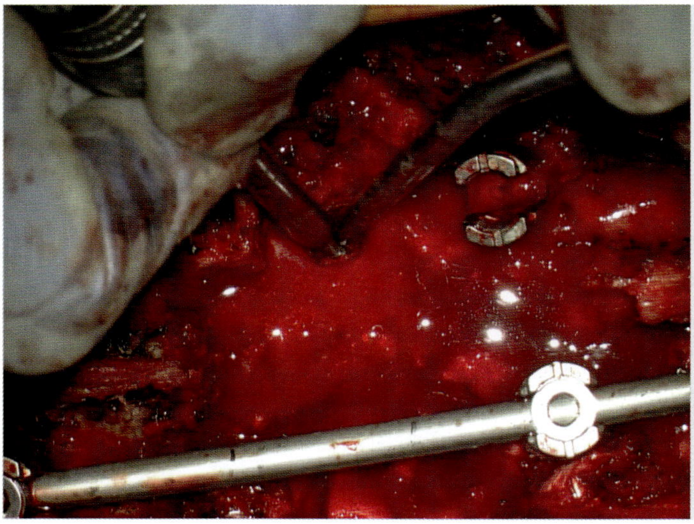

Fig. 37.1 Drilling of the pedicle after instrumentation, laminectomy, and facetectomy.

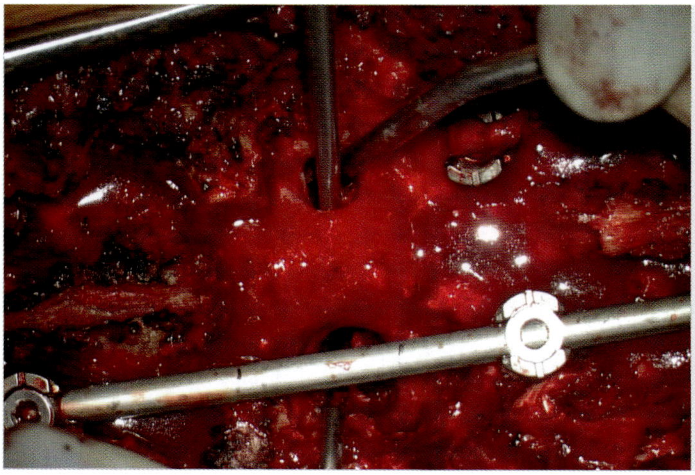

Fig. 37.2 Transpedicular removal of the vertebral body.

- Once complete and copiously irrigated, if fusion is intended, then arthrodesis is performed.
- The wound is closed in layers.

37.6 Complications

- Associated complications are similar to those related to spinal cord and/or spinal reconstructive surgery.
- These include risk of neurologic worsening either by cord injury or by reperfusion injury following decompression, infection, pseudarthrosis, or instrumentation failure.

37.7 Management Pearls

- Care should be taken to avoid direct or indirect (via retraction) injury to the spinal cord or injury (e.g., avulsion) of a nerve root.

References

[1] Patterson RH, Jr, Arbit E. A surgical approach through the pedicle to protruded thoracic discs. J Neurosurg. 1978; 48(5): 768–772

[2] Kshettry VR, Healy AT, Jones NG, Mroz TE, Benzel EC. A quantitative analysis of posterolateral approaches to the ventral thoracic spinal canal. Spine J. 2015; 15(10):2228–2238

38 Costotransversectomy

Jay I. Kumar and Gregory M. Mundis, Jr

38.1 Background

- The term costotransversectomy is derived from Latin, with *costa*, meaning rib, *transverse*, meaning transverse process, and *-ectomy*, meaning surgical removal.
- It is a technique used to remove the transverse process of a thoracic vertebra with the corresponding rib head.
- It is a less invasive alternative to thoracotomy for access to the ventral thecal sac and the anterior and middle columns of the thoracic spine.
- It is a posterior approach, which is more familiar to spine surgeons and spine operating room teams.
- It also facilitates large fusions for deformity or trauma.

38.2 Indications and Contraindications

- It was initially described for the draining of paraspinal abscesses.
- It is also used for the management of primary or metastatic tumors, thoracic disc herniations, traumatic injuries, and other pathologies of the anterior and middle columns that may exert pressure on the ventral thecal sac.
- Contraindications include conditions that require direct access to the midline ventral spinal canal.
- Indirect access, however, may be obtained through bilateral or multilevel unilateral costotransversectomy.

38.3 Patient Positioning

- The patient is typically positioned prone on a radiolucent rotating Jackson table.
- The arms are extended upward to make room for fluoroscopy equipment (C-arm) and the surgeon.
- The arms may be tucked in cases of upper thoracic pathology.
- All bony prominences are padded, and neurovascular structures are positioned without compression.
- Prepositioning and postpositioning motor-evoked potentials and somatosensory evoked potentials are obtained, and monitored throughout the procedure.

38.4 Technique

- The incision can be midline, paramedian, semilunar, or hockey stick shaped.
  - A midline incision allows for bilateral approaches and is more familiar to surgeons and allows access from both sides of the spine.
  - Paramedian and semilunar incisions may allow for better healing by avoiding bony prominences.
- Subperiosteal dissection is carried out along the spinous process down the lamina and out over the transverse process (**Video 38.1** and **Video 38.2**).
- The transverse process is fully exposed circumferentially, and resected with rongeurs or an ultrasonic bone scalpel.
- The rib head is identified and disarticulated from the vertebral body at the costovertebral joint (**Video 38.3**).
- This may be performed by inserting a narrow Cobb elevator into the costovertebral junction and slowly oscillating the paddle of the elevator to disrupt the fibrous capsule.
- The rib is then circumferentially dissected free of the parietal pleura anteriorly and the neurovascular bundle inferiorly.
- The Doyen periosteal elevator was designed to facilitate this dissection and may be used to expose 2 to 5 cm of the rib.
- The rib is divided laterally with a rib cutter or a large Leksell rongeur.
- The parietal pleura is further dissected off the anterior rib and the lateral vertebral body.
- The ipsilateral lung may be deflated by the anesthesiologist to increase direct visualization of the lateral vertebral body.
- A malleable retractor or fenestrated lung retractor may be used to control the lung anterolaterally.
- The exiting nerve root is identified at the foramen and safely preserved as it travels in the neurovascular bundle inferior to the rib.

- Special attention is paid to not handle or pull on the nerve to avoid iatrogenic spinal cord injury.

38.5 Complications

- Dermatomal numbness and paresthesia.
- Dural tear and cerebrospinal fluid (CSF) leak.
- Pneumothorax.

38.6 Management Pearls

- Some pathologies may require more than one rib to be dissected and resected. In these cases, nerve root sacrifice may be necessary.
- Patients should be counseled about this possibility and the postoperative implications including dermatomal numbness and paresthesia.
- The anterior segmental medullary arteries may pass along the midpoint of the lateral vertebral body and can be a source of blood loss and should be managed mindfully.
- Sacrifice of one vessel is generally well tolerated, but they may variably contribute to the perfusion of the spinal cord.
- The great radicular artery of Adamkiewicz (actually a segmental medullary artery) is classically described to arise between T9 and T12 on the left and provides critical supply to the spinal cord. If multiple vessels are suspected to be sacrificed, a preoperative angiogram may inform surgical planning.
- Access to the disc space generally requires resection of the rib below the corresponding disc space. For example, the T9 rib should be exposed and resected to gain access to the T8–T9 disc space.
- Dural tear and CSF leak can be difficult to manage in this approach, especially tears of the ventral thecal sac.
- Primary closure with suture of the dura is often not feasible. A circumferential repair can be performed with dural substitute wrapping around the thecal sac and sewn in place posteriorly, followed by dural sealant.
- If the parietal pleura is violated, it should be repaired. Valsalva can help determine if the pleura is violated. To avoid a pneumothorax, a chest tube may be placed during or after surgery. Alternatively, a red rubber catheter may be placed into the pleural space atraumatically and a purse stitch placed around the catheter through the parietal pleura.
- The suture is cinched tight around the catheter, Valsalva is applied to evacuate intraparietal air through the catheter, and then the catheter is removed while the purse stitch is secured to prevent new air trapping.
- Serial chest radiographs may then be used to monitor for a pneumothorax, and any pleural effusion will usually resolve without significant sequelae.
- Finally, should iatrogenic instability be expected during the procedure, temporary stabilization with contralateral pedicle screws and rod should be placed until definitive instrumented fusion can be performed.

39 Osteotomies (Thoracolumbar)

Stephen M. Bergin and Khoi D. Than

39.1 Background

- Thoracolumbar osteotomies are powerful techniques for realignment and correction of rigid spinal deformity.
- Posterior spinal osteotomy includes posterior column osteotomies, pedicle subtraction osteotomy (PSO), and vertebral column resection (VCR), as well as variations of these techniques.
- The choice of osteotomy depends on the surgical goal and correction requirement, and each osteotomy has specific advantages and limitations.
- Sagittal imbalance is directly associated with decreased health-related quality-of-life scores, and postoperative improvement in sagittal alignment improves patient outcomes.
- When combined with pedicle screw fixation, posterior spinal osteotomies can provide significant correction of regional and global sagittal as well as coronal alignment.
- Osteotomies provide surgical correction of spinal deformity in the treatment of multiple diseases including adult idiopathic scoliosis, flat back syndrome, and iatrogenic fixed sagittal imbalance.
- The SRS-Schwab osteotomy classification defines six grades of osteotomies that correspond with increased bone removal and increased degrees of spinal destabilization (▶ Fig. 39.1).
- A grade 1 osteotomy involves resection of the inferior facet and the joint capsule, and this offers 5 degrees of correction.
- A grade 2 osteotomy involves complete facet joint resection and partial resection of the posterior elements including the lamina, spinous process, and ligamentum flavum; this can accomplish 10 degrees of correction.
- Both grade 1 and 2 osteotomies require a mobile anterior column to be effective.
- A grade 3 osteotomy resects the posterior elements and creates a partial wedge resection of the posterior vertebral body. A PSO is a grade 3 osteotomy and provides 20 to 25 degrees of correction.
- A grade 4 osteotomy extends a grade 3 osteotomy to include resection of an endplate and adjacent disc.
- A VCR is a grade 5 osteotomy and removes one vertebral level and both adjacent discs. A VCR provides 35 to 60 degrees of correction.
- A grade 6 osteotomy involves resection of at least one complete vertebral body and a partial or complete second vertebra.

39.2 Indications and Contraindications

- Grade 1 and 2 osteotomies are ideal in mild to moderate sagittal plane deformity with a mobile anterior column and can be performed over multiple levels.
- Grade 3 and 4 osteotomies are performed for fixed sagittal malalignment, often in the setting of previous fusion surgery.
- VCR is the osteotomy of choice for sharp, angular kyphotic deformities.
- Significant perioperative morbidity is associated with osteotomies, and a patient's functional status and medical comorbidities should be evaluated before surgery.
- Severe osteoporosis is a relative contraindication due to the risk of instrumentation failure.

39.3 Patient Preparation

- Patients should be evaluated with standing scoliosis X-rays.
- Regional and global alignment as well as sagittal vertical axis, thoracic kyphosis, lumbar lordosis, pelvic incidence, and other spinopelvic parameters should be measured.

39.4 Patient Positioning

- The patient is positioned prone on a radiolucent frame such as a Jackson table. Intraoperative monitoring is used, including motor evoked potentials, somatosensory evoked potentials, and electromyography signals to help recognize neurologic injury.

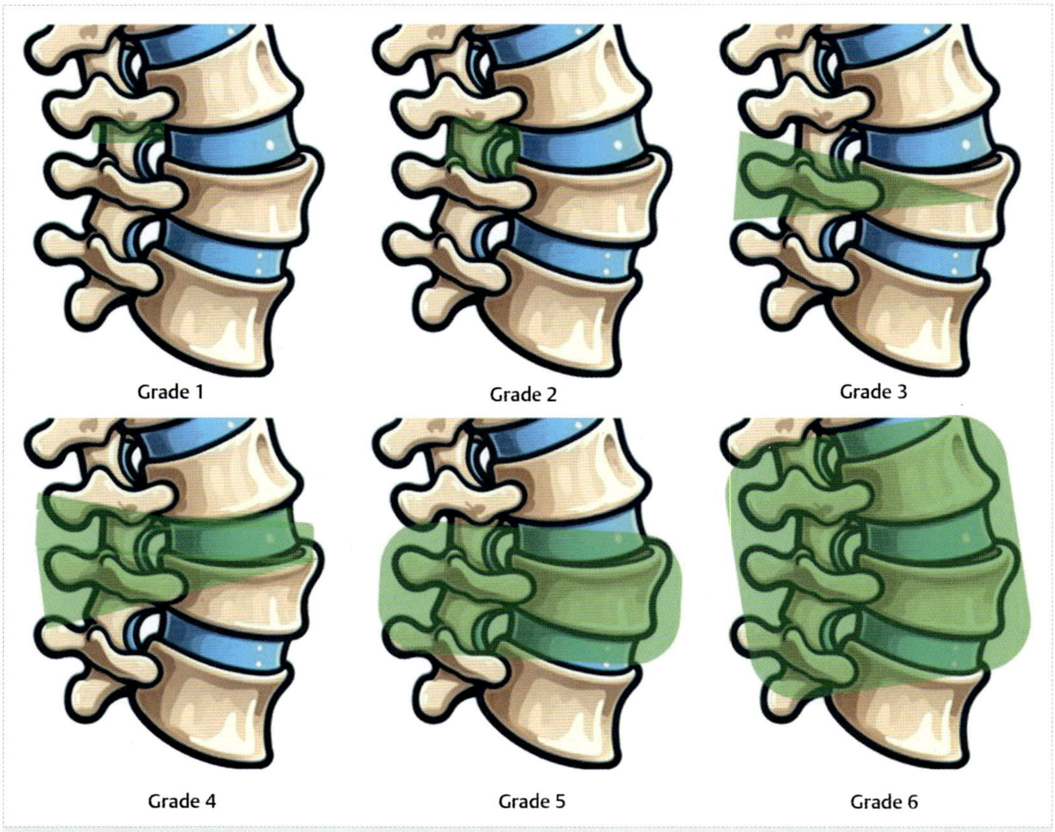

Fig. 39.1 Schwab classification of spinal osteotomies. Grade 1, partial facet; Grade 2, complete facet; Grade 3, pedicle plus partial vertebral body; Grade 4, pedicle plus partial vertebral body and disc; Grade 5, complete vertebral body and adjacent discs; Grade 6, multilevel vertebral body plus discs. (Original illustration by the author Stephen M. Bergin, inspired by Schwab et al.[1])

39.5 Technique

- For a grade 3 osteotomy (PSO), pedicle screw fixation is performed at least two levels above and below the osteotomy.
- The transverse processes are resected and soft tissue is retracted from the lateral portion of the vertebral body.
- The inferior articulating process of the level above the PSO, as well as the pars, superior and inferior facets of the PSO level are removed.
- The posterior elements are also removed. A temporary rod is placed.
- The pedicles are resected with an osteotome or drill. The lateral portion of the pedicle and vertebral body and the thin rim of the posterior vertebral body are removed last.
- Osteotomes are used to create the desired wedge of bone from the lateral aspect of the vertebral body.
- Following the removal of cancellous bone from the vertebral body, the posterior wall of the vertebral body is fractured, and bone fragments are removed.
- The osteotomy is then closed with posterior compression.
- Final rods are placed.

39.6 Postoperative Care

- Patients may require admission to the intensive care unit for blood pressure and ventilator support, as well as frequent neurologic examinations.
- Patients should mobilize early to avoid deep venous thrombosis.

39.7 Complications

- Osteotomies are associated with a high rate (~40%) of significant perioperative complications including neurologic deficit, major blood loss, and dural tears.
- Long-term complications of osteotomies include rod fracture and proximal junctional kyphosis.

39.8 Management Pearls

- Spinal osteotomies surgically correct sagittal plane deformities. Restoration of a sagittally balanced spine is crucial for clinical success of patients with spinal deformity.
- The SRS-Schwab classification[1] is an anatomically based system that defines a range of osteotomies from smaller to larger.
- A CT should be obtained to evaluate positioning of instrumentation and pseudarthrosis in patients with prior spine surgeries.
- The anesthesiologist should avoid medications that interfere with intraoperative neuromonitoring. An arterial and central line should be placed for blood pressure monitoring and volume resuscitation. Mean arterial pressure should be maintained at greater than 80 mm Hg to ensure adequate perfusion of the neural elements, especially during closure of the osteotomy. An intraoperative cell saver should be considered.
- Osteotomies can result in significant blood loss, and coagulation parameters should be monitored with early replacement of blood and coagulation factors anticipated.[2] During osteotomy closure, if there are changes in the motor evoked potentials, the closure is reversed, and further decompression is performed.

References

[1] Schwab F, Blondel B, Chay E, et al. The comprehensive anatomical spinal osteotomy classification. Neurosurgery. 2014; 74(1):112–120, discussion 120

[2] Gupta MC, Kebaish K, Blondel B, Klineberg E. Spinal osteotomies for rigid deformities. Neurosurg Clin N Am. 2013; 24(2):203–211

40 MIS (Lumbar, Microtubular Surgery)

Azeem A. Rehman, Anthony M. Alvarado, and Richard G. Fessler

40.1 Background

- A minimally invasive microtubular approach to decompression of the lumbar spine reduces trauma to the paraspinal muscles, supraspinous and interspinous ligaments, and the facet joints.

40.2 Indications and Contraindications

- The most common diseases in the lumbar spine that can be addressed through minimally invasive microtubular approaches include paracentral disc herniations, lumbar canal stenosis, lateral recess stenosis, and symptomatic lumbar synovial cysts.
- The indications for a minimally invasive microtubular approach to the lumbar spine for disc herniations and stenosis are the same as those for the open conventional approaches.
- Patient pathology at a specific spine level should always be examined in the context of any global spinal derangement. In certain cases, corrective surgery for adult spinal deformity may be indicated. However, scoliosis correction carries significant morbidity. As such, a limited minimally invasive approach for decompression may be a more suitable option, especially in the setting of older, more frail patients.[1]
- For cauda equina syndrome, some literature advocates for an open complete laminectomy and discectomy. However, minimally invasive approaches have also been adopted for this pathology with great success.[2]

40.3 Patient Preparation

- If the history and physical examination support a lumbar radicular pathology, conservative management should be pursued assuming no "red flag" symptoms or signs are present.
- After 6 weeks, if symptoms are still severe, radiographic workup with magnetic resonance imaging of the spine should be completed.
- If the patient is unable to undergo magnetic resonance imaging, then a computed tomography scan with myelography should be considered.
- In patients who have had previous lumbar spine surgery, contrast-enhanced images are helpful in differentiating scar tissue from a primary pathology.
- For patients who have had prior lumbar spine surgery, a computed tomography scan is helpful to assess for any bone defects.
- Dynamic flexion and extension radiographs should be obtained to rule out segmental instability.
- For more ambiguous cases, electromyography with nerve conduction velocity studies can be helpful.
- The surgery can be performed under general anesthesia or local anesthesia under conscious sedation. The authors prefer general anesthesia without the use of prolonged muscle relaxation.

40.4 Patient Positioning

- A table with a flat radiolucent top is utilized. The patient is positioned prone on a Wilson frame to flex the lumbosacral spine. The head can be placed in a prone view or be suspended in the air using Gardner-Wells tongs attached to a pulley-weight system.
- Gel pads are placed for the knees and pillows for the feet. Arm boards with padding for the axilla, elbows, and wrists are utilized.
- Intraoperative fluoroscopy is necessary for localization.
- A microtubular retractor system with accompanying bayoneted tools is necessary. The microtubular retractor system requires a table attachment piece, which should be placed contralaterally to the site of the surgical approach.
- Intraoperative neuromonitoring can be utilized at the surgeon's discretion.

40.5 Technique

- After positioning, the posterior lumbosacral spine is prepped and widely draped.

- The spinous processes are palpated and marked to identify the midline. Using the smallest dilator on the skin surface, lateral fluoroscopy films are obtained to center the dilator on the disc space of interest. This location is marked in the midline.
- A second mark is then made approximately one fingerbreadth lateral to this location on the ipsilateral side of the disc herniation. For decompression, this mark is made approximately 2.5 cm from the midline. This second mark is extended longitudinally approximately 2.0 to 2.5 cm to accommodate the future tubular retractor.
- Local anesthetic is administered.
- The incision is opened using a scalpel and dissection is extended to the lumbar fascia with monopolar electrocautery. Monopolar electrocautery is used to incise the fascia in line with the incision.
- The smallest dilator is then placed through the opening in the fascia. The smallest dilator is kept in a superficial plane, albeit deep to the fascia, and directed slightly medial to palpate the spinous process.
- Using palpation, the smallest dilator is moved down the spinous process to the corresponding lamina. The smallest dilator is then moved from the lamina to the inferior articulating process of the facet joint.
- Following identification of these bony landmarks, the dilator ultimately rests at the junction of the spinous process and lamina. Lateral fluoroscopy films are obtained to confirm the dilator is centered at the disc level of interest. Subsequent dilations are made and a tube of appropriate size is selected.
- Intermittently, during the dilations, lateral fluoroscopy films are obtained to confirm stable positioning (▶ Fig. 40.1).
- In addition, the smallest dilator is routinely checked to confirm the dilation system is resting on bone.
- After final positioning, lateral fluoroscopy films are obtained. Satisfied with the positioning, a final anteroposterior fluoroscopy film is obtained to confirm if the tube is resting on the ipsilateral side of the planned discectomy (▶ Fig. 40.2).
- Monopolar electrocautery is used to remove any residual paraspinal muscle.
- Subperiosteal dissection is used to identify the spinous process, lamina, and inferior

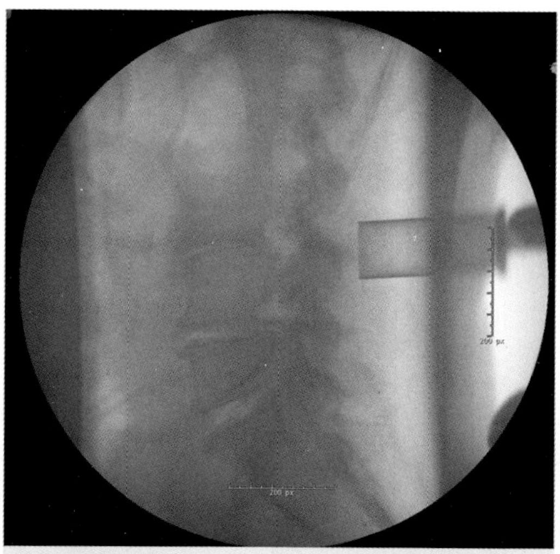

Fig. 40.1 Lateral fluoroscopy demonstrating placement of the microtubular retractor centered at the disc space of interest.

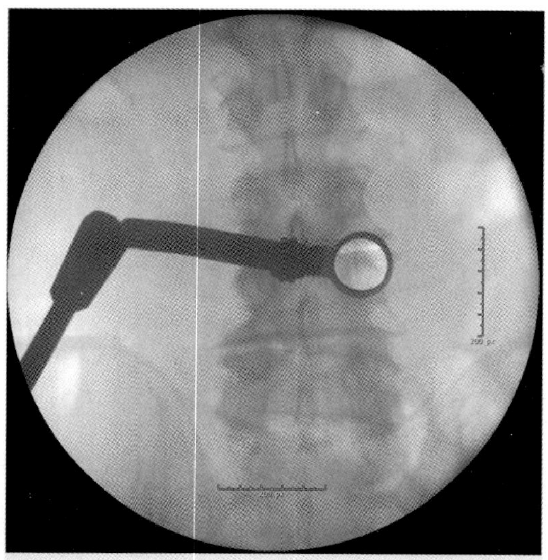

Fig. 40.2 Anteroposterior fluoroscopy confirming placement of the microtubular retractor on the appropriate side. Note that the arm affixing the retractor to the bed is contralateral to the side of the surgical approach.

articulating process. Care is taken to preserve the facet capsule.

- For a paracentral disc herniation, an upgoing curette is used to define the edge of the lamina with the spinous process. Using Kerrison rongeurs, a hemilaminotomy is performed. If necessary, this bony removal may extend to the medial facet joint. The traversing nerve root and thecal sac are retracted medially and the ventral epidural space is explored for the herniated disc. An annulotomy and discectomy are performed.
- For lumbar stenosis, Kerrison rongeurs are used to remove the superior lamina to the inferior aspect of the rostral pedicle as well as the inferior lamina to the middle of the caudal pedicle. The bony removal is extended laterally to the medial facet joint. The tubular retractor is then angled medially to undercut the ventral surface of the spinous process and contralateral lamina using a high-speed Midas Rex Legend drill (▶ Fig. 40.3). The plane between the ligamentum flavum and underlying dura is identified. The ligamentum flavum is removed using Kerrison rongeurs.
- For closure, hemostasis is achieved with bipolar electrocautery, hemostatic thrombin agents, and bone wax. The tubular retractor is removed. The fascia and subcutaneous tissue are re-approximated with stitches. The skin is re-approximated with a topical adhesive.

40.6 Postoperative Care

- Patients are routinely discharged on the same day as surgery after being monitored in the postoperative care unit. They are advised to mobilize as tolerated, but should avoid strenuous activity for 6 weeks.
- Routine follow-up is scheduled in 2 weeks for wound check. At this follow-up, outpatient physical therapy is also prescribed if indicated.

40.7 Complications

- Bleeding, wound infection, cerebrospinal fluid leak, neurologic injury, recurrent disc herniation, and future need for additional spinal surgery.
- Complications related to anesthesia should also be discussed including heart attack, stroke, and death.
- Care should be taken to dock the dilators on bone rather than the interlaminar space, which can lead to a cerebrospinal fluid leak and nerve root injury.

40.8 Management Pearls

- Higher levels (L1–L2) have a less sagittal-oriented facet articulation compared to lower levels. As such, for adequate exposure, a greater amount of the medial facet must be removed.
- When operating at the L1–L2 level, the preoperative imaging should be

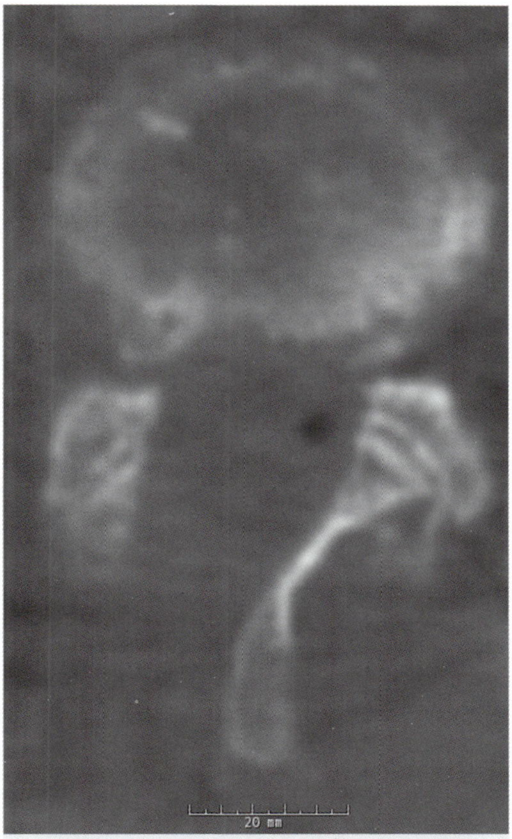

Fig. 40.3 Postoperative computed tomography axial radiographs following a unilateral right-sided approach for bilateral decompression.

reviewed to assess the location of the conus medullaris.

- The degree of facet hypertrophy should be evaluated. Significant facet hypertrophy can make dilation and subsequent medial placement of the tubular retractor difficult.
- For patients with prior lumbar spine surgery, bony defects should be evaluated on preoperative imaging. Care should be taken to ensure the initial dilators are placed on bone. Strategies to minimize this risk include palpating with a finger prior to inserting the dilator or placing the initial dilator on the lateral facet or the transverse process and carefully palpating medially. A larger diameter tube may be necessary.

References

[1] Fontes RB, Fessler RG. Lumbar radiculopathy in the setting of degenerative scoliosis: MIS decompression and limited correction are better options. Neurosurg Clin N Am. 2017; 28(3):335–339

[2] Shih P, Smith TR, Fessler RG, Song JK. Minimally invasive discectomy for the treatment of disc herniation causing cauda equina syndrome. J Clin Neurosci. 2011; 18(9):1219–1223

41 Open Sacroiliac Joint Fusion (Granite)

Jay I. Kumar and Gregory M. Mundis, Jr

41.1 Background

- The sacroiliac joint (SIJ) is subject to increased stress in the setting of long thoracolumbar fusion constructs that extend to the distal lumbar spine and the sacrum.[1]
- Subsequent SIJ arthropathy may cause significant pain, and SIJ fusion may relieve this pain.[2,3,4,5]
- In selected cases, the SIJ may be fused at the time of the lumbosacral fusion to prevent subsequent painful arthropathy, and to create a stiffer base for long constructs.[6,7]
- This may be performed from an open approach posteriorly or from a percutaneous approach.[8,9] Here, we review the technical fundamentals of an open approach.
- Familiarity with anatomy of the SIJ is of utmost importance prior to attempting this procedure.

41.2 Indications and Contraindications

- Indications for open SIJ fusion include large posterior lumbosacral or thoracolumbosacral fusions, and SIJ arthropathy causing pain.
- Dysmorphic sacral anatomy may preclude SIJ fusion. Other relative contraindications include osteoporosis and iliac defects from prior bone graft harvest.

41.3 Instruments

- Pedicle probe, ball-tipped probe, and screw tap.

41.4 Patient Positioning

- The patient is typically positioned prone on a radiolucent rotating Jackson table. The arms are extended upward to make room for fluoroscopy equipment (C-arm) and the surgeon, and to keep the hands out of the line of sight for lateral fluoroscopy.
- We discuss the use of intraoperative fluoroscopy here (▶ Fig. 41.1), but spinal navigation with intraoperative computed tomography (CT) may also be used as demonstrated in our surgical videos.
- All bony prominences are padded, and neurovascular structures are positioned without compression.
- Motor evoked potentials and somatosensory evoked potentials are not routinely monitored.
- The surgeon then stands on the side contralateral to the operative side.

41.5 Technique

- A midline incision is made or extended inferiorly from concurrent lumbosacral fusion surgery to expose the dorsal S1 and S2 foramen.
- Subperiosteal dissection with monopolar electrocautery is used to expose the sacral cortex surrounding the foramen, but it is not necessary to expose the ilium. The starting point for the SIJ implant is identified lateral to the S1 foramen.
- If an S1 pedicle screw is also performed, the starting point for the SIJ implant is below the S1 pedicle screw. If an S2 alar-iliac (S2AI) screw is performed, the starting point for the SIJ implant is above the S2AI screw (**Video 41.1** and **Video 41.2**).
- The starting point is then decorticated with a high-speed drill, rongeur, or pedicle probe per the surgeon's preference.
- The trajectory is cannulated with a pedicle probe toward the top of the greater trochanter ipsilateral to the operative side. This trajectory should be parallel and cephalad to the trajectory of an S2AI screw to minimize the risk of breaching the sciatic notch and injuring the gluteal vessels.
- To confirm correct trajectory, an obturator outlet or "teardrop" view on fluoroscopy can be used to watch the pedicle probe enter the ilium. This "teardrop" view may be roughly obtained by rotating the C-arm receiver 30 degrees over the patient toward the operative side, and canting the receiver 30 degrees toward the patient's feet, and then fine-tuning.
- Anteroposterior, pelvic inlet, and pelvic outlet views all help check for transgression across the

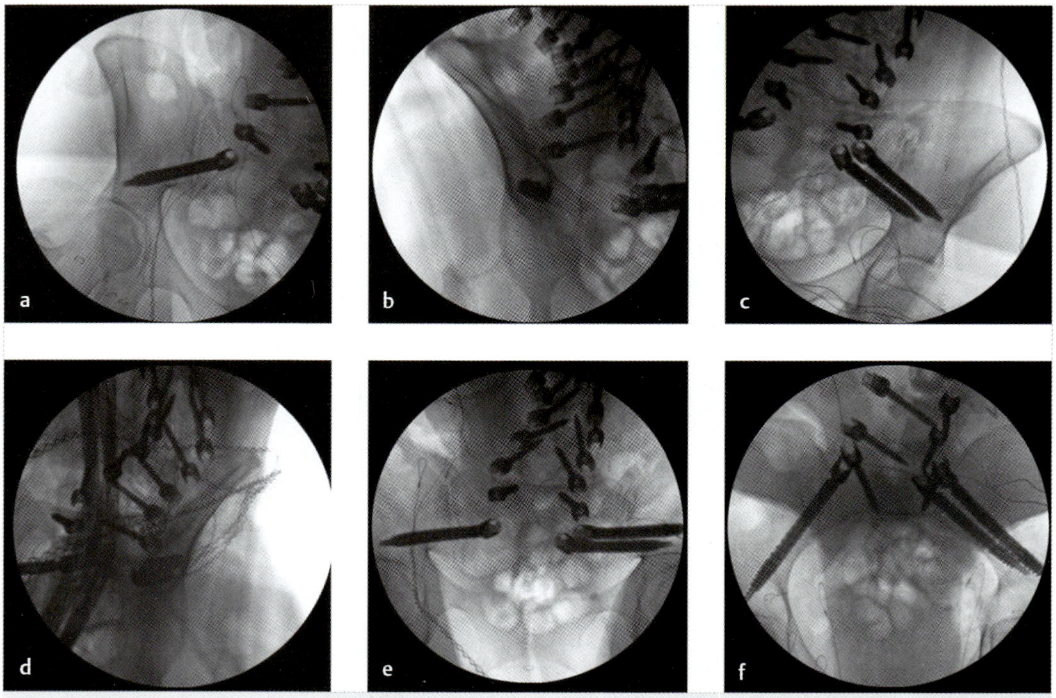

Fig. 41.1 Intraoperative fluoroscopy shots demonstrating safe implantation. **(a)** Anteroposterior (AP) image demonstrating left sacroiliac joint (SIJ) screw crossing the SIJ and running cranial to the sciatic notch. **(b)** Tear drop view demonstrating implant within the left ilium. **(c)** AP image demonstrating right SIJ screw crossing the SIJ and running cranial to the sciatic notch. **(d)** Tear drop view demonstrating implant within the right ilium. **(e)** Pelvic outlet view demonstrating implants outside of the sacral foramen. **(f)** Pelvic inlet view demonstrating implants remain outside of the pelvic viscera.

SIJ and to ensure there is no violation of the sciatic notch.

- Lateral fluoroscopy can help confirm the trajectory parallel and cephalad to the S2AI screw if present.
- The pedicle probe should cross the SIJ and enter the ilium. The pedicle probe is then removed and a ball-tipped probe is used to palpate the cannulated trajectory and inspect for any bony breaches, most commonly found laterally (**Video 41.3**).
- The ball-tipped probe is removed and a blunt guide pin is placed into the trajectory and across the SIJ.
- Fluoroscopy then confirms correct placement of the pin in the cannulated trajectory and adequate space for the implant if S1 pedicle screws or S2AI screws are also in place.
- A soft tissue protector is placed over the pin and docked on the sacrum. A pin sleeve is snapped into the tissue protector.
- The implant size is obtained by measuring the length of the pin prominent to the pin sleeve. A cannulated drill is advanced over the pin and passed across the SIJ.
- A sharp triangular broach is placed across the pin with one flat side parallel to the midline to avoid violating the S1 foramen, and a mallet is used to advance the broach across the SIJ.
- The broach is then removed over an exchange pin with a slotted reverse mallet. The implant is advanced over the pin with a mallet.
- Fluoroscopy is used to confirm placement, and the guide pin is removed.

41.6 Postoperative Care

- Special considerations discussed above should be taken in to account. Otherwise, routine postoperative spine care should be performed at the surgeon's discretion.

41.7 Complications

- Vascular and visceral injury with ventral breach and entrance into the pelvis.

41.8 Management Pearls

- Two separate diagnostic SIJ injections with immediate relief are recommended before considering SIJ fusion.
- Careful patient selection through thorough examination and history combined with two diagnostic injections is essential to a successful outcome.
- During exposure for open fusion surgery, avoid destabilizing the SIJ with periosteal dissection and electrocautery.
- While defining implant trajectory, avoid breaching the lateral ilium. If a breach occurs, remove the pedicle probe and define a new trajectory.
- The starting point may need to be moved medially. During drilling and broaching the trajectory, be mindful to not advance the guide pin.
- Check fluoroscopy as needed.
- Two fixation points across the SIJ are required for fusion (**Video 41.4** and **Video 41.5**).
- When removing the broach over the exchange pin, the guide pin may be dislodged. Downward pressure on the exchange pin, possibly exerted by a surgical assistant, can help prevent dislodgement. If the pin is dislodged, it should be replaced and confirmed under fluoroscopy.
- Implant size may also be measured by clamping the ball-tipped probe at the sacral cortex while the probe remains flush with the floor of the cannulated trajectory.
- To avoid unnecessary radiation exposure to the surgeon, long instruments such as a sponge holder or a radiolucent clamp may be used to hold the blunt guide pin while checking the trajectory.
- The implant may be packed with graft material per surgeon preference (**Video 41.6**).
- In case of suboptimal implant placement, a removal adaptor may be screwed into the proximal aspect of the implant and then extracted using a slotted mallet.

References

[1] Ivanov AA, Kiapour A, Ebraheim NA, Goel V. Lumbar fusion leads to increases in angular motion and stress across sacroiliac joint: a finite element study. Spine. 2009; 34(5): E162–E169

[2] Unoki E, Abe E, Murai H, Kobayashi T, Abe T. Fusion of multiple segments can increase the incidence of sacroiliac joint pain after lumbar or lumbosacral fusion. Spine. 2016; 41(12):999–1005

[3] Manzetti M, Ruffilli A, Barile F, et al. Sacroiliac joint degeneration and pain after spinal arthrodesis: a systematic review. Clin Spine Surg. 2023; 36(4):169–182

[4] Chen LY, Liang HD, Qin QN, et al. Sacroiliac joint fusion vs conservative management for chronic low back pain attributed to the sacroiliac joint: a protocol for systematic review and meta analysis. Medicine (Baltimore). 2020; 99 (46):e23223

[5] Katz V, Schofferman J, Reynolds J. The sacroiliac joint: a potential cause of pain after lumbar fusion to the sacrum. J Spinal Disord Tech. 2003; 16(1):96–99

[6] Noureldine MHA, Freeman TB, Alikhani P. Simultaneous sacroiliac joint fusion in patients with long lumbosacral constructs: case report and operative technique. World Neurosurg. 2020; 139:434–439

[7] Noureldine MHA, Pressman E, Kumar JI, et al. Sacroiliac joint arthropathy in adult spinal deformity patients with long constructs to the pelvis. Clin Neurol Neurosurg. 2021; 203: 106593

[8] Rudolf L. Sacroiliac joint arthrodesis-MIS technique with titanium implants: report of the first 50 patients and outcomes. Open Orthop J. 2012; 6:495–502

[9] Belanger TA, Dall BE. Sacroiliac arthrodesis using a posterior midline fascial splitting approach and pedicle screw instrumentation: a new technique. J Spinal Disord. 2001; 14 (2):118–124

42 Anterior Cervical Discectomy and Fusion

Ryan Sadjadi, Nora C. Kim, Mohamed Macki, and Lee A. Tan

42.1 Background

- This chapter reviews the relevant anatomical considerations and provides a step-by-step guide to perform a safe and effective anterior cervical discectomy and fusion (ACDF).
- A solid understanding of relevant anterior cervical surgical anatomy can help spine surgeons to perform ACDF safely and efficiently to minimize potential complications.

42.2 Indications and Contraindications

- Indications may be for cervical radiculopathy/ myelopathy, cervical spine fractures, or cervical spine instability.
- Contraindications may be for active infection, prior surgeries, or other reasons indicating poor candidacy.

42.3 Instruments

- A standard instrument layout is shown in ▶ Fig. 42.1.

42.4 Patient Preparation

- In the preoperative area, identify a natural skin crease in the neck.
  - With appropriate surgical dissection, the disc spaces from the C2 to T1 vertebral bodies can be accessed through a horizontal incision based on a skin crease closest to the intended surgical levels.
- Identify the levels of large anterior osteophytes on computed tomography (CT) or X-rays.
  - Palpation of the osteophytes intraoperatively can assist in spinal localization.
- Review the course of the vertebral artery on the magnetic resonance imaging (MRI).
  - The surgeon must note any aberrant course of the vertebral artery.

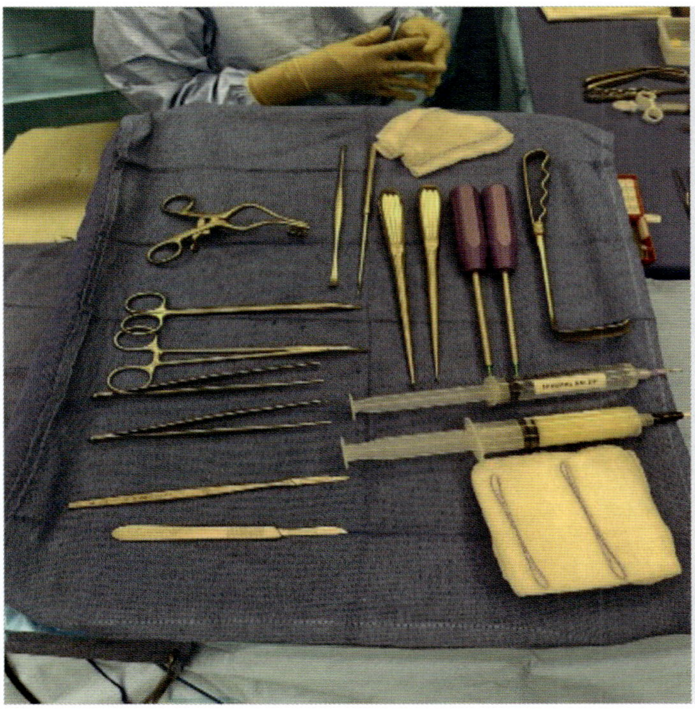

Fig. 42.1 Mayo stand setup. This arrangement includes essential instruments such as the Weitlaner retractor, Metzenbaum scissors, Penfield dissectors (no. 2 and no. 4), Schnidt tonsil forceps, toothed pickups, scalpels (no. 15, 10, or 20 blades), lateral Richardson retractor, Caspar pins, and small and medium upgoing curettes for tissue dissection, exposure, and bone preparation.

  - In over 71% of cases, the vertebral artery enters the foramen transversarium at the level of C6. The next highest frequency is C7 (18.42%), followed by C5 (5.3%), C4 (2.6%), and C3 (2.6%).[1]
  - Vertebral artery dominance, a normal congenital variation of the right and left vertebral arteries, is based on diameter. The left vertebral artery is dominant in approximately 54% of cases compared to 30% for the right vertebral artery. In 16% of cases, right and left arterial diameters are equal.
- Measure the width and depth of each vertebral body for the ACDF levels. This will provide an estimate for cervical screw length.

42.5 Patient Positioning

- The patient is placed in the supine position.
- A small shoulder roll is placed across the level of the scapula to facilitate gentle neck extension and a donut is placed under the skull to minimize head movement during surgery; taping the head is also an option to further decrease intraoperative head and neck movement from surgical manipulation.

42.6 Technique

- A demonstration of the procedure is shown in **Video 42.1**.

42.6.1 Operation

- Drape the C-arm (lateral position) into the field.
- With a left-sided approach (longer course of the recurrent laryngeal nerve and thus less potential risk of traction injury), incise at the natural neck crease, which will help make the incision site more inconspicuous and cosmetically pleasing once it heals.[2]
- Incise the neck at the incision site with a no. 10 blade scalpel.
- Use a monopolar device to cut the platysma horizontally.
- A monopolar is used to cut through the subplatysmal fascia to create a subplatysmal "pocket" cranially and caudally.
- Place a small Weitlaner retractor and dissect along the medial border of the sternocleidomastoid (SCM) and lateral border of strap muscles.
- Identify the omohyoid muscle and place the Schnidt tonsil and artery forceps around the muscle to monopolar cut.
  - After cutting the omohyoid, a corridor to the anterior spine will be apparent.
  - The oblique course (running from superomedial to inferolateral) of the omohyoid muscle helps differentiate it from the strep muscles (thyrohyoid, sternohyoid, and sternothyroid muscles), which have more vertical course.
  - *Anatomy just beyond platysma layer:* The usual neck incision reveals the position of the SCM, omohyoid, and sternohyoid strap muscles. Additionally, some of the superficial layer of the deep cervical fascia can be seen.
- Insert a finger through the corridor and palpate the carotid bundle within the carotid sheath (lateral) and the tracheoesophageal bundle (medial).
- Once the surgical plan plane is defined, retract the esophagus and trachea medially.
- Cut the prevertebral fascia by crisscrossing toothed pickup and Metzenbaum scissors.
  - In the anterior cervical exposure, the first important identification point is the coalescence of the SCM medial border, superficial layer of the deep cervical fascia, and infrahyoid fascia that allows the "danger space" between the carotid sheath, thyroid, and alar fascia to be accessed. The danger space is particularly susceptible to retropharyngeal infections, lying between the alar and the prevertebral fascia.[3,4] Because the alar fascia diverges laterally to connect with the carotid sheath, dissection that is not lateral enough will make it more difficult to reach the prevertebral fascia.[4,5]
- Palpate overhanging osteophytes to help ascertain the cervical spine level. Preoperative images that show the location of osteophytes can be used to help support level estimation.
- Confirm the level by placing a clamp on the longus colli muscle at the level of the index disc space.
  - Spinal needles are not used. A needle in the wrong intervertebral space will injure the disc and cause accelerated disc degeneration.

  - When a multilevel ACDF is planned, clamp on the higher levels will help with visualization and minimize the chance that the shoulder will block the clamp on lateral fluoroscopy images.
- Remove all other instruments from the surgical cavity and X-ray to identify the clamp relative to the intended spinal level.
- Use bipolar cautery to sever the longus colli muscle attachment at the midpoint of the vertebral body.
- *Place bed-mounted cervical retractors:* The teeth should be positioned medially against the esophagus to minimize esophageal creeping during surgery and the nonteethed portion laterally against the carotid bundle.
- Use a Leksell rongeur to remove the osteophytes above and below the endplate.
- Pilot hole at the midpoint of the disc space. Place Caspar pins parallel to the disc space and in the middle of the vertebral body. The pin site will help position the cervical plate at the end of the procedure.
- Incise the disc with a no. 15 blade.
- Use pituitary and upgoing curettes to remove the disc material and prepare the endplates. If the disc space is too collapsed to fit an upgoing curette, a Cobb retractor can break open the intervertebral space.
- A 3-mm matchstick burr is used to prep the endplates and to complete central decompression.
- The posterior longitudinal ligament (PLL) is the removed by first puncturing it with a 5-0 upgoing curette under the center of the vertebral body endplate, then gently turning the curette 90 degrees under the PLL, then lifting away from the cord to create an opening in the PLL.
- Then a 2-mm Kerrison rongeur is used to remove the PLL to achieve complete decompression of the spinal cord.

42.6.2 Uncinectomy

- An uncinectomy is a procedure conducted to treat severe bony foraminal stenosis, and should be utilized judiciously as it can be technically challenging and carries low but potential risk of vertebral artery injury.

42.6.3 Uncinate Process Anatomy

- The uncinate process is a bilateral, bony projection located on the posterolateral and superior surfaces of the cervical vertebrae C3–C7. It is adjacent to the vertebral artery and nerve root and forms the uncovertebral joint with the body of the vertebra above and forms the medial margin of the intervertebral foramen.[6] Making a window for nerve root decompression via uncinectomy depends on the height and width of the uncinate process. The average height of the uncinate process gradually increases from C3 to C6, then decreases at C7.[7,8]

42.6.4 Uncinectomy Operation

- Trace the uncinate joint with the upgoing curette from deep in the spinal canal to superficial, up to the longus colli muscle.
- With a Penfield no. 4 dissector, trace the superficial uncinate process from medial to lateral, in order to dissect the longus colli muscle, then reflect the longus colli with a Penfield no. 2 dissector.
- Remove the uncinate process as close to the lateral boarder as possible but leave a thin shelve of bone to minimize the chance of vertebral artery injury. First, burr straight down in a ventrodorsal direction about two-thirds of the way to just above the neuroforamen. Next, since the nerve root courses ventrally and laterally, the deepest part of the uncinate process is removed using a burr in a medial to lateral direction. Keep a thin layer of cortical bone to protect the nerve root. The eggshelled bone can be safely removed using a small upgoing curette to completely decompress the exiting nerve root.

42.6.5 Arthrodesis and Plating

- Place a trial to estimate the appropriate height of the interbody cage.
  - Frozen iliac crest allograft is a good alternative to cages because of its favorable effects on fusion rates.[9,10]
- Tap the interbody into place.
  - *Cage placement for C2–C3 or C3–C4 ACDF*: Standalone cages with integrated screws are preferred over plating given there is less risk of dysphagia in the former. The addition of a plate

at these levels can irritate the esophagus due to the comparatively small prevertebral space. The thickness of the prevertebral space decreases from lower cervical levels to higher levels with about 6 mm at C2 and 2 cm at the C6 level.
  - *Cage placement for C4–C7 ACDF:* Place an interbody cage and a plate.
  - *Note for three-level ACDF:* Place a titanium cage at the bottom level of the fusion construct. Do not use iliac crest bone at this level due to crushing concerns with slow healing time. The caudal level has the slowest rate of arthrodesis compared to cranial and middle levels, likely due to increased biomechanical stress at this level.[11]
- For levels C4–C7, size the plate from just above the inferior endplate of the rostral level to just below the superior endplate of the caudal level so that the top and bottom screws are placed in a diagonal trajectory and the middle screws are placed in a straight trajectory.
  - Because there is only about 15 degrees of lordosis in the subaxial cervical spine, a plate bender can be used to create a small amount of lordosis in the plate.
  - Use diagonal screws as the plate reaches the bottom of the vertebral body with a diagonal trajectory.
    - The longer the screws, the higher the pullout strength, which may lead to a higher rate of fusion. In primary two-level ACDF, a vertebral body percentage (VB%) of less than 75% is significantly associated with increased interspinous motion (≥ 1 mm) at all time points. As an intraoperative guide, spine surgeons can use the screw VB% threshold of less than 75% to avoid unnecessarily short screws. This threshold can be easily measured pre- and intraoperatively, and has been found to be strongly correlated to radiographic pseudarthrosis in the early postoperative period.[12]
  - Finally, close the wound in multiple layer and a drain is typically used for multilevel cases.

42.7 Complications

- ACDF is a common surgical technique used to treat various cervical spine pathologies, but complications such as postoperative dysphagia, recurrent laryngeal nerve injury, esophageal injury, and CSF leak can occur and negatively impact surgical outcome.

42.8 Management Pearls

- There are several important considerations for preoperative imaging when performing an ACDF.
- MRI to assess degree of neural compression (spinal cord and nerve roots) and to understand the course and dominance of the vertebral arteries (T2-weighted imaging flow voids).
- C-spine X-rays with anteroposterior, lateral, oblique, and flexion/extension views to assess the spinal alignment and rule out instability, as well as to assess bony foraminal stenosis on oblique views.
- CT to assess the degree of bony degeneration, disc–osteophyte complex, bony foraminal narrowing, as well as the presence of ossification of posterior longitudinal ligament(OPLL).
- Scoliosis X-rays in spinal deformity cases or cases where the T1 slope is abnormally elevated (> 30 degrees), suggesting the presence of thoracolumbar spine sagittal malignment.

References

[1] Sastry R, Manjunath V. The course of the V1 segment of the vertebral artery. Ann Indian Acad Neurol. 2006; 9:223–226
[2] Jung A, Schramm J, Lehnerdt K, Herberhold C. Recurrent laryngeal nerve palsy during anterior cervical spine surgery: a prospective study. J Neurosurg Spine. 2005; 2 (2):123–127
[3] Debnam JM, Guha-Thakurta N. Retropharyngeal and prevertebral spaces: anatomic imaging and diagnosis. Otolaryngol Clin North Am. 2012; 45(6):1293–1310
[4] Wong YK, Novotny GM. Retropharyngeal space - a review of anatomy, pathology, and clinical presentation. J Otolaryngol. 1978; 7(6):528–536
[5] Lee SJ, Archang M, Tubbs S, Riew KD, Janus JR, Clifton W. Identification of deep cervical fascial layers during anterior cervical spine exposure. Oper Neurosurg (Hagerstown). 2023; 24(6):e414–e420
[6] Hartman J. Anatomy and clinical significance of the uncinate process and uncovertebral joint: a comprehensive review. Clin Anat. 2014; 27(3):431–440
[7] Kim SH, Lee JH, Kim JH, Chun KS, Doh JW, Chang JC. Anatomical morphometric study of the cervical uncinate process and surrounding structures. J Korean Neurosurg Soc. 2012; 52(4):300–305
[8] Valero-Moreno F, Clifton W, Damon A, Pichelmann M. Total anterior uncinatectomy during anterior discectomy and fusion for recurrent cervical radiculopathy: a two-dimensional

operative video and technical report. Cureus. 2020; 12(3): e7466
[9] Floyd T, Ohnmeiss D. A meta-analysis of autograft versus allograft in anterior cervical fusion. Eur Spine J. 2000; 9(5):398–403
[10] An HS, Simpson JM, Glover JM, Stephany J. Comparison between allograft plus demineralized bone matrix versus autograft in anterior cervical fusion. A prospective multicenter study. Spine. 1995; 20(20):2211–2216
[11] Nichols NM, Jamieson A, Wang M, Chou D, Mummaneni PV, Tan LA. Characterizing the fusion order and level-specific rates of arthrodesis in 3-level anterior cervical discectomy and fusion: a radiographic study. J Clin Neurosci. 2020; 81: 328–333
[12] Nathan J, Lee MD, Vulapalli M. Does screw length for primary two-level ACDF influence pseudarthrosis risk? Spine J. 2020; 20(11):1752–1760

43 Odontoid Screw

Phoebe Greenwald, Bhargav Ayloo, Shailen G. Sampath, Anthony M. DiGiorgio, and Andrew K. Chan

43.1 Background

- Odontoid fractures are a common type of upper cervical spine fracture in the elderly and in patients following high-velocity trauma. Patients commonly present with neck pain and restricted cervical range of motion. The most common type of odontoid fracture is the type II fracture that occurs at the base of the odontoid process and C2 vertebral body.[1] These fractures also carry the highest rate of nonunion in part due to the region's poor vascularization, which can be further compromised by injury.[2,3] Although neurological deficits from odontoid fractures are rare, their presence is associated with a poor prognosis.[4] Prompt evaluation of suspected odontoid fracture patients is helpful to avoid complications such as nonunion and spinal cord injury.
- Both surgical and conservative methods are viable treatment options depending on the odontoid fracture type, patient-specific risk factors, and presence of cervical instability. The primary goals of treatment include restoring spinal alignment, promoting fracture healing, and providing neural decompression if needed. Typically, type I and III odontoid fractures are treated conservatively, while surgical intervention is often reserved for type II odontoid fractures.[5] In this chapter, we discuss the use of anterior odontoid screw fixation in the treatment of a patient who sustained a type II odontoid fracture following a motor vehicle accident. ▶ Fig. 43.1 shows a representative preoperative computed tomography (CT) image demonstrating a type II odontoid fracture. Additionally, we have provided a supplemental surgical video (**Video 43.1**) that demonstrates the key steps of anterior odontoid screw fixation, from patient positioning and fracture reduction to drilling, K-wire placement, and final screw insertion. This video serves as a comprehensive guide and can be viewed alongside the written description and images.

43.2 Indications and Contraindications

- *Indications*:
  - Type II fracture.[6,7]
  - Good bone quality.[8]
  - Chest anatomy or body habitus that allows for low trajectory of screws.[9]
  - Acute fractures.
    - It is best to operate at least within 6 months of injury[5] and ideally within 1 to 2 weeks.[6,9]
  - Reducible fractures.
  - Minimal comminution.[9]
- *Contraindications*:
  - Any characteristic that compromises appropriate screw trajectory or fixation, including the following[10]:
    - Comminuted fracture.
    - Severe osteoporosis.
    - Severe cervicothoracic kyphosis.
    - Fracture line from anteroinferior to posterosuperior of the odontoid[3] wherein

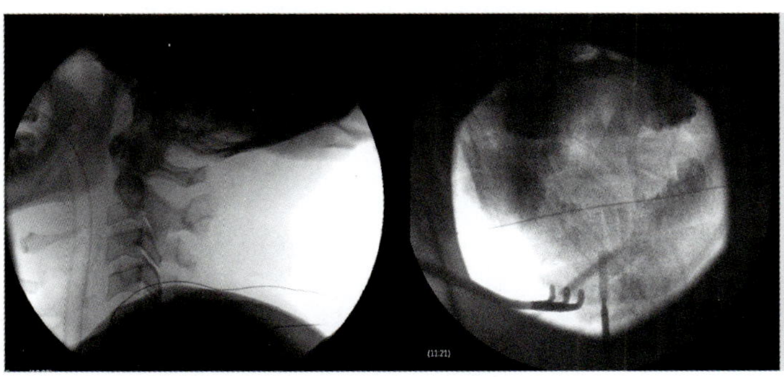

Fig. 43.1 Computed tomography (CT) image demonstrating an odontoid fracture. These sagittal and coronal CT images (respectively) demonstrate a type II odontoid fracture. The patient in these and subsequent images is a 47-year-old man who presented with neck pain status post motor vehicle accident.

the fracture line is parallel to the trajectory of the odontoid screw.
  - Nonreducible fractures.
- Transverse ligament rupture because of difficulty capturing the odontoid and persistent instability after procedure.
- Remote fracture (> 18 months) because progressive sclerotic changes may impede bony union.[11]
- Body habitus, which prevents appropriate trajectory, approach, or reliable fluoroscopic assessment.
- Older patients in whom the exposure and retraction predisposes severe postoperative dysphagia.

43.3 Instruments

- Personnel:
  - Surgeon.
  - Scrub nurse.
  - Anesthesiologist.
- Instruments:
  - Retraction system.
  - Drill guide.
  - A 20-cm-long, 1.2-mm K-wire with sharp tip.
  - Depth gauge.
  - Cannulated countersink.
  - Self-drilling, odontoid-type cannulated lag screw.
- Other equipment:
  - Fluoroscopy with two image intensifiers (anteroposterior [AP] and lateral).
  - Radiolucent mouth gag.
  - Local epinephrine anesthetic.
  - Absorbable sutures and sterile adhesive strips.

43.4 Patient Preparation

- The patients should be evaluated preoperatively with the following:
  - Neurological examination.
  - AP and lateral radiographs.
  - CT.
  - Magnetic resonance imaging (MRI) to assess the integrity of the transverse ligament.

43.5 Patient Positioning

- **Position the patient** supine with a folded sheet under the shoulders, with the head extended.
  - Head extension may help reduce the fracture and facilitate screw insertion.
  - Stabilization of the head in a Mayfield can assist with positioning and reduction of the fracture.
  - Placing the articulating arm off-center to ensure AP fluoroscopy is unobstructed.

43.6 Technique

43.6.1 Setup and Exposure

- Use **two image intensifiers** to identify the odontoid process in the AP and lateral views.
  - Place a radiolucent bite block to keep the jaw open in order to have a clear AP odontoid shot.
  - Proper placement of these two C-arms (biplanar fluoroscopy) is illustrated in ▶ Fig. 43.2.
- Note: The surgical team may use intraoperative motor and somatosensory evoked potential monitoring.[6,7]
- Additional note: The use of two screws is recommended when the odontoid has sufficient diameter to accommodate both.
- **Reduce the fracture** prior to surgical access[12]:
  - This can be accomplished by using halo traction preoperatively as well as intraoperative head flexion or extension as necessary.
  - Note that you may need to reduce the fracture intraoperatively as well.
  - Make use of frequent visualization with C-arm fluoroscopy while reducing the fracture along with frequent checks of neuromonitoring (▶ Fig. 43.3).
- **Plan the incision** by estimating the intended direction of the screws:
  - Do this by using a K-wire, holding it alongside the neck, and viewing its position on fluoroscopy (the incision should be where the K-wire will exit the skin).
    - You may also use another straight hyperdense marker instead of a K-wire.
    - In most cases, this is at the C4–C5 level.[3,11]
    - Make your 2-cm incision at the medial edge of the sternocleidomastoid.
    - *Practical tip*: You can use anatomical landmarks to help facilitate the correct trajectory. The tip of the nose, suprasternal notch, and xiphisternum should be in the same anatomical line.[7]

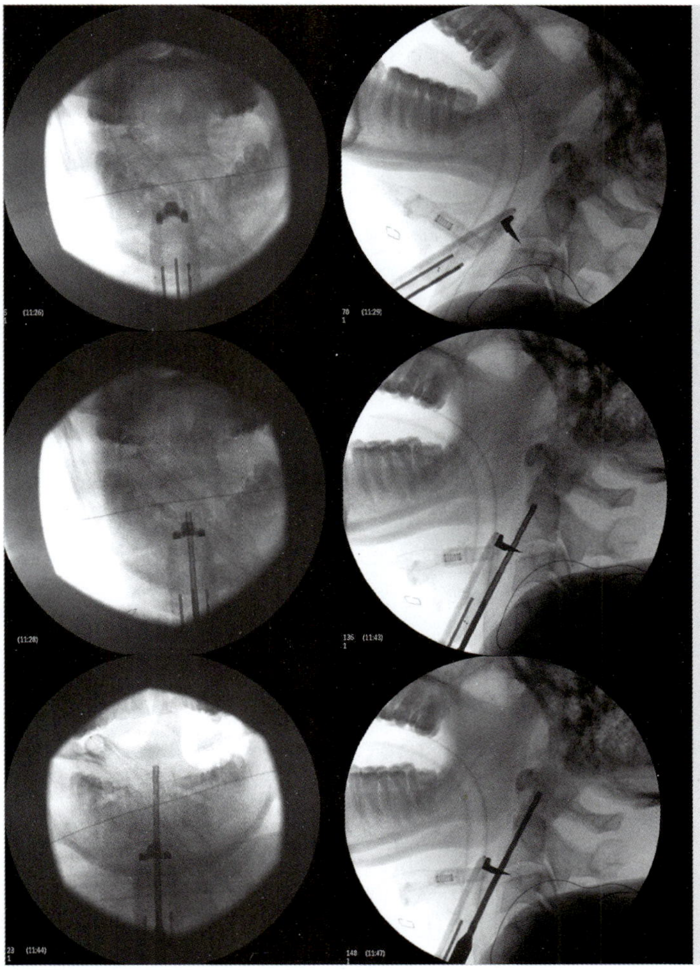

Fig. 43.2 Biplanar fluoroscopy. This picture demonstrates the appropriate orientation of the two C-arms in order to facilitate biplanar fluoroscopy.

- Once satisfied with patient positioning and fracture reduction, and the incision is planned, **prep and drape** the patient.
- **Inject local** epinephrine for hemostasis.
- Make the 2-cm **transverse incision**:
  - **Exposure** and **retraction** are accomplished next.
  - Use a standard anterior cervical spinal approach and dissection to expose the prevertebral fascia of C2–C3.
  - Maintain adequate exposure using the Apfelbaum or other similar retraction systems.[5]
  - Take another fluoroscopic image prior to dissection of the prevertebral fascia to ensure accurate localization.

43.6.2 Cannulated Screw Insertion

- **Plan** the screw **entry point**(**s**) at the anteroinferior lip of the C2 body, that is, plan to drill into the inferior C2 endplate.
  - In order to optimize the entry point, some authors recommend first **creating a "gutter"** in the anterior body of C3[12,13] and removing some of the C2–C3 disc.

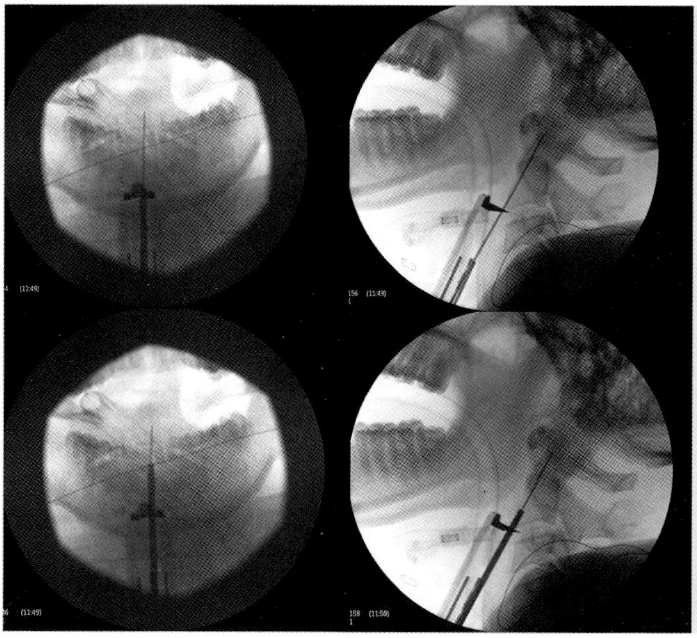

Fig. 43.3 Biplanar fluoroscopic imaging of the odontoid. These lateral and AP images were taken while the patient was on the operating table and before surgical access. The lateral view demonstrates reduction of the fracture, and the AP view shows good visualization of the odontoid.

    - If you choose to remove the disc, plan to remove the anterior aspect (one-third to one-half) of the annulus.[8]
- **Place** the **drill guide instrument** on the exposed inferior C2 endplate.
  - For reference, both screws should be angled slightly posteriorly in order to exit at the posterior half of the odontoid tip.[12]
  - In order to insert two screws, position each screw at a paramedian site 2 to 3 mm off the midline.[11]
- **Drill** a **trajectory** through the tip of the odontoid (▶ Fig. 43.4).
- **Insert** a 20-cm-long, 1.2-mm **K-wire** into the corridor and advance it through the tip of the odontoid[6,12,14]:
  - Confirm positioning with frequent fluoroscopic visualization.
  - Advance the K-wire through the tip of the dens.
  - During this step, you may need to optimize the alignment of the C2–C3 complex and odontoid.
    - If so, prior to advancing past the fracture site, you may use the drill guide to depress or elevate the C2–C3 complex as needed.
    - The patient's head may also need to be manipulated at this time.[11]
    - Take care not to skive off the anterior odontoid at this step. We recommend live lateral fluoroscopy as the drill passes the fracture line.
    - Alternating AP and lateral fluoroscopic shots are necessary to ensure proper trajectory as well as to gauge safe depth of drilling.
  - See ▶ Fig. 43.5 for a demonstration of K-wire placement.
- **Measure** the length of the **K-wire** in the bone:
  - This measurement indicates the length of screw required (typically 38–42 mm).[12]
- Before inserting the screw, **perforate the cortex** with a special cannulated countersink.
- Next, use a cannulated tap to tap the trajectory (see ▶ Fig. 43.5).
- **Insert** a self-drilling, odontoid-type, partially threaded, cannulated lag **screw** (with threads distal to the fracture) of appropriate length:
  - Insert the screw directly over the K-wire.
  - Observe on live lateral fluoroscopy to ensure that the K-wire does not advance superiorly as this could injure the spinal cord or brainstem.

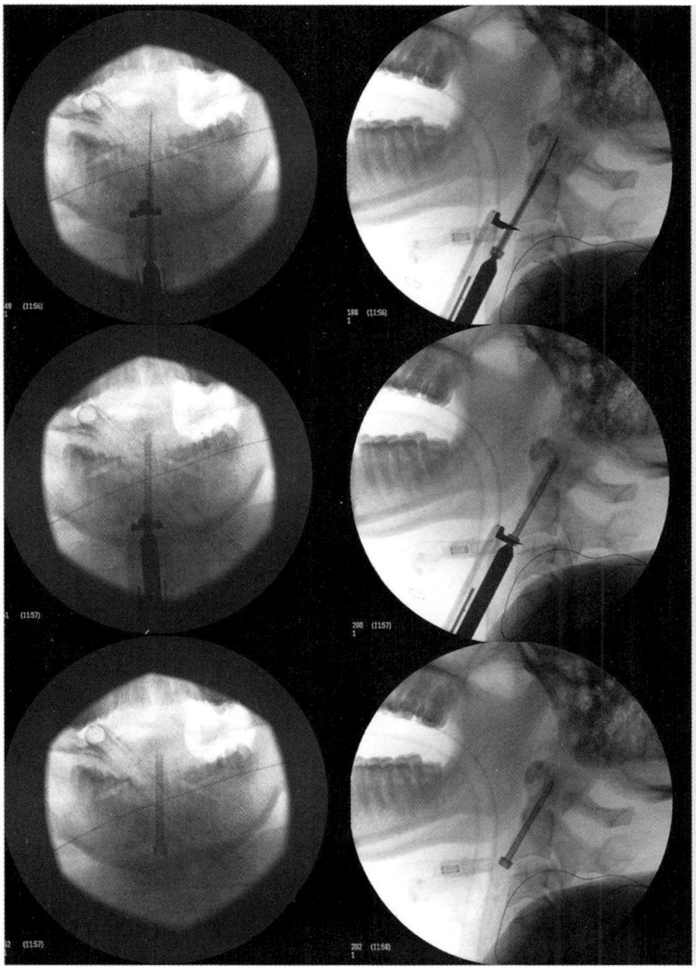

Fig. 43.4 Drill guide placement and corridor drilling. These images are intraoperative fluoroscopic shots. The top panel shows docking of the drill guide; note the spike, which helps fix the guide in place in the C2–C3 disc space. The middle panel shows the drill advancing into the odontoid. The bottom panel shows the drill advanced further, past the fracture line.

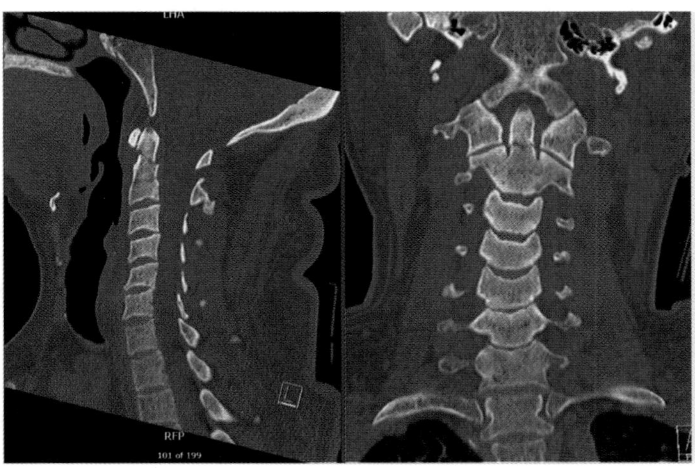

Fig. 43.5 K-wire and tap placement. These images are intraoperative fluoroscopic shots. The top panel shows K-wire insertion into the drilled trajectory through the tip of the odontoid. The bottom panel shows the cannulated tap as it starts to advance along the K-wire.

- Tighten the screw until the head is countersunk with respect to the C2 body and one or two threads of the screw penetrate through the tip of the dens.[6]
- See ▶ Fig. 43.6 for a demonstration of screw placement.

- Once the screw is fully inserted, **remove** the **K-wire.**
- Use the same technique to **insert a second screw.**
- The surgeon or assistant may **flex and extend the head** under fluoroscopic visualization to confirm that there is no C1/C2 instability.
- Complete **irrigation** and ensure **hemostasis.**
- **Closure:**
  - Closure should be done in layers; you may use interrupted absorbable sutures in the platysma muscle and subcutaneous layer, with adhesive strips on the skin.[11]

43.7 Postoperative Care

- Early mobilization is ideal and, if possible, patients are instructed to stand and walk on the day of surgery.
- Patients are often followed with periodical radiographs beginning on the first postoperative day, as well as at 6 weeks, 3 months, 6 months, and 1 year, or until bony union is achieved.[12] A postoperative CT image demonstrating successful odontoid screw placement is shown in ▶ Fig. 43.7.
- Use of a collar is optional.

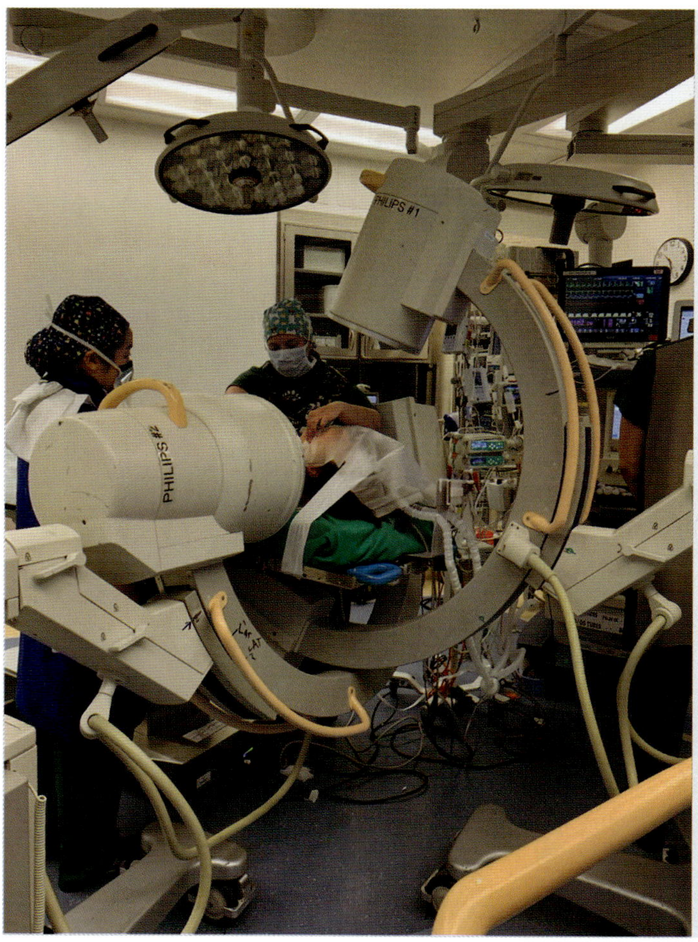

Fig. 43.6 Placement of cannulated screw: These images are intraoperative fluoroscopic shots. The top panel shows the cannulated screw as it advances past the fracture line. The middle panel shows the lag screw at its final position. The bottom panel shows the screw in position after removal of the drill guide.

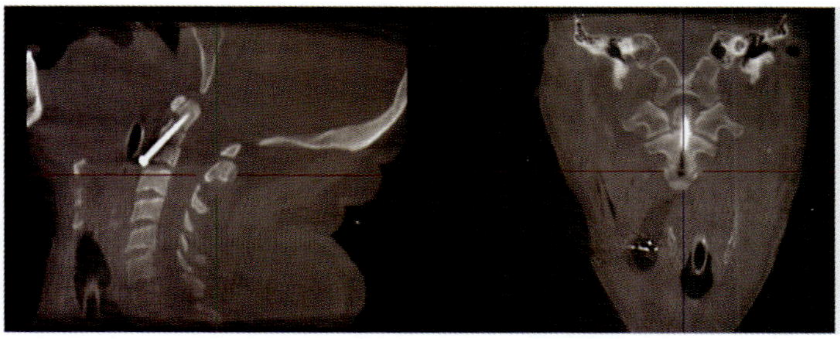

Fig. 43.7 CT images status post screw insertion. These postoperative sagittal and coronal CT images (respectively) demonstrate successful odontoid screw placement.

43.8 Complications

- Critical structures can be damaged during insertion of K-wires and drilling; therefore, liberal use of fluoroscopy is essential during this procedure. In particular, the spinal cord (and vertebral arteries) may be injured due to instrument malpositioning.[7] Bleeding is another intraoperative risk and should be mitigated with careful hemostasis.[6]
- Some patients experience difficulty swallowing after this procedure due to intraoperative manipulation and the presence of a screw head at the C2–C3 interspace.[7] Several measures may prevent dysphagia, including the following:
  - Creation of a gutter on the anterior surface of C3.
  - Countersinking the screw.
  - Minimizing retropharyngeal retraction and dissection.
  - Avoiding this procedure in elderly patients.
- Other complications may include the following:
  - Screw loosening.
  - Nonunion.
  - Reoperation.
  - Vocal cord dysfunction.[10]
  - Respiratory dysfunction.
  - Wound infection.
  - Hematoma.

43.9 Management Pearls

- Be wary of instability in extension and, if necessary, employ fiberoptic guidance or nasotracheal intubation. Skull traction may also be useful to maintain fracture reduction during intubation.[10]
- Some surgeons do not use cannulated screw systems. An alternate approach makes use of a drill bit to make a pilot hole.[12] The creation of a pilot hole may or may not[8] be preceded by the insertion of a K-wire through to the odontoid tip. Following creation of a pilot hole, the surgeon may choose to overdrill the proximal odontoid fragment in order to create a guide hole, and then tap the distal fragment. A partially threaded, cancellous lag screw can then be inserted.[6,11,12]
- For patients with osteoporotic bone, the surgeon can consider the following:
  - Bone cement, which can be injected into the C2 body to increase screw anchorage.
  - Anterior transarticular C1–C2 fixation.[12,15]
- Posterior C1–C2 fusion can be a reasonable alternative for patients with contraindications to anterior odontoid fixation, but this approach eliminates normal C1–C2 rotary motion.

References

[1] Robinson AL, Möller A, Robinson Y, Olerud C. C2 fracture subtypes, incidence, and treatment allocation change with age: a retrospective cohort study of 233 consecutive cases. BioMed Res Int. 2017; 2017:8321680

[2] Chapman J, Smith JS, Kopjar B, et al. The AOSpine North America Geriatric Odontoid Fracture Mortality Study: a retrospective review of mortality outcomes for operative versus nonoperative treatment of 322 patients with long-term follow-up. Spine. 2013; 38(13):1098–1104

[3] Cloney M, Thirunavu V, Roumeliotis A, et al. Odontoid fracture type and angulation affect nonunion risk, but comminution and displacement do not: a propensity score matched analysis of fracture morphology. Clin Neurol Neurosurg. 2023; 231:107855

[4] Patel A, Smith HE, Radcliff K, Yadlapalli N, Vaccaro AR. Odontoid fractures with neurologic deficit have higher mortality and morbidity. Clin Orthop Relat Res. 2012; 470(6): 1614–1620

[5] Nouri A, Da Broi M, May A, et al. Odontoid fractures: a review of the current state of the art. J Clin Med. 2024; 13(20):6270

[6] Konstantinou D, Levi ADO, Sonntag VKH, Dickman CA. Odontoid Screw Fixation. Barrow Neurological Institute.

Accessed October 7, 2022 at https://www.barrowneuro.org/for-physicians-researchers/education/grand-rounds-publications-media/watch-neuroscience-grand-rounds/odontoid-screw-fixation/

[7] Munakomi S, Tamrakar K, Chaudhary PK, Bhattarai B. Anterior single odontoid screw placement for type II odontoid fractures: our modified surgical technique and initial results in a cohort study of 15 patients. F1000 Res. 2016; 5:1681

[8] Sasso RC. Odontoid Screw Fixation. 2015. Accessed October 7, 2022 at: https://www.youtube.com/watch?v=LO_w9yTYI7A

[9] Jacobs BW. Anterior Odontoid Screw Fixation for Type II Odontoid Fracture. Congress of Neurological Surgeons. 2021. Accessed October 7, 2022 at: https://www.cns.org/nexus/case/detail/anterior-odontoid-screw-fixation-type-ii-odontoid-

[10] Wang Y, Li M, Cui G, et al. A new tool in percutaneous anterior odontoid screw fixation. BMC Musculoskelet Disord. 2021; 22(1):87

[11] Apfelbaum RI, Lonser RR, Veres R, Casey A. Direct anterior screw fixation for recent and remote odontoid fractures. J Neurosurg. 2000; 93(2) Suppl:227–236

[12] Lehman R, Riew D, Schnake K, Vialle L. Odontoid screw fixation for Anderson d'Alonzo Type III. AO Foundation Surgery Reference. Accessed October 7, 2022 at: https://surgeryreference.aofoundation.org/spine/trauma/occipitocervical/anderson-dalonzo-type-iii/odontoid-screw-fixation

[13] Mazur MD, Mumert ML, Bisson EF, Schmidt MH. Avoiding pitfalls in anterior screw fixation for type II odontoid fractures. Neurosurg Focus. 2011; 31(4):E7

[14] Sawarkar DP, Singh PK, Agrawal D, et al. Anterior odontoid screw fixation for pediatric and adolescent odontoid fractures: single-center experience over a decade. World Neurosurg. 2021; 153:e153–e167

[15] Dickman CA, Foley KT, Sonntag VKH, Smith MM. Cannulated screws for odontoid screw fixation and atlantoaxial transarticular screw fixation. Technical note. J Neurosurg. 1995; 83(6):1095–1100

44 Anterior Lumbar Interbody Fusion

Ayush Arora, Rafid Kasir, Jay Kaushik Shah, and Sigurd Berven

44.1 Background

- There is an increasing recognition of the functional and clinical importance of lumbar lordosis in the healthy and pathologic spine.[1] It has been found that the intervertebral disc shape contributes to almost 90% of lordosis in the lumbar spine,[2] and it is therefore no surprise that degenerative pathologies of the spine are associated with changes in lumbar lordosis.[3] The loss of normal lordosis often results in sagittal spinal imbalance, persistent back pain, and increased muscle fatigue.[4,5,6,7]
- The anterior approach to reconstruction of the lumbar spine is important for restoration of spinal alignment in the sagittal and coronal planes and to achieve a reliable fusion, especially in cases of long fusion. The approach provides excellent access to the lumbar spine extending from the L2–L3 disc to the first sacral segment (S1). The fusion achieved by an interbody fusion is robust, and the restoration of disc height is especially effective in restoring the intervertebral foraminal height. With the release of anterior soft tissues and the addition of an interbody device, the loss of lordosis that often accompanies the degeneration of the lumbar spine may be restored and alignment improved. Furthermore, with its anterior column support, anterior lumbar interbody fusion (ALIF) is especially effective in cases of coronal malalignment involving the lumbosacral junction. The purpose of this chapter is to provide an overview of the technique for anterior lumbar surgery using a retroperitoneal approach, and to illustrate specific examples in which anterior surgery is useful including management of pseudarthrosis and in the correction of sagittal and coronal plane deformity.

44.2 Indications and Contraindications

- Restoration of lumbar lordosis:
  - Restoring sagittal alignment is an independent predictor of good outcome after spine surgery.[8] Furthermore, the load distribution on the spine is significantly dependent on its shape and curvature in the sagittal plane.[9] Sagittal alignment after the treatment of degenerative disc disease has been found to play a significant role in predicting adjacent segment disease.[10,11] With all this in mind, the involvement of sagittal alignment in most spinal pathologies is pervasive and should be respected when treating the scope of surgical pathologies.[7] Multiple studies have shown that restoring the natural intervertebral shape through ALIF is an effective method of restoring physiologic alignment.[12,13]
  - The physiologic distribution of lordosis within the lumbar spine is an important consideration in reconstructive surgery when addressing spinal deformity. Understanding the distribution of natural lordosis is essential in its restoration, and Burkert and Bridwell examined the normal segmental alignment of the spine in asymptomatic volunteers and demonstrated that more than 60% of lumbar lordosis comes from the segments at L4 to S1.[14] Building on this, Roussouly et al classified spinal alignment into four distinct patterns based upon sacral slope and the apex of lordosis.[15] In general, a sacral slope less than 35 degrees and a low pelvic incidence are associated with a relatively flat, short lumbar lordosis with a low apex at L5. A sacral slope greater than 45 degrees and a high pelvic incidence are associated with long, curved lumbar lordosis with the curve apex above L4. When addressing spinal deformity, the surgeon must assess global alignment as well

as the distribution of alignment within the curve according to these observations.
  - Most recently, the global alignment and proportion (GAP) score has been developed and has been shown as an effective predictor of mechanical complication after spinal reconstruction for thoracolumbar deformity.[9,16] The score is calculated by adding scores of relative pelvic version, relative lumbar lordosis, lordosis distribution index, relative spinopelvic alignment, and an age factor, and can range from 0 to 13 points. Yilgor et al showed that postoperatively, patients with a proportioned spinopelvic state according to the GAP score had a mechanical complication rate of 6%, while those with moderately or severely disproportioned spinopelvic states had failure rates of 47 and 95%, respectively.[9] Besides being a significant component of the GAP score, the appropriate restoration of lordosis, especially from L4 to S1, is paramount in deformity surgery and has been shown to predict favorable outcomes after surgery.[17]
- Realignment of the fractional curve:
  - In addition to sagittal alignment, the configuration of the spine in the coronal plane poses certain considerations prior to and during surgery. Bao et al introduced a classification to examine the relationship of curve direction to the coronal vertical axis.[18] Type A describes a coronally aligned spine with a less than 3 cm shift of the C7 plumb line from the center sacral vertical axis. Type B describes a scoliosis in which a plumb line from C7 falls along the convexity of the curve. In these cases, correction of the main curve will lead to correction of the coronal vertical axis. On the other hand, type C describes a curve in which the C7 plumb line falls along its concavity. Without careful surgical considerations, correction of the main curve in type C patients would lead to worsening of the coronal alignment. This is due to a fractional curve that usually involves L4, L5, and S1 and creates an oblique lumbosacral takeoff angle. The fractional curve must be addressed in these deformities. Obeid et al expanded on this concept and created an algorithmic approach toward treating coronal malalignment using a similar classification scheme.[19]
  - As mentioned, difficulty arises when attempting to correct Bao type C curves or Obeid type 2 curves with a posterior only approach due to the forces required to restore the fractional curve along such a short segment. In fact, posterior only approaches to type C curves have been found to have unchanged or even worsened coronal malalignment in over 60% of cases.[20] Studies have found ALIF to be more effective than posterior only approaches in correcting the fractional curve.[21] The anterior approach to the fractional curve at the lower segments is effective in releasing the rigid fractional deformity, and as a result, indirectly decompressing the foramen with thicker cages than transforaminal lumbar interbody fusion (TLIF).[22] The large forces required to correct a fractional curve are better absorbed by a larger cage in compression along the anterior column, which decreases the tension on the posterior-based rod, evidenced by a decrease in rod fracture rates when utilizing ALIF.[22] ALIF provides large structural graft with surface area for fusion, a greater anterior column load distribution, indirect decompression of neural foramen, and release of the anterior longitudinal ligament for increased lordosis and greater control in coronal and sagittal balance. We have found a combined anterior and posterior approach to be especially effective in the realignment of an Obeid type 2 or Bao type C deformity.
- Obtaining solid fusion:
  - In addition to the pathologies and indications we have already discussed, ALIF is an effective tool when used with the goal of achieving a fusion.[23] This is especially helpful in cases of pseudarthrosis, as ALIF can give the surgeon a large fusion surface area without further disruption of the paraspinal musculature.[24] Having a wide available footprint for the cage ensures low subsidence rates and solid anterior support.[25] When combined with a

posterior approach, it offers the most reliable chance of fusion.[26] At our institution, we have found ALIF to be a safe and effective technique for the treatment of pseudarthrosis after a previous TLIF and also after long fusions to the sacrum, with a favorable risk profile.[27]

- Long fusions for deformity ending at S1 can be an unfortunately common reason for pseudarthrosis, with more recent symptomatic nonunion rates reported anywhere from 19 to 41% depending on diagnosis, surgical approaches, and instrumentation techniques.[4] In these long constructs, especially when extending above L3, the large cantilever forces can overpower the biomechanical stability that even tricortical fixation to the sacrum can provide.[28,29] These can be exceptionally challenging to revise and to successfully achieve a solid fusion given that these patients are usually older, have poor bone quality, and present with large sagittal deformities and mismatch. Most importantly, it has been clearly demonstrated in the literature that a nonunion in these situations leads to significantly worse patient outcomes and quality of life, and is a large burden on the health care system and costs.[30]
- ALIF becomes an essential technique to tackle these issues for several reasons. One, anterior interbody support has consistently been shown to reduce S1 screw strain by 30 to 57% in several biomechanical studies.[31,32] When combined with posterior iliac fixation such as iliac bolts or S2 alar-iliac screws, there is an even more pronounced decrease in both S1 screw and posterior rod strain and improvement in rigidity in the sagittal plane, axial rotation, and lateral bending.[32] Second, persistent sagittal imbalance is a large risk factor for pseudarthrosis in long constructs to the sacrum.[33] As discussed earlier, ALIF, with its natural release of the ALL, anterior positioning, and large footprint, reliably restores physiologic lordosis. This not only allows for restoration of sagittal alignment in primary deformity cases, significantly decreasing the risk of construct failure and pseudarthrosis, but is also essential in revision cases.[34] Patients in the revision setting often present with significant sagittal imbalance requiring a large correction. However, they commonly have failed implants posteriorly with poor bone purchase and real estate, making ALIF and anterior column reconstruction the best option to restore sagittal parameters, aside from complex posterior-based osteotomies, which often can be morbid and have a higher complication profile.[25] By decreasing strain on the posterior construct, providing rigid anterior column support, and recreating proper sagittal alignment, ALIF can enhance the rate of successful spinal arthrodesis, especially in the revision setting.

44.3 Instruments

- The surgical approach to the anterior lumbar spine is commonly performed by or with the assistance of a vascular surgeon. This interdisciplinary approach may result in lower risk of vascular injury and shorter operative time.[35] A pulse oximeter should be attached to the patient's foot on the side of retraction of the common iliac vessels for intraoperative monitoring of peripheral blood flow, which can identify excessive retraction or a thromboembolic event. An abdominal retractor system should be available to retract the abdominal contents and great vessels. The anterior lumbar interbody cages and trials should be available for use along with allograft bone. Intraoperative fluoroscopy is useful to confirm levels. If posterior instrumentation is to be performed as well, then this should also be available.

44.4 Patient Positioning

- The patient is positioned supine and may be hyperextended with a bump either placed under the lumbosacral junction or placed over a break in the table with subsequent extension of the lumbosacral junction.

44.5 Technique

- Typically, a left-sided retroperitoneal incision is utilized, but may be modified in the setting of prior abdominal, gynecologic, urologic, or anterior spinal surgery. A transperitoneal approach may be used, but is generally avoided due to its association with an increased complications rate of retrograde ejaculation due to injury of the superior hypogastric plexus.[36,37]
- The incision may be transverse, oblique, or vertical in nature depending on patient factors and surgeon preferences. A longitudinal incision of the anterior rectus sheath is made, and an approach to the retroperitoneum at the midline, medial to the rectus muscle, preserves its segmental innervation. As the epigastric vessels are encountered dorsal to the rectus, they are preserved and retracted along with the muscle. The arcuate line is palpated, and below this line the peritoneum may be separated from the psoas muscle to approach L5–S1. Above the arcuate line, the posterior rectus sheath must be divided longitudinally to access the upper lumbar spine. The ureter is elevated with the peritoneum and retracted medially.
- The L5/S1 segment is approached between the common iliac vessels, and the middle sacral vessels should be ligated to facilitate access to the disc. The discs from L2–L3 to L4–L5 are approached lateral to the common iliac vessels and the great vessels. The iliolumbar vessels branching laterally should be ligated to allow mobilization of the common iliac vessels and great vessels medially.
- Intraoperative fluoroscopy is useful to confirm levels. We prefer to not place a needle in the disc space in order to avoid unwanted disc injury. The great vessels can be held in a retracted position using stainless steel vein retractors fixed to an abdominal retractor system.
- The disc is incised along its periphery using electrocautery or a no. 10 blade always moving away from the vessels to avoid accidental iatrogenic injury. A large sharp Cobb elevator may be used to elevate the disc from the bottom and top endplate. The disc is removed in its entirety using a combination of curettes and rongeurs, taking the dissection all the way to the posterior longitudinal ligament. Systematic removal of endplate cartilage with curettes and a rasp enhances thorough removal. Thrombin-soaked gel may be used to control bleeding, which may be brisk with posterior disc removal.
- Interbody trials are then sequentially placed into the disc space to serially dilate and increase height and lordosis. In general, gaining posterior height first is useful followed by the use of progressively increasing lordotic trials. Once an appropriately sized implant is selected, autograft material or a bone morphogenetic protein 2 (BMP-2) impregnated collagen sponge may be used to fill the final implant. Fixation of the implant with screw fixation may prevent migration. Screw fixation limited to only one endplate can facilitate further posterior deformity correction if this is planned. Although it may not be necessary in all cases, augmentation with posterior transpedicular screws has been found to increase construct stiffness.[38]
- Cases:
    - *Case 1:* A 70-year-old man status post L1–S1 posterior spinal fusion approximately 18 months prior presented with continued debilitating back pain. Anteroposterior (AP) and lateral full-length standing films demonstrating previous hardware and sagittal imbalance are shown in ▶ Fig. 44.1. Axial and sagittal CT cuts demonstrating haloing around loose L1 and S1 screws with pseudarthrosis are shown in ▶ Fig. 44.2. Postoperative AP and lateral full-length standing films demonstrating final construct with L5–S1 ALIF, T10 to pelvis revision posterior fusion with bilateral S2AI and supplemental sacroiliac joint fixation, and T10 cement augmentation vertebroplasty are shown in ▶ Fig. 44.3.

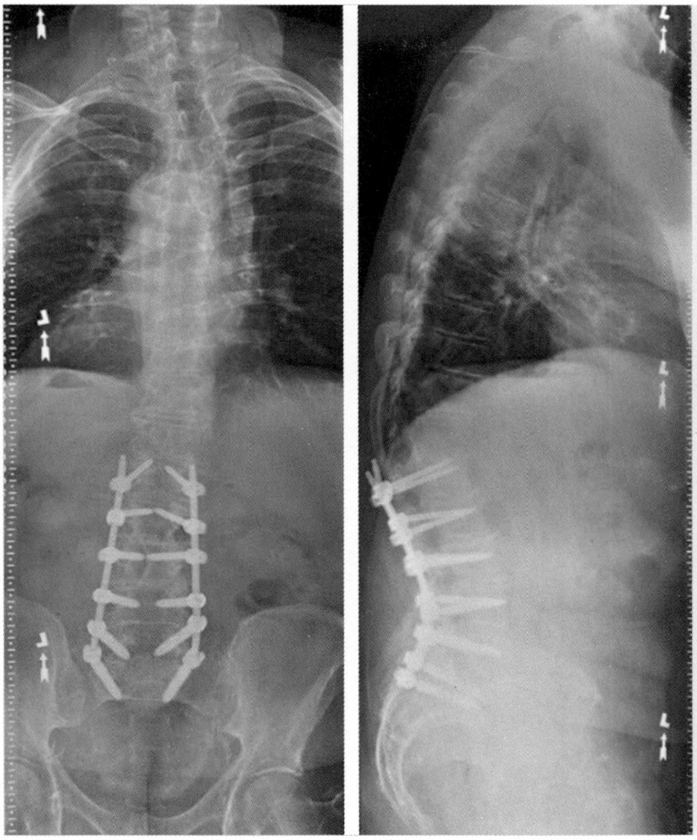

Fig. 44.1 Anteroposterior (AP) and lateral full-length standing films demonstrating previous hardware and sagittal imbalance.

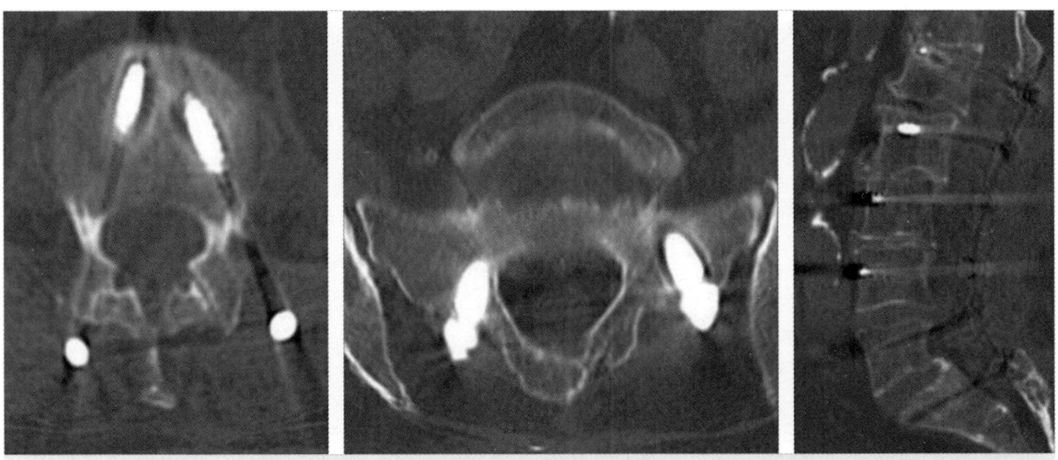

Fig. 44.2 Axial and sagittal CT cuts demonstrating haloing around loose L1 and S1 screws with pseudarthrosis.

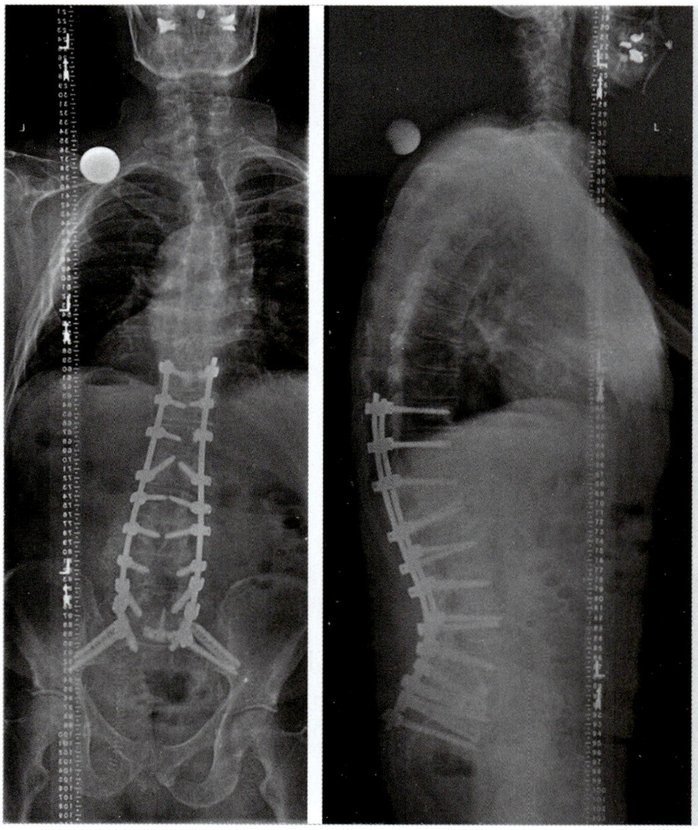

Fig. 44.3 L5–S1 anterior lumbar interbody fusion (ALIF), T10 to pelvis revision posterior fusion with bilateral S2 alar-iliac (S2AI) and supplemental sacroiliac joint fixation, and T10 cement augmentation vertebroplasty.

- *Case 2:* A 72-year-old woman presented with debilitating back pain and right-sided foot drop. AP and lateral full-length standing films demonstrating coronal (Bao type C and Obeid type 2) and sagittal malalignment are shown in ▶ Fig. 44.4. Postoperative AP and lateral full length standing films demonstrating final construct with L4/L5 and L5/S1 TLIF and T11 to pelvis posterior spinal fusion with persistent coronal malalignment and positive sagittal vertical axis are shown in ▶ Fig. 44.4.
- *Case 3:* A 64-year-old woman presented with debilitating back pain and neurogenic claudication. AP and lateral X-rays (▶ Fig. 44.5) show malalignment in the sagittal and coronal plane (Bao type C and Obeid type 2). Correction was performed with ALIF at L3–S1 and a posterior fusion of T10 to the pelvis, showing a well-aligned spine (▶ Fig. 44.6).

44.6 Complications

- In a study of 1,315 patients undergoing an anterior retroperitoneal lumbar approach, 6 patients were identified to have left iliac artery

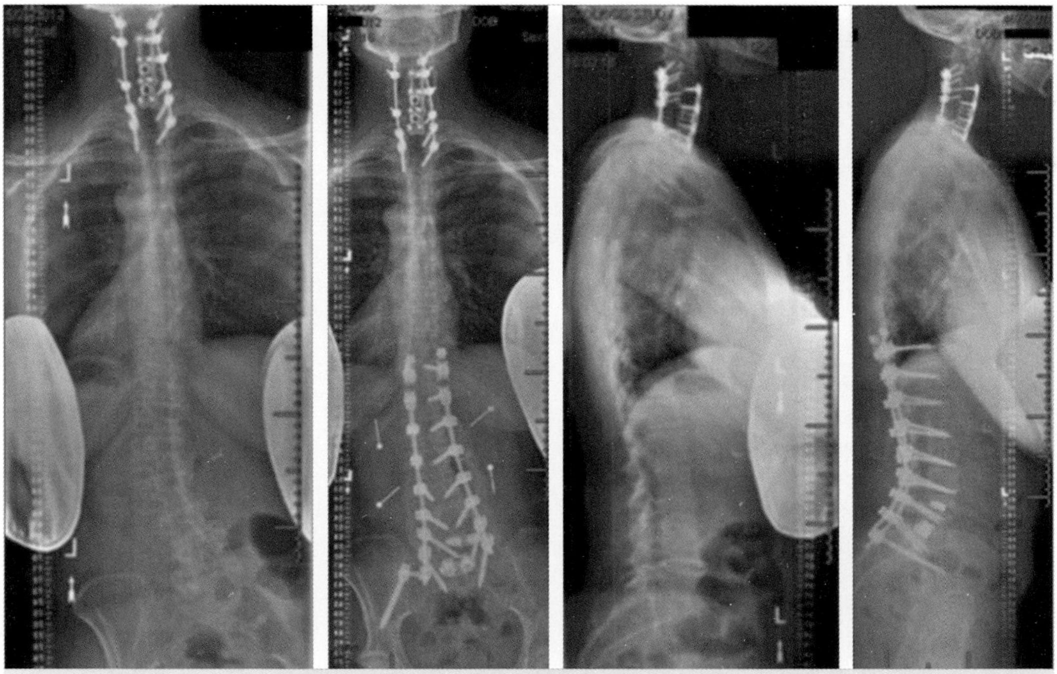

Fig. 44.4 L4/L5 and L5/S1 transforaminal lumbar interbody fusion (TLIF) and T11 to pelvis posterior spinal fusion with persistent coronal malalignment and positive sagittal vertical axis.

thrombosis (0.45%), and 19 had major vein lacerations (1.4%).[39]

- Ureteral injuries occur much less frequently in the literature.[40]
- Retrograde ejaculation may occur in men and, more commonly, with transperitoneal approaches due to damage to the hypogastric plexus.[41]
- Other complications may include bowel or bladder injury, lumbosacral plexus injury, wound infection, and deep vein thrombosis.
- During the anterior lumbar approach, the abdominal contents are retracted to expose the great vessels overlying the spine. The preoperative lumbar MRI should be evaluated to assess the vascular anatomy. The renal vessels limit the proximal extension of the exposure. At the upper lumbar spine, an aberrant lower pole renal artery may be encountered and should be preoperatively evaluated. The left ureter is retracted with the peritoneal contents and can be identified by stimulated peristalsis or intraoperative administration of intravenous indigo carmine. The sympathetic chain is anterior and medial to the psoas, and the presacral plexus lies directly over the sacrum. The genitofemoral nerve lies anterior to the psoas and the lumbosacral plexus lies within the psoas muscle.

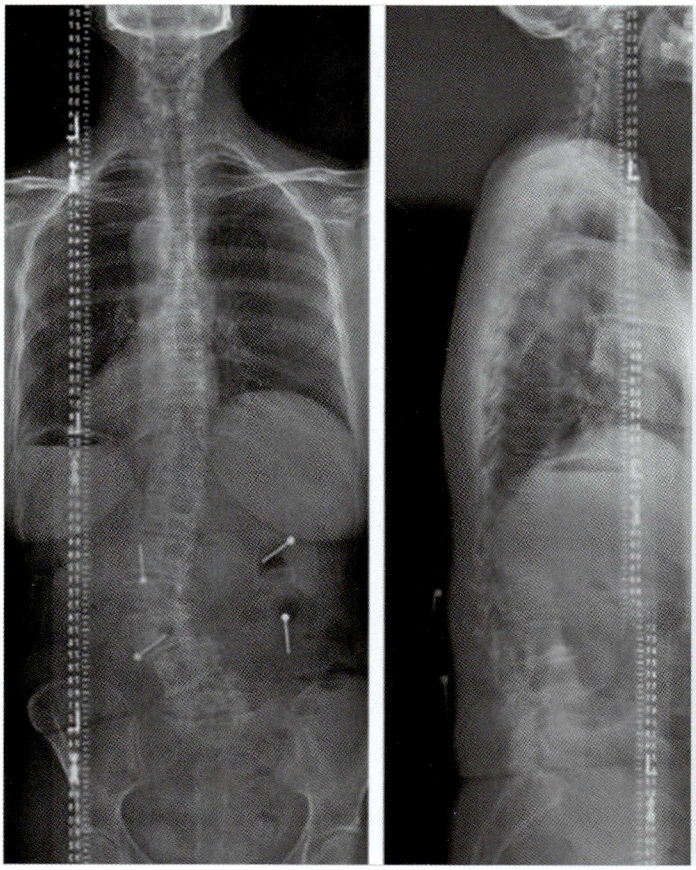

Fig. 44.5 Malalignment in the sagittal and coronal plane (Bao type C and Obeid type 2).

- Relative contraindications include prior anterior approach or other abdominal surgery, fascial mesh, colostomy, pelvic radiation, low great vessel bifurcation, obesity due to depth of exposure, and severe atherosclerosis or aneurysms preventing vascular mobilization.

44.7 Management Pearls

- ALIF is an effective tool when used with the goal of restoration of lumbar lordosis, realignment of the fractional curve, and obtaining a solid fusion.

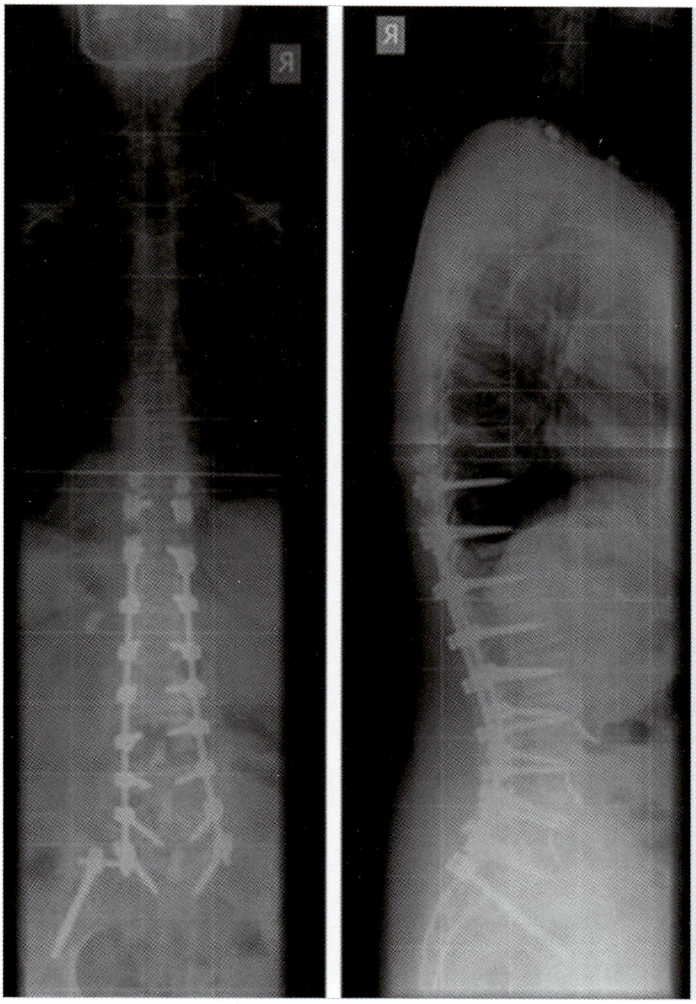

Fig. 44.6 Anterior lumbar interbody fusion (ALIF) at L3–S1 and a posterior fusion of T10 to the pelvis, showing a well-aligned spine.

- A wide available footprint for the cage ensures low subsidence rates and solid anterior support.
- ALIF combined with a posterior approach offers the most reliable chance of fusion.

References

[1] Been E, Kalichman L. Lumbar lordosis. Spine J. 2014; 14(1): 87–97

[2] Been E, Barash A, Pessah H, Peleg S. A new look at the geometry of the lumbar spine. Spine. 2010; 35(20):E1014–E1017

[3] Łebkowski WJ, Łebkowska U, Niedźwiecka M, Dzieciol J. The radiological symptoms of lumbar disc herniation and degenerative changes of the lumbar intervertebral discs. Med Sci Monit. 2004; 10 Suppl 3:112–114

[4] Emami A, Deviren V, Berven S, Smith JA, Hu SS, Bradford DS. Outcome and complications of long fusions to the sacrum in adult spine deformity: Luque-Galveston, combined iliac and sacral screws, and sacral fixation. Spine. 2002; 27(7):776–786

[5] Glassman SD, Berven S, Bridwell K, Horton W, Dimar JR. Correlation of radiographic parameters and clinical symptoms in adult scoliosis. Spine. 2005; 30(6):682–688

[6] Schwab F, Patel A, Ungar B, Farcy JP, Lafage V. Adult spinal deformity-postoperative standing imbalance: how much can you tolerate? An overview of key parameters in assessing alignment and planning corrective surgery. Spine. 2010; 35 (25):2224–2231

[7] Diebo BG, Varghese JJ, Lafage R, Schwab FJ, Lafage V. Sagittal alignment of the spine: what do you need to know? Clin Neurol Neurosurg. 2015; 139:295–301

[8] Le Huec JC, Thompson W, Mohsinaly Y, Barrey C, Faundez A. Sagittal balance of the spine. Eur Spine J. 2019; 28(9):1889–1905

[9] Yilgor C, Sogunmez N, Boissiere L, et al. European Spine Study Group (ESSG). Global alignment and proportion (GAP) score: development and validation of a new method of analyzing spinopelvic alignment to predict mechanical complications after adult spinal deformity surgery. J Bone Joint Surg Am. 2017; 99(19):1661–1672

[10] Kumar MN, Baklanov A, Chopin D. Correlation between sagittal plane changes and adjacent segment degeneration following lumbar spine fusion. Eur Spine J. 2001; 10(4):314–319

[11] Umehara S, Zindrick MR, Patwardhan AG, et al. The biomechanical effect of postoperative hypolordosis in instrumented lumbar fusion on instrumented and adjacent spinal segments. Spine. 2000; 25(13):1617–1624

[12] Ajiboye RM, Alas H, Mosich GM, Sharma A, Pourtaheri S. Radiographic and clinical outcomes of anterior and transforaminal lumbar interbody fusions: systematic review and meta-analysis of comparative studies. Clin Spine Surg. 2018; 31(4):E230–E238

[13] Chan AK, Mummaneni PV, Shaffrey CI. Approach selection: multiple anterior lumbar interbody fusion to recreate lumbar lordosis versus pedicle subtraction osteotomy: When, why, how? Neurosurg Clin N Am. 2018; 29(3):341–354

[14] Bernhardt M, Bridwell KH. Segmental analysis of the sagittal plane alignment of the normal thoracic and lumbar spines and thoracolumbar junction. Spine. 1989; 14(7):717–721

[15] Roussouly P, Gollogly S, Berthonnaud E, Dimnet J. Classification of the normal variation in the sagittal alignment of the human lumbar spine and pelvis in the standing position. Spine. 2005; 30(3):346–353

[16] Jacobs E, van Royen BJ, van Kuijk SMJ, et al. Prediction of mechanical complications in adult spinal deformity surgery: the GAP score versus the Schwab classification. Spine J. 2019; 19(5):781–788

[17] Ohba T, Ebata S, Oba H, Koyama K, Yokomichi H, Haro H. Predictors of poor global alignment and proportion score after surgery for adult spinal deformity. Spine. 2019; 44(19): E1136–E1143

[18] Bao H, Yan P, Qiu Y, Liu Z, Zhu F. Coronal imbalance in degenerative lumbar scoliosis: prevalence and influence on surgical decision-making for spinal osteotomy. Bone Joint J. 2016; 98-B(9):1227–1233

[19] Obeid I, Berjano P, Lamartina C, Chopin D, Boissière L, Bourghli A. Classification of coronal imbalance in adult scoliosis and spine deformity: a treatment-oriented guideline. Eur Spine J. 2019; 28(1):94–113

[20] Theologis AA, Lertudomphonwanit T, Lenke LG, Bridwell KH, Gupta MC. The role of the fractional lumbosacral curve in persistent coronal malalignment following adult thoracolumbar deformity surgery: a radiographic analysis. Spine Deform. 2021; 9(3):721–731

[21] Geddes BJ, Glassman S, Mkorombindo T, Gardner J, Carreon LY. 105. ALIF generates better correction of the fractional lumbar curve vs posterior instrumentation alone in spinal deformity fusion to the pelvis. Spine J. 2020; 20(9):S52

[22] Buell TJ, Shaffrey CI, Bess S, et al. International Spine Study Group. Multicenter assessment of outcomes and complications associated with transforaminal versus anterior lumbar interbody fusion for fractional curve correction. J Neurosurg Spine. 2021; 35(6):729–742

[23] Chun DS, Baker KC, Hsu WK. Lumbar pseudarthrosis: a review of current diagnosis and treatment. Neurosurg Focus. 2015; 39(4):E10

[24] Owens RK, II, Djurasovic M, Crawford CH, III, Glassman SD, Dimar JR, II, Carreon LY. Impact of surgical approach on clinical outcomes in the treatment of lumbar pseudarthrosis. Global Spine J. 2016; 6(8):786–791

[25] Formica M, Quarto E, Zanirato A, et al. ALIF in the correction of spinal sagittal misalignment. A systematic review of literature. Eur Spine J. 2021; 30(1):50–62

[26] Albert TJ, Pinto M, Denis F. Management of symptomatic lumbar pseudarthrosis with anteroposterior fusion. A functional and radiographic outcome study. Spine. 2000; 25 (1):123–129, discussion 130

[27] Safaee MM, Tenorio A, Haddad AF, et al. Anterior lumbar interbody fusion with cage retrieval for the treatment of pseudarthrosis after transforaminal lumbar interbody fusion: a single-institution case series. Oper Neurosurg (Hagerstown). 2021; 20(2):164–173

[28] Lee CS, Chung SS, Choi SW, Yu JW, Sohn MS. Critical length of fusion requiring additional fixation to prevent nonunion of the lumbosacral junction. Spine. 2010; 35(6):E206–E211

[29] Shono Y, Kaneda K, Abumi K, McAfee PC, Cunningham BW. Stability of posterior spinal instrumentation and its effects on adjacent motion segments in the lumbosacral spine. Spine. 1998; 23(14):1550–1558

[30] Raizman NM, O'Brien JR, Poehling-Monaghan KL, Yu WD. Pseudarthrosis of the spine. J Am Acad Orthop Surg. 2009; 17 (8):494–503

[31] Cho W, Wang W, Bucklen B, de la Garza Ramos R, Yassari R. The role of biological fusion and anterior column support in a long lumbopelvic spinal fixation and its effect on the S1 screw: an in silico biomechanics analysis. Spine. 2021; 46(4):E250–E256

[32] Cunningham BW, Sefter JC, Hu N, Kim SW, Bridwell KH, McAfee PC. Biomechanical comparison of iliac screws versus interbody femoral ring allograft on lumbosacral kinematics and sacral screw strain. Spine. 2010; 35(6):E198–E205

[33] Kim YJ, Bridwell KH, Lenke LG, Rhim S, Cheh G. Pseudarthrosis in long adult spinal deformity instrumentation and fusion to the sacrum: prevalence and risk factor analysis of 144 cases. Spine. 2006; 31(20):2329–2336

[34] Lee KY, Lee JH, Kang KC, et al. Strategy for obtaining solid fusion at L5-S1 in adult spinal deformity: risk factor analysis for nonunion at L5-S1. J Neurosurg Spine. 2020; 33(3):323–331

[35] Garg J, Woo K, Hirsch J, Bruffey JD, Dilley RB. Vascular complications of exposure for anterior lumbar interbody fusion. J Vasc Surg. 2010; 51(4):946–950, discussion 950

[36] Sasso RC, Kenneth Burkus J, LeHuec JC. Retrograde ejaculation after anterior lumbar interbody fusion: transperitoneal versus retroperitoneal exposure. Spine. 2003; 28(10):1023–1026

[37] Lindley EM, McBeth ZL, Henry SE, et al. Retrograde ejaculation after anterior lumbar spine surgery. Spine. 2012; 37(20): 1785–1789

[38] Udby PM, Bech-Azeddine R. Clinical outcome of stand-alone ALIF compared to posterior instrumentation for degenerative disc disease: a pilot study and a literature review. Clin Neurol Neurosurg. 2015; 133:64–69

[39] Brau SA, Delamarter RB, Schiffman ML, Williams LA, Watkins RG. Vascular injury during anterior lumbar surgery. Spine J. 2004; 4(4):409–412

[40] Migliorini F, de Maria N, Tafuri A, et al. Late diagnosis of ureteral injury from anterior lumbar spine interbody fusion surgery: case report and literature review. Urol J. 2023; 90 (3):579–583

[41] Feeley A, Feeley I, Clesham K, Butler J. Is there a variance in complication types associated with ALIF approaches? A systematic review. Acta Neurochir (Wien). 2021; 163(11): 2991–3004

45 Retropleural

Omar Sorour, Hannah L. Tetreault, Nitin Agarwal, and Dean Chou

45.1 Background

- Thoracic disc herniations occur around T8–L1 and are calcified in approximately 40% of cases.[1] These herniations are termed "giant" when they occupy more than 40% of the canal.[1] These large, calcified discs, particularly centrally located ones, present a unique surgical challenge. Structures such as the aorta, lungs, vena cava, and ribs add anatomical complexity.[2,3] The retropleural approach to the thoracic spine is uniquely suited for large, central, and calcified thoracic discs, with less risk of pleural violation compared to the more traditional transthoracic approach.[4,5]

45.2 Indications and Contraindications

45.2.1 Indications

- Severe, refractory[6] thoracic myelopathic signs such as gait imbalance and lower extremity weakness, especially if explained by a large, central, and calcified disc.
- If the patient has preexisting pulmonary conditions, the retropleural approach would be preferred over the transthoracic route.
- The retropleural approach is also indicated for other thoracic pathology including tumors and infections.
- Refractory radiculopathy greatly diminishing quality of life.

45.2.2 Contraindications

- Pulmonary comorbidities may preclude a transthoracic or retropleural approach altogether.
- A relative contraindication includes a hostile thorax secondary to radiation or prior surgery.[7]
- Additionally, the retropleural approach may be technically challenging above T5,[7] especially due to the proximity of the scapula and mediastinal structures.[8]

45.3 Instruments

- Neuronavigation.[9]
- Intraoperative computed tomography (CT).[9]
- Microsurgical thoracic spine instruments.
- Minimally invasive retractors.
- Operative microscope.
- High-speed drill.
- Doyen rib raspatory.
- Rib shears.

45.4 Patient Preparation

- Magnetic resonance imaging (MRI) T2 sagittal and axial sequences of the thoracic spine allow visualization of disc herniations, cord signal change, and ligamentous injury.
- CT scan helps outline calcifications in disc fragments, as well as a calcified aorta, which would preclude operating from the left side.[7]
- Anteroposterior and lateral radiographs identify rib pathology.[10]
- Some recommend preoperatively identifying the artery of Adamkiewicz—found from T9 to T12—via MR angiography, and approaching the spine contralaterally to avoid cord ischemia.[11]
- Intubation with general anesthesia is particularly important for this approach, along with decreasing the volume of oxygen flow to decrease the risk of pleural injury.[10]

45.5 Patient Positioning

- A lateral decubitus positioning with a preoperative long cassette localizer is necessary for safe exposure.

45.6 Technique

45.6.1 Exposure

- The chest, abdominal region, and ipsilateral iliac crest should be draped in the usual sterile fashion, with a reference arc placed into the iliac crest if guidance is used.
- Once the rib is exposed, a microscope should be utilized to dissect away its anterior portion to further identify the retropleural space.
  - It has been demonstrated that one could reduce the risk of pleural violation by resecting this short piece of rib followed by tracing along

the rib curvature to access the vertebrae of interest.[12] The rib piece should be saved as autograft for arthrodesis.
- Once the rib head is dissected, the pleura can be identified (▶ Fig. 45.1 and ▶ Fig. 45.2). The spine can then be exposed through a minimally invasive approach using special retractors and navigated dilators.
- With microdissection and navigation,[9] one can identify the disc space, canal, and vertebral bodies, and localizing the depth of ventral and dorsal dissection (▶ Fig. 45.3).

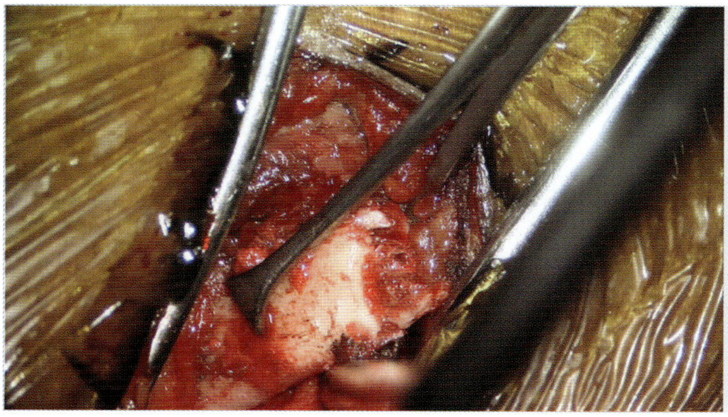

Fig. 45.1 Resection of the anterior rib head to expose the parietal pleura.

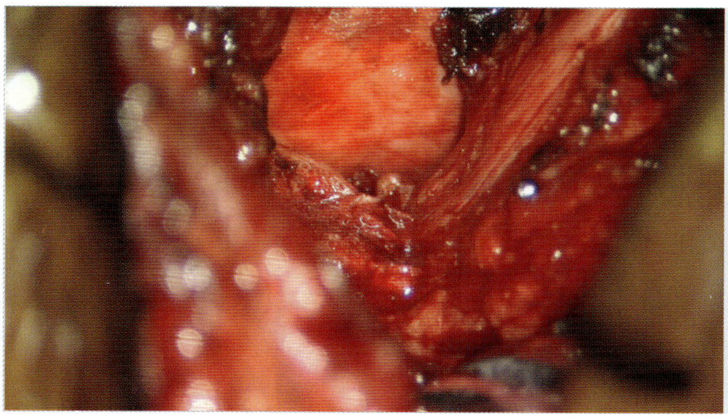

Fig. 45.2 Exposure of the parietal pleura.

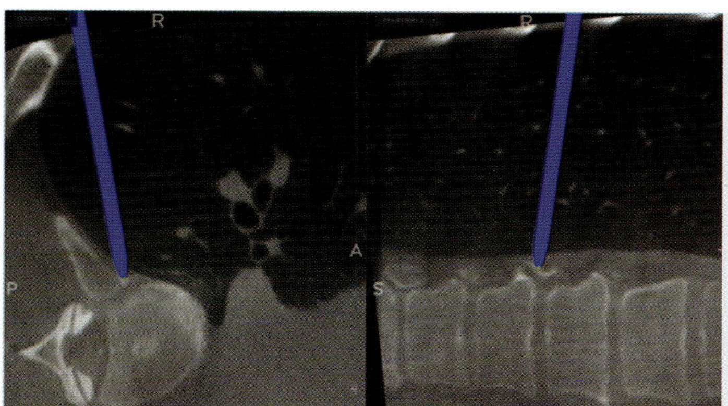

Fig. 45.3 Localizing depth of ventral and dorsal dissection using navigation.

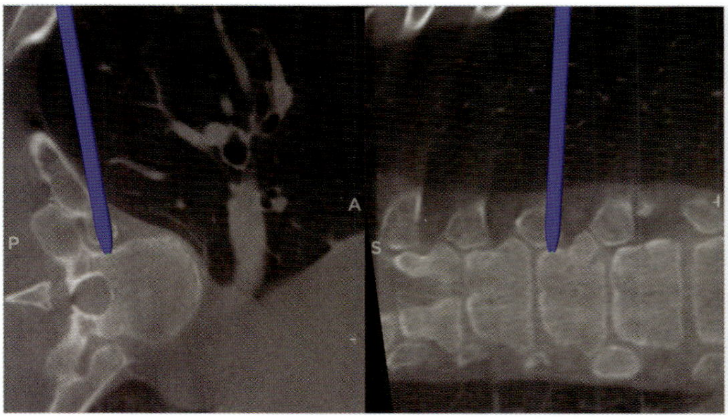

Fig. 45.4 Use of navigation to confirm the anatomical location during spinal cord decompression.

- Spinal cord decompression can then be performed safely (▸ Fig. 45.4). Navigation allows for partial pedicle preservation, avoiding the need for instrumentation or fusion extension.

45.6.2 Closure

- Although the risk of pleural violation is minimized with the retropleural approach, re-inspection is preferred.
- Valsalva should be performed to evaluate for CSF egress.
- Finally, a retropleural drain should be placed prior to closure.

45.7 Postoperative Care

- The main postoperative concern with a retropleural approach is the rare but serious side effect of pleural injury.
- If not noticed intraoperatively, one way to determine this complication is if the retropleural drain placed postoperatively fills up with air. This should prompt immediate thoracic surgery consultation.[7]
- A postoperative X-ray would also rule out pneumothorax.[13]

45.8 Complications

- Retropleural approaches share similar risks as other approaches such as potential reoperation and possible extension of fusion.
- Other complications include lung injury, spinal cord ischemia, and injury to mediastinal structures.
- Although the retropleural approach reduces risk of pleural injury, placing a chest tube may still be a possibility.
  - However, in one study, none of the 33 patients who underwent a mini-open retropleural approach required tube placement.[14] This suggests that this complication can be avoided with careful maneuvers.

45.9 Management Pearls

- Neuronavigation should be considered to identify the correct level, disc, and pedicle. Navigation in the thoracic spine is especially useful for visualizing the aorta and vena cava.[15]
- In addition to better visualization of the canal, neuronavigation better identifies the extent of resection to the contralateral side.
- While the aorta, vena cava, ribs, and mediastinal structures pose complexity in the thoracic spine, the diaphragm is especially relevant in thoracolumbar pathology, including its attachments to both the 12th rib and the transverse process of L1.[16]

References

[1] Court C, Mansour E, Bouthors C. Thoracic disc herniation: surgical treatment. Orthop Traumatol Surg Res. 2018; 104 1S:S31–S40

[2] Angevin PD, McCormick PC. Retropleural thoracotomy. Technical note. Neurosurg Focus. 2001; 10(1):1–5

[3] Laws MT, von Glinski A, Halalmeh DR, Moisi MD, Oskouian RJ. Lateral approaches to the thoracic spine. In: Tubbs RS, Iwanaga J, Oskouian RJ, Moisi M, eds. Surgical Anatomy of the Lateral Transpsoas Approach to the Lumbar Spine. Philadelphia, PA: Elsevier; 2020:199–209

[4] McCormick PC. Retropleural approach to the thoracic and thoracolumbar spine. Neurosurgery. 1995; 37(5):908–914

[5] Soda C, Faccioli F, Marchesini N, et al. Trans-thoracic versus retropleural approach for symptomatic thoracic disc herniations: comparative analysis of 94 consecutive cases. Br J Neurosurg. 2021; 35(2):195–202

[6] Chen TC, Khoo LT, Benzel EC, McCormick PC, Stillerman CB. Thoracic discectomy. In: Steinmetz MP, Berven SH, Benzel EC, eds. Benzel's Spine Surgery. 2-Volume Set. Philadelphia, PA: Elsevier; 2017:783–798.e1

[7] Tender G, Serban D, Florea M, Constantinescu A, Parikh K. Thoracic lateral retropleural discectomy. In: Tender G, eds. Minimally Invasive Spine Surgery Techniques. Cham: Springer; 2018:173–182

[8] Christiansen PA, Huang S, Smith JS, Shaffrey ME, Uribe JS, Yen CP. Mini-open lateral retropleural/retroperitoneal approaches for thoracic and thoracolumbar junction anterior column pathologies. Neurosurg Focus. 2020; 49(3):E13

[9] Pojskić M, Bopp M, Saß B, Kirschbaum A, Nimsky C, Carl B. Intraoperative computed tomography-based navigation with augmented reality for lateral approaches to the spine. Brain Sci. 2021; 11(5):646

[10] Menezes CM, Fernandes FMM, Arruda ADO, Bringel ML. Minimally invasive lateral retropleural approach to the thoracolumbar junction: review & experience. Coluna/ Columna. 2020; 19(4):236–242

[11] Sharma SB, Kim JS. A review of minimally invasive surgical techniques for the management of thoracic disc herniations. Neurospine. 2019; 16(1):24–33

[12] Li B, Kuzmik GA, Shabani S, et al. Short segment rib resection to mitigate risk of pleural violation during retropleural lateral thoracic interbody fusion. Neurosurg Focus Video. 2022; 7(1):V4

[13] Uribe JS, Katsevman GA, Morgan CD, Paisan GM, Snyder LA. Mini-open lateral retropleural thoracic discectomy approach. Neurosurg Focus Video. 2022; 7(1):V2

[14] Noureldine MHA, Pressman E, Krafft PR, et al. Management of thoracic disc herniation using the mini-open retropleural approach: technique illustration and clinical outcomes of 33 patients from a single academic center. Oper Neurosurg (Hagerstown). 2020; 19(5):567–581

[15] Chou Saman Shabani D, Mummaneni PV, Chan A, et al. The management of thoracic disc pathology via the lateral approach: advances using the minimally invasive approach and navigation. Int J Spine Surg. 2022; 60504 S1:S44–S52

[16] Dakwar E, Ahmadian A, Uribe JS. The anatomical relationship of the diaphragm to the thoracolumbar junction during the minimally invasive lateral extracoelomic (retropleural/ retroperitoneal) approach. J Neurosurg Spine. 2012; 16(4): 359–364

46 Oblique Lumbar Interbody Fusion

Joseph R. Linzey, Hannah L. Tetreault, Ayobami Ward, Paul Park, and Neel Anand

46.1 Background

- Oblique lateral interbody fusion (OLIF) is a minimally invasive approach to the lumbar spine that utilizes the anatomical window between the great vessels and the psoas muscle to access the intervertebral disc space for placement of an interbody cage. OLIF minimizes injury to the lumbar plexus and psoas muscle compared to the classic trans-psoas lateral lumbar interbody fusion (LLIF) approach. The traditional OLIF procedure is indicated for surgical treatment of spinal degeneration or deformity from L2 to L5 and can be particularly effective in correcting lumbar deformity. More recently, a modification of OLIF has allowed access to L5–S1.[1]
- Multiple other procedures exist to access the anterior or lateral lumbar spine, including anterior lumbar interbody fusion (ALIF) and trans-psoas LLIF–extreme lateral interbody fusion (LLIF/XLIF). An ALIF traditionally involves the patient lying in a supine position for a retroperitoneal approach to the spine via the abdomen. This approach is often limited to lower lumbar levels given the difficulty in safely mobilizing the great vessels more proximally along the lumbar spine.[2] The ALIF approach typically involves collaboration with a vascular or general surgeon to assist in creating the surgical corridor and mobilizing the vasculature. A disadvantage of the LLIF/XLIF is potentially increased risk of injuring the lumbar plexus and causing an intra-psoas hematoma compared to OLIF.[3]

46.2 Indications and Contraindications

46.2.1 Indications

- The OLIF procedure was originally promoted to provide access to the L2–L5 disc levels.[1]
- More recently, it has been used in the surgical treatment of spinal degeneration or deformity from L1 to S1.[3]
- Given the ability to place a large cage with resultant distraction, OLIF can be particularly effective in treating stenosis via indirect decompression.[4] In addition, OLIF is effective in treating spondylolisthesis with improved lordosis compared to transforaminal lumbar interbody fusion.[5]
- The OLIF technique also offers the ability to treat deformity with minimal invasiveness.[6,7] Typically, percutaneous fixation is used with OLIF for increased stability and fusion.

46.2.2 Contraindications

- Retroperitoneal surgery.
- Aberrant psoas anatomy.
- Aberrant vascular anatomy.
- High-grade spondylolisthesis.
- Certain types of stenosis due to bony growth rather than ligamentous hypertrophy may not be as amenable to the indirect decompression afforded by OLIF.

46.3 Instruments

- Basic spine tray.
- High-speed drill.
- Interbody support.
- Headlight.
- Loupes or microscope.
- Bipolar cautery and insulated-tip Bovie cautery.
- Intraoperative X-ray and/or fluoroscopy.
- Anterior retractor system.

46.4 Patient Preparation

- X-rays.
- Magnetic resonance imaging (MRI).
- Computed tomography/myelogram.

46.5 Patient Positioning

- The patient should be placed in the right lateral decubitus position.
- The patient's top leg should be slightly flexed to relax the psoas muscle and the bottom leg relatively straight to optimize lumbar lordosis.[8]
- A left-side-up approach is favored to prevent possible damage to the vena cava and iliac veins,

which are more difficult to repair than the aorta or iliac arteries if damaged.
- A large gel roll should be placed superior to the iliac crest in addition to a smaller axillary gel roll.
- The patient should be securely taped to the table to ensure that the back remains perpendicular to the floor.
- Slight flexion can be applied to the table to allow greater access to the vertebral column between the iliac crest and the rib cage.[8]
- The appropriate level is confirmed with fluoroscopy or navigation before an incision is made (**Video 46.1**).

46.6 Technique

- The external and internal abdominal oblique and transverse muscle fibers should be spread with tonsils or blunt dissection until the retroperitoneal fat is encountered.[2]
- Blunt dissection can be performed within the retroperitoneal space with a finger and lighted blade retractors to release the retroperitoneal fat.
- Once the psoas is identified, the left iliac artery should be palpated to assist in guiding the retractor blades between the psoas muscle and left iliac artery at the appropriate intervertebral level.[9]
- The intervertebral level should be confirmed with fluoroscopy.
- Once the correct level is identified, sequentially larger tubes are inserted to dilate the soft tissue opening to allow for final, lighted retractor placement (**Video 46.2**).
- Once the correct level is identified, the disc is accessed (**Video 46.3**) and a discectomy is performed along with endplate preparation (**Video 46.4**).
  - The discectomy should include disruption of the contralateral annulus to allow for appropriate mobilization and correction of the level with the interbody cage.
- Trial cages are inserted for appropriate sizing. Before the cage is placed, graft should be placed within the interbody space.
- The interbody cage is inserted obliquely and then turned orthogonal by shifting the cage inserter dorsally (**Video 46.5**).[9]
- Once the cage is placed and correction is verified with fluoroscopy, the external abdominal oblique fascia is closed.

46.7 Postoperative Care

- Remove dressing after 48 hours.
- I let patient advance to regular diet immediately after surgery.
- I do not recommend postoperative antibiotics.
- The patient has nothing by mouth until evidence of gastrointestinal motility has returned.
- Mobilize as appropriate.
- Routine wound care.
- Intensive care unit stay not necessary unless there was significant blood loss or there are other concerns.
- Postoperative antibiotics, two to three doses.

46.8 Complications

- Infection.[10]
- Bleeding and hematoma formation.
- Bowel injury, ureter injury, kidney injury.
- Injury to the vasculature or retroperitoneal organs.
- Endplate damage.
- nerve injury.
- Psoas weakness.
- Hardware failure.
- Pseudohernia development.

46.9 Management Pearls

- Initial dissection can be performed with the Bovie; however, the use of the Bovie should stop once the external abdominal oblique is encountered.

References

[1] Li R, Li X, Zhou H, Jiang W. Development and application of oblique lumbar interbody fusion. Orthop Surg. 2020; 12(2): 355–365

[2] Allain J, Dufour T. Anterior lumbar fusion techniques: ALIF, OLIF, DLIF, LLIF, IXLIF. Orthop Traumatol Surg Res. 2020; 106 1S:S149–S157

[3] Mobbs RJ, Phan K, Malham G, Seex K, Rao PJ. Lumbar interbody fusion: techniques, indications and comparison of interbody fusion options including PLIF, TLIF, MI-TLIF, OLIF/ATP, LLIF and ALIF. J Spine Surg. 2015; 1(1):2–18

[4] Shimizu T, Fujibayashi S, Otsuki B, Murata K, Matsuda S. Indirect decompression via oblique lateral interbody fusion for severe degenerative lumbar spinal stenosis: a comparative study with direct decompression transforaminal/posterior lumbar interbody fusion. Spine J. 2021; 21(6):963–971

[5] Chandra VVR, M Prasad BC, Hanu TG, Kale PG. BC MP, Hanu TG, Kale PG. Comparison between oblique lumbar interbody fusion (OLIF) and minimally invasive transforaminal lumbar interbody fusion (MISTLIF) for lumbar spondylolisthesis. Neurol India. 2022; 70(1):127–134

[6] Chou D, Lafage V, Chan AY, et al. International Spine Study Group (ISSG). Patient outcomes after circumferential minimally invasive surgery compared with those of open correction for adult spinal deformity: initial analysis of prospectively collected data. J Neurosurg Spine. 2021; 36(2):203–214

[7] Lee JS, Son DW, Lee SH, et al. Surgical outcome of minimal invasive oblique lateral interbody fusion with percutaneous pedicle screw fixation in the treatment of adult degenerative scoliosis. Medicine (Baltimore). 2022; 101(48):e31879

[8] Swiatek PR, McCarthy MH, Weiner J, Bhargava S, Vaishnav AS, Iyer S. Intraoperative image guidance for lateral position surgery. Ann Transl Med. 2021; 9(1):90

[9] Pham MH, Gupta M, Stone LE, Osorio JA, Lehman RA. Minimally invasive L5–S1 oblique lumbar interbody fusion with simultaneous robotic single position posterior fixation: 2-dimensional operative video. Oper Neurosurg (Hagerstown). 2021; 21(6):E543

[10] Zeng ZY, Xu ZW, He DW, et al. Complications and prevention strategies of oblique lateral interbody fusion technique. Orthop Surg. 2018; 10(2):98–106

47 Transpsoas (Lateral Spine)

Katriel E. Lee, Nima Alan, Luke K. O'Neill, Krishna P. Nayak, and Juan S. Uribe

47.1 Background

- Lateral lumbar interbody fusion (LLIF) via a transpsoas approach is a safe and effective way to treat a variety of spinal pathologies.
- LLIF is a favorable approach because it avoids the great vessels and preserves the posterior ligamentous and paraspinous musculature.[1]
- In addition, the interbody used in LLIF can span the vertebral body, making contact with the stronger apophyseal ring and thus increasing the likelihood of fusion and biomechanical stability.[2]

47.2 Indications and Contraindications

- Indications include degenerative spondylolisthesis,[3] foraminal stenosis,[4] trauma, and scoliosis.[5,6,7,8]
- If the psoas morphology is unfavorable (see "Patient Preparation" section), LLIF should not be attempted.
- Great vessel location is also important for determining the suitability of LLIF and the laterality of approach.

47.3 Informed Consent

- Risks, benefits, and alternatives should be discussed with the patient. Specific risks of the LLIF include abdominal pseudohernia, incisional hernia, and femoral nerve palsy.

47.4 Instruments

- C-arm fluoroscopy
- Radiolucent operative bed that can break or flex
- Scalpel
- Cautery
- Long tonsillar hemostats
- Dilators
- Intraoperative neuromonitoring including electromyography (EMG)
- Fluoroscopy
- Kirschner wire (K-wire)
- Lateral interbody fusion retractors
- Light source to attach to the retractor blades
- Pituitary rongeur
- Cobb elevator
- Box cutter disc shaver
- Curettes
- Rasp
- Trial cage
- Shims
- 0 polyglactin 910 sutures
- 20 or 30 polyglactin 910 sutures
- 30 or 40 poliglecaprone 25 sutures

47.5 Patient Preparation

- Magnetic resonance imaging (MRI) is used to evaluate psoas morphology, vasculature, and retroperitoneal content.
  - Psoas morphology is favorable when the anterior border of the psoas on axial view does not extend beyond the anterior aspect of the vertebral body (▶ Fig. 47.1). Anteriorly displaced psoas, commonly referred to as "Mickey Mouse ears," can place the lumbar plexus in the path of the approach, especially at L4–L5, where femoral nerve injury is most likely to occur.[9]
  - The great vessels (descending aorta, inferior vena cava, and iliac arteries and veins) may be translated posteriorly, increasing the likelihood of vascular injury.
- Computed tomography (CT) also provides indispensable information:
  - With distinct visualization of bony anatomy, tentative sizing of the interbody cage and screw sizes and trajectories can be planned.
  - In addition, vacuum disc phenomenon could be identified easily on CT, which is a harbinger of potential for disc height restoration, extent of indirect decompression, and improvement of segmental lordosis.[10]
- Standing long-cassette radiography is mandatory for preoperative planning. It provides a view of segmental, regional, and global alignment in both the sagittal and coronal planes.
  - At L4–L5, the height of the iliac crest plays a significant role in preoperative planning. It will dictate whether the iliac crest blocks

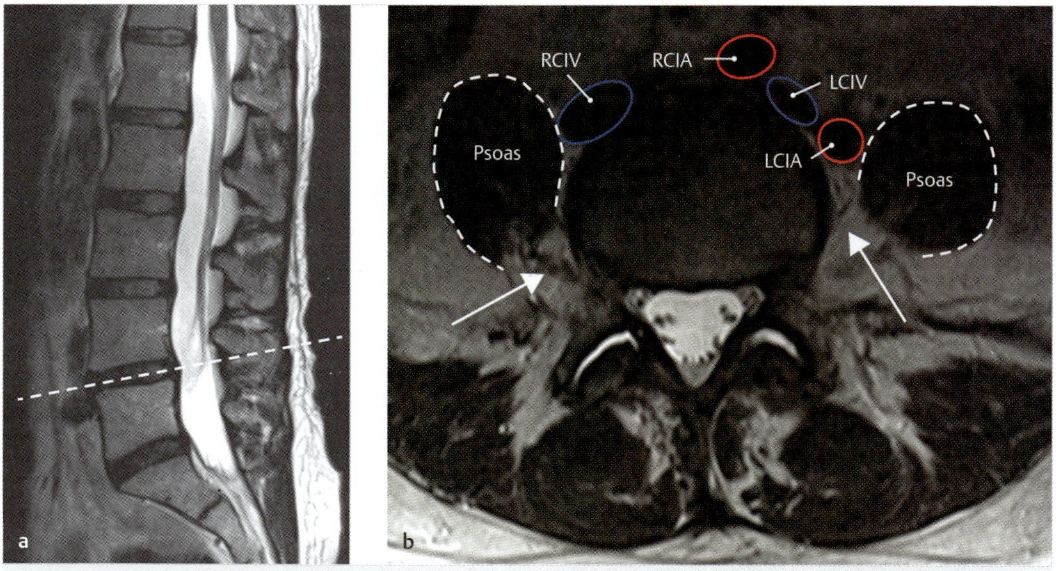

Fig. 47.1 **(a)** Sagittal and **(b)** axial T2-weighted magnetic resonance imaging showing an L4–L5 (*dashed line* in **a**) spondylolisthesis with unfavorable anatomy. Great vessels have split early into the common iliac arteries and veins and are lateral on the vertebral body, and the risk of vascular injury is high. Additionally, the psoas muscles have the classic "Mickey Mouse ear" (*dashed lines* in **b**), with ventral displacement of the lumbar plexus (*white arrows*). Arteries are circled in *red*. Veins are circled in *blue*. LCIA, left common iliac artery; LCIV, left common iliac vein; RCIA, right common iliac artery; RCIV, right common iliac vein. (Used with permission from Barrow Neurological Institute, Phoenix, Arizona.)

access to the L4–L5 disc altogether or whether the use of angled instruments is necessary.
- In the presence of scoliosis, which results in rotational deformity, it is favorable to approach the side of concavity to address multiple levels with one incision, if necessary.

47.6 Patient Positioning

- The patient is placed in the lateral decubitus position, with the approach side up. The knees and hips should be flexed, with a pillow between the knees (▶ Fig. 47.2).
- Axillary rolls are placed. Rolls can also be utilized anteriorly and posteriorly to the patient's back and abdomen for additional support when positioning.
- The iliac crest is aligned with the operative bed break.
- The disc space is localized with C-arm fluoroscopy with a radiopaque instrument. There should be an orthogonal angle with respect to the disc space. Patient and bed positioning (e.g., rotation, [reverse] Trendelenburg position, head and leg up or down) may be utilized to ensure proper positioning.
- The patient is secured with 5- to 10-cm silk tape wrapped circumferentially under and over the bed, with foam padding as needed. Typically, wrapping around the chest, pelvis, and legs is required. Taping is performed after the patient has been fully positioned, ensuring any necessary adjustments can be made beforehand.
- Anterior, posterior, superior, and inferior borders of the disc level are mapped with a skin marker to best guide the optimal trajectory.
- There should be no metal bars or any other objects that may interfere with intraoperative fluoroscopy when positioning and before sterile preparation.

47.7 Technique

47.7.1 Exposure

- A 3- to 4-cm linear transverse incision is made along the lateral abdominal wall. If multiple levels

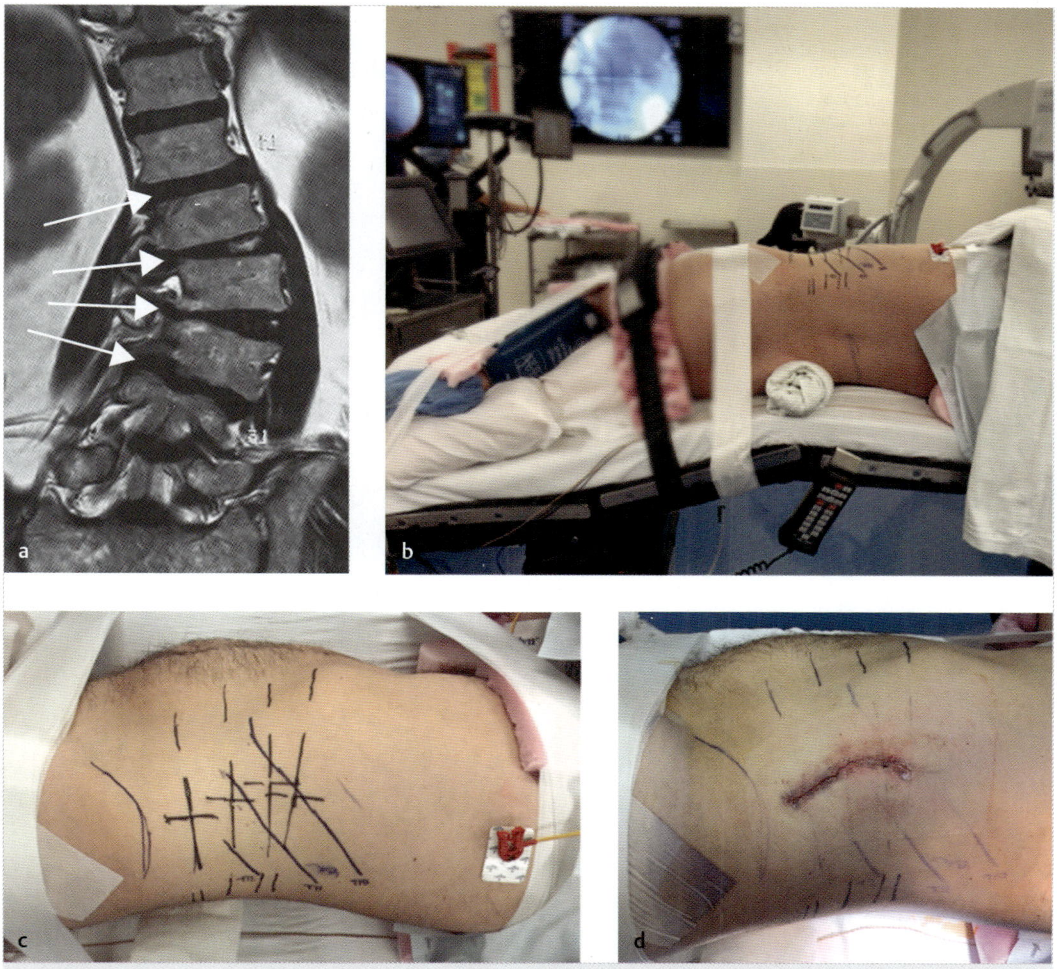

Fig. 47.2 **(a)** Coronal T2-weighted magnetic resonance imaging revealing degenerative scoliosis and the convergence of disc space entry points by approaching from the concavity of the lumbar curve from L1 to L5 (*white arrows*). **(b)** The patient is placed in the lateral decubitus position. The break in the bed is used to open up the space between the iliac crest and the ribs for entry at each level. **(c)** Levels are marked with fluoroscopy before sterile prepping. **(d)** The postoperative closure is shown. Preoperative positioning allowed for use of a single incision to incorporate all entry points. (Used with permission from Barrow Neurological Institute, Phoenix, Arizona.)

are planned, then an incision along the rostral-to-caudal axis is optimal, with a slightly oblique angle following the lordotic curvature of the spine. This incision should intersect the center of the disc space, as mapped out previously.

- A transverse incision is made with cautery at the external oblique fascia.
- The abdominal musculature is bluntly dissected with the use of long tonsillar hemostats.
- After the muscle layers of the abdominal wall are dissected, the transversalis fascia is bluntly penetrated, signifying entrance into the fatty retroperitoneal space.
- Using blunt finger dissection, the surgeon mobilizes the peritoneal contents anteriorly to access the lateral spine.
- ▸ Fig. 47.3[11] highlights the abdominal layers traversed during the approach.

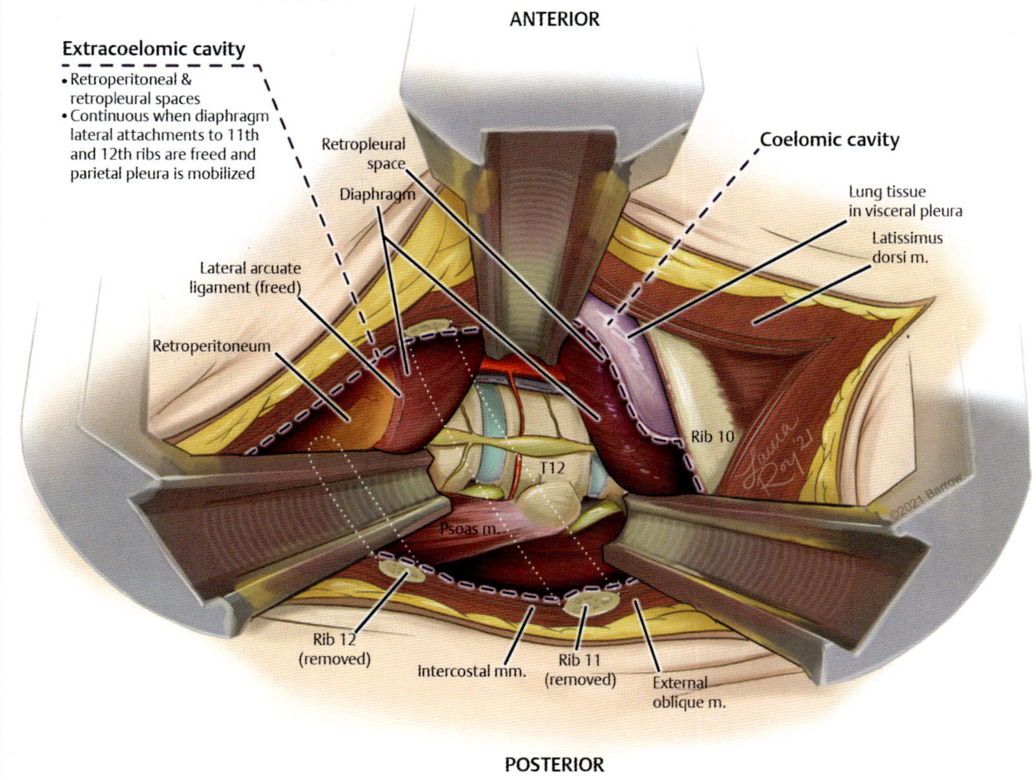

Fig. 47.3 Illustration showing the layers of the anterolateral abdomen traversed during the lateral approach. m., muscle; mm., muscles. (Used with permission from Barrow Neurological Institute, Phoenix, Arizona.)

47.7.2 Docking of the Tubular Retractor and Dilation

- The transverse process of the spinal column and muscle attachments are palpated, and the disc space is identified.
- With the finger guiding its position, the initial dilator is docked onto the posterior third quartile of disc space without penetrating through the psoas.
- Directional EMG is used to map the lumbar plexus. The absence of any motor signal at 10 mA on directional EMG indicates a generally safe working distance from the lumbar plexus.
- Fluoroscopy is used to confirm the correct position, and adjustments are made as needed. Once the position is confirmed, the K-wire is advanced through the dilator and into the disc.
- Each sequential dilator is then placed, with the rotation of the directional EMG repeated. If a signal is identified, the K-wire should be repositioned, and the dilator should be placed again.
- With the final dilator placed, the tubular retractors are inserted, and a light source is attached to the blades.
- The annulus of the disc space is directly visualized through the barrel of the retractor system. The K-wire should be at the center of the retractor.
- Lateral fluoroscopy is used to confirm the correct docking position. Slight adjustments are possible and can be made with the K-wire in place. Care should be taken to not displace the K-wire out of the disc space, as this will necessitate removal of the retractor and repeating the steps from the beginning.

47.7.3 Discectomy

- A rectangle annulotomy is performed using a scalpel on a long handle, followed by the removal of the large disc fragments with a pituitary rongeur.
- Under anteroposterior fluoroscopy, a Cobb elevator is used to scrape the disc off the top and bottom endplates, ensuring the contralateral annulus is released.
- The box cutter disc shaver is placed flush against the endplate and, with visualization under fluoroscopy, is malleted along the length of the endplates.
- A pituitary rongeur, ringed curettes, upbiting curette, rasp, and various scraping instruments are used to remove all remaining disc fragments and prepare the endplates for arthrodesis.

47.7.4 Interbody Graft Placement

- A trial cage is inserted into the disc space. The tensile feedback and fluoroscopy guide the choice of the optimal interbody graft size to restore disc height.
- An interbody graft is then selected. Aim for graft size that contacts the lateral endplates on both sides of the vertebral body. Biologics can then be used to promote fusion.
- With the optimal disc cage selected, the graft is malleted in position, with anteroposterior and lateral fluoroscopy used to confirm the position within the disc space and crossing the apophyseal ring borders.
- The graft is released, and the retainment device is removed.

47.7.5 Closure

- The operative corridor is thoroughly irrigated.
- The shims are removed, and the retractor is slowly withdrawn. At each tissue plane, the tissue is closely monitored for areas of active hemorrhage; any areas of hemorrhage are cauterized as needed.
- With the retractor withdrawn, 0 polyglactin 910 sutures are used to close the external oblique and Scarpa fascia.
- The subcutaneous layer is closed with 20 or 30 polyglactin 910.
- The dermis is closed with subcuticular 30 or 40 poliglecaprone 25 suture and surgical glue.

47.8 Postoperative Care

- Standing can usually be achieved by the first day after surgery.[12]
- Brace should be worn to reduce lumbar spine movement for the first month after surgery.[12]
- Physical therapy can be beneficial but is not necessary.[12]

47.9 Complications

- There is risk of vascular injury[13] or injury to abdominal organs, such as the bowel, kidney, and ureter.[14]
- Injury to the lumbar nerves and neurological complications such as iliopsoas weakness, anterior thigh numbness, quadriceps weakness, and radiculopathy can occur.[13]
- Failure of vertebrae to fuse, hardware fracture, or bone graft migration can occur, which may necessitate additional surgery.[14]
- As with all spinal fusions, there is a risk of adjacent segment disease.[14]
- General complications of surgery can occur, including infection, bleeding, and anesthesia-related complications.[13]

47.10 Management Pearls

- Operative anatomy:
  - *Abdominal wall:* The layers of the abdominal wall, in order from superficial to deep, are the skin, Camper fascia, Scarpa fascia, external oblique muscle, internal oblique muscle, transverse fascia, and extraperitoneal tissue.
  - *Vasculature:* The aorta courses along the anterior aspect of the vertebral bodies, paramedian toward the left side, and bifurcates into the common iliac arteries at L4–L5. Bifurcation into the internal and external iliac arteries typically occurs at L5–S1. The common iliac veins ascend bilaterally to form the inferior vena cava at L5 along the right side of the vertebral column (▶ Fig. 47.4).[1]
  - *Sympathetic trunk:* The ganglia of the sympathetic nervous system course bilaterally along the vertebrae from the base of the skull

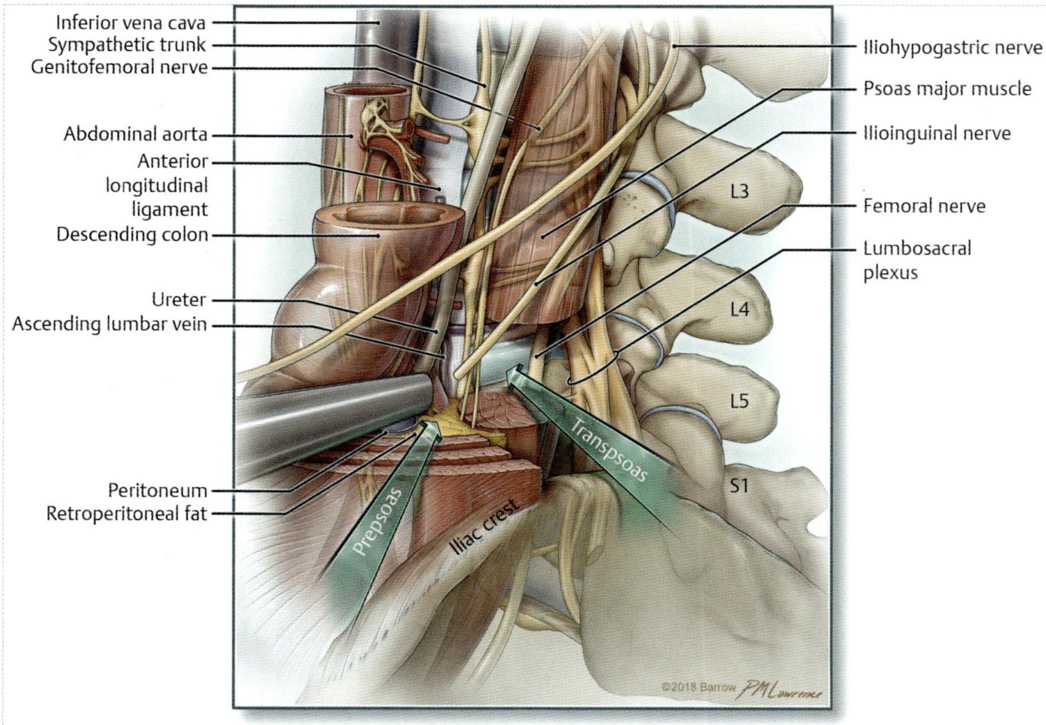

Fig. 47.4 Illustration of the anatomy of the approach for lateral minimally invasive surgeries for the lumbar spine. (Used with permission from Barrow Neurological Institute, Phoenix, Arizona.)

to the coccyx and are at risk of injury, although such complications are rare.[15,16]

- *Lumbar plexus:* The exiting nerve roots of the lumbar and sacral spine coalesce to form the lumbosacral plexus. The plexus travels intertwined with the psoas major and is at risk of injury during this procedure. The iliohypogastric (T12–L1), ilioinguinal (L1), and lateral femoral cutaneous (L2–L3) nerves are contained within the abdominal wall. At the level of the psoas, the genitofemoral nerve can be encountered anteriorly (L1–L2), and the femoral and obturator nerves can be encountered posteriorly (L2–L4). When placing the tubular retractor, it is important not to land the tubular retractor system on or immediately adjacent to these nerves.

- Care must be taken to avoid disruption of the anterior longitudinal ligament (ALL). Once the position of the retractor blades is confirmed on lateral fluoroscopy (before any discectomy is performed), the "working zone" is functionally defined by the retractor blades. Thus, confining oneself to the confirmed barriers of the retractor blades and maintaining an orthogonal angle to the disc space ensures the ALL is not violated. Violation of the ALL could cause catastrophic vascular injury, necessitating the use of a lateral plate to avoid cage migration and/or pedicle screws to stabilize the segment.
- Care must be taken to not violate the endplates. Any instrument during the discectomy has the potential, to a varying degree, to violate the endplate. Maintaining an orthogonal angle to the disc space and the judicious use of fluoroscopy to confirm a near-parallel angle to the endplates ensures a meticulous discectomy technique. Intraoperative violation of the endplate sets the stage for postoperative cage subsidence, defeating the purpose of the indirect decompression.

47.11 Disclosures

- Juan S. Uribe receives royalties from NuVasive Medical, Inc., and is a consultant for SI-BONE, Inc.; Mainstay Medical, Inc.; Viseon, Inc.; and Misonix, Inc. All other authors have no personal, financial, or institutional interest in any of the drugs, materials, or devices described in this chapter.

Acknowledgments

- We thank the staff of Neuroscience Publications at Barrow Neurological Institute for assistance with manuscript preparation.

References

[1] Walker CT, Farber SH, Cole TS, et al. Complications for minimally invasive lateral interbody arthrodesis: a systematic review and meta-analysis comparing prepsoas and transpsoas approaches. J Neurosurg Spine. 2019; 30(4):446–460

[2] Marchi L, Abdala N, Oliveira L, Amaral R, Coutinho E, Pimenta L. Radiographic and clinical evaluation of cage subsidence after stand-alone lateral interbody fusion. J Neurosurg Spine. 2013; 19(1):110–118

[3] Aichmair A, Alimi M, Hughes AP, et al. Single-level lateral lumbar interbody fusion for the treatment of adjacent segment disease: a retrospective two-center study. Spine. 2017; 42(9):E515–E522

[4] Kepler CK, Sharma AK, Huang RC, et al. Indirect foraminal decompression after lateral transpsoas interbody fusion. J Neurosurg Spine. 2012; 16(4):329–333

[5] Castro C, Oliveira L, Amaral R, Marchi L, Pimenta L. Is the lateral transpsoas approach feasible for the treatment of adult degenerative scoliosis? Clin Orthop Relat Res. 2014; 472(6):1776–1783

[6] Ahmadian A, Bach K, Bolinger B, et al. Stand-alone minimally invasive lateral lumbar interbody fusion: multicenter clinical outcomes. J Clin Neurosci. 2015; 22(4):740–746

[7] Lehmen JA, Gerber EJ. MIS lateral spine surgery: a systematic literature review of complications, outcomes, and economics. Eur Spine J. 2015; 24 Suppl 3:287–313

[8] Pimenta L, Oliveira L, Schaffa T, Coutinho E, Marchi L. Lumbar total disc replacement from an extreme lateral approach: clinical experience with a minimum of 2 years' follow-up. J Neurosurg Spine. 2011; 14(1):38–45

[9] Davis TT, Bae HW, Mok JM, Rasouli A, Delamarter RB. Lumbar plexus anatomy within the psoas muscle: implications for the transpsoas lateral approach to the L4-L5 disc. J Bone Joint Surg Am. 2011; 93(16):1482–1487

[10] Yen CP, Beckman JM, Vivas AC, Bach K, Uribe JS. Effects of intradiscal vacuum phenomenon on surgical outcome of lateral interbody fusion for degenerative lumbar disease. J Neurosurg Spine. 2017; 26(4):419–425

[11] Xu DS, Walker CT, Farber SH, et al. Surgical anatomy of minimally invasive lateral approaches to the thoracolumbar junction. J Neurosurg Spine. 2021; 36(6):937–944

[12] Balsano M, Härtl R, Hussain I. Lateral lumbar interbody fusion (LLIF). AO Surgery Reference. Accessed April 25, 2025 at: https://surgeryreference.aofoundation.org/spine/-degenerative/lumbar/degenerative-spondylolisthesis/lateral-lumbar-interbody-fusion

[13] Sofianos DA, Briseño MR, Abrams J, Patel AA. Complications of the lateral transpsoas approach for lumbar interbody arthrodesis: a case series and literature review. Clin Orthop Relat Res. 2012; 470(6):1621–1632

[14] Mayfield Clinic. Spinal Fusion: Lateral Lumbar Interbody Fusion (LLIF). Mayfield Brain & Spine. Accessed April 25, 2025 at: https://mayfieldclinic.com/pe-llif.htm

[15] Brickman B, Tanios M, Patel D, Elgafy H. Clinical presentation and surgical anatomy of sympathetic nerve injury during lumbar spine surgery: a narrative review. J Spine Surg. 2022; 8(2):276–287

[16] Rutter G, Phan K, Smith A, Stewart F, Seex K, Gragnaniello C. Morphometric anatomy of the lumbar sympathetic trunk with respect to the anterolateral approach to lumbar interbody fusion: a cadaver study. J Spine Surg. 2017; 3(3): 419–425

48 Percutaneous Sacroiliac Joint Fusion: Indications and Technique

Erin Thomson and Peter Carlos Gerszten

48.1 Background

- Sacroiliac joint (SIJ) pain is a common and underdiagnosed cause of lower back pain. The surgical treatment for SIJ dysfunction traditionally has been an open fusion with a significant dissection and disruption of normal tissues in order to expose the joint and allow for arthrodesis. More recently, minimally invasive percutaneous techniques have been developed for SIJ fusion. A substantial body of evidence now supports the benefits of percutaneous SIJ fusion compared to nonoperative management for decreasing pain and improving quality of life. SIJ pain has been demonstrated to be responsible for 22% of low back pain and is found in 43% of patients who have previously undergone lumbar fusion. Because of the growing patient population with SIJ pain, as well as an increased recognition of its diagnosis, percutaneous SIJ fusion has become a more utilized surgical technique. This overview will help define the indications and minimally invasive techniques utilized for the treatment of SIJ dysfunction.[1,2,3]
- The SIJ is the largest axial joint in the human body with an average surface area of 17.5 cm^2. The joint is important for weight bearing, functioning as a triplanar shock absorber. The intricate design of ligamentous structures allows for little motion within the SIJ. The anterior ligaments are short and strong, allowing little movement while at the same time providing significant stability. The posterior ligaments follow a basket weave pattern for increased strength as well as stability. The primary motion of the SIJ is referred to as nutation, which is a nodding type of motion. Rotation is usually limited to 1 to 2 degrees in males and 2 to 4 degrees in females.
- SIJ pain is common, causing chronic low back pain, and groin, buttocks, and even sciatic pain. SIJ dysfunction may be related to degenerative and inflammatory arthritis, posttraumatic arthritis, postpartum instability, iatrogenic from iliac graft harvest, an infectious etiology, and previous lumbar fusion (most commonly at L5–S1). It is more often diagnosed in women versus men, and primarily posttraumatic with a mechanical fall being the inciting event, followed by motor vehicle accident (MVA) and heavy lifting. Symptomatic SIJ pain can mimic discogenic or radicular back pain related to the lumbar spine, which can lead to misdiagnosis and mistreatment.[1]
- The diagnosis of SIJ dysfunction requires an exclusion of lumbar spine and hip pathology and includes a triad history of low back, hip, groin, and gluteal pain, without associated neurological deficits. Lower extremity pain, paresthesias, and weakness may be present and are typically unilateral and can cause leg instability. Patients commonly complain of discomfort while sitting or standing for an extended amount of time.
- Physical examination findings include a positive Fortin finger test with tenderness to palpation of the SIJ at Fortin's point or sacral sulcus, as well as the reproduction of pain with provocative maneuvers such as Gaenslen's maneuver, Patrick's maneuver, distraction, compression tests, and thigh thrust.
- There is no single diagnostic imaging study for the diagnosis of SIJ pathology. Magnetic resonance (MR) imaging of the lumbar spine is completed to rule out other pathologies. A noncontrast computed tomography (CT) of the pelvis is useful in demonstrating degeneration of the SIJ and for preoperative planning purposes. Generalized pain behavior such as somatoform disorders and fibromyalgia must also be ruled out.
- The gold standard for diagnosis of sacroiliitis is an image-guided SIJ injection, performed for both diagnostic and therapeutic purposes. If the patient notes ≥ 75% relief of low back pain within 15 to 30 minutes of the injection on two separate occasions, it confirms the SIJ as the source of symptoms and is considered a positive response. Therapeutic benefit is achieved with the injection of steroids that may confer long-standing pain relief.[4]

48.2 Indications and Contraindications

- Indication: Intractable SIJ pain, not amenable to be relieved with conservative therapy.
- Medical contraindications.

48.3 Patient Positioning

- SIJ fusion is performed under general anesthesia on a bumpy Jackson table in a straight prone position. No Foley catheter is used. Somatosensory evoked potential (SSEP) neurophysiological monitoring is employed. Fluoroscopic image guidance is used for the entirety of the procedure.

48.4 Technique

The following technique is an overview employing the TriCor Sacroiliac Fusion System (Zimmer Biomet, Denver, CO) with only minor variations in technique using other systems.[5,6]

A 2-cm-long incision is made using a no. 15 scalpel blade based upon fluoroscopic guidance on the lateral border of the buttocks (▶ Fig. 48.1, ▶ Fig. 48.2, ▶ Fig. 48.3, and ▶ Fig. 48.4). The subcutaneous tissue is coagulated using bipolar electrocautery, without violation of the fascia. A lateral image is obtained with focal alignment of the greater sciatic notch and ala, considered a true lateral. A Steinmann pin is placed through the fascia and guided in a needle-eye view to approximately 1 cm caudal from the S1 superior endplate and 1 cm anterior to the posterior sacral cortex into the ileum. This trajectory is parallel to the sacral ala. After the pin is stabilized at its entry point within the outer cortical bone of the ileum, an outlet view is obtained in order to assess the pin's trajectory. In the outlet view, the anterior wall of the sacrum and S1 foramen should be in a single line. This view allows for the identification of the soft tissue ventral to the sacrum that must be avoided. If the Steinmann pin is too anteriorly placed, it can breach the pelvic brim and lead to potential bowel or vascular injury. If the trajectory of the pin is posteriorly placed, the pin might penetrate the sacral canal causing neural injury. The pin should be angled 10 to 15 degrees toward the middle of the sacrum to maximize a safe trajectory.

The inlet view is then used to assess the first two sacral foramen. The pubic symphysis should

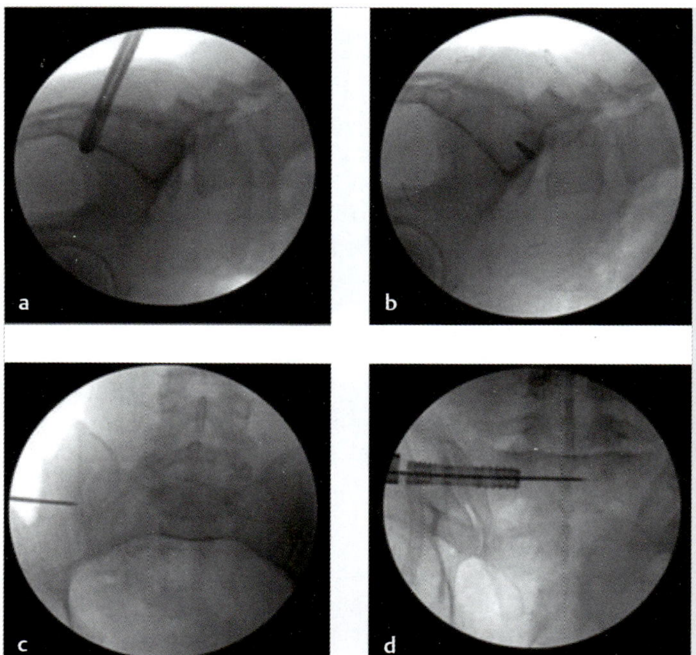

Fig. 48.1 This is a representative case of 45-year-old man with complaints of right sacroiliac (SI) joint pain. He had a positive reduction of pain after an SI joint injection. **(a)** The location of the incision is determined by using a metallic marker on the skin. There has been a careful demarcation of the L5 and S1 endplates, ala, and greater sciatic notch. **(b)** The Steinmann pin is placed 1 cm caudal from the S1 endplate and 1 cm anterior to the posterior cortex, parallel to the sacral ala. **(c)** In the pelvic outlet view, the ventral sacrum is well delineated. **(d)** The inlet view is demonstrated after the drilling and tapping have been completed and a 55-mm-long implant packed with autograft and allograft is placed. Note the placement of the first implant 1 cm superior to the S1 foramen. The implant should be placed approximately 50% past the SI joint.

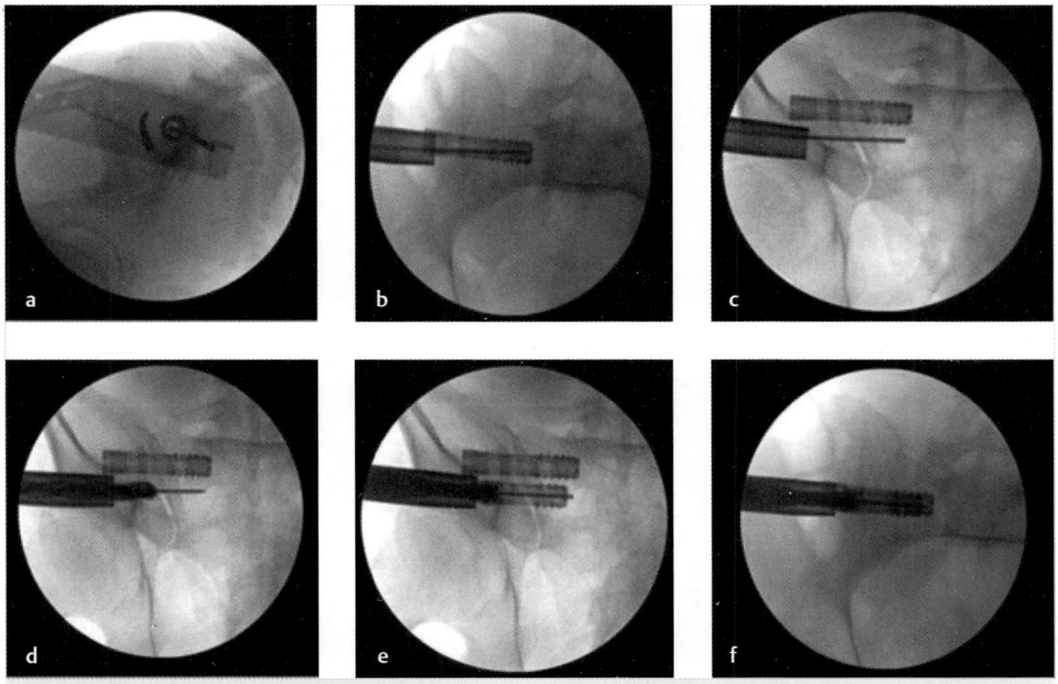

Fig. 48.2 **(a)** Lateral, **(b)** pelvic outlet, and **(c)** pelvic inlet views are demonstrated. The second Steinmann pin is placed in a lateral image with the assistance of a parallel pin guide 20 mm caudal to the first implant **(a)**. In an outlet view, there is no breach of the pelvic brim and the pin is parallel to the first implant **(b)**. In an inlet view, the dilators are placed, and the pin does not breach the S1 foramen **(c)**. **(d)** The drill is advanced in an inlet projection. **(e)** A 40-mm-long implant is placed over the pin, ending just lateral to the S1 foramen. **(f)** The inlet view confirms the safe placement of the implant parallel to the first implant and not breaching the pelvic brim.

be covering the S3 and S4 foramen. The first pin/implant is placed slightly rostral to the S1 neural foramen. The second implant is placed at the level of or just caudal to the S1 foramen and the third implant is placed between the S1 and S2 foramen. A handheld battery-powered drill is used to advance the Steinman pin through the ileum, SIJ, and sacrum without advancing through the foramen or bending the pin as it traverses the bony structures.

Once the first pin is advanced to its final position superior and slightly lateral to the S1 foramen toward the S1 pedicle (Denis zone 1), a depth gauge is used to determine the length of the implant that will be placed. As a rule of thumb, the implant is 5 mm longer than the measurement indicated on the depth gauge to allow the screw to sit slightly proud to the ileum. Using frequent fluoroscopic imaging in an inlet view, a battery-operated handheld drill is placed over the Steinmann pin. A path through the ileum, SIJ, and sacrum is drilled that will allow for the final position of the implant.

Following the drilling of the path and with the Steinmann pin still in place, three sequential dilators are placed such that a final working channel dilator is placed against the ileum. The trajectory is tapped over the pin and through the final working channel. The implant is screwed into the final position over the pin in an inlet projection. A parallel pin guide is placed to guide the next implant into the appropriate trajectory 20 mm caudal to the first implant. This ensures enough distance such that the two implants will be parallel and not touch one another within the body. For smaller patients, a third smaller diameter screw can be inserted.

The TriCor system employs threaded compression titanium plasma–coated implants that come

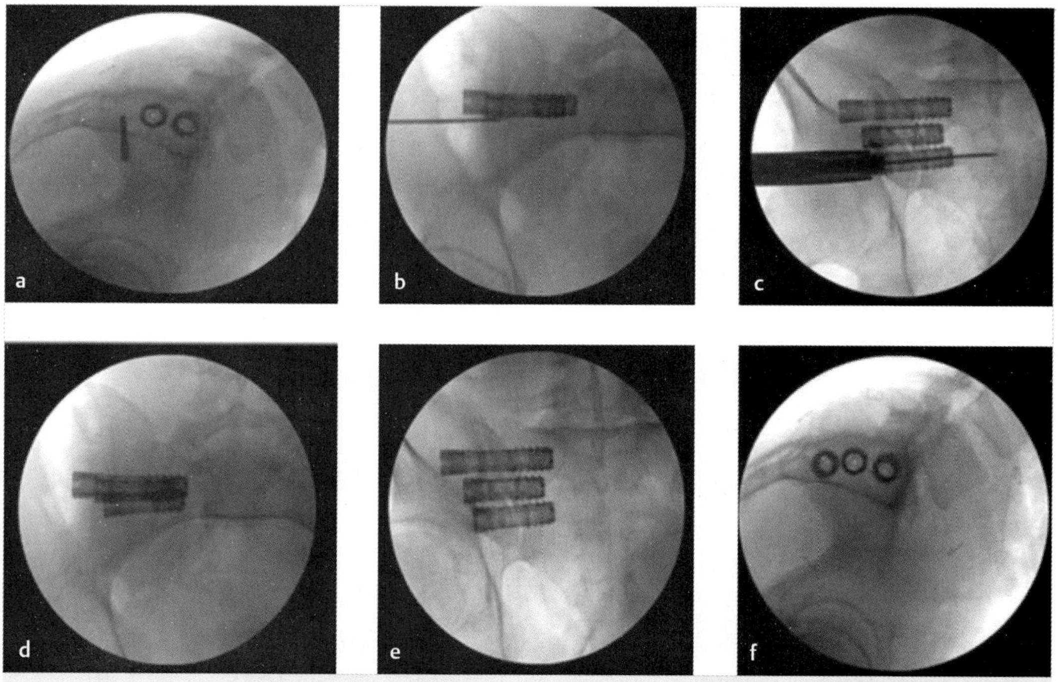

Fig. 48.3 **(a)** Lateral, **(b)** pelvic outlet, and **(c)** pelvic inlet views are demonstrated. The lateral image is useful to determine if a third larger implant can be placed **(a)**. The outlet view confirms that no breach to the pelvic brim has occurred by the pin, which is parallel to the other implants **(b)**. In the inlet view, a third implant is placed caudal to the S1 neural foramen and superior to the S1 foramen **(c)**. **(d)** Final outlet, **(e)** inlet, and **(f)** lateral projections illustrate the appropriate placement of the sacroiliac joint implants.

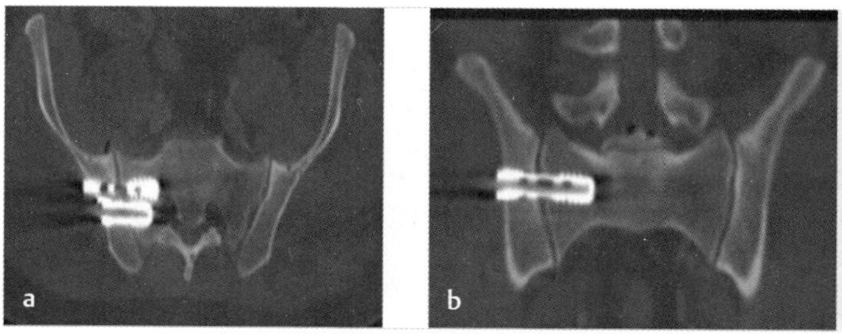

Fig. 48.4 **(a)** Axial and **(b)** coronal projections illustrate 6-month post-operative CT imaging, demonstrating well-placed sacroiliac joint implants. The patient had complete resolution of their preoperative pain symptoms.

in multiple diameters (▶ Fig. 48.5). The dual threaded implant design allows for a lag compression to fixate the SIJ, providing controlled insertion. The implants are hollow, and local autograft bone is harvested from the drill and tap and manually packed into the implant prior to insertion. This autograft bone may be augmented with allograft bone as well. The implants are fenestrated to allow for bony ingrowth and the titanium plasma coating is designed to facilitate bony incorporation.

Once all implants have been inserted and placement is confirmed in the final lateral, inlet, and outlet radiographic views, a standard closure of the fascia, deep dermal layer, and subcuticular skin layer is performed. Steri-Strips are placed over the surgical wound and a Primapore dressing is applied.

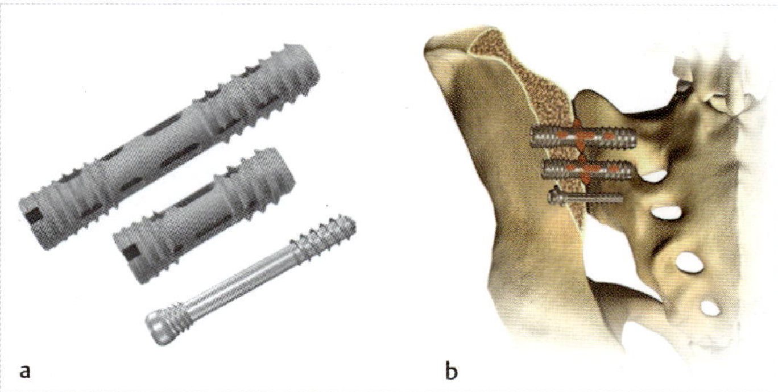

Fig. 48.5 **(a)** The TriCor Sacroiliac Fusion System (Zimmer-Biomet) demonstrating the dual threaded design of the implants that allows for lag compression across the SIJ. **(b)** The implants are hollow, which allows for bone graft insertion and arthrodesis.

48.5 Postoperative Care

- The patient is admitted for a 23-hour observation status. All patients are evaluated by the physical therapy service on postoperative day 1 and discharged with crutches or a walker based upon preference. They are instructed to partially weight bear for 3 weeks until their first postoperative visit. After 3 weeks, they may return to full weight bearing and activity as tolerated. A pelvic X-ray is performed at 3 months to ensure proper hardware placement and evolving fusion. Home and outpatient physical therapy programs are avoided in the immediate postoperative period.

48.6 Complications

- Excess intraoperative bleeding, postoperative infection, and pain.

48.7 Management Pearls

- Nonsurgical treatment options include nonsteroidal anti-inflammatory drugs (NSAIDs), pelvic floor physical therapy for stabilization of the SIJ, external fixation with a sacral belt, or radiofrequency ablation of the SIJ following successful SIJ injection. Most patients will stabilize with appropriate nonsurgical care within 8 weeks of initiating treatment. However, when a patient has failed 6 months of conservative management, they may be considered a surgical candidate.
- The purpose of SIJ fusion surgery is to minimize SIJ motion and reduce tissue irritation by stabilizing the joint through fixation while facilitating arthrodesis with implant–bone integration. The literature in support of open arthrodesis includes a lengthy hospital admission with non-weight-bearing to the affected side for several months with higher rates of complications such as deep wound infection, iliac crest fractures, pulmonary embolism, and reoperation rates. For this reason, the current trend is a less invasive percutaneous approach to SIJ fusion.[4]

48.8 Emerging Technologies

- Pain that originates from SIJ dysfunction may be difficult to diagnose and successfully treat despite it being responsible for a large subset of patients complaining of lower back pain. Patients should be considered as surgical candidates for percutaneous SIJ fusions when other nonsurgical treatments fail to decrease their pain and the patient's quality of life is significantly adversely affected. A growing body of literature supports the efficacy of percutaneous SIJ fusion surgery over both traditional open surgical procedures and nonsurgical management. These techniques are an important addition to the surgical management of patients with SIJ-mediated pain.

References

[1] Rudolf L. Sacroiliac joint arthrodesis: MIS technique with titanium implants—report of the first 50 patients and outcomes. Open Orthop J. 2012; 6(1):495–502

[2] North American Spine Society. Coverage Policy Recommendations. Percutaneous Sacroiliac Joint Fusion.

2015. Accessed November 13, 2016 at: https://www.spine.org/PolicyPractice/CoverageRecommendations/AboutCoverageRecommendations.aspx
[3] Zaidi HA, Montoure AJ, Dickman CA. Surgical and clinical efficacy of sacroiliac joint fusion: a systematic review of the literature. J Neurosurg Spine. 2015; 23(1):59–66
[4] Miller LE, Reckling WC, Block JE. Analysis of postmarket complaints database for the iFuse SI Joint Fusion System®: a minimally invasive treatment for degenerative sacroiliitis and sacroiliac joint disruption. Med Devices (Auckl). 2013; 6:77–84
[5] Polly DW, Cher DJ, Wine KD, et al. INSITE Study Group. Randomized controlled trial of minimally invasive sacroiliac joint fusion using triangular titanium implants vs nonsurgical management for sacroiliac joint dysfunction: 12-month outcomes. Neurosurgery. 2015; 77(5):674–690, discussion 690–691
[6] Polly DW, Swofford J, Whang PG, et al. INSITE Study Group. Two-year outcomes from a randomized controlled trial of minimally invasive sacroiliac joint fusion vs. non-surgical management for sacroiliac joint dysfunction. Int J Spine Surg. 2016; 10:28

49 Endoscopic Spine Approaches

Yuping Derek Li, Andrew T. Coxon, Daniel M. Hafez, and John Ogunlade

49.1 Background

- Endoscopic spine surgery approaches can largely be divided into two categories: interlaminar and transforaminal.
- The interlaminar endoscopic approach is well suited for lumbar disc herniations, synovial cyst, central stenosis, and lateral recess stenosis.
- The transforaminal endoscopic approach can generally be used to treat radiculopathy due to impingement of the extraforaminal nerve root. Etiologies of this may include far lateral disc herniation, far out syndrome, osteophytes, or displaced interbody spacers.

49.2 Indications and Contraindications

- Indications include unilateral or bilateral radiculopathy due to disc herniation, lateral recess stenosis, facet arthropathy, synovial cyst, hypertrophied/redundant ligamentum flavum, compressive osteophyte, or interbody cage subsidence.[1]
- Contraindications include extensive disc migration and calcification, instability on dynamic X-rays or high-grade spondylolisthesis, and nerve root abnormalities.[1]
- Relative contraindications include multilevel disease and vertical neuroforaminal stenosis.

49.3 Instruments

- The instruments and equipment required for transforaminal endoscopic decompression are similar to those use in interlaminar endoscopic decompression cases. The patient is positioned prone on a Wilson frame on a flat top spine table (can use open spine table with hip pads and legs in a sling). Other necessary equipment include endoscopic tower (radiofrequency ablator, endoscopic drill, irrigation pump, high-definition camera), endoscopic instrument trays (± trephines), transforaminal endoscope, neuromonitoring, fluoroscopy ± intraoperative neuronavigation system.

49.4 Patient Preparation

- After obtaining a complete history and physical examination, a magnetic resonance imaging (MRI) without contrast is important for planning the transforaminal endoscopic approach.
- A computed tomography (CT) scan may also be helpful with surgical planning, especially if bony anatomy or hardware is implicated in the pathology.
- In patients with multilevel radiographic disease, electromyography (EMG)/nerve conduction velocity (NCV) and/or diagnostic nerve blocks can help confirm the level of radiculopathy.
- Endoscopic approaches require significantly less tissue mobilization and manipulation than conventional approaches. Owing to the decreased morbidity, lumbar endoscopic techniques can be done awake with regional/local anesthesia, under monitored anesthesia care (MAC)/conscious sedation, or under general anesthesia.[2]
- Avoiding general anesthesia can expedite recovery from sedation and promote early mobilization. If general anesthesia is used, neuromonitoring should be considered and the proper anesthesia considerations should be followed.[2]

49.5 Patient Positioning

- The patient is positioned prone on a Wilson frame to flex the lumbar spine and increase the neuroforaminal height and open the interlaminar window.

49.6 Technique

- **Transforaminal approach[3] —incision**:
  - The patient should be prepped and draped in the standard sterile fashion. A wide sterile field should be prepped in case a conversion to open decompression is necessary. Once the patient is prepped and draped, a true anteroposterior (AP) and lateral X-ray using intraoperative fluoroscopy are used to plan the skin incision. The true midline is marked on

the AP X-ray, best achieved by airplaning the bed to achieve a true AP while the C-arm remains at 0 degrees. The rostrocaudal approach trajectory can vary depending on the location of the targeted pathology, but in general, the inclination angle of 5 to 15 degrees can be used. With regard to the mediolateral dimension, the skin incision is roughly 8 to 12 cm off the true midline, depending on the size of the patient. The goal of the approach trajectory is to follow the lateral border of the facet joint toward the neuroforamen.[4,5]

- **Transforaminal approach—targeting**:
  - A long 18-gauge spinal needle or Jamshidi needle is passed through the incision and advanced toward the superolateral aspect of the caudal pedicle under AP and lateral fluoroscopic guidance (▶ Fig. 49.1). The location of the exiting nerve root within the foramen and the extraforaminal area should be carefully assessed on the preoperative MRI to minimize the risk of injury during this approach. A guidewire is then left in place and the needle is removed.[4,5]
- **Transforaminal approach—endoscope placement**:
  - Sequential soft tissue dilators are placed over the guidewire. The final working tubular retractor is placed over the final dilator with the bevel open to the exiting nerve root. Once docked, the bevel is rotated to face the caudal pedicle and an AP and lateral X-ray confirms the intended position and level prior to bringing in the endoscope. At the conclusion of the approach, the superolateral aspect of the caudal pedicle, the superior articulating process (SAP), and the posterosuperior endplate of the caudal vertebral body should be visualized with the endoscope.[4,5]
- **Transforaminal approach—decompression**:
  - By following the superior aspect of the caudal pedicle and the posterosuperior endplate rostrally, the annulus of the intervertebral disc can be readily identified. A grasper can be used to carefully remove any free-floating remnant soft tissue. The ligamentum flavum can be identified given its characteristic yellow color. Resecting the yellow ligament along its attachment on the SAP will uncover the traversing nerve root medially and exiting nerve root cranially. In some cases, it may be necessary to perform a foraminoplasty, or widen the neuroforamen. This can be done by removing some or all of the tip of the SAP with a diamond burr. The disc herniation should now be identifiable and can be removed with endoscopic graspers (▶ Fig. 49.2). If the annular defect is seen, it should be thoroughly probed for remaining loose fragments, then ablated with the radiofrequency probe to prevent further disc herniation. After decompression, the traversing nerve will return to a ventral position in the canal and the exiting nerve root will descend into the foramen. A thorough foraminal decompression is complete when the traversing nerve is pulsatile and free floating and the exiting

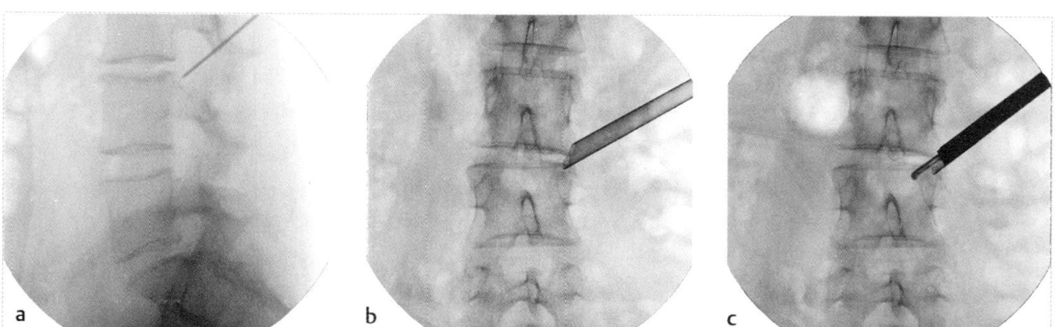

Fig. 49.1 Localization for a right-sided transforaminal approach to L3–L4. **(a)** Placement of localizing spinal needle. **(b)** Placement of tubular retractor. **(c)** Kerrison on the superior surface of the caudal pedicle.

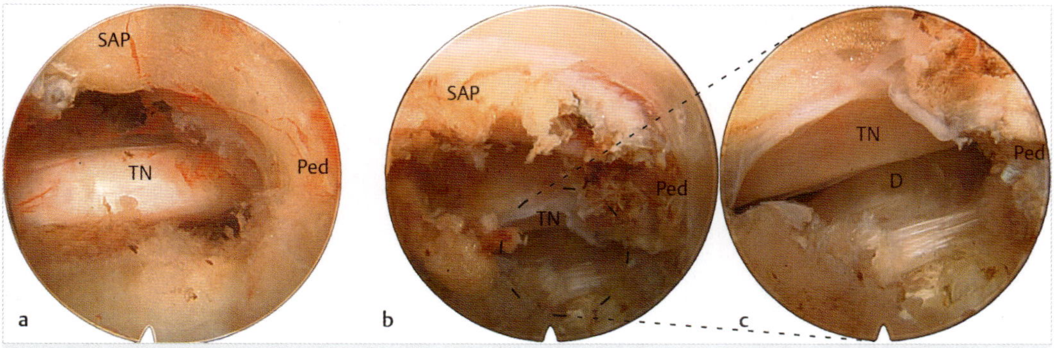

Fig. 49.2 Left-sided transforaminal decompression for central disc herniation. **(a)** Transforaminal view of the SAP, pedicle, and traversing nerve with the ligamentum flavum removed. **(b)** Left transforaminal view before discectomy. **(c)** View before discectomy with the endoscope advanced to show anterior pathology. D, disc; Ped, pedicle; SAP, superior articulating process; TN, traversing nerve.

nerve root has been decompressed from the medial aspect of the caudal pedicle to the lateral aspect of the SAP.[4,5]

- **Interlaminar approach**[3]:
  - As with any endoscopic spine approaches, the approach angle is extremely important. Initially, an endplate view of the caudal vertebral body is obtained on AP fluoroscopy. The interlaminar window is optimized by adding approximately 0 to 5 degrees of caudal C-arm tilt in the upper lumbar segments and approximately 10 to 15 degrees in the lower lumbar segments. This maneuver utilizes the patient's interlaminar window and centers the interlaminar corridor over the disc space.[6] A blunt-tipped tissue dilator is advanced under fluoroscopy until it reaches the target edge of the lamina (▸ Fig. 49.3). Serial dilation is performed until the final working tube is resting on the inferior medial edge of the rostral lamina. The endoscope is brought in and soft tissue resection/cautery is done to expose the bony lamina edge. The ligamentum flavum is removed by drilling along its attachment to the ventral surface of the rostral lamina. Once the ligamentum flavum has been removed, it is important to identify the epidural fat and the lateral edge of the thecal sac. In most cases, the outer working tube can be utilized to retract the traversing nerve medially to isolate the disc fragment and annular defect. Once the decompression is complete, the traversing nerve should be visibly free of compression at the shoulder and axilla (▸ Fig. 49.4).[4]

49.7 Postoperative Care

- Patients should be followed up in 2 weeks for a routine wound check. Patients should refrain from heavy lifting, pushing, or pulling, and avoid forceful bending or twisting for 6 weeks.

49.8 Complications

- Although rare, a durotomy can occur when grasping fragments of disc, using the burr, or taking bites with the Kerrison rongeurs; therefore, it is imperative to always view the tip of the instrument and to slowly resect fragments to ensure that the dura is not adherent.
- If a durotomy occurs, it can often by remedied by using a dural substitute to plug the defect, followed by applying fibrin sealant through the tubular retractor, just prior to removal at the end of the case.[7]

49.9 Management Pearls

- Different approaches in endoscopic spine surgery often share similar principles, and many pathologies treated with a transforaminal approach may also be accessible through an interlaminar approach. See ▸ Fig. 49.5 for target

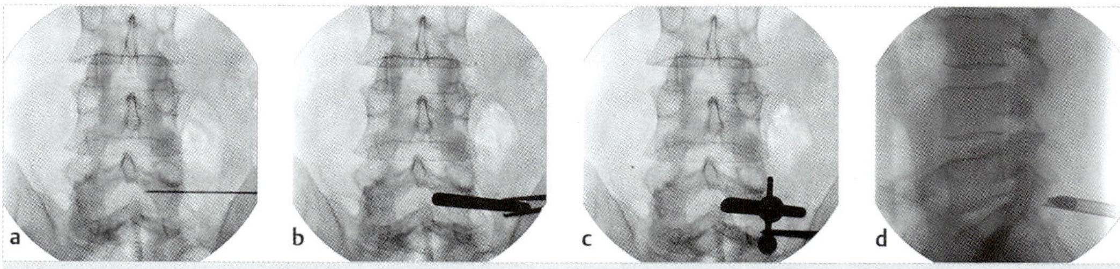

Fig. 49.3 Localization for a right-sided interlaminar approach to L4–L5. **(a)** Placement of localizing spinal needle. **(b–d)** Placement of sequential tubular retractors.

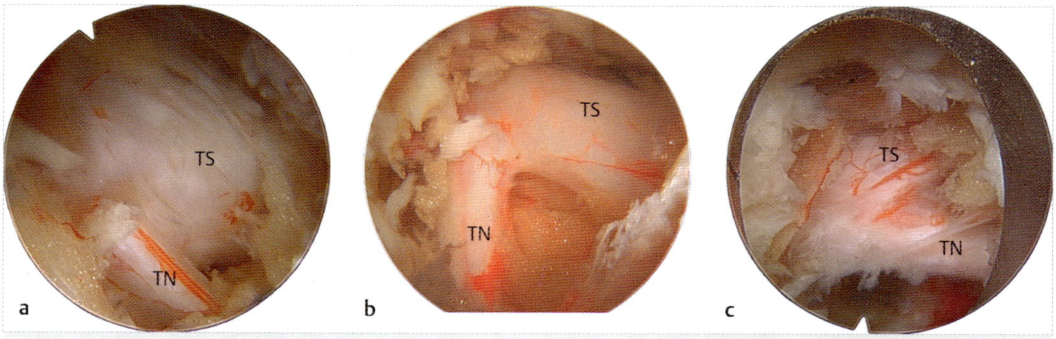

Fig. 49.4 Left-sided interlaminar decompression. **(a)** View prior to decompression. **(b, c)** Views after decompression. TN, traversing nerve root; TS, thecal sac.

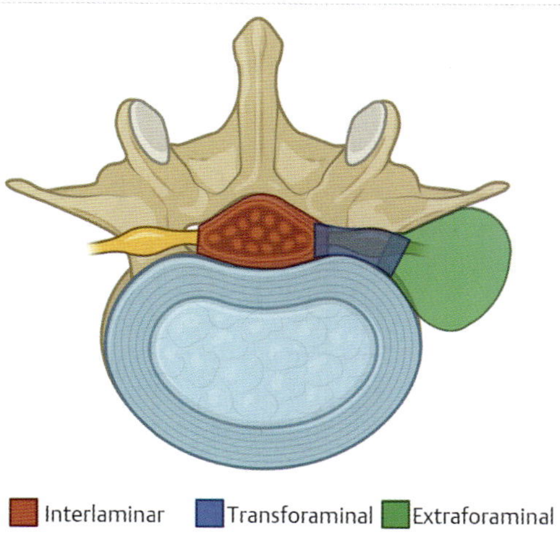

Fig. 49.5 Areas of pathology that can be addressed by interlaminar and transforaminal endoscopic spine approaches.

regions for various endoscopic spine approaches. Decreased morbidity and improved recovery are benefits of all endoscopic spine approaches when applied to the correct patients.

- Owing to decreased morbidity of endoscopic spine surgery approaches, patients are able to mobilize and recover rapidly after surgery.
- It is critical to have a comprehensive understanding of the anatomy, specifically with regard to the patient's pathology, in order to best choose the optimal approach and minimize risk of nerve injury.
- During transforaminal approaches, caution must be exercised to avoid injury to the exiting nerve root. Neuromonitoring should be used to help identify when the exiting nerve is being irritated. Docking onto the SAP and partial resection of the lateral aspect of the SAP can often mitigate this risk. The surgeon should

always be aware of the direction of the bevel opening to avoid inadvertent injury to the exiting nerve root.

- During interlaminar approaches, the surgeon should maintain constant awareness of the edge of the working tube to avoid inadvertent injury to the nerves or thecal sac. Using the working tube as a nerve root retractor can be quite useful but requires clear identification of the lateral edge of the traversing nerve root as well as mobilization of the traversing nerve root medially. Care should be taken to avoid excessive and prolonged traction on the traversing nerve root to avoid injury.

References

[1] Ahn Y. Endoscopic spine discectomy: indications and outcomes. Int Orthop. 2019; 43(4):909–916

[2] Hasan S, Härtl R, Hofstetter CP. The benefit zone of full-endoscopic spine surgery. J Spine Surg. 2019; 5 Suppl 1:S41–S56

[3] Hofstetter CP, Ahn Y, Choi G, et al. AOSpine consensus paper on nomenclature for working-channel endoscopic spinal procedures. Global Spine J. 2020; 10(2) Suppl:111S–121S

[4] Hofstetter C, Ruetten S, Zhou Y, Wang M. Atlas of Full-Endoscopic Spine Surgery. 1st ed. New York, NY: Thieme; 2019

[5] Khandge AV, Sharma SB, Kim JS. The evolution of transforaminal endoscopic spine surgery. World Neurosurg. 2021; 145:643–656

[6] Shepard NA, Protopsaltis T, Kim Y. Lumbar endoscopic spine surgery: a comprehensive review. Bull Hosp Jt Dis. 2021; 79(1):35–42

[7] Sivakanthan S, Hasan S, Hofstetter C. Full-endoscopic lumbar discectomy. Neurosurg Clin N Am. 2020; 31(1):1–7

50 Interlaminar

Harmon S. Khela, Hasan S. Ahmad, Yohannes Ghenbot, and Jang Won Yoon

50.1 Background

- Interlaminar endoscopic spine surgery is a versatile minimally invasive technique that can be used to address a wide variety of spinal pathologies such as central, paracentral, or foraminal disc herniation, spinal stenosis with and without instability (interlaminar lumbar interbody fusion can be utilized here), facet joint synovial cysts, and even epidural abscess evacuation.
- Interlaminar routes for discectomy, decompression, or fusion are especially advantageous at the L5–S1 level due to the iliac crest hindering transforaminal access.
- Under intraoperative fluoroscopic guidance, surgeons can create a small skin incision at the level of the interlaminar window, enter the epidural space through the ligamentum flavum, retract the traversing nerve root, and approach the pathology for surgical intervention.
- It can be used to treat most lumbar, as well as many cervical and thoracic, pathologies including disc herniations, central/lateral recess stenosis, synovial cyst rupture, foraminal stenosis, and lumbar spondylolisthesis.
- With limited collateral tissue damage, this technique can potentially allow for a more favorable approach than open discectomies of the spine.
- It began as an alternate approach to transforaminal endoscopic lumbar discectomy (TELD), especially in patients with anatomical obstruction by the iliac crest at the L5–S1 level.[1,2,3,4,5,6] At this level, the interlaminar window is large enough to allow the discectomy to be completed without drilling of any bony structures (lamina, facet joints), which are typically partially removed in a traditional open decompression or TELD.
- As the development of endoscopic instruments progressed, interlaminar endoscopic lumbar discectomy (IELD) also became a valuable technique for decompressions when the herniated disc is significantly migrated, or the herniated disc itself is large enough to occupy a majority of the spinal canal, as full visualization and disc removal with TELD may be difficult in these situations and can lead to neural injury.[7,8,9,10,11,12]
- Postoperatively, multiple studies have found that, for the most part, objective and patient-reported surgical outcomes, recovery time, and frequency of adverse events are relatively similar between interlaminar and transforaminal endoscopic techniques.[13,14,15,16,17] However, some reports indicate longer operative time and greater intraoperative radiation exposure with TELD compared to IELD.[14,16,17]
- More recently, interlaminar approaches have also been used for decompression with instrumented fusion, synovial cyst resection, and epidural abscess evacuation.[18,19,20]

50.2 Indications and Contraindications

- It is indicated for the treatment of sequestered or nonsequestered lumbar disc herniations at all levels (most advantageous at the L5–S1 level), a large or highly migrated lumbar disc herniation that comprises more than half the spinal canal at any level, recurrent disc herniations after initial endoscopic operations, lumbar canal and lateral recess stenoses, calcified discs, foraminal pathologies, and ruptured synovial cysts.[21,22]
- Interlaminar endoscopic spine techniques can be especially advantageous for evacuating epidural abscesses, as reduced tissue disruption can decrease the risk of secondary wound dehiscence or direct tissue extension of the infection.[20] Endoscopic surgery including the interlaminar approach can also be helpful in patients undergoing revision after prior posterior spine surgery, as an interlaminar channel can avoid the effects of adhesions and iatrogenic instability.
- Interlaminar endoscopy is relatively contraindicated in the cases where there may be compressive foraminal pathologies, extreme central spinal canal stenoses, severe fibrotic adhesions from prior surgery and prior history of CSF leak/pseudomeningocele, multisegmental

stenosis, emergent cauda equina syndrome, and multilevel spinal infection with neurological compromise.[21,22]

50.3 Instruments

- Endoscopy camera and tower, interlaminar endoscope, blunt dissector, micropunch, pituitary rongeur, C-arm, radiofrequency tissue ablator, Kerrison rongeur, burr, Wilson frame (decompression), open Jackson table (fusion), tissue dilator, beveled working channel, dissector (short and long tips), retractable nerve root probe, endoscopic scissors, endoscopic grasper, and endoscopic drills.

50.4 Patient Preparation

- Routine preoperative workup is required to properly select patients undergoing spine endoscopy.
- Spine imaging (magnetic resonance imaging [MRI], computed tomography [CT], X-rays) should be obtained prior to surgery.
- For far lateral disc herniations causing exiting nerve root compression, a diagnostic injection can sometimes be helpful in identifying the pain generator.

50.5 Patient Positioning

- Interlaminar endoscopic spine surgery is generally performed with the patient lying in the prone position while being provided local, epidural, or general anesthesia.

50.6 Technique

- Create an 8-mm incision through the skin and lumbar fascia above the interlaminar window on the ipsilateral side.
- Insert a dilator at a slight medial angle to locate the inferomedial laminar edge. Verify that the tip of the dilator is located at the appropriate level using fluoroscopy.
- Insert subsequent dilators onto this location followed by the introduction of a beveled working tube, with the open side of the tube facing medially. The endoscope should then be introduced into this working tube and fluoroscopy can be utilized to confirm correct placement of the working tube.
- Once the endoscope has been inserted, the radiofrequency ablator and pituitary rongeurs can be used to dissect tissue until the ligamentum flavum has been identified. At this point, a laminotomy and/or medial facetectomy may be required depending on the lumbar level or if it is a posterolateral disc herniation.
- Once the ligamentum flavum has been clearly identified, the micropunch can be used to cut through the ligamentum flavum from the midline to the medial part of the facet joint. Epidural fat should then appear, which should then be removed to successfully locate the thecal sac and traversing nerve root.
- Identify the lateral border of the traversing nerve root and use the working sleeve to mobilize the neural elements medially. The working sleeve can be rotated clockwise or counterclockwise 180 degrees such that the long end of the bevel shields the nerve root medially.
- Disc pathologies (e.g., herniation, degeneration) should now be visible, and the appropriate surgery (e.g., discectomy, fusion) can be executed. Discectomy can be achieved using a pituitary rongeur to perform an annulotomy. For sequestered lumbar disc herniations, fragments may be readily visible and can be removed with pituitaries.
- After successful surgery, ensure that there is no significant free disc tissue, bleeding, or dural sac damage. Once hemostasis has been achieved, remove the endoscopic system and close the skin with standard sutures.
- For a visual demonstration of a single-level endoscopic TLIF using fluoroscopy-based instrument tracking, see **Video 50.1**.

50.7 Postoperative Care

- For routine IELD without intraoperative complications, patients should return for a routine postoperative clinic visit 4 to 6 weeks after surgery.
- For those who required instrumentation or interbody fusion, longer follow-up may be needed with X-rays and CT scans at regular intervals.

50.8 Complications

- Potential complications of interlaminar endoscopy include traversing nerve root irritation, dural tears, epidural hematomas, untreated pain, motor weakness, and surgical site infections.
- Exiting nerve roots can be aggravated if the working sleeve and serial dilators do not carefully contact the nerve, which can lead to severe pain, neural injury, postoperative dysesthesia, or other neurological complications.
- During tissue dissection and subsequent discectomy, an intraoperative dural tear may occur and not be detected, largely due to the continuous irrigation associated with endoscopic surgery.
- Although rare when compared to open surgery, surgical site infections (e.g., epidural abscess or discitis) may occur in interlaminar endoscopy, which places patients at a risk of postoperative spondylodiscitis and associated back pain, radicular pain, wound swelling, etc.
- Continuous irrigation with preventive antibiotics and the maintenance of sterility in the operating room can help preclude these issues.
- Additionally, the sheer pressure of the irrigation fluid in endoscopy may elevate epidural pressure and lead to vascular complications, such as epidural hematomas; however, postoperative epidural hematomas are relatively uncommon in interlaminar endoscopy compared to open surgery and can be self-limiting or subclinical in many cases.
- Although there is a learning curve that surgeons must overcome to avoid complications during endoscopic treatment, the accumulation of operative experience and improvement in surgical skill and technical proficiency can substantially improve patient outcomes and prevent such issues.

50.9 Management Pearls

- There is currently no formal certification process for interlaminar endoscopic spine surgery through a national or an international professional organization, nor is there a dedicated educational curriculum endorsed by neurosurgical or orthopaedic societies. Since spinal endoscopy is a relatively new technique that is being embraced by minimally invasive spine surgeons within the United States, there are only few academic centers and fellowship programs around the country that offer spinal endoscopy as a part of their educational curriculum. Most spine endoscopists have learned the technique on their own by partaking in cadaver courses being offered at national meetings or at industry-sponsored courses. There are also informal shadowing and observership opportunities offered at certain institutions. There is a clear need for the development of a formal educational curriculum so that the residency and fellowship programs can integrate spine endoscopy into their neurosurgical and/or orthopaedic training.
- There are limited reports in peer-reviewed literature comparing interlaminar endoscopic spine surgery with traditional open spine surgery, though available studies indicate endoscopic techniques were noninferior to open surgery when evaluating subjective postoperative pain, quality of life, and functional status.[23,24]
- Endoscopic techniques such as interlaminar approaches to the spine have also been compared to other traditional minimally invasive spine techniques (i.e., tubular), with recent reports indicating reduced risk of surgical site infections in endoscopic surgeries.[25]

References

[1] Kambin P, Sampson S. Posterolateral percutaneous suction-excision of herniated lumbar intervertebral discs. Report of interim results. Clin Orthop Relat Res. 1986; 207:37–43

[2] Mathews HH. Transforaminal endoscopic microdiscectomy. Neurosurg Clin N Am. 1996; 7(1):59–63

[3] Reulen HJ, Müller A, Ebeling U. Microsurgical anatomy of the lateral approach to extraforaminal lumbar disc herniations. Neurosurgery. 1996; 39(2):345–350, discussion 350–351

[4] Ebraheim NA, Xu R, Huntoon M, Yeasting RA. Location of the extraforaminal lumbar nerve roots. An anatomic study. Clin Orthop Relat Res. 1997; 340:230–235

[5] Choi G, Lee SH, Raiturker PP, Lee S, Chae YS. Percutaneous endoscopic interlaminar discectomy for intracanalicular disc herniations at L5-S1 using a rigid working channel endoscope. Neurosurgery. 2006; 58(1) Suppl:ONS59–ONS68, discussion ONS59–ONS68

[6] Ruetten S, Komp M, Godolias G. A New full-endoscopic technique for the interlaminar operation of lumbar disc herniations using 6-mm endoscopes: prospective 2-year results of 331 patients. Minim Invasive Neurosurg. 2006; 49(2):80–87

[7] Kim CH, Chung CK, Woo JW. Surgical outcome of percutaneous endoscopic interlaminar lumbar discectomy for highly migrated disk herniation. Clin Spine Surg. 2016; 29(5):E259–E266

[8] Kim CH, Chung CK, Jahng TA, Yang HJ, Son YJ. Surgical outcome of percutaneous endoscopic interlaminar lumbar diskectomy for recurrent disk herniation after open diskectomy. J Spinal Disord Tech. 2012; 25(5):E125–E133

[9] Khandge AV, Kim JS. Modified interlaminar endoscopic lumbar discectomy for highly upmigrated disc herniation: a proctorship description of the technique via translaminar route. Neurospine. 2020; 17 Suppl 1:S66–S73

[10] Choi KC, Lee DC, Shim HK, Shin SH, Park CK. A strategy of percutaneous endoscopic lumbar discectomy for migrated disc herniation. World Neurosurg. 2017; 99:259–266

[11] Choi KC, Kim JS, Ryu KS, Kang BU, Ahn Y, Lee SH. Percutaneous endoscopic lumbar discectomy for L5-S1 disc herniation: transforaminal versus interlaminar approach. Pain Physician. 2013; 16(6):547–556

[12] Lee S, Kim SK, Lee SH, et al. Percutaneous endoscopic lumbar discectomy for migrated disc herniation: classification of disc migration and surgical approaches. Eur Spine J. 2007; 16(3): 431–437

[13] Huang Y, Yin J, Sun Z, et al. Percutaneous endoscopic lumbar discectomy for LDH via a transforaminal approach versus an interlaminar approach: a meta-analysis. Orthopade. 2020; 49(4):338–349

[14] Wu R, Liao X, Xia H. Radiation exposure to the surgeon during ultrasound-assisted transforaminal percutaneous endoscopic lumbar discectomy: a prospective study. World Neurosurg. 2017; 101:658–665.e1

[15] Nie H, Zeng J, Song Y, et al. Percutaneous endoscopic lumbar discectomy for L5-S1 disc herniation via an interlaminar approach versus a transforaminal approach: a prospective randomized controlled study with 2-year follow up. Spine. 2016; 41 Suppl 19:B30–B37

[16] Gao A, Yang H, Zhu L, et al. Comparison of interlaminar and transforaminal approaches for treatment of L_5/S_1 disc herniation by percutaneous endoscopic discectomy. Orthop Surg. 2021; 13(1):63–70

[17] Jitpakdee K, Liu Y, Kotheeranurak V, Kim JS. Transforaminal versus interlaminar endoscopic lumbar discectomy for lumbar disc herniation: a systematic review and meta-analysis. Global Spine J. 2023; 13(2):575–587

[18] Nakajima Y, Takaoki K, Akahori S, Motomura A, Ohara Y. A review of fully endoscopic lumbar interbody fusion. Journal of Minimally Invasive Spine Surgery and Technique. 2023; 8(2):177–185

[19] Hellinger S, Lewandrowski KU. Clinical outcomes with endoscopic resection of lumbar extradural cysts. J Spine Surg. 2020; 6 Suppl 1:S133–S144

[20] Ghenbot Y, Arena J, Wathen C, et al. Endoscopic-assisted evacuation of lumbar epidural abscess: 2-dimensional operative video. Oper Neurosurg (Hagerstown). 2024; 26 6:754

[21] Ruetten S. The full-endoscopic interlaminar approach for lumbar disc herniations. In: Mayer HM, eds. Minimally Invasive Spine Surgery. Berlin: Springer-Verlag; 2006: 346–355

[22] Wagner R, Haefner M. Indications and contraindications of full-endoscopic interlaminar lumbar decompression. World Neurosurg. 2021; 145:657–662

[23] Gadjradj PS, Rubinstein SM, Peul WC, et al. Full endoscopic versus open discectomy for sciatica: randomised controlled non-inferiority trial. BMJ. 2022; 376:e065846

[24] Page PS, Ammanuel SG, Josiah DT. Evaluation of endoscopic versus open lumbar discectomy: a multi-center retrospective review utilizing the American College of Surgeons' National Surgical Quality Improvement Program (ACS-NSQIP) Database. Cureus. 2022; 14(5):e25202

[25] Mahan MA, Prasse T, Kim RB, et al. Full-endoscopic spine surgery diminishes surgical site infections: a propensity score-matched analysis. Spine J. 2023; 23(5):695–702

Part V

Stereotactic and Functional Neurosurgery

V

51 Frame-Based Stereotactic Radiosurgery

Prateek Agarwal, Anthony J. Schulien, Joseph Hudson, Ajay Niranjan, and L. Dade Lunsford

51.1 Background

- Frame-based stereotactic radiosurgery (SRS), more commonly known as frame-based Gamma Knife radiosurgery, is used to treat brain tumors, both primary and metastatic, vascular malformations, and functional or pain disorders.
- Primary brain tumors that can be treated with Gamma Knife include vestibular schwannomas, meningiomas, pituitary adenomas, and craniopharyngiomas, among others. High-grade glioma may also be considered for treatment if progression occurs despite standard of care with surgical resection and conventional chemoradiation.[1]
- Vascular malformations amendable to treatment with Gamma Knife include arteriovenous malformations (AVMs), dural arteriovenous fistulas (dAVFs), and cerebral cavernous malformations. It is important to note that AVMs and dAVFs cannot be treated with frameless SRS, given the requirement to obtain images from a cerebral angiogram that is defined in stereotactic space using the Leksell Coordinate Frame G.[2]
- Functional or pain disorders that can be treated with Gamma Knife include trigeminal neuralgia, movement disorders such as essential tremor, and treatment-resistant epilepsy.[3,4,5]

51.2 Indications and Contraindications

- Frame-based SRS can be employed to treat many intracranial pathologies as outlined above. However, the advent of frameless technologies that improve patient comfort necessitates appropriately tailored indications. We have already noted that treatment of AVMs and dAVFs requires frame placement.
- The need for precision with solid cranial fixation due to the location of targets near critical structures is another important reason to use frame-based SRS. Such targets may include sellar or clinoidal lesions near the optic nerves, cerebellopontine angle targets adjacent to the brainstem and cranial nerves, and the thalamic ventral intermediate nucleus near sensorimotor fibers of the internal capsule.
- Other key reasons to use frame-based SRS are length of single treatment session greater than 30 minutes and patients factors such as anxiety, claustrophobia, or cognitive issues. Frameless SRS using a thermoplastic mask necessitates that patients remain as immobile as possible for precise targeting, which is generally not possible in our experience beyond approximately 30 minutes or for patients with aforementioned issues.
- One of the few, if only, absolute contraindications to frame-based SRS are targets that are located below the base of the coordinate Frame G, generally at the level of the C2 odontoid process. More relative contraindications include multisession treatment and extensive cranial defects that preclude four points of fixation.

51.3 Informed Consent

- As per ethical guidelines, the primary surgeon will confirm that the patient has the cognitive capacity to make informed decisions for their medical care; if not, they will find the legal representative for the patient and disclose all risks and benefits associated with the procedure, including the operative procedures, goals for the operation, and potential peri- and postoperative complications.

51.4 Instruments

- Standard equipment for frame placement includes the Leksell Coordinate Frame G with four fixed posts, bilateral ear bars with sliding adaptors, frame pin set, pin wrenches, and local anesthetic loaded in two 10-mL syringes. In our institutional practice, we have found it most efficient to use ear bars with sliding adaptors to position the frame symmetrically. Unless limited by the patient's shoulders or short neck, we place the ear bars in the uppermost hole of the sliding adaptors to lower the frame as caudally as possible. We also use angled anterior posts, as we have found they best allow for pin placement at the level of the superior temporal line. More recently, the Leksell Vantage (known as the "blue frame") system can be used with the recent generation Gamma Knife technologies. This composite material has reduced imaging artifact and has both magnetic resonance imaging (MRI) and computed tomography (CT) fiducial systems. The blue frame cannot be used for cases that require angiography.

51.5 Patient Preparation

- In order to use Gamma Knife radiosurgery, the appropriate imaging must be obtained and defined in stereotactic space. While this usually involves obtaining an MRI of the brain after frame placement and fiducial box application, the latest Leksell Gama Knife ICON and Esprit systems from Elekta allow for definition of the brain stereotactic space by obtaining a cone beam computed tomography (CBCT) scan. As mentioned above, treatment of AVMs and dAVFs requires a stereotactic cerebral angiogram.
- In order to ensure patient comfort and compliance, frame placement for SRS requires the use of both conscious sedation and local anesthetic. Our institution uses a combination of intravenous midazolam and fentanyl to achieve adequate conscious sedation while simultaneously monitoring heart rate, blood pressure, and oxygen saturation. Approximately 5 mL of local anesthetic is also injected at each of the pin sites.

51.6 Patient Positioning

- The patient is positioned sitting up near 90 degrees with a pillow placed between the shoulder blades to create space between the cranium and the stretcher. Mild intravenous sedation is administered. For most cases, we initially place the sliding ear bar adaptors at 95 mm to center the G frame in the anteroposterior axis. The frame is lowered over the cranium with the curved side facing anteriorly by two individuals standing on either side of the patient. The ear bars are advanced into the external auditory canal bilaterally and adjusted to achieve symmetry in the lateral–medial axis.

51.7 Technique

- While supporting the frame with one hand, approximately 5 mL of local anesthetic is injected to create a wheal at each of the pin entry sites at the level of the superior temporal line. Pin lengths are then chosen based on approximate scalp thickness and distance between the skin and the outer aspect of the fixed posts. Pins are inserted by hand first until the sharp tip engages the skin, with care taken not to cross-thread. Then, pin wrenches are used to tighten the pins across from each other simultaneously. After the four pins are tightened, the frame is gently lifted to confirm adequate fixation, indicated by the cranium and frame moving together.
- Frame cap and the adaptor to dock to the Gamma Knife couch are placed to verify adequate fit. Skull bubble measurements are taken, which serve as a backup to skull measurements calculated from MRI/CT images. The heights of the four fixed posts are measured along with the distance that pins protrude from the outer aspect of the posts, which serve as a backup to the frame cap fitting. At this point, the patient is ready for necessary preparatory imaging.
- There are two important considerations to bear in mind during frame application. First, the surgeon must avoid any cranial defects, cranioplasties, or shunts when placing pins, which may require shifting frame location or using one or two short fixed posterior posts. Second, the surgeon must think critically about adjusting the frame depending on the location of brain targets to avoid collisions with the internal frame cap. Targets anterior to the pituitary fossa often require using short fixed posterior posts or shifting the frame anteriorly by moving the sliding ear bar adaptors posteriorly. Analogously, extremely posterior targets often require shifting the frame posteriorly by moving the sliding ear bar adaptors anteriorly. One can also shift the frame in the lateral–medial axis (**Video 51.1**).
- After G frame placement is complete and cranial imaging is obtained, the Gamma Knife treatment may be planned. Typically, MRI or digital subtraction angiography (DSA)—in the case of AVM treatment—is completed following frame

placement, to allow for stereotactic co-registration of the frame fiducials with MRI. In the cases where a recent and adequate MRI is available, a CBCT scan can be performed to co-register with a prior MRI. When relevant images have been uploaded to Leksell GammaPlan software, a unique patient chart and treatment date is created. MRI/DSA imaging is then uploaded, and each sequence is co-registered to the stereotactic reference frame. Next, a dose matrix containing the pathology to be treated may be created and relevant volumes can be defined for both irradiation targets and eloquent anatomy for which the surgeon wishes to limit dose to.

- Gamma Knife treatments can be planned on Leksell GammaPlan software utilizing two different theoretical strategies: (1) manual planning or (2) inverse/automatic planning. Manual planning refers to the surgeon placing individually chosen radiation shots from 4-, 8-, or 16-mm collimators in the dose matrix and building an isodose falloff that appropriately treats the target pathology while sparing nearby eloquent structures. To complete a manual plan, individual shots are placed, and an isodose line is automatically calculated that displays the whole treatment in stereotactic space. Advantages of manual planning include advanced control over shot placement and typically reduced treatment time given the relative simplicity of this planning method. Manual planning is effective for small, spherical lesions, such as metastases, and may be less advantageous for complex and irregularly shaped lesions. Inverse planning refers to an automatically generated plan that GammaPlan calculates relative to the surgeon defining the lesional volume that they wish to treat. To complete a reverse plan, the surgeon manually defines an outline of each slice of lesion or tissue to be treated with a "paintbrush" or "pencil" tool, then defines a marginal dose (Gy) and the program computes an ideal plan based on the lesion volume, with an automatically generated isodose. Advantages of the inverse plan include ease of use, treatment of complex or irregularly shaped lesions, and the ability to automatically limit dose to eloquent anatomical structures. This planning method allows selection of "hazard" volumes that can be fine-tuned to limit radiation dose to these defined structures.

Table 51.1 Common prescription isodoses for common pathologies

Pathology	Typical marginal prescription (Gy)
Meningioma	12–14
Vestibular schwannoma	12–12.5
Trigeminal neuralgia	40 (80-Gy central dose)
Arteriovenous malformation	18–22
Metastatic brain tumors	16–20
Nonfunctioning pituitary adenoma	12–14
Functional pituitary adenoma	14–25 (based on relationship to optic system)

- Several common pathologies that are managed with Gamma Knife SRS include meningiomas, vestibular schwannomas, AVMs, metastatic brain tumors, and trigeminal neuralgia cases. While prescription isodose recommendations are impacted by lesion size and vicinity to eloquent surrounding structures, general dose ranges for common lesions are overviewed in ▶ Table 51.1.

51.8 Postoperative Care

- Postoperatively, the frame is removed by using the pin wrench to unscrew all four pins. Once the frame is removed, gentle pressure with gauze is held over the pin sites for minor bleeding. Rarely a suture may be needed for pin sites near an arterial branch. Band-aids are placed at each of the pin sites and the head is wrapped with Kerlix gauze. In the relatively rare event that pulsatile arterial bleeding is encountered upon pin removal, a simple absorbable figure-of-eight or purse-string stitch may be placed.

51.9 Complications

- Potential complications and special risks associated with frame-based SRS as opposed to

frameless SRS are related to pin placement. These include frame dislodgment with possible pin laceration, ventricular shunt perforation, cranial vault penetration through defect, cranioplasty deformation, and pin site infection.[6]
- In our 43-year institutional experience over 25,000 frame-based procedures, we have only had two complications related to frame application, one delayed frame dislodgement and one cranial vault penetration via an unrecognized burr hole.

51.10 Management Pearls

- Frame-based SRS is critical for treatment of AVMs/dAVFs, targets near critical structures, treatment sessions greater than 30 minutes, and patients who are unable to remain relatively immobile.
- Contraindications to frame-based SRS include targets below the base of the frame (i.e., approximately at the level of the C2 odontoid process), multisession treatment, and extensive cranial defects.
- Important considerations during frame application include avoiding cranial defects, cranioplasties, or shunts when placing pins and shifting frame location or using short fixed posterior posts depending on target location to avoid collisions.

51.11 Emerging Technologies

- The main two variants to frame-based SRS are thermoplastic mask-based Gamma Knife radiosurgery using the ICON or ESPRIT system and frameless SRS systems using linear particle accelerator (LINAC) technology, such as CyberKnife. Although patient comfort may be superior with these variants, there are certain features of frame-based SRS that render it more appropriate for many indications.

References

[1] Niranjan A, Monaco EA, III, Kano H, Flickinger JC, Lunsford LD. Stereotactic radiosurgery in the multimodality management of residual or recurrent glioblastoma multiforme. Prog Neurol Surg. 2018; 31:48–61

[2] Lunsford LD, Niranjan A, Kano H, Kondziolka D. The technical evolution of Gamma Knife radiosurgery for arteriovenous malformations. Prog Neurol Surg. 2013; 27:22–34

[3] Kondziolka D, Flickinger JC, Lunsford LD. Stereotactic radiosurgery for epilepsy and functional disorders. Neurosurg Clin N Am. 2013; 24(4):623–632

[4] Mureb M, Golub D, Benjamin C, et al. Earlier radiosurgery leads to better pain relief and less medication usage for trigeminal neuralgia patients: an international multicenter study. J Neurosurg. 2020; 135(1):237–244

[5] Niranjan A, Raju SS, Kooshkabadi A, Monaco E, III, Flickinger JC, Lunsford LD. Stereotactic radiosurgery for essential tremor: retrospective analysis of a 19-year experience. Mov Disord. 2017; 32(5):769–777

[6] Safaee M, Burke J, McDermott MW. Techniques for the application of stereotactic head frames based on a 25-year experience. Cureus. 2016; 8(3):e543

52 Frameless Gamma Knife Stereotactic Radiosurgery

Alexandros Bouras, Daniel Rivera, Sakibul Huq, Greg Bednarz, Serah Choi, John C. Flickinger Sr, L. Dade Lunsford, Ajay Niranjan, and Constantinos G. Hadjipanayis

52.1 Background

- Gamma Knife stereotactic radiosurgery (GKSRS) involves the use of a Gamma Knife, which is a specialized neurosurgical device that delivers conformal high dose of radiation to a precise anatomical location in the brain. "Frameless" refers to the fact that instead of using a stereotactic guiding device (frame) that is attached to the patient's head (with fixation pins) during treatment, this approach uses a thermoplastic mask molded to the patient's head and coupled to the head cradle and then affixed to the patient positioning system. In combination with advanced imaging technology (cone beam computed tomography [CBCT] image guidance), a 3D map of the patient's skull and brain is created in order to accurately (on the order of 0.1–0.5 mm) position the patient's head and target the radiation to the lesion of interest.[1] This allows for extreme precision and accuracy in treating intracranial lesions, while also minimizing the side effects that can occur with traditional open surgery or other forms of conventional fractionated radiation therapy.[2] This form of securing the head during GKSRS offers certain advantages over frame-based immobilization in properly selected patients. Understanding the principles of frameless fixation can improve patient workflow and comfort, without compromising patient outcomes and safety.[1]
- Frame-based and frameless GKSRS are two approaches used to deliver highly precise radiosurgery to the brain. Frame-based GKSRS uses a head frame to provide stereotactic precision and to stabilize the patient's head during the procedure, which is secured to the patient's outer table of the skull using titanium pins. Frameless GKSRS does not use a head frame. Instead, a thermoplastic mask with head support is used to immobilize the patient's head during the procedure and a CBCT scan is used to provide stereotactic coordinates. Movement of the patient's head within the immobilization mask is tracked during treatment and the treatment is given (gated) only if the head position is within prescribed limits.[1]
- Both frame-based and frameless GKSRS have their advantages and disadvantages.[2] Frame-based GKSRS is potentially more precise than frameless GKSRS since the head frame rigidly attaches to the head and thereby virtually eliminates the risk of target movement during the procedure.[1,3]
- However, some patients may find the head frame uncomfortable in the absence of mild sedation, and preexisting surgical cranial defects may preclude four-point frame pin placement.[2] Frameless GKSRS is more tolerable for patients who are not claustrophobic since the mask covers the face. Head movement is monitored continuously by cameras, which track the position of a reflective marker on the tip of the nose. When the system detects the movement of this marker beyond a user-set threshold (typically 1–1.5 mm), the radiation beams (Co-60 radiation sources) are retracted, and the treatment is paused.[4] The treatment resumes when the system indicates that the marker is again within the set limits. If the marker position remains beyond the set limits and the preset time, the beams remain retracted, the robotic patient couch returns to its base, and the radiation shielding doors close. In order to resume the treatment, a new positioning CBCT is performed, the remaining planned treatment is co-registered to the new CBCT head coordinates, and treatment is restarted.[5,6] Additionally, in the cases where two to five sessions of multifraction GKSRS are required, frameless GKSRS is preferred due to the ability to easily reuse the mask, reduced treatment times per session, and increased patient comfort.

52.2 Indications and Contraindications

52.2.1 Indications

- Both frameless and frame-based GKSRS can be effective treatment options for certain neurological disorders.[7]
  - Benign brain tumors such as meningiomas, pituitary adenomas, vestibular schwannomas, and craniopharyngiomas.[7,8]
  - Malignant brain tumors including metastases and primary brain tumors such as glioblastomas, and other gliomas.[7]
  - Vascular malformations such as arteriovenous malformations (AVMs), cavernous malformations, and dural arteriovenous fistulas.[1]
- Even though both frame-based and frameless GKSRS can be used to treat the above disorders, there are some indications for when frameless GKSRS may be preferred over frame-based GKSRS:
  - *Patient preference:* Some patients may prefer frameless GKSRS as it does not require the attachment of a rigid frame to the skull, which can be uncomfortable and may not be tolerated by some patients since it typically requires local anesthesia and intravenous (IV) sedation.
  - *Fractionated GKSRS:* There is growing evidence supporting the use of multiple sessions of multifraction GKSRS in several instances (e.g., large meningiomas and multiple brain metastases, larger postoperative surgical resection cavities, reirradiation of brain metastases that previously underwent SRS, and tumors adjacent to the optic nerves/chiasm). In these instances, mask-based GKSRS is preferred due to the more favorable balance of tumor control and treatment toxicity that multifraction SRS provides compared to single-fraction SRS.[9,10]
  - Patients who have large head circumference, or skull deformities, which preclude frame-based GKSRS.[2]

52.2.2 Contraindications

- The contraindications for frameless GKSRS may include the following:
  - Inability to tolerate the thermoplastic mask, which can cause discomfort or claustrophobia.[4]
  - When GKSRS treatment time is long (typically over 45 minutes), which may be difficult for the patient to tolerate the mask and may likely require multiple repositioning CBCTs. This situation may arise when multiple tumors need to be treated during the same GKSRS treatment session.[4]
  - Inaccurate imaging due to patient motion or movement of the thermoplastic mask during the procedure, which can lead to treatment errors.[4]
  - Tumors or lesions to be treated in a single session of GKSRS, which require more extensive immobilization for precision that is difficult to be achieved with a thermoplastic mask.[5]
  - Certain anatomical structures involving or adjacent to the target lesion, such as the brainstem, which are close to the target area and could be inadvertently affected by the radiation beam with minimal patient motion.[5]
  - Patients who have metal implants or dental fillings in their head or neck, as these can cause image distortions that can affect the accuracy of the treatment.[5]
  - High body mass index (BMI) patients whose weight, short neck, or large chest prevents tracking of the nasal marker as it compares its movement to the positions of the reference reflective markers imbedded in the mask cradle.[5]

    It is important to note that both frame-based and frameless GKSRS have their own advantages and limitations. The choice of the technique should be based on the patient's preferences, lesion characteristics (size, number, shape, location, etc.), and the expertise of the treating team. A comprehensive evaluation by a multidisciplinary team is essential to determine the most appropriate treatment approach for each patient.
  - Some patients with large heads and extremely anterior or posterior targets might be unable to have those targets treated without changing the angle of their head and neck. With a frame-based technique, the gamma angle (angle of the base frame in relation to the angle of the table) can be changed from a

neutral position (at a 90-degree gamma angle) to a hyperextended or flexed position (at a 70- or 110-degree gamma angle) to avoid collision of the machine with the patient's head or frame. With the masked-based frameless technique, the patient's headrest and mask can be remade with the head positioned differently, but it often is more difficult to accomplish than changing the angle with a frame-based treatment setup.

52.3 Instruments

- In addition to personnel, the necessary materials and technology for frameless GKRS typically include the following:
  - *CBCT image guidance:* CBCT allows acquisition of brain imaging while the patient is in a mask. This is done immediately before GKSRS treatment to confirm localization of the head and lesion targeting. Patients can undergo a volumetric magnetic resonance imaging (MRI) scan of diagnostic CT scan prior to mask placement. These images can then be co-registered with the CBCT scan to complete the computer planning.[5]
  - *Radiosurgery delivery system:* This system includes the Gamma Knife technology that uses 192 high-energy gamma rays generated by the decay of cobalt-60 to deliver radiation to a localized target area in the brain.[2]
  - *Computerized treatment planning system:* This system is used to develop and optimize the treatment plan based on the lesion location, patient anatomy, critical structures surrounding the lesion, and tumor characteristics.[2]
  - *Monitoring equipment:* This includes audiovisual devices to visualize and communicate with the patient as well as devices to monitor the patient's vital signs during the procedure.[4]

52.4 Patient Preparation

- The patient's medical record should include the history and physical examination, the patient's functional status, and a description of current performance status, as well as the necessity and frequency of treatment. Documentation should also include the date and treatment dose. A neurosurgeon and a radiation oncologist must evaluate the clinical aspects of the treatment, and document and sign this evaluation. A radiation oncologist and medical physicist must evaluate the technical aspects of the treatment and document and sign this evaluation.[1]

52.5 Patient Positioning

- Referenced in the "Technique" section.

52.6 Technique

- The frameless GKSRS procedure includes the following steps (see **Video 52.1** for additional details):
  1. Imaging for localization (CT, MRI, angiography, magnetoencephalography, etc.) based on the lesion treated
  2. Face mask and head support cushion preparation.
  3. Computer-assisted tumor localization/image guidance (CBCT).
  4. Treatment planning (number of beams, beam size and weight, etc.).
  5. Patient positioning.
  6. Setup and accuracy verification testing.
  7. Radiation treatment delivery.
- Face mask and head support cushion preparation:
  - The patient is counseled about the face mask and head support preparation and is then positioned on the Gamma Knife couch. The Klarity oven is turned on for 5 minutes. When the temperature reaches 73 °C, the thermoplastic mask is taken out of its packet and placed in the Klarity oven for 8 minutes. In the meantime, a head support cushion is prepared. The head support cushion material is taken out from its packet. Head cushion is made of polystyrene beads with hydrourethane resin. The cover material is polypropylene. Some water is injected into the head cushion, and it is placed under the patient's head. It gradually starts to harden and molds to support the patient's head.[6] After about 8 minutes, the face mask is taken out of oven. At this point, the mask is very soft and warm and is placed over the patient's face. After placing it over the patient's face, the top edge of the mask is

attached to the top edge of the head holder (the cradle) and the side attachments are fixed to the designated sites of head holder. The mask is then molded gently around the patient's face. The patient remains in the same position without moving the head. The edges of the mask are everted around the nose for the patient's comfort. The patient is instructed to stay with the mask in the same position for the next 10 minutes. After 10 minutes, when the mask becomes hard, the CBCT scan setup is initiated.

- *CBCT scan:* The tilt arm is brought into the position first. After that, a CBCT scan arm is positioned. The entire team is then moved out of the Gamma Knife room. From outside of the room, a CBCT scan is initiated. When the CBCT scan images appear on the treatment console, they are accepted and transferred to the planning computer. Afterward, the preplan is co-registered to the CBCT scan to obtain the stereotactic coordinates and the dose plan is reevaluated.[5] Once the treating team is satisfied and agrees with the margin dose as well as the treatment plan, the dose plan is approved and printed. The patient's ID is checked, and the patient is then counseled that the treatment is about to start. A second CBCT scan is performed, and the dose plan is rechecked. The treatment is then initiated. Once the treatment is completed, the face mask is released from the patient's face. The patient is removed from the unit and observed in the Gamma Knife suite for the next 45 minutes.

52.7 Postoperative Care

- There are several ways to avoid or mitigate the potential complications of frameless GKSRS that may arise after being discharged. Here are some general guidelines:
  - *Headaches:* Some patients may experience mild to severe headaches after GKSRS that may last from a few days to a few weeks. Patients can take over-the-counter pain medications like acetaminophen or ibuprofen. However, it is important to consult with the treating physician before taking any medications. In some cases, the headaches may be related to dehydration, so drinking plenty of fluids can also help.[9]
  - *Nausea and vomiting:* Some patients may experience nausea and vomiting after GKSRS, usually related to medications used during the treatment. Patients can take antinausea medications prescribed by their treating physician. Eating small, frequent meals and avoiding fatty or spicy foods may also help.[9]
  - *Neurological symptoms:* In rare cases, GKSRS can lead to late-onset neurological symptoms such as weakness, numbness, or vision changes depending on the target location. Patients should inform their treating physician immediately. In some cases, medications may be prescribed to help manage the symptoms.[9]
  - *Infection:* Patients should follow the posttreatment instructions provided by their health care team carefully, including proper hygiene practices to avoid infection. If the patient experiences pain, redness, or swelling at the site of the mask, the treating physician must be informed.[1]
  - *Adverse radiation effect (ARE):* ARE is a rare but serious complication that can occur after GKSRS. It is caused by damage to healthy brain tissue surrounding the treated area. Symptoms can include seizures, headaches, and neurological deficits. In some mild cases, steroids may be prescribed to help reduce inflammation and swelling. In severe cases, surgery may be necessary.[10]
- It is important for patients to communicate openly with their treating physician and to follow their instructions carefully to reduce the risk of complications after being discharged from the GKSRS clinic.

52.8 Complications

- There are some possible complications of frameless GKSRS that are different from those of frame-based GKRS, including the following:
  - *Inaccuracy in targeting:* Frameless GKSRS relies on imaging guidance, and any errors in the acquisition of images or the registration process can result in inaccurate targeting of the radiation beams, leading to potential complications. Without the frame to immobilize the head, there is a higher chance of head movement during the procedure, which can increase the risk of radiation exposure to healthy brain tissue. This could

cause damage to healthy tissue surrounding the target area and potentially lead to side effects such as headaches, nausea, or neurological symptoms.[4]
  - *Potentially longer treatment time:* Frameless GKRS may require additional time if the patient moves during treatment, requiring reacquisition of imaging. Studies have shown that patients with head rotations exceeding 0.47 degrees or extended planned treatment times typically experience treatment interruptions. In these cases, frame-based GKSRS or fractionated mask-based GKSRS should be considered to lessen the total treatment time.[4]
  - *Discomfort or pain during treatment:* Some patients may experience discomfort or pain during the procedure due to the need for a tight-fitting mask or headrest.[2]
- Most of these complications are overall relatively rare, and the majority of patients do not experience adverse effects from frameless GKSRS. The multidisciplinary treating team is responsible for discussing the potential risks and complications of the procedure with the patient before informed consent is obtained.

52.9 Management Pearls

- Radiosurgery is a rapidly expanding field that requires a unique set of trained skills. Focused training in GKSRS during residency in the form of a formal rotation in radiosurgery is necessary to ensure that trainees are proficient in this procedure.[1] After residency, recent graduates with strong interest in radiosurgery may also choose to pursue a fellowship in stereotactic image-guided neurosurgery, functional surgery, and radiosurgery, ranging in length from 6 months to 2 years, to be better equipped and become future leaders in the field.
- The personnel involved in frameless GKSRS may vary depending on the specific center and procedure. However, a typical team may include a neurosurgeon, radiation oncologist, medical physicist (a specialist in medical radiation physics who works together with the radiation oncologist and neurosurgeon to develop and implement the treatment plan), anesthesiologist (for pediatric cases that require general anesthesia), and a nurse and/or advanced practice provider who assists with patient positioning and immobilization.[2]
- *Special features in pregnant women*:
  - GKSRS is generally not recommended for pregnant women, especially during the first trimester, as even scattered radiation exposure during this time may increase the risk of birth defects.[1]
- *Special features in children and adolescents*:
  - It is essential to carefully consider the risks and benefits of GKSRS for children/adolescents on an individual basis, and to use the lowest effective radiation dose possible. Additionally, children/adolescents may require specialized immobilization devices that are appropriately sized and comfortable to ensure accurate treatment delivery.[1]
- *Special features in older patients*:
  - In all cases, it is important to consult with a multidisciplinary team, including a radiation oncologist, neurosurgeon, and other specialists as necessary, to carefully evaluate the risks and benefits of GKSRS in specific patient populations and to develop a personalized treatment plan that takes into account the individual needs and characteristics of each patient.[1]
- *Special features for other groups of people*:
  - There are some other patient populations that may require special consideration when undergoing frameless GKSRS. These include the following:
    - *Patients with prior radiation therapy:* Patients who have previously received brain radiation therapy may have a higher risk of developing complications after GKSRS given the doses initially received by surrounding normal structures. It is important to carefully evaluate the risks and benefits of GKSRS in these patients and to use the lowest effective radiation dose possible and/or consider multifraction GKSRS.[10]
    - *Patients with large or irregularly shaped tumors:* Patients with large or irregularly shaped tumors may require specialized immobilization devices or image guidance to ensure accurate treatment delivery.[10]
    - *Patients with multiple brain metastases:* Patients with multiple brain metastases may require more complex treatment planning to ensure that all tumors are adequately treated while minimizing the risk of complications.[7]

- *Patients with cognitive or behavioral issues:* Patients with cognitive or behavioral issues, such as dementia or psychiatric disorders, may require additional support and monitoring to ensure that they understand the treatment and can comply with posttreatment instructions. In some cases, sedation or anesthesia may be necessary to ensure accurate treatment delivery.[7]

References

[1] Lunsford LD, Niranjan A, Fallon K, Kim JO. Frame versus frameless Leksell stereotactic radiosurgery. Prog Neurol Surg. 2019; 34:19–27

[2] Liu J, Goenka A, Calugaru E, et al. Retrospective analysis of treatment workflow in frame-based and frameless Gamma Knife radiosurgery. Cureus. 2022; 14(8):e28606

[3] Grimm MA, Köppen U, Stieler F, et al. Prospective assessment of mask versus frame fixation during Gamma Knife treatment for brain metastases. Radiother Oncol. 2020; 147:195–199

[4] Wegner RE, Xu L, Horne Z, et al. Predictors of treatment interruption during frameless Gamma Knife Icon stereotactic radiosurgery. Adv Radiat Oncol. 2020; 5(6):1152–1157

[5] Carminucci A, Nie K, Weiner J, Hargreaves E, Danish SF. Assessment of motion error for frame-based and noninvasive mask-based fixation using the Leksell Gamma Knife icon radiosurgery system. J Neurosurg. 2018; 129 Suppl1:133–139

[6] Kutuk T, Kotecha R, Tolakanahalli R, et al. Zero setup margin mask versus frame immobilization during Gamma Knife® Icon™ stereotactic radiosurgery for brain metastases. Cancers (Basel). 2022; 14(14):14

[7] Bhatnagar AK, Flickinger JC, Kondziolka D, et al. Stereotactic radiosurgery for four or more intracranial metastases. Int J Radiat Oncol Biol Phys. 2006; 64(3):898–903

[8] Kondziolka D, Mathieu D, Lunsford LD, et al. Radiosurgery as definitive management of intracranial meningiomas. Neurosurgery. 2008; 62(1):53–58; discussion 58–60

[9] McTyre E, Helis CA, Farris M, et al. Emerging indications for fractionated Gamma Knife radiosurgery. Neurosurgery. 2017; 80(2):210–216

[10] Kirkpatrick JP, Soltys SG, Lo SS, Beal K, Shrieve DC, Brown PD. The radiosurgery fractionation quandary: single fraction or hypofractionation? Neuro-oncol. 2017; 19 suppl_2:ii38–ii49

53 Spinal Stereotactic Radiosurgery

Ria Mulherkar, Zaid Siddiqui, John C. Flickinger Sr, and Peter Carlos Gerszten

53.1 Background

- Spinal stereotactic radiosurgery (SRS) is used to treat primary and malignant tumors of the spine, most commonly metastatic extradural malignancy. This treatment modality is made possible by advances in the field of radiotherapy that allow for high doses of radiation in one to five fractions to be delivered precisely and accurately using a highly conformal plan and steep fall-off dose gradients to protect adjacent organs at risk (OAR). In this chapter, we summarize the details of spine SRS in the treatment of metastatic spine tumors.
- SRS to the spine is a radiotherapy technique used to accurately deliver high-dose radiation in one to five fractions to tumor using a highly conformal plan and steep fall-off dose gradients to protect adjacent OAR. SRS was first described for treatment of intracranial tumors,[1] but advances in patient immobilization, precise targeting of radiation using image-guided radiation therapy (IGRT), and intensity-modulated radiotherapy (IMRT) have made radiosurgery feasible for extracranial targets.[2,3] The major advantages of spine SRS compared to conventional external beam radiation (cEBRT) include delivery of higher therapeutic dose in fewer fractions to allow for improved pain control and local control.[4] Applications of spine SRS include definitive or adjuvant postoperative therapy for metastatic spine tumors, as well as neoadjuvant therapy for benign or malignant primary spine tumors.[5] Most commonly, spine SRS has been used for treatment of metastatic extradural spine tumors.[6,7,8,9,10]
- In this chapter, we discuss patient selection, technique, normal tissue dose constraints, and complications of spine SRS.

53.2 Indications and Contraindications

- Definitive or adjuvant postoperative therapy for metastatic spine tumors, as well as neoadjuvant therapy for benign or malignant primary spine tumors.[5]
- Most commonly, spine SRS has been used for treatment of metastatic extradural spine tumors.
- Contraindications may include larger spinal tumors, instability, or tumors closer to the cord.

53.3 Instruments

- BodyFix (Elekta).
- Vac-Lok (Civco).
- Computed tomography (CT) scanner/magnetic resonance imaging (MRI) or positron emission tomography (PET) CT fusion.
- Linear accelerator.
- Planning software.

53.4 Technique

- Treatment planning for radiation therapy begins with the simulation process, where the patient is immobilized, and CT images are obtained for delineation of target volumes and OAR. Immobilization should be reliable, so that patient position at the time of CT simulation can be reproduced and maintained for the duration of each treatment. Commercially available immobilization systems including BodyFix (Elekta) and Vac-Lok cushions (Civco) have been shown to create reproducible setups with both inter- and intrafraction motion less than 2.5 mm.[11,12,13] Treatment planning CT images are fused to thin-slice axial T1 postcontrast and T2 noncontrast MRI for target delineation when possible.
- Target volumes are contoured on CT images within radiation treatment planning system, though MRI or PET CT fusion may be used to assist in visualization of tumor and OAR. Consensus guidelines for target volume definition in spine SRS have been published by the International Spine Radiosurgery Consortium.[14] The clinical target volume (CTV) contains the gross tumor volume (GTV) with an additional expansion into physiologic bone marrow spaces that might harbor subclinical disease. Each vertebra is divided into

compartments including the vertebral body, pedicle, transverse process, lamina, and spinous process. Any compartment that contains GTV is included in its entirety, with additional expansion to include adjacent normal compartments as per consensus recommendations (▶ Fig. 53.1). In cases of postoperative spine SRS, CTV expansions should take into account extent of both preoperative and postoperative disease to adequately cover epidural space.[15] The planning target volume (PTV) includes CTV plus a margin of ≤ 3 mm to account for inter- and intrafraction motion. Planning risk volume (PRV) structures may also be created as necessary, adding an additional margin to account for inherent motion of mobile organs such as the spinal cord and small bowel. A PRV margin of 1.5 to 2 mm on the cord is strongly recommended.[16]

- Several dose fractionation schedules for spine SRS have been described, including 12 to 24 Gy in one fraction, 24 Gy in two fractions, and 27 to 30 Gy in three to five fractions, with fractionated approach favored for tumors that are very large or have previously received significant irradiation.[4,17,18,19] Radiation planning techniques have evolved significantly since the three-dimensional planning era. Spine SRS is possible due to technological advances including IMRT and later volumetric intensity-modulated arc radiotherapy (VMAT), which allow more accurate and conformal delivery of higher radiation dose to target volume while sparing adjacent OAR.[20] VMAT technology involves placement of a linear accelerator on a rotating gantry that continuously delivers radiation while rotating around the patient. A VMAT spine SRS plan may involve one or more such rotations,

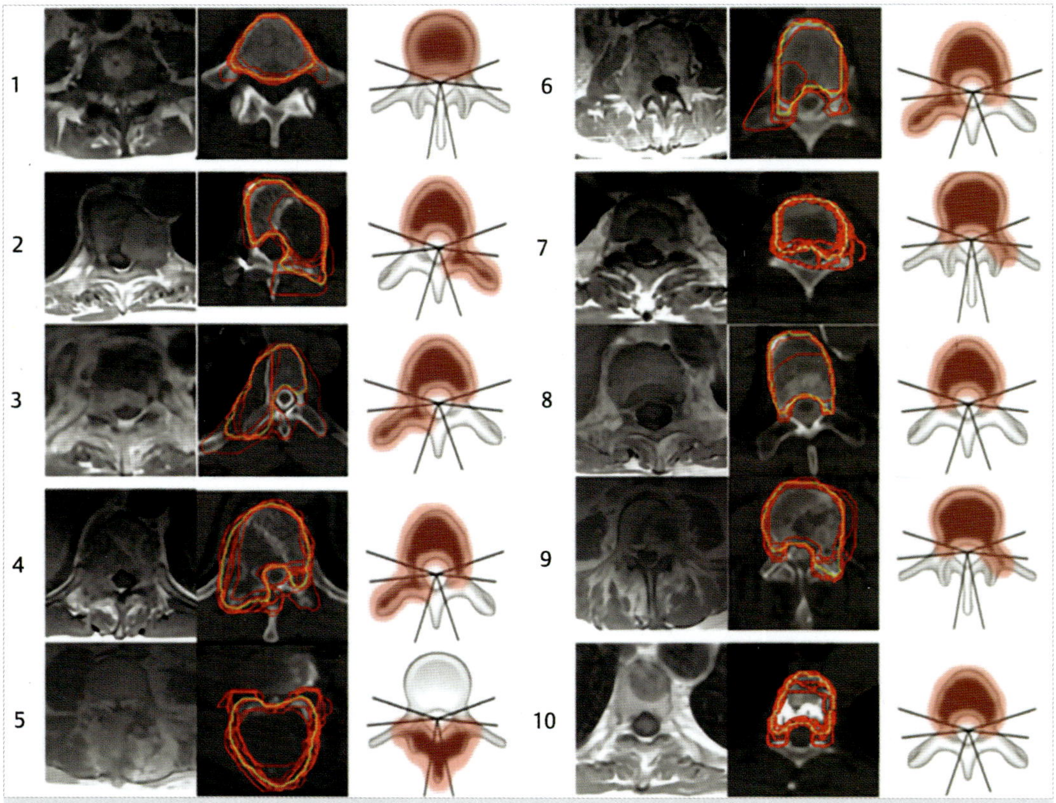

Fig. 53.1 Consensus clinical target volume (CTV) contour recommendation from the International Spine Radiosurgery Consortium. (This article was published in Int J Radiat Oncol Biol Phys, 83(5), Cox BW, Spratt DE, Lovelock M et al, International Spine Radiosurgery Consortium consensus guidelines for target volume definition in spinal stereotactic radiosurgery, e597–605, Copyright Elsevier 2012.)

known as arcs. Within each arc, various components of the radiation beam are modulated including dose rate, speed of the rotating gantry, and beam shape via multileaf collimator leaves.[21] VMAT plans maintain adequate target coverage and OAR sparing and have been shown to improve delivery efficiency by an average of 53% compared to traditional "step and shoot" IMRT plans.[22]

- Representative examples of VMAT plans for spine SRS with arc configuration, dose cloud, and dose-volume histograms to evaluate target coverage and OAR constraints are shown in ▶ Fig. 53.2 and ▶ Fig. 53.3.

53.5 Normal Tissue Dose Constraints in Spine SRS

- Target coverage for spine SRS is limited by dose constraints of normal organs adjacent to the treatment volume, including spinal cord, esophagus, heart, and small bowel. It is important to realize that the biologically effective dose (BED) to a particular tissue at any given dose of radiation is a function of the total dose, dose per fraction, and a complicated radiobiological principal of tissue response to radiation known as the alpha/beta ratio, which is typically assumed to be higher for early-responding tissues such as tumors (alpha/beta 10) and lower for late-responding tissues such as normal OAR (alpha/beta 1–3).[23,24] The High Dose per Fraction, Hypofractionated Treatment Effects in the Clinic (HyTEC) project includes a series of publications with data regarding tissue and OAR response to SRS and stereotactic body radiotherapy (SBRT) treatments for various disease sites in one to five fractions. The tolerances for OAR in spine SRS have been published as part of this project and should be abided in all treatment plans to reduce risk of complications.[25,26]

53.6 Complications

- Acute toxicities of spine SRS may include pain flare, which is defined as a temporary increase in pain in the period immediately following radiation treatment. A prospective study in patients treated with spine SRS revealed that pain flare occurred in 68% of patients, most commonly 1 day following radiation treatment, and that patients rescued with dexamethasone experienced significant decrease in their pain scores over time.[27] Other retrospective reviews of patients who underwent spine SRS demonstrated potential risk factors for pain flare including number of treatment fractions, higher prescription dose, higher performance status, female gender, and cervical or thoracic spine location.[28,29] Many institutions will deliver prophylactic dose of steroids to prevent pain flare, and a short steroid taper can be utilized to treat pain flare if it occurs. Other common acute toxicities of spine SRS include grade 1 or 2 skin toxicity or toxicity to the esophagus. Strategies to obtain favorable therapeutic ratio and mitigate risk of common toxicities associated with SRS and SBRT have been previously published.[30]
- Potential late toxicities of spine SRS include radiation myelopathy (RM) and vertebral compression fracture (VCF). RM is a rare but potentially devastating complication of radiation to the spine, which can occur due to microvascular damage and oligodendroglial cell depletion; symptoms can manifest transiently approximately 3 to 4 months following radiation, which self-resolve, or as a progressive complication 12 to 14 months after treatment that may ultimately result in complete paralysis and loss of bowel and bladder control.[31] In a retrospective review of 562 patients treated with spine SRS in the setting of primary treatment or reirradiation, 7.4% of patients experienced long-term grade 2 neuropathy, and 5.6% of patients, all of whom had received prior cEBRT, experienced grade 3 neuropathy.[32] Logistic regression analyses have been used to correlate spinal cord dose to risk of RM in spine SRS; less than 5% risk of RM has been observed with thecal sac point dose less than 12.4 Gy in 1 fraction, 17.0 Gy in 2 fractions, 20.3 Gy in 3 fractions, 23.0 Gy in 4 fractions, and 25.3 Gy in 5 fractions.[33]
- Another more frequent toxicity associated with spine SRS is VCF. Like RM, VCF can be seen after cEBRT, but incidence is higher following spine SRS. Bone metastases directly impair the integrity of vertebral bone and increase the risk of pathologic fracture; radiation to the bone can

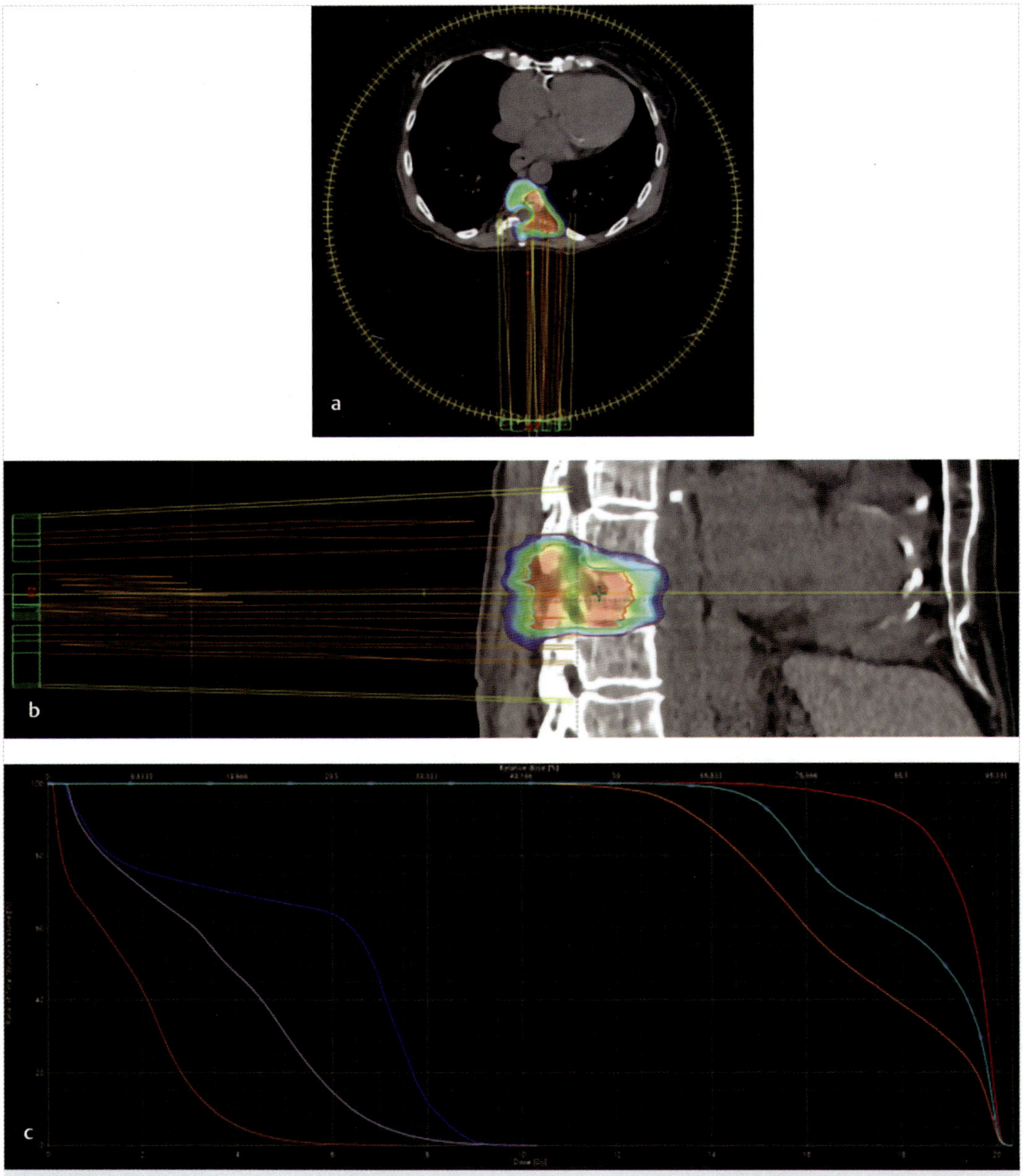

Fig. 53.2 Example case of a 65-year-old woman with metastatic sarcoma of the uterus involving the vertebral bodies and transverse processes of the T8–T9 vertebrae. She was treated with 12 Gy in one fraction prescribed to the planning target volume (PTV), 14 Gy in one fraction prescribed to clinical target volume (CTV), and 18 Gy in one fraction prescribed to gross tumor volume (GTV). A stereotactic ablative radiotherapy plan was created using two full arc rotations. **(a)** Axial view of the spine stereotactic radiosurgery (SRS) plan with GTV outlined in *red*, CTV outlined in *cyan*, and PTV outlined in *orange*, dose cloud depicting the area that receives 12 Gy, and depiction of two arcs oriented around the same isocenter, one rotating clockwise and the other counterclockwise. **(b)** Sagittal view of the spine SRS plan with GTV outlined in *red*, PTV outlined in *orange*, dose cloud depicting the area that receives 12 Gy, and depiction of starting point of each arc. **(c)** Dose-volume histogram for the spine SRS plan that plots total dose in gray against relative percent volume of each structure for GTV (*red*), CTV (*cyan*), PTV (*orange*), spinal cord (*dark blue*), esophagus (*lavender*), and heart (*brown*).

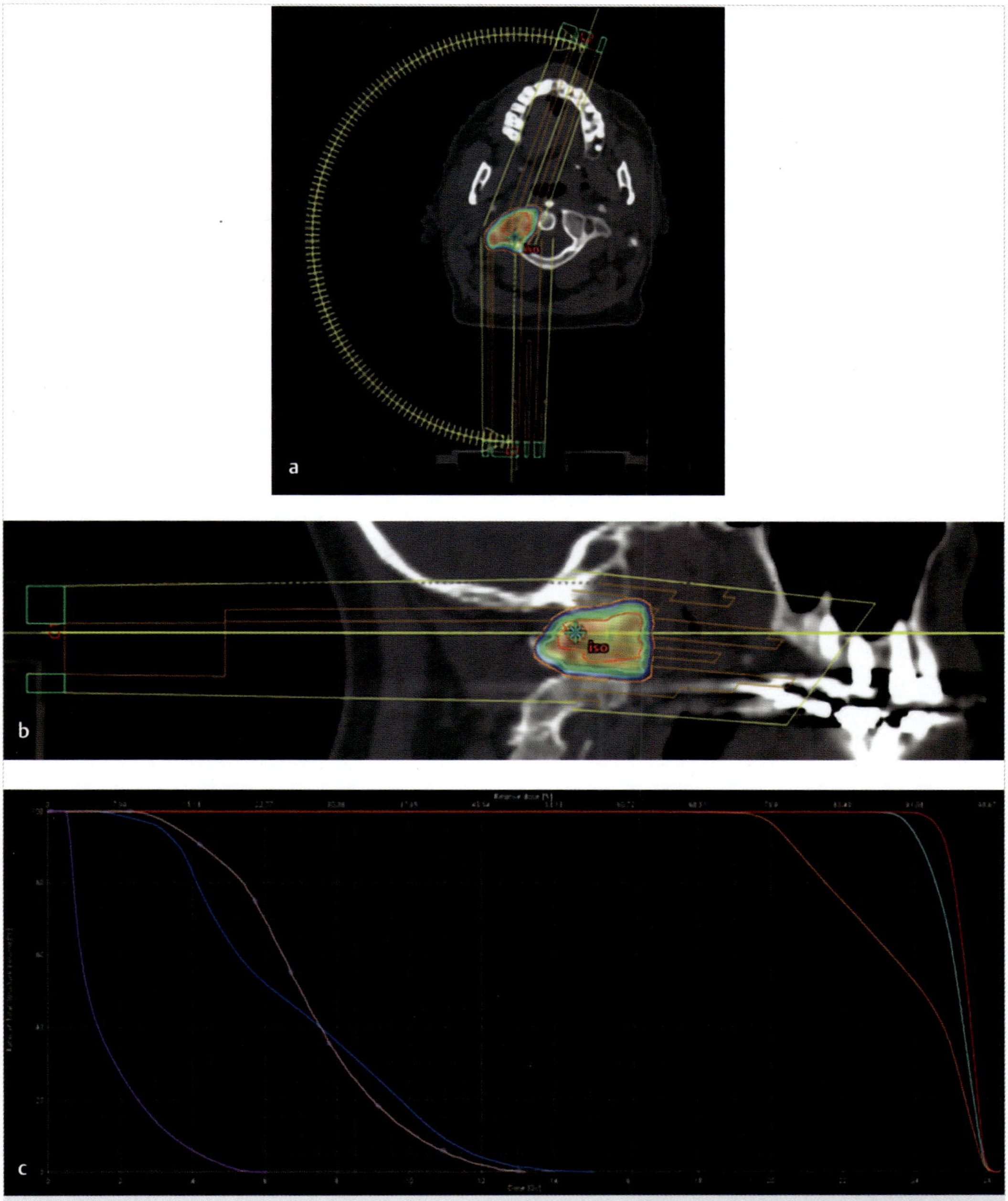

Fig. 53.3 Example case of a 66-year-old man with oligometastatic hepatocellular carcinoma involving the right transverse process of the C1 vertebra. He was treated with 20 Gy in two fractions prescribed to the planning target volume (PTV), and 24 Gy in two fractions prescribed to the clinical target volume (CTV). A stereotactic ablative radiotherapy plan was created using two partial arcs. **(a)** Axial view of the spine stereotactic radiosurgery (SRS) plan with gross tumor volume (GTV) outlined in *red*, CTV outlined in *cyan*, and PTV outlined in *orange*, dose cloud depicting the area that receives 20 Gy, and depiction of two partial arcs oriented around the same isocenter, one rotating clockwise and the other counterclockwise. **(b)** Sagittal view of the spine SRS plan with GTV outlined in *red*, PTV outlined in *orange*, dose cloud depicting the area that receives 20 Gy, and sagittal depiction of each partial arc. **(c)** Dose-volume histogram for the spine SRS plan that plots total dose in gray against relative percent volume of each structure for GTV (*red*), CTV (*cyan*), PTV (*orange*), spinal cord (*pink*), pharynx (*dark blue*), and brainstem (*purple*).

further reduce bone strength via collagen damage and potentially cause osteoradionecrosis, leading to increased risk of fracture.[34] Recursive partitioning analysis has been used to generate a stratification system to predict risk of VCF following spine SRS, and the key predictors for increased risk of fracture include GTV > 10 mL, lumbar location, epidural extension of tumor, and spinal instability neoplastic score greater than 6.[35] Based on retrospective dosimetric analysis for single-fraction spine SRS, the recommended maximum point dose to vertebra is recommended to be less than 24.0 Gy, with less than 24% of the vertebral volume receiving greater than 20 Gy to reduce risk of VCF.[36]

53.7 Management Pearls

- Suitability for spine SRS is dependent on numerous considerations including patient factors (performance status, neurologic status, pain level, life expectancy, and ability to tolerate treatment), oncologic factors (tumor histology and radiosensitivity, disease burden, and options for systemic therapy), and treatment-specific factors (radiographic appearance, size and location of tumor, spinal instability, and history of prior irradiation).[37] The NOMS (Neurologic, Oncologic, Mechanical Instability, Systemic Disease) decision framework integrates recommendations for surgery and radiation to provide a modern paradigm for treatment of spine metastases.[38] In general, appropriate candidates for spine SRS are patients with histologically proven malignancy, oligometastatic disease, Karnofsky performance status 70% or higher, disease involving no more than three contiguous vertebral levels, and without high-grade spinal cord or cauda equina compression.
- Spine SRS represents a major advance in the field of radiotherapy and has become integral in the treatment of malignant spine tumors, particularly in the setting of oligometastatic disease. Appropriate patient selection for use of spine SRS is paramount, and treatment planning should incorporate modern techniques such as VMAT to obtain optimal target coverage while respecting normal tissue constraints. Efficacy of spine SRS in controlling residual tumor in the postoperative adjuvant setting has led to increased use of minimally invasive surgical treatments. Radiosurgery for treatment of spine metastases in the definitive setting is also well tolerated and has shown improved palliation of symptoms and superior local control compared to cEBRT. The treatment paradigm for metastatic spinal tumors continues to evolve, and spine SRS is at the forefront of this change.

References

[1] Leksell L. The stereotaxic method and radiosurgery of the brain. Acta Chir Scand. 1951; 102(4):316–319

[2] Yenice KM, Lovelock DM, Hunt MA, et al. CT image-guided intensity-modulated therapy for paraspinal tumors using stereotactic immobilization. Int J Radiat Oncol Biol Phys. 2003; 55(3):583–593

[3] Ryu S, Fang Yin F, Rock J, et al. Image-guided and intensity-modulated radiosurgery for patients with spinal metastasis. Cancer. 2003; 97(8):2013–2018

[4] Sahgal A, Myrehaug SD, Siva S, et al. trial investigators. Stereotactic body radiotherapy versus conventional external beam radiotherapy in patients with painful spinal metastases: an open-label, multicentre, randomised, controlled, phase 2/3 trial. Lancet Oncol. 2021; 22(7):1023–1033

[5] Bilsky MH, Angelov L, Rock J, et al. Spinal radiosurgery: a neurosurgical perspective. J Radiosurg SBRT. 2011; 1(1):47–54

[6] Gerszten PC, Burton SA, Ozhasoglu C, Welch WC. Radiosurgery for spinal metastases: clinical experience in 500 cases from a single institution. Spine. 2007; 32(2):193–199

[7] Gerszten PC, Burton SA, Belani CP, et al. Radiosurgery for the treatment of spinal lung metastases. Cancer. 2006; 107(11): 2653–2661

[8] Gerszten PC, Burton SA, Ozhasoglu C, et al. Stereotactic radiosurgery for spinal metastases from renal cell carcinoma. J Neurosurg Spine. 2005; 3(4):288–295

[9] Gerszten PC, Burton SA, Welch WC, et al. Single-fraction radiosurgery for the treatment of spinal breast metastases. Cancer. 2005; 104(10):2244–2254

[10] Gerszten PC, Burton SA, Quinn AE, Agarwala SS, Kirkwood JM. Radiosurgery for the treatment of spinal melanoma metastases. Stereotact Funct Neurosurg. 2005; 83(5–6):213–221

[11] Hyde D, Lochray F, Korol R, et al. Spine stereotactic body radiotherapy utilizing cone-beam CT image-guidance with a robotic couch: intrafraction motion analysis accounting for all six degrees of freedom. Int J Radiat Oncol Biol Phys. 2012; 82(3):e555–e562

[12] Copeland A, Barron A, Fontenot J. Analytical setup margin for spinal stereotactic body radiotherapy based on measured errors. Radiat Oncol. 2021; 16(1):234

[13] Finnigan R, Lamprecht B, Barry T, et al. Inter- and intra-fraction motion in stereotactic body radiotherapy for spinal and paraspinal tumours using cone-beam CT and positional correction in six degrees of freedom. J Med Imaging Radiat Oncol. 2016; 60(1):112–118

[14] Cox BW, Spratt DE, Lovelock M, et al. International Spine Radiosurgery Consortium consensus guidelines for target volume definition in spinal stereotactic radiosurgery. Int J Radiat Oncol Biol Phys. 2012; 83(5):e597–e605

[15] Chan MW, Thibault I, Atenafu EG, et al. Patterns of epidural progression following postoperative spine stereotactic body radiotherapy: implications for clinical target volume delineation. J Neurosurg Spine. 2016; 24(4):652–659

[16] Oztek MA, Mayr NA, Mossa-Basha M, et al. The dancing cord: inherent spinal cord motion and its effect on cord dose in spine stereotactic body radiation therapy. Neurosurgery. 2020; 87(6):1157–1166

[17] Sprave T, Verma V, Förster R, et al. Randomized phase II trial evaluating pain response in patients with spinal metastases following stereotactic body radiotherapy versus three-dimensional conformal radiotherapy. Radiother Oncol. 2018; 128(2):274–282

[18] Nguyen Q-N, Chun SG, Chow E, et al. Single-fraction stereotactic vs conventional multifraction radiotherapy for pain relief in patients with predominantly nonspine bone metastases: a randomized phase 2 trial. JAMA Oncol. 2019; 5(6):872–878

[19] Chang EL, Shiu AS, Mendel E, et al. Phase I/II study of stereotactic body radiotherapy for spinal metastasis and its pattern of failure. J Neurosurg Spine. 2007; 7(2):151–160

[20] Guckenberger M, Sweeney RA, Flickinger JC, et al. Clinical practice of image-guided spine radiosurgery: results from an international research consortium. Radiat Oncol. 2011; 6(1):172

[21] Kuijper IT, Dahele M, Senan S, Verbakel WFAR. Volumetric modulated arc therapy versus conventional intensity modulated radiation therapy for stereotactic spine radiotherapy: a planning study and early clinical data. Radiother Oncol. 2010; 94(2):224–228

[22] Marchand EL, Sahgal A, Zhang TJ, et al. Treatment planning and delivery evaluation of volumetric modulated arc therapy for stereotactic body radiotherapy of spinal tumours: impact of arc discretization in planning system. Technol Cancer Res Treat. 2012; 11(6):599–606

[23] Jones B, Dale RG, Deehan C, Hopkins KI, Morgan DA. The role of biologically effective dose (BED) in clinical oncology. Clin Oncol (R Coll Radiol). 2001; 13(2):71–81

[24] Williams MV, Denekamp J, Fowler JF. A review of α/β ratios for experimental tumors: implications for clinical studies of altered fractionation. Int J Radiat Oncol Biol Phys. 1985; 11(1):87–96

[25] Sahgal A, Chang JH, Ma L, et al. Spinal cord dose tolerance to stereotactic body radiation therapy. Int J Radiat Oncol Biol Phys. 2021; 110(1):124–136

[26] Soltys SG, Grimm J, Milano MT, et al. Stereotactic body radiation therapy for spinal metastases: tumor control probability analyses and recommended reporting standards. Int J Radiat Oncol Biol Phys. 2021; 110(1):112–123

[27] Chiang A, Zeng L, Zhang L, et al. Pain flare is a common adverse event in steroid-naïve patients after spine stereotactic body radiation therapy: a prospective clinical trial. Int J Radiat Oncol Biol Phys. 2013; 86(4):638–642

[28] Pan HY, Allen PK, Wang XS, et al. Incidence and predictive factors of pain flare after spine stereotactic body radiation therapy: secondary analysis of phase 1/2 trials. Int J Radiat Oncol Biol Phys. 2014; 90(4):870–876

[29] Balagamwala EH, Naik M, Reddy CA, et al. Pain flare after stereotactic radiosurgery for spine metastases. J Radiosurg SBRT. 2018; 5(2):99–105

[30] Lo SS, Sahgal A, Chang EL, et al. Serious complications associated with stereotactic ablative radiotherapy and strategies to mitigate the risk. Clin Oncol (R Coll Radiol). 2013; 25(6):378–387

[31] Siker ML, Bovi J, Alexander B. Spinal cord tumors. In: Gunderson LL, Tepper JE, eds. Clinical Radiation Oncology. 4th ed. Philadelphia, PA: Elsevier; 2016:521–540.e5

[32] Ling DC, Flickinger JC, Burton SA, et al. Long-term outcomes after stereotactic radiosurgery for spine metastases: radiation dose-response for late toxicity. Int J Radiat Oncol Biol Phys. 2018; 101(3):602–609

[33] Sahgal A, Weinberg V, Ma L, et al. Probabilities of radiation myelopathy specific to stereotactic body radiation therapy to guide safe practice. Int J Radiat Oncol Biol Phys. 2013; 85(2):341–347

[34] Sahgal A, Whyne CM, Ma L, Larson DA, Fehlings MG. Vertebral compression fracture after stereotactic body radiotherapy for spinal metastases. Lancet Oncol. 2013; 14 (8):e310–e320

[35] Kowalchuk RO, Johnson-Tesch BA, Marion JT, et al. Development and assessment of a predictive score for vertebral compression fracture after stereotactic body radiation therapy for spinal metastases. JAMA Oncol. 2022; 8(3):412–419

[36] Lee MY, Ouyang Z, LaHurd D, et al. A volumetric dosimetry analysis of vertebral body fracture risk after single fraction spine stereotactic body radiation therapy. Pract Radiat Oncol. 2021; 11(6):480–487

[37] Tseng C-L, Eppinga W, Charest-Morin R, et al. Spine stereotactic body radiotherapy: indications, outcomes, and points of caution. Global Spine J. 2017; 7(2):179–197

[38] Laufer I, Rubin DG, Lis E, et al. The NOMS framework: approach to the treatment of spinal metastatic tumors. Oncologist. 2013; 18(6):744–751

54 Robotic Fundamentals (Functional)

Matthew J. Recker, Steven Blake Housley, and Jonathan Riley

54.1 Background

- Stereotactic accuracy is paramount to the modern practice of functional neurosurgery. This foundational principle has been enhanced by years of technological advancement. Current generation robotic platforms have added to the surgeon's armamentarium.
- Various robotic systems are available for clinical use with applications in the diagnosis and treatment of epilepsy, movement disorders, psychiatric disorders, pain, tumors, and vascular malformations.
- The benefits of robotic platforms for functional neurosurgical applications are best achieved with an increasing number of trajectories. This occurs because (1) robotic techniques cognitively offload the surgical team by reducing the number of factors to account for (e.g., with frame programming during frame-based stereotaxy) and (2) the initial time investment for setup becomes progressively offset with each subsequent trajectory due to the short time per trajectory compared to frame-based techniques.
- For these reasons, most studies of robotics in functional neurosurgery describe the utilization of this technology for depth electrode placement in epilepsy.
- This chapter will focus on the fundamentals and technical aspects of one common application of robotics in stereotactic and functional neurosurgery: stereoelectroencephalography (SEEG).

54.2 Indications and Contraindications

- The indications for the use of robotics in functional neurosurgery vary based on the pathology at hand, with applications in the treatment of epilepsy, movement disorders, psychiatric disorders, pain, tumors, and vascular malformations.
  - For example, robotic-assisted SEEG is used in patients with medically refractory epilepsy to better delineate the epileptogenic network and define an epileptogenic zone that may be amenable to surgical intervention.
- Patients typically will have noninvasive studies, such as electroencephalography (EEG), positron emission tomography (PET), or magnetic encephalography (MEG), or neuropsychiatric testing that does not precisely identify the epileptogenic zone but suggests there may be a focal onset.

54.3 Patient Preparation

- A stereotactic protocol magnetic resonance imaging (MRI) study that can be integrated into the planning software must be obtained to plan the anticipated trajectories. Some form of contrast imaging is necessary to visualize the vascular structures and plan the trajectories accordingly. The stereotactic protocol MRI can be used to accomplish this goal. Alternatively, a supplementary computed tomography (CT) angiogram may be considered. These images can be co-registered to those of the stereotactic MRI for planning purposes.

54.4 Patient Positioning

- The patient's head must be placed in a head holder. A Mayfield head holder (Integra LifeSciences, Princeton, NJ) or stereotactic frame base may be used for this. Our preference is the latter as four points of fixation are utilized as opposed to three. The head holder should be thoughtfully applied to avoid interfering with the planned trajectories. This can be evaluated prior to draping the patient and robot by "driving" the robot's working arm to the planned trajectories to ensure they are feasible with the applied head fixation strategy. The patient is positioned supine on an operating room table with the head of the bed elevated. The patient's head is appropriately positioned for access to the desired entry sites and the head holder is secured to the robot. Stereotactic registration is performed using fiducials or laser registration. Registration is confirmed using anatomical landmarks. The patient's scalp is prepared and draped.

54.5 Technique

- *Anesthesia*:
  - Patients will typically be placed under general anesthesia for robotic cases. On the basis of the indication and specific surgery to be performed, some surgeons may perform awake surgery during which the patient will be placed under conscious sedation and aroused for specific portions of the case. For example, at some centers, deep brain stimulator implantation is performed while the patient is awake and can be examined during the implantation to evaluate for efficacy and side effects. Routine monitoring performed by the anesthesiologist includes pulse oximetry, electrocardiography, intra-arterial blood pressure monitoring, and temperature probe. A Foley catheter may be placed. Prophylactic antibiotics should be administered prior to the first skin incision.
- *Personnel, material, and equipment*:
  - Representatives from the robot manufacturer are often present to assist in the operation of the robot. Implants specific to the procedure to be performed must be available. For example, for SEEG implantation, SEEG electrodes, anchor bolts, an anchor bolt driver, anchor bolt caps, a slide rule, and a stylet are required. A representative from the implant manufacturer is typically present as well. The acquisition of image sets with the patient in a head holder for co-registration to the preoperative images can be done in a variety of ways, including with an intraoperative three-dimensional (3D) imaging system or in a formal CT scanner. A multidisciplinary team is necessary for the surgical management of patients with epilepsy. Although the entire team does not directly participate in SEEG surgery itself, epileptologists, neurosurgeons, radiologists, neuropsychologists, social workers, and clinical nurse specialists are all critical to the preoperative and postoperative care of these patients.
- *Technique*:
  - The following technical description focuses on the application of robotics for the placement of SEEG depth electrodes (**Video 54.1**), one of the most common uses. The principles and technical nuances described are similar for other applications of robotics in functional neurosurgery.
  - The SEEG electrode trajectories are planned in advance based on the patient's specific noninvasive data and the regions of interest. Common structures targeted for SEEG recording include the amygdala, hippocampus, insula, cingulum, thalamic nuclei, and neocortical structures (particularly the temporal lobe). The trajectories should be planned to avoid any dural or sulcal blood vessels. Some surgeons choose to avoid crossing pial boundaries to minimize risk of bleeding and deflections, whereas others feel that orthogonal trajectories that cross pial boundaries give a better spatial representation of EEG data and provide more contact with gray matter.
  - Several techniques exist for registering the robot to the patient. A stereotactic registration image may be acquired to co-register to the preoperative plan. This can be performed in the operating room with intraoperative CT, 3D fluoroscopic imaging, or in a formal CT scanner. Some surgeons choose to place bone fiducials in the scalp to optimize registration accuracy. Alternatively, laser co-registration can be used, which does not require additional imaging. After the patient is positioned, the robotic arm is draped in a sterile fashion and its sterile attachment is secured.
  - The robotic arm is navigated to the first planned trajectory. The drill guide is applied and an anchor bolt driver is passed through the drill guide to contact the skin. The skin is marked at this location, and a stab incision is made with a no. 11 blade.
  - A high-speed drill is passed through the drill guide and through the stab incision. The bit is feathered to pass through soft tissue until contact is made with the skull. The drill stop is adjusted based on the skull thickness to prevent unintentional plunging. The drill is advanced at full speed through the skull. The dura can be opened with the drill by intentionally driving

slightly past the depth of the inner table or by removing the drill and coagulating the dura percutaneously with a stylet.

- It is imperative to evaluate the preoperative images to ensure that no traversing blood vessels are present in the immediate vicinity, which could be injured during this step. The anchor bolt length is chosen based on the thickness of the skull and soft tissues.
  The anchor bolt is inserted through the robotic guidance arm and tightened until good bony purchase is achieved. The stereotactic trajectory is now encoded in the anchor bolt.
- Care must be taken to not overtighten the anchor bolts, especially in areas of thin bone, as this can lead to fracture and instability or driving of the threads past the inner table. Coaxial alignment of the anchor bolt is confirmed by passing the anchor bolt driver back through the robotic arm to ensure the driver meets the anchor bolt as expected. The anchor bolt cap is applied, and the robotic arm is advanced in a coaxial trajectory until contact is just made with the anchor bolt cap. The robotic device can then calculate the distance to the target from this point.
- This distance to the target is measured on the stylet using a slide rule and marked with a marking pen. The robotic guidance arm is navigated away from the field. The stylet is advanced through the anchor bolt to the marked depth. The electrode is measured to the same depth and marked with a cut Steri-Strip (3 M, St. Paul, MN), which remains in place and can be used as a reference during recording to indicate if the lead position has moved. The stylet is removed and compared antiparallel to the electrode to ensure that the depths of the stylet and electrode match. The electrode is inserted to the prescribed depth through the anchor bolt and the anchor bolt cap is tightened. This process should occur rather quickly to minimize cerebrospinal fluid (CSF) loss.
- The robotic guide arm is navigated to the next trajectory, and the above steps are repeated until all leads are placed. The anchor bolt exit site is wrapped with Xeroform gauze (Cardinal Health, Dublin, OH). The head holder is removed and the head is carefully wrapped with sterile gauze.

54.6 Postoperative Care

- After implantation, a head CT scan is obtained to identify any postoperative hemorrhage and to determine the accuracy of electrode placement. The patient is then taken to the epilepsy monitoring unit for surveillance and recording. Antibiotics should be prescribed perioperatively to minimize the risk of infection. Once in the epilepsy monitoring unit, the leads are connected to the monitoring cables. The bundle of cables is secured to the patient in a tension-free manner to prevent tugging on the leads. Dressing changes are minimized to prevent exposure and contamination of the exit sites and reduce risk of displacement of the leads. If the dressing becomes soiled, the neurosurgical team should perform the dressing change. At the conclusion of the study, the anchor bolts and electrodes are removed, and the stab incisions are closed with a single suture at each site.
- Postexplant head CT is recommended to evaluate for hemorrhage, pneumocephalus, or other complications. Typically, the patient is able to be discharged to home on postexplant day 1. The patient should return to the office for further discussion regarding definitive management based on the results of the study after an intentional delay to allow time for the multidisciplinary team to analyze and interpret the study findings in conference. Ideally, wound healing should be achieved without any signs or symptoms of infection or other complications before proceeding with any ensuing therapeutic surgical intervention.

54.7 Complications

- The procedure is carried out through a series of craniostomies without direct visualization of the underlying brain. Intracranial hemorrhage has been reported at a rate of up to approximately 0.5%[1] per electrode placed or a rate of 19.1% per patient implantation,[2] although a need for surgical evacuation of hemorrhage or the occurrence of a permanent neurologic deficit is rare. The quoted rate of hemorrhage is considered the upper bound in the reported literature. During surgery, if bloody return is encountered from a craniostomy site after the stylet is removed, irrigation through the anchor

bolt should be utilized until the return clears. If continued bloody return is evident, the surgeon may consider expanding the incision and performing a burr hole adjacent to the entry site to evaluate for epidural or subdural hemorrhage.
- Infection at the implantation site is possible, and the risk increases the longer the electrodes are in place. CSF leak is also possible after lead explantation.

54.8 Management Pearls

- Maintaining coaxial alignment is critical to ensure accuracy and should be confirmed at every step.
- Trajectories that are orthogonal to the skull pose the least risk of skiving while drilling the craniotomy. Trajectory angles that deviate greatly from orthogonal to the skull should be avoided as feasible.
- The most challenging anchor bolts to place are in the thin bone of the squamous temporal bone. Care should be taken to not overtighten the anchor bolts in this location in order to minimize the risk of fracturing the bone or driving the bolt entirely through the bone. New-generation undersized drill bits can help improve purchase.
- Several stereotactic methods are utilized in functional neurosurgery. Robotic technology helps improve workflow efficiency while maintaining the high level of precision required.[3] Current robotic systems utilize a working arm that maintains a preplanned trajectory through which the surgeon can implant a variety of intracranial devices. The gold standard of stereotactic neurosurgery is frame-based stereotaxy, which allows for an accuracy of 1 to 3 mm or less to be achieved at the target.[4] Robotic-assisted surgery has resulted in an accuracy similar to that of frame-based stereotaxy while offering improved operative times in the cases where several trajectories will be utilized.[3,5,6,7,8]
- Patients should understand that SEEG is a diagnostic tool and that the severity of their epilepsy is not expected to be improved by the procedure. The goal of SEEG is to identify an epileptogenic focus considered amenable to surgical intervention; thus, a positive outcome would be the ability to offer the patient a surgical treatment as the next step. It is important to stress this expectation to patients such that they are eager to proceed with not only the SEEG procedure but also any therapeutic intervention that may be offered as a result.
- There is the possibility of a negative SEEG study, meaning no clear epileptogenic focus was defined and the risk of undergoing surgery was without apparent benefit. Moreover, the hospital course after implantation can be prolonged as the goal is to record the necessary data to make further decisions, which often means waiting until multiple clinical and electrographic seizures are captured. The patient should be advised that due to the open-ended nature of the study, the duration of recording may be only a few days but may also last more than a week.
- Special risks include intracerebral hemorrhage, infection, CSF leak, and loosening of the anchor bolts used during SEEG over time. The surgical risk is minimized by careful planning of trajectories to avoid blood vessels.

References

[1] Triano MJ, Schupper AJ, Ghatan S, Panov F. Hemorrhage rates after implantation and explantation of stereotactic electroencephalography: reevaluating patients' risk. World Neurosurg. 2021; 151:e100–e108

[2] McGovern RA, Ruggieri P, Bulacio J, Najm I, Bingaman WE, Gonzalez-Martinez JA. Risk analysis of hemorrhage in stereo-electroencephalography procedures. Epilepsia. 2019; 60(3): 571–580

[3] González-Martínez J, Bulacio J, Thompson S, et al. Technique, results, and complications related to robot-assisted stereoelectroencephalography. Neurosurgery. 2016; 78(2): 169–180

[4] Roth A, Buttrick SS, Cajigas I, Jagid JR, Ivan ME. Accuracy of frame-based and frameless systems for deep brain stimulation: a meta-analysis. J Clin Neurosci. 2018; 57:1–5

[5] Mei S, Yu K, Ren Z, et al. Techniques of frameless robot-assisted deep brain stimulation and accuracy compared with the frame-based technique. Brain Sci. 2022; 12(7):906

[6] Ahmed SI, Javed G, Mubeen B, et al. Robotics in neurosurgery: a literature review. J Pak Med Assoc. 2018; 68(2):258–263

[7] Gonzalez-Martinez J, Mullin J, Vadera S, et al. Stereotactic placement of depth electrodes in medically intractable epilepsy. J Neurosurg. 2014; 120(3):639–644

[8] Fomenko A, Serletis D. Robotic stereotaxy in cranial neurosurgery: a qualitative systematic review. Neurosurgery. 2018; 83(4):642–650

55 Stereoelectroencephalography Using a Stereotactic Cranial Robotic Platform

Ali Reza Tafreshi and Philip S. Lee

55.1 Background

- Stereoelectroencephalography (SEEG) is widely used in the workup of patients with medically refractory epilepsy[1,2] to localize an epileptogenic focus.[1,2]
- A 10th to a 3rd of epilepsy cases are drug resistant, defined as the failure of two tolerated, appropriately chosen and used antiepileptic drug schedules, whether as monotherapies or in combination, to achieve sustained seizure freedom.[3]
- Prior to SEEG implantation, preparatory diagnostic testing includes scalp video electroencephalographic (EEG) monitoring, magnetic resonance imaging (MRI), positron emission tomography (PET) scan, ictal single photon emission computed tomography (CT), neuropsychological studies, and functional monitoring.
- A multidisciplinary committee including epileptologists, neurosurgeons, psychologists/ psychiatrists, and neuroradiologists will then determine the utility of SEEG based on these metrics.[4]

55.2 Indications and Contraindications

55.2.1 Indications

- Medically refractory epilepsy.
- No detectable structural abnormalities on imaging.
- Discrepancy between radiologic, EEG, and clinical findings.
- Visible lesion on imaging, but evidence suggests the epileptogenic zone extends beyond it.
- Large lesion partially involving an eloquent cortical area, with signs that limited resection may still be beneficial.
- Clinical or EEG findings indicate potential involvement of deep, functionally critical brain regions.[5]

55.2.2 Contraindications

- Contraindications to undergo general anesthesia.
- Patients with uncorrectable coagulopathy may be at increased risk of complications.

55.3 Informed Consent

- The primary surgeon is responsible for ensuring informed consent is obtained before any procedure. This involves a discussion tailored to the patient's level of understanding, which must cover the following: the indication for surgery, why the patient is a candidate, any planned modifications to the standard procedure, risks and benefits, types and likelihood of complications, and what to expect during recovery. Informed consent reflects evolving ethical and legal standards that uphold patient autonomy.
- Decision-making capacity must be assessed before obtaining consent. Only patients with clear capacity can provide valid consent. If capacity is lacking, a legally designated surrogate, such as a power of attorney or the next of kin, as defined by law, must make decisions on the patient's behalf.

55.4 Instruments

- Robotic surgical platform (e.g., ROSA ONE Brain, Zimmer Biomet).
  - Most widely used stereotactic robotic system for SEEG, with demonstrated safety and efficacy.
  - Each case typically includes manufacturer support for nonsterile software guidance.
- Instrument holder (robot arm mounted).
- Drill (for marking and skull drilling).
- Drill bit (2.4-mm diameter, longest available length > 200 mm).
- Drill stop.
- Powered drill handpiece (e.g., Medtronic TRITON, Stryker System 7).
- Electrocautery pen (monopolar).

- Electrosurgical generator.
- Ruler (for measuring drill depth).
- Dural puncture needle.
- Stylet (or obturator stylet).
- Monopolar cautery used with a stylet.
- Anchor bolt (e.g., PMT, Dixi).
- Anchor bolt driver/screwdriver.
- Obturator (rigid stylet to create electrode tract).
- Flexible depth electrodes:
  - Most common options include the following:
    - Depthalon electrodes (PMT Corporation, United States).
    - MICRODEEP electrodes (Dixi Medical, France).
  - The workflow described here is primarily with PMT electrodes, though both are similar.
- Inner flexible stylet (within the electrode).
- Friction cap (electrode locking mechanism).
- Sterile surgical marker (pen).
- Steri-Strip (3M) or tape.
- Sterile connecting cable.
- Mobile EEG workstation.
- Betadine-soaked gauze.
- Nonabsorbable sutures.
- Kerlix wrap.
- Stockinette.

55.5 Patient Preparation

- Patients undergo general anesthesia with special consideration, as particular anesthetics may dampen EEG signaling, compromising the procedure.
- Hair shaving prior to surgery can be minimized by doing so in patches; however, cosmesis may be improved with one or two larger shaves.[6] The surgeon should consider the surgeries that are likely to follow (i.e., lobectomy, responsive neurostimulation [RNS], responsive neurostimulation [DBS]). In addition, cosmesis influences overall psychosocial health, which is both a motivation for epilepsy surgery and critical for recovery.[7,8,9]
- The patient is then prepped and draped in the standard sterile fashion. A sterile instrument holder attachment is affixed to the robotic arm using thumb screws, and then the robotic arm is covered with a clear sterile drape from the manufacturer.[10]

55.6 Patient Positioning

- Head fixation strategy varies significantly depending on the range of trajectories chosen. Head fixation should be thoughtful to account for the inclusion of all trajectory entry points and the clearance needed for the robotic arm.
- In the case of the ROSA ONE robot, registration is typically performed with laser-based surface matching of facial reference points (▶ Fig. 55.1).[10]
- The software automatically verifies the robotic arm's ability to align itself with all trajectories after registration. The software calculates whether the arm joints can bend to place the instrument holder along the planned trajectory at each entry point without colliding with the patient's rendered image.
- If the software deems a trajectory to be inaccessible, you can sometimes achieve accessibility by directing the software to

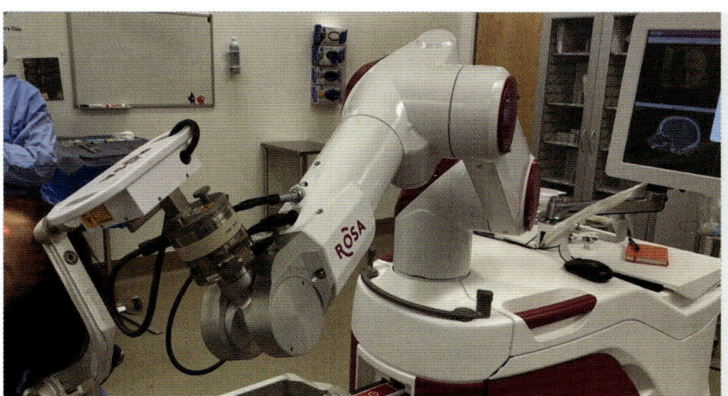

Fig. 55.1 Automated laser registration of the patient to preoperative imaging.

rotate the instrument holder to a different angle.

- If the trajectory is still unachievable, the robot is typically either too close or far from the patient's head. This requires repositioning of the head relative to the robot and re-registration to correct.
- The software is not able to account for potential collisions with the cranial fixation method (e.g., Mayfield clamp or Leksell or CRW frame). Therefore, it is useful to drive to points that appear close to the fixation pins to verify adequate clearance prior to proceeding with subsequent steps (▶ Fig. 55.2).

55.7 Technique

55.7.1 Incision

- Select the trajectory on the robot and step on the pedal to allow alignment of the robot arm along the chosen trajectory. The arm will move along the axis of the trajectory (axial mode), and you can manually advance it as close as desired to the entry point on the skin. You may select "fast" or "slow" speed for moving the arm.
- Mark the entry point by placing the drill through the instrument holder to make a small indentation on the skin using the tip of the drill (▶ Fig. 55.3).

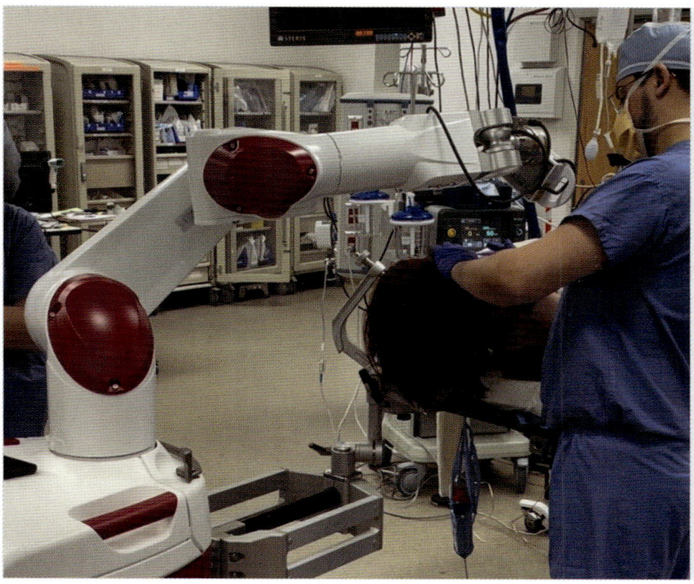

Fig. 55.2 Verifying adequate clearance for trajectories and marking entry points on the skin for hair clipping and sterile preparation.

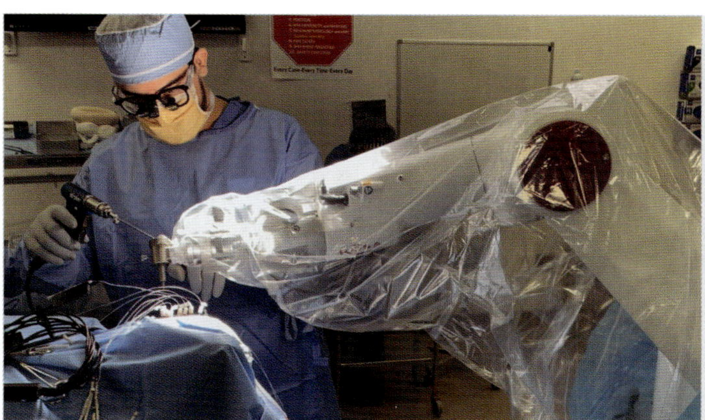

Fig. 55.3 Moving the robotic arm to a given trajectory and marking the entry point.

- In axial mode, pull the robot arm away from the scalp insertion site to give yourself enough clearance to administer local anesthetic, fit a blade, and use an electrocautery pen.
- Using a no. 15 blade, make a stab incision at the entry point. The orientation of the blade should be such that the long axis of the blade is oriented along the superior inferior (craniocaudal) axis. This is to minimize the risk of transversely cutting a scalp blood **vessel**, which is most likely to run from inferior to superior.[11] Moreover, such an incision will be parallel with the lines of minimum tension (Langer lines), maximizing healing potential and minimizing scarring.[12]
- Insert the electrocautery pen into the stab incision and coagulate. The goal is to dissect a small window in the periosteum and coagulate subcutaneous bleeders. Avoid excessive burning of tissue, which can compromise wound healing and cause postoperative pain.[13]

55.7.2 Drilling

- The bone thickness can be estimated using the software for each trajectory.
- The drill bit and stop are supplied by the electrode manufacturer and have a diameter compatible with the necessary anchor bolt. The drill bit is typically used with a standard powered handheld drill (e.g., Medtronic TRITON, Stryker System 7 rotary handpiece, etc.). The bit should be affixed to the drill handle with the shortest necessary length to pass through the instrument holder and skull; this minimizes wobble at the distal end of the bit during use. Place the drill stop onto the proximal end of the drill bit.
- Insert the drill through the instrument holder and advance the tip of the drill to the bone. This can efficiently be achieved by leaving your foot on the robot's vigilance pedal (in axial movement mode), placing the drill in the instrument holder, and pushing the robotic arm and drill tip forward together until the drill tip hits bone. Then, using the axial movement again, push the tip of the instrument holder to the surface of the skin.
- With the drill tip touching the bone, adjust the drill stop to the estimated bone thickness. This can be done with a ruler or can be approximated, as the stop is only meant as a rough guide. Remember to keep the tip of the instrument holder pushed to the skin surface in the prior step.
- Begin drilling at full speed until you have breached the inner table, being careful not to plunge into the brain (▶ Fig. 55.4). Ensure that your foot is off the vigilance pedal during this step so the instrument holder does not move closer to the patient while drilling. As with any other drill used in neurosurgery, the operator must attend to the tactile perception of the bone density. Recognizing the distinct feel of the outer table, cancellous bone, and inner table of the skull comes with experience and is the key to this step in the surgery. Be aware that the retention screw for the drill stop may loosen with the vibration of the drill. This should be recognized by the operator by observing the

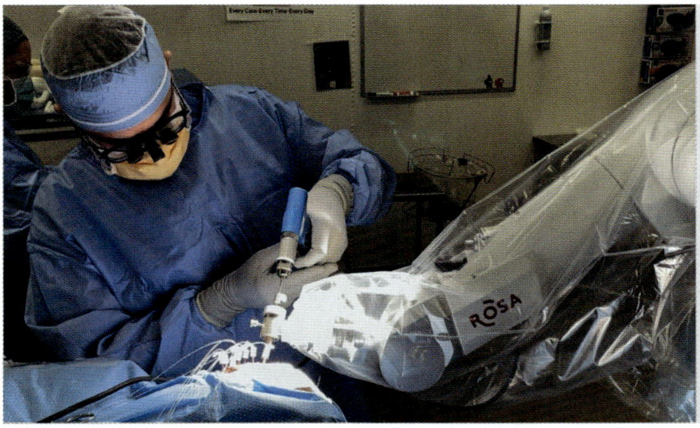

Fig. 55.4 Drilling through the instrument holder. Note the drill stop proximal to the instrument holder.

motion of the drill stop relative to the drill bit and the motion of the operator's hand. Drilling at that point should be paused and the drill should not be removed from the instrument holder to preserve the estimated depth of drilling. The drill stop is then retightened. Do not rely on the drill stop to prevent plunging after the inner table has been breached. The drill stop should be thought of as nothing more than a warning of the rough distance to the end of the inner table. It is possible that a dural opening is made with the drill, which is generally acceptable, provided there is no damage/hemorrhage caused to the underlying brain.

- Remove the drill and confirm that the inner table has been successfully breached by inserting a dural puncture needle or an obturator stylet through the instrument holder and bony opening. The length of the stylet inserted should be roughly equivalent to the length from the tip of the drill to the drill stop. This can be estimated by placing the stylet against the drill with the drill stop in place and moving your fingers to hold the stylet at the correct distance. Add a few millimeters to this length to account for the thickness of the dura. Then, insert the stylet through the instrument holder and bony opening to make a durotomy. This step can be aided with the use of monopolar cautery in contact with the stylet. The electrode manufacturers also have sharp stylets or coagulating stylets that can be used at this step as well. If any residual bone is felt with the stylet, then the drilling step must be repeated with a longer drill length.

55.7.3 Anchor Bolt Placement

- Pull the robotic arm back about 1 cm to allow room to visualize the anchor bolt. Of note, this is the first point at which the arm is moved since being placed into position for drilling.
- Load an anchor bolt on its driver and pass it through the instrument holder until it contacts the outer opening in the bone (▶ Fig. 55.5). Note that not all manufacturers' anchor bolts pass through the instrument holder. If so, the robot arm must be slightly withdrawn on axial mode, the screwdriver is passed through the instrument holder, the anchor bolt is placed on the end of the screwdriver, and then threaded into the burr hole. It is important to visualize the anchor bolt as it is susceptible to plunging. Even with minimal force, the anchor bolt may plunge through the burr hole into the brain, as unforeseeable factors such as defects or hollow areas in the bone may compromise the borders of the bony window, allowing the bolt to slip in.
- Screw in the anchor bolt. The bolt should be finger tight. Keep in mind that screws going through certain locations, such as the thin squamosal temporal bone, may feel loose even when screwed in the appropriate depth. Care must be taken not to screw in too deeply, as this

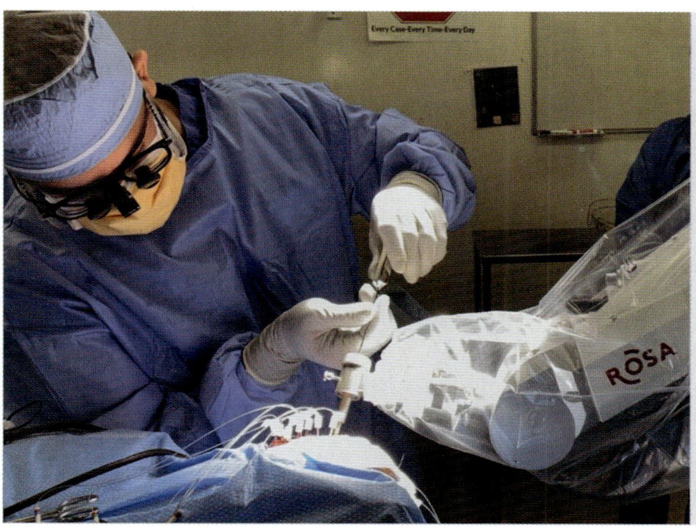

Fig. 55.5 Placing the anchor bolt through the instrument holder. Note that the arm is moved slightly away from the patient's head on the axial mode to visualize the bolt.

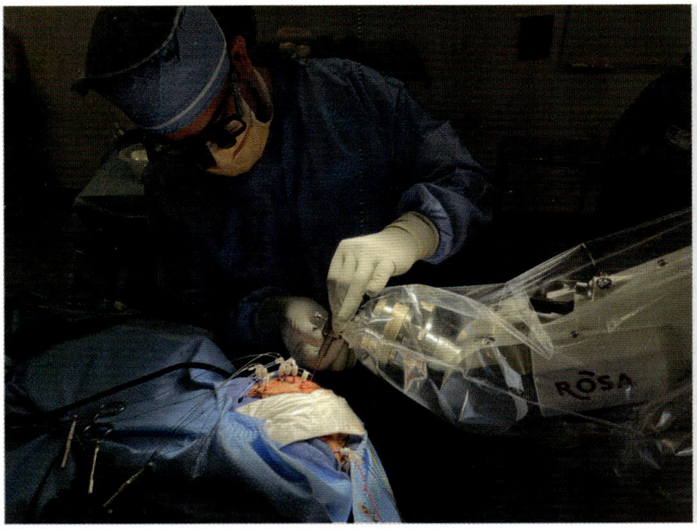

Fig. 55.6 Measurement of the electrode length. The instrument holder is moved on the axial mode to the top of the bolt; the software then provides a measurement.

may breach the inner table. Again, it is critical to visualize the depth of the anchor bolt due to the risk of plunging. After placing the bolt, move the robot arm on axial mode away from the patient and check that the bolt is securely placed by gently pressing on the side of the bolt.

- Bring the tip of the instrument holder to the top of the anchor bolt (▶ Fig. 55.6). This allows the robot's software to measure the distance from the top of the anchor bolt to the target. This distance is the electrode length.

55.7.4 Lead Placement and Electrophysiological Confirmation

- The PMT electrode has an inner stylet but is not sufficiently rigid to prevent deflections and deviations from a straight path. Therefore, an obturator stylet is used to create a tract for the subsequent electrode. Measure the obturator and place a stop at the measured length to target.
- Gently insert the obturator to depth. This will open the pial planes that will allow the flexible electrode to pass through, helping assure that the appropriate trajectory is followed. As with any step that involves passage of instruments through the brain, the obturator should be advanced slowly and carefully. Leave the obturator in place in the brain until the electrode is ready for placement.
- While inserting the obturator, an assistant should measure the length of the electrode to be inserted. This is done by moving the friction cap on the electrode to the bolt-to-target distance. Because the cap may slide on the electrode, a marker can be used to indicate the correct length. An effective method is to use a small cut piece of Steri-Strip (3 M, Saint Paul, MN) tape folded around the electrode at the distal end of the cap, preventing the cap from sliding distal to the measured length. Thus, from distal to proximal, you have the tape, the cap, and then a length of electrode equal to the measured bolt-to-target distance.
- Carefully remove the obturator from the anchor bolt, and slowly pass the electrode through the anchor bolt. It is helpful to hold the electrode at the interface of the screw cap and the tape, so that all the components are advanced as a unit.
- Tighten the friction cap while holding the electrode in place and remove the inner flexible stylet of the electrode prior to fully securing the cap. When the cap is tightened, friction will prevent the electrode from sliding in the anchor bolt. The inner stylet is typically removed after a few turns of the cap but before full tightening, as compression of the electrode will prevent removal of the stylet. The electrode should not be advanced into the brain without the inner stylet, as this "soft pass" would increase the likelihood of deflection. The electrode may need to be advanced a millimeter or two to the proper distance as the cap is tightened.

- Plug in the electrode to the sterile connecting cable connected to the mobile EEG workstation. This is to capture a short tracing to check the proper function of the electrode. In some instances, the information acquired intraoperatively can be used to guide additional electrode placement or indicate a nonfunctional electrode that should be replaced.

55.7.5 Closure

- Wrap the base of the anchor bolts with thin strips of betadine-soaked gauze. Electrode wires are clustered together with a tension relief loop and sutured to the scalp.
- A Kerlix wrap and stockinette can be used to cover the head, and the electrode plugs can be threaded out of a hole cut in the top.

55.8 Postoperative Care

- The patient should be extubated at the end of the case.
- A postoperative CT scan is obtained to determine the presence of any major electrode deflection or complication and to reconstruct final electrode positions.
- The patient is transferred to an epilepsy monitoring unit suited for constant monitoring of seizure activity.
- There will be a decrease in antiseizure medication to induce a seizure for monitoring.
- Monitor electrode insertion sites for signs of bleeding, cerebrospinal fluid (CSF) leak, or infection.
- After a week or longer, if needed, and one or more seizure instances, electrodes will be removed under localized anesthesia in the operating room.

55.9 Complications

55.9.1 Intraoperative

- CSF leak and loss.
- Hemorrhage with subsequent brain shift.

55.9.2 Postoperative

- CSF leak.
- Cerebritis.
- Hemorrhage.
- Confusion and behavioral symptoms.
- Infection at insertion sites.
- Electrode breaking.

55.9.3 Special Risks

- Incomplete bone drilling causes the electrode to deflect off of this in an unintended trajectory, potentially damaging other structures.
- Compromised electrode accuracy and weakened bone resulting from redrilling and placement of a rescue bolt.
- An anchor bolt may slip into the cranium, rendering the bolt unusable. This may increase the risk of CSF loss and brain shift with hemorrhage.

55.10 Management Pearls

- Omitting or incompletely achieving a single step can lead to multiplicative downstream consequences, including harmful complications or inaccurate data. This may contribute to SEEG's failure rate in localizing the seizure focus.[5]
- There are opportunities to maximize efficiency, particularly when there are two operators present. The soonest you can ask for the bone thickness of the next trajectory is after completion of the drilling step, so that an assistant can prepare the drill with the stop in the appropriate position while waiting. The soonest an assistant can make an incision on the next trajectory is after measuring the distance to the target of the prior trajectory, at which point the robotic arm is then free for use.
- The longer end of the same cannula used to create the pial/parenchymal tract for the electrode can likely be used to check for bone clearance and to make a durotomy without needing to change the position of the stop, provided that the prior trajectory was not significantly longer.

References

[1] Jobst BC, Cascino GD. Resective epilepsy surgery for drug-resistant focal epilepsy: a review. JAMA. 2015; 313(3): 285–293

[2] Ryvlin P, Cross JH, Rheims S. Epilepsy surgery in children and adults. Lancet Neurol. 2014; 13(11):1114–1126

[3] Kwan P, Arzimanoglou A, Berg AT, et al. Definition of drug resistant epilepsy: consensus proposal by the ad hoc Task Force of the ILAE Commission on Therapeutic Strategies. Epilepsia. 2010; 51(6):1069–1077

[4] Miller KJ, Fine AL. Decision-making in stereotactic epilepsy surgery. Epilepsia. 2022; 63(11):2782–2801

[5] Méreaux J-L, Gilard V, Le Goff F, et al. Practice of stereo electroencephalography (sEEG) in drug-resistant epilepsy: retrospective series with surgery and thermocoagulation outcomes. Neurochirurgie. 2020; 66(3):139–143

[6] Pereira JLB, Vieira G, Jr, de Albuquerque LAF, et al. Skin closure in vascular neurosurgery: a prospective study on absorbable intradermal suture versus nonabsorbable suture. Surg Neurol Int. 2012; 3:94

[7] Azuma H, Akechi T. Effects of psychosocial functioning, depression, seizure frequency, and employment on quality of life in patients with epilepsy. Epilepsy Behav. 2014; 41:18–20

[8] Ratanalert S, Sriplung H. Social attitudes toward shaving for cranial neurosurgery. Br J Neurosurg. 2001; 15(2): 132–136

[9] McDowell MM, Ortega Peraza D, Abel TJ. Development and implementation of a novel child life protocol to enhance psychosocial support for pediatric awake craniotomies: technical note. Neurosurg Focus. 2020; 48(2):E5

[10] Zimmer_Biomet. ROSA ONE® Brain SEEG Demo. 2023. Available at: https://www.zimmerbiomet.eu/en/products/rosa-one-r-brain?videoId=6277781091001

[11] Ellis H, Mahadevan V. The surgical anatomy of the scalp. Surgery (Oxf). 2014; 32:e1–e5

[12] Seery GE. Surgical anatomy of the scalp. Dermatol Surg. 2002; 28(7):581–587

[13] Massarweh NN, Cosgriff N, Slakey DP. Electrosurgery: history, principles, and current and future uses. J Am Coll Surg. 2006; 202(3):520–530

56 ROSA-Assisted Deep Brain Stimulation Surgery in Awake Patient

Khaled Taghlabi, Sibi Rajendran, Rijul Nanda, Isuru Somawardana, Jesus G. Cruz-Garza, and Amir H. Faraji

56.1 Background

- Deep brain stimulation (DBS) is a neurosurgical procedure utilized to treat neurological disorders, including Parkinson's disease,[1] essential tremor,[2] epilepsy,[3] dystonia,[4] and in obsessive-compulsive disorder[5] and depression[6] that is refractory to pharmacological treatment.[7] ROSA One (Robotic Stereotactic Assist; Zimmer Biomet, Warsaw, IN) is a stereotactic tool used to precisely locate and target specific areas of the brain. It can be utilized in DBS surgery to place electrodes under the direction of the surgeon, often in conjunction with motor testing in an awake operation.[8]
- In this procedure, specific deep areas of the brain are targeted, including the subthalamic nucleus (STN) or globus pallidus internus (GPi) in Parkinson's disease, and the ventral intermediate nucleus (VIM) of the thalamus in essential tremor. Electrodes can be stimulated with variable parameters. In Parkinson's disease, for example, this procedure may help treat tremor, rigidity, and bradykinesia. A programmable internal pulse generator (IPG) is implanted (often in a second-stage procedure in the chest) to help deliver constant therapy.

56.2 Indications and Contraindications

- DBS is utilized in the United States for the treatment of several conditions, including essential tremor, Parkinson's disease, epilepsy, dystonia, and obsessive-compulsive disorder that is refractory to treatment.[7] DBS with robotic assistance is indicated for all the same procedures in which DBS is indicated. DBS has also been utilized for the treatment of pain disorders, Tourette's syndrome, and experimentally for the treatment of major depressive disorder.[9,10]
- There are few contraindications for DBS, and these contraindications are most often related to the inability to properly operate the implanted IPG.[11] The presence of advanced cognitive deficits, based on neuropsychological testing, and psychiatric comorbidities are the major nonmedical contraindications for DBS. These patients include those with dementia and psychiatric disorders, psychogenic movement disorders, and asymptomatic Parkinson's disease. Active infections may also represent a contraindication, as with many operations involving implanted hardware.

56.3 Instruments

- Robotic stereotactic assistance device:
  - The ROSA One robot is a cutting-edge system used in various neurosurgical procedures, including DBS.[8,12,13] The ROSA robot was developed to provide a high level of precision, accuracy, and safety in neurosurgical procedures.[8,12,13] In DBS, it allows for the precise placement of electrodes by smoothly integrating with various imaging modalities, such as computed tomography (CT) and magnetic resonance imaging (MRI).[8,12,13] The system features a robotic arm that can be controlled by the surgeon to mark entry points, create burr holes, and assist in electrode implantation.[8,12,13]
  - While workflow may vary by surgeon preference, an intraoperative CT scan is often obtained and fused to preoperatively acquired MRI in ROSA imaging software.[8,13] Robot registration is completed based on fiducial or frame-based landmarks after the patient's skull is secured. Trajectories are created based on this fused image. The secure robotic arm can identify and move to planned trajectories—with a variety of attachments that can facilitate burr hole creation, lead insertion, and microelectrode recording when applicable.[8,13]
- Leksell stereotactic frame:
  - The Leksell frame is an essential instrument in neurosurgery, particularly in DBS surgery. Its primary purpose is to provide surgeons with a stable and highly precise reference system to

accurately target specific brain regions.[14,15] It is an arc-shaped lightweight structure composed of sturdy materials like carbon fiber or aluminum and it is attached to the patient's skull with pins and screws. It reduces the risk of damaging healthy tissue by enabling surgeons to navigate the brain with remarkable accuracy.[15]
  - The Leksell frame is attached to the patient's head before surgery, and a three-dimensional (3D) brain map is produced using stereotactic imaging methods such as CT or MRI scans.[16] This map is then aligned with the frame's coordinates allowing the surgeon to precisely guide their instruments.
- Alpha Omega Microdrive:
  - The Alpha Omega microelectrode drive system (NeuroFortis, Alpha Omega Engineering, Nof HaGalil, Israel) is a motorized and automatic drive system that allows for microelectrode recording, macrostimulation, and recording of local field potentials.[8] These techniques can be combined with awake neurological testing to confirm proper lead placement, therapeutic success, and avoidance of off-target effects.

56.4 Patient Preparation

- The initial diagnostic phase begins with a thorough evaluation of the patient's medical history, physical examination, and clinical symptoms. The selection process for appropriate patient candidates considers factors such as the patient's medical comorbidities, cognitive function, and suitability for awake surgery. A comprehensive neurological assessment is conducted to identify the exact targets for stimulation within the brain, aligning them with the patient's specific disease profile, and assessing the patient's Unified Parkinson's Disease Rating Scale (UPDRS) and Hoehn and Yahr scores. Certain other diagnostics including dopamine transporter scan may be used as an adjunct in diagnosis, with the bulk of this workup completed by the neurology team.
- To ensure the patient's cognitive and emotional well-being throughout the procedure, comprehensive neuropsychological assessments are performed preoperatively.
- In summary, robot-assisted DBS surgery in an awake patient demands meticulous preparatory diagnostics. This comprehensive approach, encompassing patient selection, neuroimaging, target localization, preoperative planning, neuropsychological assessments, and anesthesia consultation, sets the stage for a successful surgical intervention. By tailoring these diagnostics to the patient's unique disease profile, the surgical team can optimize the outcomes of the DBS procedure, ultimately improving the patient's quality of life.

56.5 Patient Positioning

- Supine with the head of the bed elevated.

56.6 Technique

- The following section provides a detailed account of the technical steps involved in a typical DBS surgery for Parkinson's disease using ROSA robotic assistance in an awake patient (**Video 56.1**).
- Preoperative preparation:
  - The patient, in stable condition, is transported from the holding area to the operating room. Intravenous sedation is administered by the anesthesia team to ensure patient comfort and immobility. The patient's scalp is prepared for surgery (**Video 56.1**). The Leksell frame is mounted on the patient's head. Pin sites are anesthetized with a mixture of 0.5% Marcaine, 2% lidocaine, and 1:100,000 epinephrine. Four pins are placed (two in the frontal bone and two in the occipital bone) per the standard mounting procedure (**Video 56.1**).
- Stereotactic planning:
  - The patient is transported to the CT scanner, where a stereotactic volumetric fine-cut scan of the brain is obtained (**Video 56.1**). The acquired CT scan images are transferred to the ROSA workstation. These images are merged with a volumetric MRI scan of the brain on the ROSA intraoperative system. A 3D fused reconstruction is created, facilitating precise targeting (**Video 56.1**).
  - *Coordinate determination:* The white matter commissures are identified, and the anterior commissure–posterior commissure (AC-PC) line is established, along with its midpoint. In consultation with the patient's neurologist, the clinical target is determined. Entry points are

carefully chosen, considering factors such as the patient's hairline, vasculature, and ventricles, to minimize pial transgressions. Once the patient is positioned and the head frame secured to the robot, the ROSA system is registered using four fiducial Leksell pin sites, ensuring precise alignment (**Video 56.1**). The ROSA root mean square error is minimized and a tolerance of ≤ 0.50 mm is generally accepted. To minimize the risk of injury, bed controls are unplugged, and the ROSA is locked securely to the Leksell frame head holder. DBS entry points are marked on the patient's skin. A minimal head shave is performed, followed by degreasing and sterilization. Proposed incision sites are anesthetized using local anesthesia. Sterile drapes, including a clear drape, are placed to maintain aseptic conditions (**Video 56.1**).

- Surgical procedure:
  - Small coronally oriented incisions are made at the entry points using a no. 10 blade. Self-retaining retractors are placed, and hemorrhage is controlled using monopolar and bipolar electrocautery. The ROSA arm is introduced to mark bone entry sites, and burr holes are created on both sides of the midline using a perforator drill (**Video 56.1**). The device locking cap systems are carefully placed and tested to ensure proper function. The ROSA system verifies the absence of collisions along the potential implantation tracts.
- Intraoperative steps:
  - The patient is allowed to awaken from sedation, and a baseline neurological examination is conducted. The dura is cauterized on the left side, opened in a cruciate fashion using a no. 11 blade, and a small corticectomy is performed using bipolar cautery and a no. 11 blade (**Video 56.1**). The ROSA navigates to the left side and is set to 160 mm from the target for microelectrode recordings. The Alpha Omega microelectrode drive is mounted, and three simultaneous guide tubes and microelectrodes are passed down different trajectories (**Video 56.1**). Microelectrode recordings are obtained, and brain physiological mapping is performed while macrostimulation is applied at increasing currents. The patient's neurological examination is monitored for any off-target effects. Once a satisfactory tract is identified, the microelectrodes are removed, but the guide tubes remain in place. The DBS electrode is lowered to the target along the appropriate guide tube tract (**Video 56.1**). A microlesion effect and good efficacy are often observed with the leads activated at standard parameters and through the range of standard programming currents.
- Electrode placement and closure:
  - Once passed down the appropriate guide tube tract, the electrode is secured using the standard device burr hole system and marked distally with a long uncut protecting boot (**Video 56.1**). The same process is repeated on the opposite side. The DBS electrode is marked distally with a protecting boot or marking. The distal aspect of the electrode from one side is brought through a subgaleal tunnel to a pocket at the parietal boss site. Redundant coils are placed in a subgaleal fashion. Copious amounts of antibiotic irrigation are used for infection prevention. Vancomycin powder is applied to further reduce infection risk. All bleeding points are meticulously controlled using bipolar cautery. Monopolar cautery is avoided after lead placement.
- Closure and postoperative care wound closure:
  - The galea is closed using the usual inverted interrupted fashion, followed by skin closure with suture or skin staples. The wounds are cleaned with hydrogen peroxide and dried. Bacitracin ointment is applied, and sterile dressings are placed.

56.7 Postoperative Care

- Wound care is essential.
- Engage in physical activities/activities of daily living as tolerated; do not strain.

56.8 Complications

- While uncommon, hemorrhage, infection, and hardware malfunction or failure remain the most frequently encountered complications. Intracerebral hemorrhage rates vary across literature, typically cited as approximately 2.3% of cases.[17] Infection is also uncommon, cited as 5% or so of cases, but often requires explanation of one or more system components.[18] Hardware malfunctions (typically requiring revision) are thought to occur in less than 2% of cases.[19] Decline in verbal fluency has been reported as a long-term side effect in Parkinson's disease patients who underwent DBS surgery[20,21,22] with a significant medium effect size of $d = -0.47$ for letter fluency when comparing STN-DBS patients versus those in the nonsurgical comparison group.[23]

56.9 Management Pearls

- Careful attention should be given to patient selection, choosing those without advanced neurocognitive deficits or serious neuropsychiatric comorbidities that could complicate awake surgery and successful stimulation.
- Awake, robot-guided DBS with microelectrode recording and macrostimulation, where applicable, increases both precision and accuracy, with a widely adoptable workflow.
- Effective communication and collaboration between neurosurgeons, neurophysiology staff, device representatives, anesthesia, and neurology teams are critical to successful therapy, both during and after surgery.
- DBS is an FDA-approved treatment for Parkinson's disease and other neurological disorders.[24] Initially, it evolved from early surgical lesioning procedures such as thalamotomy and pallidotomy, which were among the first treatments for Parkinson's disease in the 1950s.[25] However, it was not until the 1980s that modern DBS, involving midbrain and basal ganglia electrical stimulation, was introduced to suppress intention tremor. Over the years, DBS has shown a more favorable side effect profile compared to thalamotomy and pallidotomy procedures, including offering greater adjustability and safety.[26] Additionally, DBS has also become a valuable research tool, shedding light on the basal ganglia, including the anatomy and electrical properties, as well as neural network interactions.[27]
- The field of DBS has rapidly grown, with over 160,000 patients worldwide receiving DBS, and new patients treated at a rate exceeding 12,000 per year.[28] Advances in DBS technology have been notable, including improvements in preoperative and intraoperative imaging, surgical techniques, and device enhancements. The development of noninvasive DBS techniques, although currently less temporally precise and anatomically specific than traditional DBS, is an area of active research.[29,30] Finally, future DBS developments are aimed at disease modification, seeking to address the underlying neurological disorder or circuit abnormality rather than just alleviating symptoms. The potential for gene therapy, immunotherapy, and cell transplantation, combined with emerging techniques like optogenetics, magnetogenetics, and sonogenetics, offers the prospect of a more targeted and effective approach to neurological and psychiatric disorders.[28]
- Additional resources on ROSA-assisted DBS in awake patients can be found in the following:
  - Faraji AH, and Richardson RM. Deep brain stimulation in early Parkinson's disease may slow rest tremor progression. Neurosurgery 2019;84(1): E13–E14.
  - Peña CE, Faraji AH, Richardson RM. Deep brain stimulation for Tourette syndrome. Neurosurgery 2018;83(1):E13.
  - Jin H, Gong S, Tao Y, et al. A comparative study of asleep and awake deep brain stimulation robot-assisted surgery for Parkinson's disease. NPJ Parkinson's Dis 2020;6:27.
  - Merola A, Singh J, Reeves K, et al. New frontiers for deep brain stimulation: directionality, sensing technologies, remote programming, robotic stereotactic assistance, asleep procedures, and connectomics. Front Neurol 2021;12:694747.
  - Schulder M, Mishra A, Mammis A, et al. Advances in technical aspects of deep brain stimulation surgery. Stereotact Funct Neurosurg 2023;101(2):112–134.

56.10 Emerging Technologies

- One variant of robot-assisted DBS for Parkinson's disease is extradural motor cortex stimulation, which is a less invasive operation for some patients.[31] Other patients may be indicated for pallidotomy, a procedure that creates a lesion in the globus pallidus interna if they have levodopa toxicity, dystonia, or bradykinesia and tremor.[32] Thalamotomy, an operation in which the thalamus is cauterized, is another option for patients for the treatment of tremors.[32] Focused ultrasound ablation is also being utilized for the treatment of essential tremors[33] and Parkinson's disease.[34] DBS, however, remains the most used procedure for patients with Parkinson's disease, dystonia, and essential tremor due to the ability to modulate therapy over the course of many years.[35] Outside of surgery, medical management is recommended.[36]

References

[1] Faraji AH, Richardson RM. Deep brain stimulation in early Parkinson's disease may slow rest tremor progression. Neurosurgery. 2019; 84(1):E13–E14

[2] Wong JK, Hess CW, Almeida L, et al. Deep brain stimulation in essential tremor: targets, technology, and a comprehensive review of clinical outcomes. Expert Rev Neurother. 2020; 20 (4):319–331

[3] Peltola J, Colon AJ, Pimentel J, et al. MORE Study Group. Deep brain stimulation of the anterior nucleus of the thalamus in drug-resistant epilepsy in the MORE multicenter patient registry. Neurology. 2023; 100(18):e1852–e1865

[4] Dietz N, Neimat J. Neuromodulation: deep brain stimulation for treatment of dystonia. Neurosurg Clin N Am. 2019; 30(2): 161–168

[5] Sheth SA, Mayberg HS. Deep brain stimulation for obsessive-compulsive disorder and depression. Annu Rev Neurosci. 2023; 46:341–358

[6] Figee M, Riva-Posse P, Choi KS, Bederson L, Mayberg HS, Kopell BH. Deep brain stimulation for depression. Neurotherapeutics. 2022; 19(4):1229–1245

[7] Fariba K, Gupta V. Deep Brain Stimulation. Treasure Island, FL: StatPearls Publishing; 2020

[8] Faraji AH, Kokkinos V, Sweat JC, Crammond DJ, Richardson RM. Robotic-assisted stereotaxy for deep brain stimulation lead implantation in awake patients. Oper Neurosurg (Hagerstown). 2020; 19(4):444–452

[9] Sugiyama K, Nozaki T, Asakawa T, Koizumi S, Saitoh O, Namba H. The present indication and future of deep brain stimulation. Neurol Med Chir (Tokyo). 2015; 55(5):416–421

[10] Peña CE, Faraji AH, Richardson RM. Deep brain stimulation for Tourette syndrome. Neurosurgery. 2018; 83(1):E13

[11] Kocabicak E, Temel Y, Höllig A, Falkenburger B, Tan SKh. Current perspectives on deep brain stimulation for severe neurological and psychiatric disorders. Neuropsychiatr Dis Treat. 2015; 11:1051–1066

[12] Liu L, Mariani SG, De Schlichting E, et al. Frameless ROSA® robot-assisted lead implantation for deep brain stimulation: technique and accuracy. Oper Neurosurg (Hagerstown). 2020; 19(1):57–64

[13] Giridharan N, Katlowitz KA, Anand A, et al. Robot-assisted deep brain stimulation: high accuracy and streamlined workflow. Oper Neurosurg (Hagerstown). 2022; 23(3): 254–260

[14] Bot M, van den Munckhof P, Bakay R, Sierens D, Stebbins G, Verhagen Metman L. Analysis of stereotactic accuracy in patients undergoing deep brain stimulation using Nexframe and the Leksell frame. Stereotact Funct Neurosurg. 2015; 93(5):316–325

[15] Phillips KR, Mackel CE, Alterman RL. Targeting accuracy of the Leksell Vantage Stereotactic System for deep brain stimulation surgery: a retrospective review. Oper Neurosurg (Hagerstown). 2023; 24(6):602–609

[16] Simon SL, Douglas P, Baltuch GH, Jaggi JL. Error analysis of MRI and Leksell stereotactic frame target localization in deep brain stimulation surgery. Stereotact Funct Neurosurg. 2005; 83(1):1–5

[17] Jung I-H, Chang KW, Park SH, Chang WS, Jung HH, Chang JW. Complications after deep brain stimulation: a 21-year experience in 426 patients. Front Aging Neurosci. 2022; 14: 819730

[18] Tabaja H, Yuen J, Tai DBG, et al. Deep brain stimulator device infection: the Mayo Clinic Rochester Experience. Open Forum Infect Dis. 2023; 10(1):ofac631

[19] Rolston JD, Englot DJ, Starr PA, Larson PS. An unexpectedly high rate of revisions and removals in deep brain stimulation surgery: analysis of multiple databases. Parkinsonism Relat Disord. 2016; 33:72–77

[20] Tripoliti E, Zrinzo L, Martinez-Torres I, et al. Effects of subthalamic stimulation on speech of consecutive patients with Parkinson disease. Neurology. 2011; 76(1):80–86

[21] Skodda S. Effect of deep brain stimulation on speech performance in Parkinson's disease. Parkinson's Disease. 2012; 2012:850596

[22] Baudouin R, Lechien JR, Carpentier L, Gurruchaga JM, Lisan Q, Hans S. Deep brain stimulation impact on voice and speech quality in Parkinson's disease: a systematic review. Otolaryngol Head Neck Surg. 2023; 168(3):307–318

[23] Wyman-Chick KA. Verbal fluency in Parkinson's patients with and without bilateral deep brain stimulation of the subthalamic nucleus: a meta-analysis. J Int Neuropsychol Soc. 2016; 22(4):478–485

[24] Bell E, Mathieu G, Racine E. Preparing the ethical future of deep brain stimulation. Surg Neurol. 2009; 72(6):577–586, discussion 586

[25] Okun MS, Foote KD. Parkinson's disease DBS: what, when, who and why? The time has come to tailor DBS targets. Expert Rev Neurother. 2010; 10(12):1847–1857

[26] Brice J, McLellan L. Suppression of intention tremor by contingent deep-brain stimulation. Lancet. 1980; 1(8180): 1221–1222

[27] Dostrovsky JO, Lozano AM. Mechanisms of deep brain stimulation. Mov Disord. 2002; 17 Suppl 3:S63–S68

[28] Lee DJ, Lozano CS, Dallapiazza RF, Lozano AM. Current and future directions of deep brain stimulation for neurological and psychiatric disorders. J Neurosurg. 2019; 131(2):333–342

[29] Grossman N, Bono D, Dedic N, et al. Noninvasive deep brain stimulation via temporally interfering electric fields. Cell. 2017; 169(6):1029–1041.e16

[30] Liu X, Qiu F, Hou L, Wang X. Review of noninvasive or minimally invasive deep brain stimulation. Front Behav Neurosci. 2022; 15:820017

[31] Wolters Kluwer Health: Lippincott Williams & Wilkins. Less-invasive method of brain stimulation helps patients with Parkinson's disease. ScienceDaily. 2012. Accessed April 26, 2025 at: www.sciencedaily.com/releases/2012/10/121016103413.htm

[32] Fukuda M, Kameyama S, Yoshino M, Tanaka R, Narabayashi H. Neuropsychological outcome following pallidotomy and thalamotomy for Parkinson's disease. Stereotact Funct Neurosurg. 2000; 74(1):11–20
[33] Torii J, Maesawa S, Nakatsubo D, et al. Cutoff values for the best management strategy for magnetic resonance-guided focused ultrasound ablation for essential tremor. J Neurosurg. 2022; 138(1):38–49
[34] Schrag A. Focused ultrasound ablation of the globus pallidus internus for Parkinson's disease. N Engl J Med. 2023; 388(8): 759–760
[35] Limousin P, Foltynie T. Long-term outcomes of deep brain stimulation in Parkinson disease. Nat Rev Neurol. 2019; 15(4):234–242
[36] Schapira AH. Treatment options in the modern management of Parkinson disease. Arch Neurol. 2007; 64(8):1083–1088

57 Stereotactic Thermal Ablation for Temporal Lobe Epilepsy

Ryan T. Cleary, Salil Bhole, and Jon T. Willie

57.1 Background

- Open temporal lobe surgery is effective and has been considered the gold standard for treatment of medically refractory temporal lobe epilepsy (TLE). However, the introduction of stereotactic laser interstitial thermal therapy (LITT) as a minimally invasive alternative has challenged the primary role of open surgery, especially for medial or deep-seated seizure onset zones (SOZs). Below we will discuss the workup for TLE, compare advantages and disadvantages of open surgery versus LITT, and outline our recommendations on operative planning and technique for LITT.
- TLE is the most common cause of medically refractory epilepsy in adults. TLE can be further divided into subtypes based on the predominant location of the SOZ: mesial TLE (MTLE), neocortical lateral TLE (LTLE), temporopolar epilepsy (TPE), and temporal plus epilepsy (TE+) in which the SOZ extends to extratemporal lobe structures (e.g., operculoinsular, orbitofrontal, and cingulate cortices). Proper understanding and identification of these subtypes has important implications for treatment strategies and outcomes. Common characteristics associated with these four subtypes are outlined in ▶ Table 57.1.
- The 2001 randomized controlled trial by Wiebe et al demonstrated that rates of seizure freedom in patients with MTLE undergoing anterior temporal lobectomy (ATL) are superior to medical management alone.[1,2] Although the benefits of seizure freedom generally outweigh adverse effects,[3] open temporal lobe surgery is nevertheless associated with undesirable neurocognitive deficits.[1] Subsequent

Table 57.1 Clinical features of temporal lobe epilepsy subtypes

	MTLE	LTLE	TPE	TE+
Mesial temporal sclerosis	Often	No	Often	Variable
Auras	Epigastric sensation, smell, fear, déjà vu	Auditory, vertiginous, complex visual hallucinations	Similar to MTLE	Gustatory, auditory, vertiginous hallucinations
Seizure semiology	Behavior arrest, oral automatisms	Behavior arrest, clonic movements	Similar to MTLE with earlier LOC; hypermotor	Eye/head contraversion, piloerection, tonic movement
Video EEG/SEEG	Unilateral anteromesial temporal lobe onset	Unilateral lateral temporal lobe onset	Involvement of TP in seizure onset; typically requires SEEG	Extratemporal involvement; typically requires SEEG
FDG-PET	Mesial temporal lobe hypometabolism	Neocortical hypometabolism, normal mesial metabolism	Similar to MTLE	Variable
Postoperative outcomes	Engel I: 75% ATL, 57–64% SLAH	Engel I: 69–79% ATL	Engel I: 90% ATL (data from single series)	Variable

Abbreviations: ATL, anterior temporal lobectomy; FDG-PET, positron emission tomography with ^{18}F-fluorodeoxyglucose; LOC, loss of consciousness; LTLE, neocortical lateral temporal lobe epilepsy; MTLE, mesial temporal lobe epilepsy; SLAH, stereotactic laser amygdalohippocampectomy; TE+, temporal plus epilepsy; TP, temporopolar; TPE, temporopolar epilepsy.

development of selective amygdalohippocampectomy (SAH) was proposed to decrease the incidence of naming and verbal memory deficits by preserving lateral and temporopolar structures, leading to some marginal neurocognitive benefits compared to ATL.[4,5,6,7] Meta-analyses comparing open ATL with SAH showed rates of seizure freedom of 69 to 75% for ATL and 66 to 67% for SAH.[8,9]

- Stereotactic laser amygdalohippocampectomy (SLAH), a minimally invasive procedure in which LITT is used to treat MTLE, further minimizes collateral damage. SLAH is better tolerated than analogous open surgeries, with briefer hospitalizations, less discomfort, fewer and less serious complications, and earlier return to work.[9,10,11,12,13,14,15,16,17,18] SLAH further lends itself to staged procedures and does not preclude subsequent open surgery to treat recurrent or persistent seizures, if needed.[11,19,20]
- Early published series of SLAH reported rates of seizure freedom to be lower than traditional open surgeries, with an average rate of 57% in one meta-analysis.[9] Seizure outcomes continue to improve, however, with advances in surgical technique, patient selection, and definitive SOZ localization with SEEG.[21,22,23,24,25,26,27,28] A compilation of seizure outcomes after SLAH from prior studies can be found in ▶ Table 57.2 .[10,11,12,13,14,15,18,28,29,30,31,32]
- From a surgical perspective, imaging is key to initial assessment of an SOZ. In cases of discrete epileptogenic lesions, such as mesial temporal sclerosis (MTS; defined on MRI as hippocampal atrophy, loss of internal architecture, and increased T2/FLAIR intensity), cerebral cavernous malformation, focal cortical dysplasia, or tumor, surgical approach may rely on lesionally or anatomically defined borders. By contrast, MRI-negative TLE or cases with discordant findings in noninvasive workup typically require invasive stereoelectroencephalography (SEEG) to physiologically define an SOZ, understand seizure semiology, and map functional networks to delineate surgical targets.
- Indeed, there is increasing evidence that treatment failures in lesional TLE may be due to insufficient understanding of the SOZ(s), which can extend beyond visible lesions. Indeed, while the presence of MTS has traditionally been associated with favorable surgical outcomes,[11,14,33] more recent studies suggest that SEEG guidance may be a critical predictor of efficacy.[10,18,22]
- Deficits of naming, object recognition, and verbal memory, as well as exacerbation of psychiatric burden, are common after ATL and SAH, particularly after resection in the dominant hemisphere.[34] Although reductions in seizure frequency after temporal lobe surgery provide significant improvements in quality of life,[35] even subtle declines in naming, object recognition, and verbal memory can negatively impact daily life and return to work.[36,37] Comparisons of neurocognitive outcomes after SLAH have demonstrated superior naming and verbal memory outcomes compared to ATL and SAH.[9,36,38] The stereotactic approach to mesial temporal lobe structures may be associated with improved cognitive outcomes by relative sparing of injury to the temporal pole, lateral neocortices, parahippocampal gyrus, and temporal stem white matter tracts.[39,40] Furthermore, SLAH has been suggested to stabilize and improve postoperative depression and anxiety.[41]
- There is some evidence that rates of seizure freedom after ATL may be slightly higher in suspected TPE compared to MTLE.[42,43] Rates of seizure freedom in LTLE are similar to MTLE, ranging between 69 and 79% after ATL, with the best outcomes seen in patients with neoplastic lesions.[44,45,46,47]
- Treatment of TE + remains difficult, owing in part to the need to adequately assess deep and medial structures, and failure to recognize TE + is likely a frequent cause of TLE surgery failure.[48] SEEG is particularly useful in these cases for careful SOZ mapping, but complete resection of the SOZ remains challenging due to the risk of extending resection into adjacent extratemporal regions, especially around the sylvian fissure. Although studies directly comparing LITT to open surgery are lacking for each TLE subtype, several studies indicate that LITT may be safe and effective for treating SOZs involving the insula, cingulate, and other medial frontal/parietal structures.[19,49,50,51] Likewise, preliminary studies using LITT to address TPE associated with encephaloceles are also encouraging.[52,53]

Table 57.2 Select review of case series results of stereotactic laser amygdalohippocampotomy for MTLE, minimum 12 months of follow-up

Study	Patients	Age range, (y)	Mean follow-up (mo)	Engel I seizure outcomes, *n* (%)			Mean hospital stay (d)
				MTS	Non-MTS	All	
Willie et al[54]	13	16–64	14	6/9 (67%)	4	7/13 (54%)	1
Waseem et al[16]	5	54–67	12	NR	NR	4/5 (80%)	1.6
Kang et al[13]	11	11–66	13.1	4/10 (40%)	0/1 (0%)	4/11 (36.4%)	1.2
Jermakowicz et al[12]	23	12–37	22.4	11/15 (73.3%)	5/8 (62.5%)	16/23 (69.6%)	~1.3
Gross et al[11]	58	16–67	> 12	26/43 (60.5%)	5/15 (33.3%)	31/58 (53.4%)	1.4
Donos et al[10]	43	18–73	20.3	23/34 (67.6%)	6/9 (66.7%)	29/43 (67.4%)	1
Greenway et al[30]	15	22–66	17	4/11 (36.3%)	1/4 (25%)	5/15 (33.3%)	NR
Grewal et al[31]	23	20–60	36	13/18 (72.2%)	2/5 (40%)	15/23 (65.2%)	NR
Tao et al[15]	21	20–65	24	8/11 (72.7%)	3/10 (30%)	11/21 (52.3%)	1.2
Le et al[14]	29	17–70	18	16/22 (72.7%)	2/7 (28.5%)	18/29 (62%)	~1.3
Vakharia et al[28]	19	14–66	> 12	11/19 (57.8%)	NR	11/19 (57.8%)	NR
Youngerman et al[18]	30	19–69	17	10/18 (56%)	7/12 (58.3%)	17/30 (57%)	1.1
Cajigas et al[29]	26	21–66	> 24	13/19 (68%)	3/7 (42.8%)	16/26 (61.5%)	NR

Abbreviations: MTS, mesial temporal sclerosis; n, number of patients; NR, not recorded.

57.2 Indications and Contraindications

- LITT is indicated for treating defined lesions or SOZs of size, shape, and location amenable to a stereotactic approach. LITT is particularly useful for deep or hard-to-reach locations (e.g., medial temporal and frontal cortices) in which an open approach would require larger exposures, greater discomfort, or risk to collateral structures, but LITT may also be used to treat superficial targets. Large volumes (e.g., > 50 mL), lobectomies, and topectomies intended to preserve white matter may be more pragmatically accomplished with open surgery.
- All epilepsy surgery candidates should undergo a standard workup and exhibit sufficient concordance of noninvasive and/or invasive diagnostic studies. A careful history confirms medically refractory epilepsy, defined as "failure of adequate trials of two tolerated, appropriately chosen, and used antiepileptic drug schedules

(whether as monotherapies or in combination) to achieve sustained seizure freedom."[55] Attention is given to patient descriptions of ictal semiology (the signs and symptoms associated with seizures), risk factors (e.g., abnormal birth history, physical and psychosocial trauma, febrile seizures, etc.), and current seizure triggers (e.g., sleep deprivation, stress, substance intoxication/abuse, missed medications, etc.). A summary of available evaluations and a typical decision tree is outlined in ▶ Fig. 57.1.

- Long-term video electroencephalographic (EEG) monitoring (LTVM) using scalp electrodes not only confirms the diagnosis of epilepsy but also provides primary clinical–anatomical–electrophysiological correlation of semiology, interictal epileptiform discharges, and first approximation of the SOZ. Seizure semiology should be consistent with temporal lobe onset, although it should be emphasized that (1) semiology reflects symptomatic zone more strictly than SOZ, (2) it is possible for a seizure isolated to an SOZ to be relatively asymptomatic (e.g., an isolated hippocampal seizure without spread to wider temporal and/or extratemporal lobe structures may be clinically "silent"), and (3) semiologies can differ based on the TLE subtype, seizure spread patterns (▶ Table 57.1), and/or other factors such as abnormal anatomy. Atypical clinical or electrographic features consistent with extratemporal involvement, multiple distinct semiologies, bilateral/multifocal electrographic onsets, or other discordant findings typically warrant intracranial SEEG monitoring to guide further surgical decision-making.
- High field strength (≥ 3 T) anatomical magnetic resonance imaging (MRI) is typically the next step in surgical workup and can identify the presence or absence of epilepsy-associated lesions, especially MTS, focal cortical dysplasia, heterotopias, hamartomas, gliomas, gliosis, encephaloceles, or cerebral cavernous malformations. MTS is most commonly associated with MTLE and/or TPE, whereas LTLE is more typically associated with discrete (albeit possibly occult) lesions, including neoplastic lesions (e.g., low-grade gliomas) and non-neoplastic lesions (e.g., focal cortical dysplasia, cavernous malformations, infarcts).[44,56]
- Most patients should undergo preoperative neuropsychological evaluation. This information can be used prognostically and as additional confirmation of laterality of an SOZ. Lateralization and extent of preoperative neurocognitive deficits (e.g., verbal vs. visuospatial memory, other language or fine motor deficits) not only is localizing but also can help stratify risks of deficits associated with different surgical approaches.[57,58,59,60] Concordance between areas of neurocognitive deficit and presumed SOZ strengthens the diagnostic accuracy, whereas discordance should prompt additional workup. Task-based functional MRI can also help lateralize language dominance, especially in the setting of left-handedness and/or potentially discordant neuropsychological results.
- Additional workup is typically required for non-MTLE, MTLE cases without MTS or other lesions, and whenever clearly discordant findings are present. Interictal positron emission tomography with ^{18}F-fluorodeoxyglucose (FDG-PET) is frequently used, and findings of hypometabolism in the suspected area of seizure onset can corroborate clinical history and LTVM findings. Ultimately, SEEG or other invasive EEG techniques are the gold standard for localizing seizure onset and spread when above data are insufficiently lateralizing, localizing, or otherwise discordant.
- Some contraindications specific to LITT for TLE may include poor seizure localization, independent bilateral SOZs (e.g., bilateral hippocampal seizures), deemed need for larger volume (> 50 mL) extirpations (e.g., lobectomy), need for superficial topectomy sparing underlying white matter (better served by open surgery), and need for awake ablation (LITT without general anesthesia and intubation is technically feasible but impractical).

57.3 Informed Consent

- Expected rates of seizure freedom from ablation alone depends upon multiple patient and surgical factors. Unilateral MTS with concordant noninvasive studies, or non-MTS but with

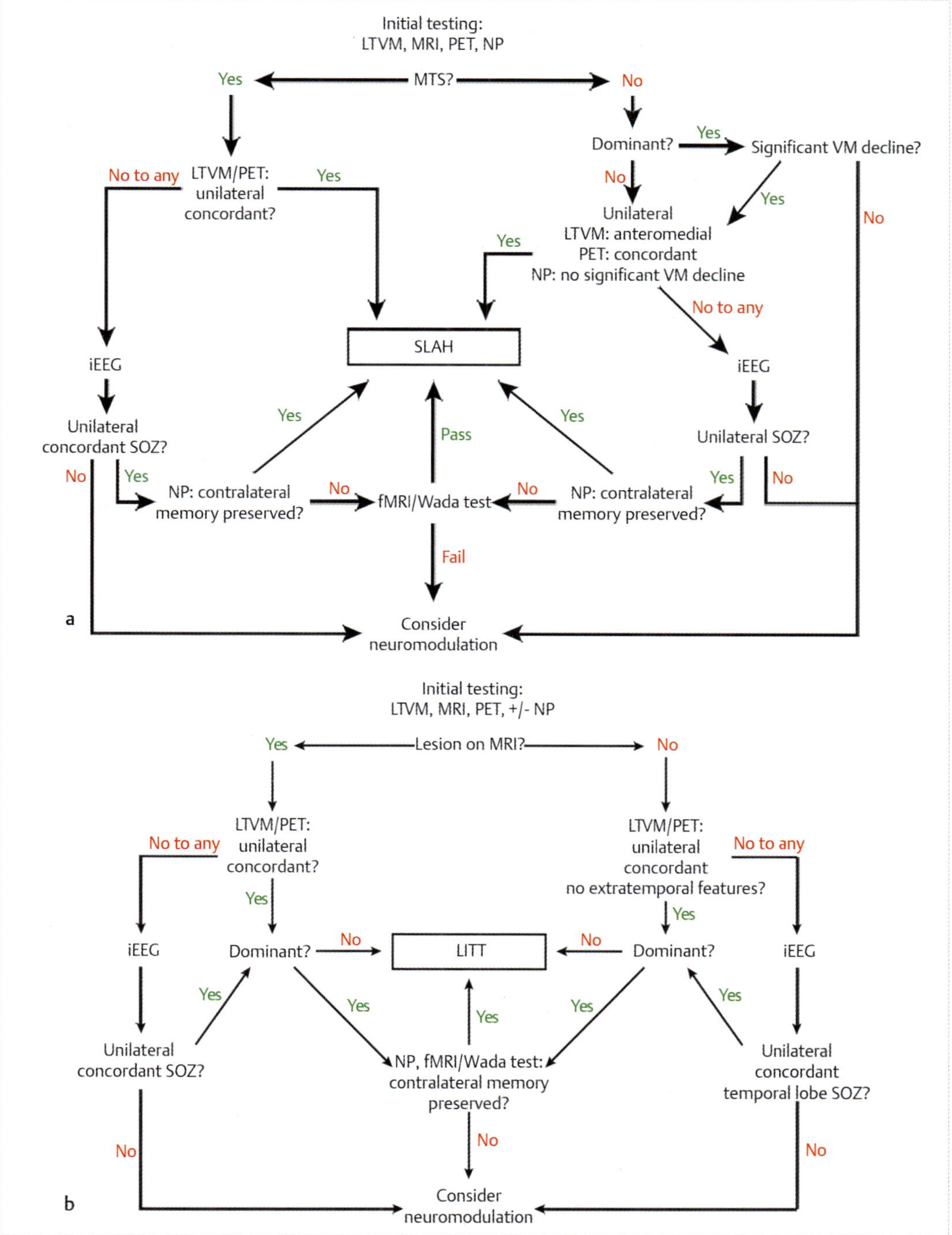

Fig. 57.1 Surgical decision tree for LITT in **(a)** MTLE and **(b)** non-MTLE. iEEG, intracranial electroencephalogram; fMRI, functional magnetic resonance imaging; LTVM, long-term video electroencephalographic monitoring; MTLE, mesial temporal lobe epilepsy; MTS, mesial temporal sclerosis; NP, neuropsychiatric testing; PET, positron emission tomography; SLAH, stereotactic laser amygdalohippocampotomy; SOZ, seizure onset zone; VM, verbal memory.

rigorous SEEG-proven definition of SOZ (and which excludes other hypotheses) followed by technically adequate hippocampal, entorhinal, and uncal ablation should approach effectiveness of open selective surgery (> 65% Engel I). Poorer localization/concordance may reduce rates of seizure freedom to less than 50%. General consent discussion includes risks of stereotactic procedures including need for multiple trajectories, intracranial hemorrhage, incomplete ablation, transient or persistent cranial nerve dysfunction (e.g., double vision or facial numbness), neurocognitive deficits, persistent or recurrent seizures, discomfort, cosmetic deformity, and need for additional procedures.

57.4 Instruments

- Exact instrumentation varies by workflow using either an intraoperative MRI or a diagnostic MRI and surgeon preferences.
- Stereotactic device such as traditional stereotactic frame, stereotactic robot, 3D-printed frame, or direct MRI guidance device and compatible twist drill.
- Commercially available laser device system (Medtronic Visualase, Monteris NeuroBlate, ClearPoint Prism, etc.).
- Minimal instrumentation: hand or power twist drill. MRI-compatible instruments (needle drivers, forceps, suction, bipolar coagulation).

57.5 Patient Preparation

- SLAH should be performed under general anesthesia with endotracheal intubation. The approximate entry point for typical transoccipital approach SLAH is approximately 5 cm above inion and approximately 5 cm lateral to midline. If using MRI-incompatible clippers, it may be necessary to clip this vicinity of hair prior to nearing the magnetic field, especially if using an interventional MRI suite to perform all surgical procedures. Broad-spectrum antibiotic, antiseizure medication, and dexamethasone are routinely administered prior to surgery.

57.6 Patient Positioning

- Positioning depends upon selected workflow. In most cases, the head will be fixed in pins with an appropriate head clamp. Supine with the head end of the bed elevated, supine shoulder bump and head turned, or prone with chin tuck are all acceptable based on surgeon preference, stereotactic device, and specific surgical workflow.
- Particular care must be taken to ensure head positioning allows for orientation of the laser probe down the barrel of the MRI bore. Probes aligned at or near perpendicular to the floor may not fit within the MRI bore and require patient repositioning.

57.7 Technique

- The mesial temporal lobe consists of a complex network of structures with broad connections to the surrounding brain. Surgical technique and ablation targets within the temporal lobe are important determinants of seizure outcomes after SLAH.[21,22] While many early studies emphasized extent of hippocampal resection as a key determinant of seizure freedom,[8,61,62,63] this understanding ignores the contribution of other mesial structures in seizure generation and does not account for patients with continued seizures despite adequate hippocampal resection.[23,64,65,66,67,68]
- Removal of the parahippocampus, amygdala–piriform complex, and rhinal cortices have recently been emphasized to contribute to seizure freedom after open temporal lobe surgery or SLAH.[21,22,24]
- However, since sparing of these structures might account in part for improved naming and verbal memory outcome after SLAH compared to open TL surgery,[36,38,39] careful definition of the SOZ should be undertaken when deciding whether or not to target these areas, especially in the language-dominant hemisphere.
- Below we will outline different approaches for targeting the mesial temporal lobe, including typical trajectories, the use of SEEG to guide ablation, and possible adjunctive use of radiofrequency thermal ablation (RFA; **Video 57.1**). Trajectory planning should account for desired extent of ablation and relevant surrounding anatomy. Since MTLE is the most common TLE subtype and principles for SLAH can be applied to other targets, we

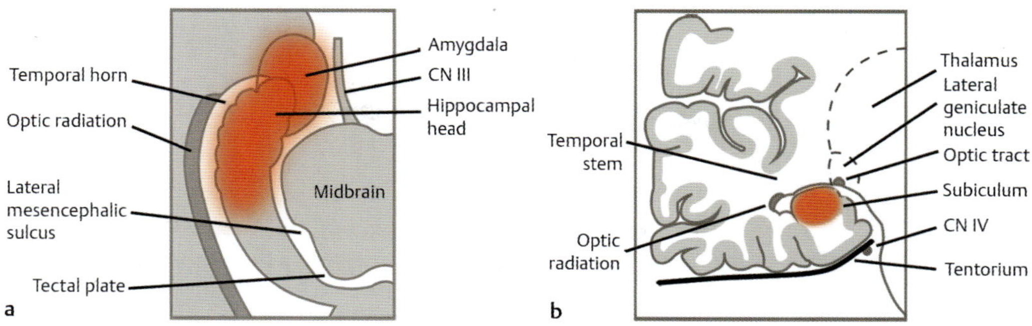

Fig. 57.2 Relevant anatomy in stereotactic laser amygdalohippocampotomy for mesial temporal lobe epilepsy (MTLE). **(a)** Axial and **(b)** sagittal schematics demonstrating target ablation area (*red area*) and important surrounding anatomy at risk of injury with improper laser probe placement. CN, cranial nerve.

will confine our discussion to SLAH. Improper trajectories can lead to insufficient ablation of target anatomy, as well as injury to surrounding structures (► Fig. 57.2). As always, ideal stereotactic trajectories are modified as needed to avoid cortical vessels, sulci, and the ventricle, when possible, to minimize risks of defection and bleeding.

- *Transoccipital approach:*
  - Traditional SLAH uses a single laser probe running along the long axis of the hippocampus and terminating in the uncus (► Fig. 57.3a; Box 57.1). Maximal ablation diameters with LITT generally extend from 18 to 25 mm but in this application are relatively restricted by the pial borders inferomedially and by the ependyma of the temporal horn superolaterally. Proceeding from anterior to posterior, ablated structures from an idealized single trajectory should include the uncinate gyrus, basal-lateral amygdala, hippocampus inversus, pes hippocampus, subiculum, and body of the hippocampus.
  - Routine targeting of the hippocampal tail posterior to the tectal plate has not been associated with benefit and additionally risks injury to the adjacent optic radiations or posterior parahippocampal cortices critical to spatial memory.[21,54,69]
  - The addition of a second approximately parallel transoccipital trajectory may be used to further envelope the entorhinal and anterior parahippocampal cortices if implicated in the SOZ (► Fig. 57.3b).[25]
  - In general, care must be taken to avoid thermal injury near the course of the optic tract, above the body of the hippocampus, or adjacent to cranial nerves such as near the deep aspect of the uncus (CN III), the lateral cavernous sinus (CN IV), foramina rotundum and ovale (CN V), and petrous bone (CN VII; ► Table 57.3).
  - While thermal image monitoring is generally used to protect off-target structures, this modality suffers relatively poorer signal near cerebrospinal fluid cisterns and the skull base, requiring a high index of suspicion and thorough familiarity of regional anatomy.
- *Transoccipital plus lateral approach*:
  - The addition of a lateral trajectory has been advocated in patients with normal hippocampal volume, to improve ablation of the superior uncus amygdala–piriform complex, or if the initial transoccipital trajectory was not ideal due to anatomical restrictions (e.g., unfavorable vasculature or hippocampal curvature).[25,70] Lateral trajectories typically traverse the superior or middle temporal gyri to target amygdala–piriform complex, entorhinal, and perirhinal cortices (► Fig. 57.3c).

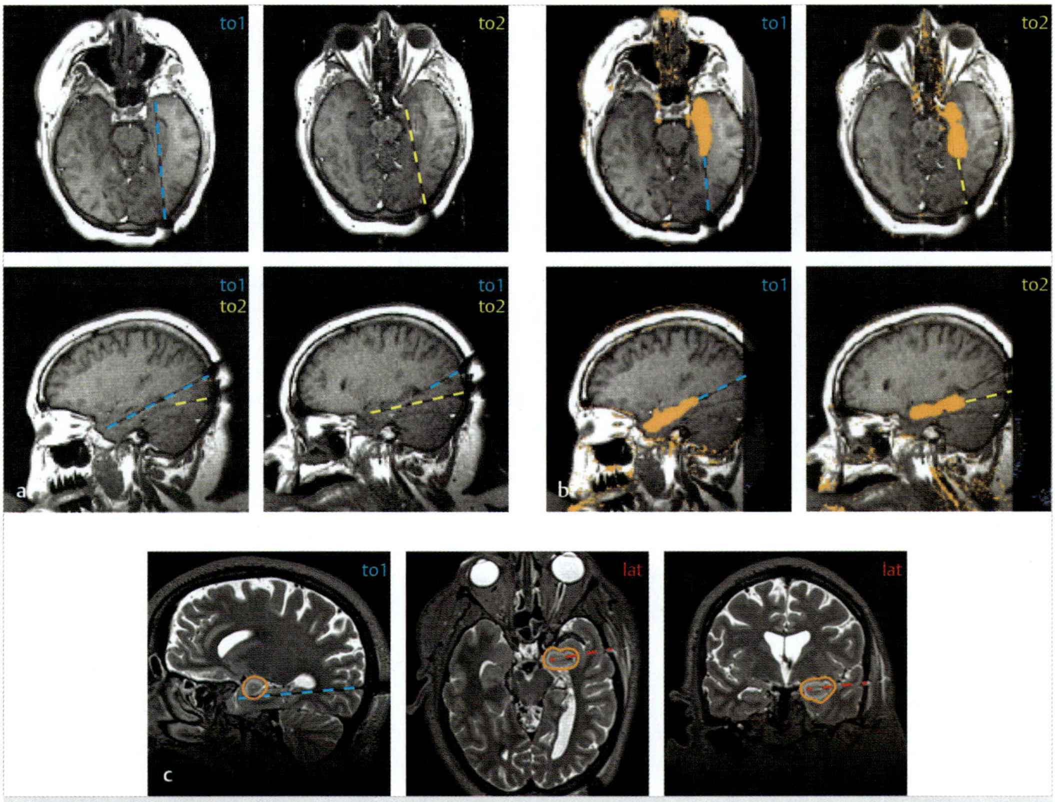

Fig. 57.3 Example trajectories for stereotactic laser amygdalohippocampotomy. **(a, b)** T1-weighted magnetic resonance (MR) images from a case using two transoccipital laser probes. Sagittal and axial views demonstrate laser probe placement **(a)** and the final estimated region of ablation (**b**; *orange-shaded area*) along a standard transoccipital trajectory (to1; *dotted blue line*) targeting the hippocampus, and a modified transoccipital trajectory (to2; *dotted yellow line*) targeting the entorhinal cortex, uncus, and parahippocampal gyrus medially. **(c)** T2-weighted MR images obtained after initial radiofrequency ablation (*ablation area outlined in orange*) and prior to laser interstitial thermal therapy (LITT) hippocampal ablation. A sagittal view of the transoccipital trajectory (to1; *dotted blue line*) targeting the hippocampus is shown on the left. Axial (middle) and coronal (right) MR images demonstrate the lateral trajectory (lat; *red dotted line*) used for radiofrequency ablation targeting the amygdala and uncus.

Table 57.3 Risks and pitfalls associated with improper trajectories for stereotactic laser amygdalohippocampectomy (SLAH)

Trajectory	Risks
Too medial	Injury to CN III, CN IV, and cerebral peduncle. Insufficient ablation of the lateral hippocampus
Too lateral	Injury to optic radiation and temporal stem. Insufficient ablation of the pes hippocampus
Too superior	Injury to optic tract, lateral geniculate nucleus. Insufficient ablation of the subiculum
Too inferior	Insufficient ablation of the amygdala or body of the hippocampus

Table 57.4 Comparison of laser interstitial thermal therapy (LITT) and radiofrequency thermal ablation technology and clinical uses

	Radiofrequency thermal ablation	LITT
Active tip dimensions (diameter × length)	1.6 × 2 mm 1.6 × 10 mm	1.65 × 3 mm 1.65 × 10 mm
Expendable cost	$	$$$
Pairs well with biopsy	Yes	Yes
Patient or MRI transport	No	Yes
Time from placement to begin ablation	~1–2 min	> 30 min (IMRIS) > 60 min (diagnostic MRI)
Temperature monitoring	Tip thermistor only	MR thermography
Real-time imaging, lesion modeling	No	Yes
Neuromonitoring/awake procedures	Yes	No
Maximum ablation diameter	8–12 mm	18–25 mm
Best uses	Unlimited trajectories, smaller diameter ablations, awake or asleep, insurance denials	Generally 1–2 trajectories, larger ablations, asleep
CPT codes	61735	61736 (one trajectory), 61737 (≥ 2 trajectories)

Abbreviations: IMRIS, intraoperative magnetic resonance imaging system; MRI, magnetic resonance imaging.

  - With lateral-to-medial trajectories targeting above the hippocampus, particular care must be taken to avoid thermal injury to the optic tract superior to the amygdala and CN III medial to the uncus.
- *RFA as a substitute for LITT*:
  - The use of RFA for destruction of epileptogenic foci has been reported in a number of case series dating back to the 1960s.[71,72,73] The technique has not been widely adopted in the United States, but at least one European group has published extensively on the use of RFA for stereotactic amygdalohippocampotomy in MTLE with reported seizure-free rates of 78%.[74,75] While the particular RFA probe used in that series is not currently available in the United States, these data indicate that RFA can be a viable alternative to LITT with comparable rates of seizure freedom if optimal targeting and ablation volumes are achieved. The main disadvantages of RFA relative to LITT are absence of real-time thermal imaging and smaller ablation diameters, necessitating additional trajectories. RFA can be a useful adjunct to LITT in certain circumstances (▶ Table 57.4), and multitrajectory RFA can replace LITT in cases of insurance denial or other resource limitations.
  - Furthermore, RFA can also be applied directly through existing SEEG leads (on- or off-label depending upon the specific devices used) by connecting the end of the lead to a radiofrequency lesion generator. Owing to the small electrode size, individual ablation diameters around each contact are small (8–10 mm) but can be additive by ablating contiguous contacts, and surrounding edema transiently mimics a larger ablation. This approach is well tolerated and has the distinct advantage of being performed awake with neurological testing during ongoing SEEG

monitoring in targets of particular functional concern. Although overall less effective, the temporary duration of seizure reduction with this approach allows better risk assessments and predicts success with subsequent LITT. This method can thus be used as further confirmation of adequate delineation of SOZs and functional implications prior to definitive ablation.[26]

Box 57.1 Recommended steps for transoccipital trajectory planning

- *Initial target:* Geometric center of the head (pes) of the hippocampus on coronal view.
- *Initial entry:* Geometric center of the posterior hippocampal body on coronal view, which is located between the lateral mesencephalic sulcus and tectal plate on axial view.
- Using reformatted trajectory views on a stereotactic workstation, extend the target anteriorly through the inferior aspect of the amygdala into the medial temporal pole and posteriorly to the skull.
- A typical scalp entry is approximately 5 cm above the inion and approximately 5 cm lateral to midline.
- Adjust the trajectory as needed to avoid blood vessels, sulci, ventricles, and choroid plexus. The corridor between the lateral ventricle and collateral sulcus posterior to the hippocampal body is often the most restrictive.
- Enter the posterior hippocampus from the underlying parahippocampal gyrus to avoid traversing the ventricle and minimize risks of deflection and intraventricular hemorrhage. Avoid the posterior cerebral artery branches within the sulcus associated with the parahippocampal gyrus.

57.8 Postoperative Care

- As a minimally invasive procedure, LITT abrogates many risks of open surgery. Whereas ATL and SAH require a large incision and craniotomy, LITT trajectories are performed through stab incisions and small twist drill hole craniostomies, which can be closed with single dissolvable sutures. Our pooled analysis of available case series found an average length of stay of 1.2 days after SLAH (▶ Table 57.2). A propensity-matched observational study comparing LITT to open surgery for epilepsy in a pediatric population found that the mean hospital stay after LITT (3.1 days) was significantly shorter than after open surgery (7.2 days).
- Patients should continue antiseizure medications without fail. Additional intravenous levetiracetam or lorazepam may be used to supplement in cases of missed oral medication. Oral or intravenous dexamethasone is often tapered in the perioperative period to ameliorate headaches, nausea, or transient cranial neuropathy per surgeon preferences. Patients with a history of headaches or migraines may experience greater perioperative discomfort.

57.9 Complications

- Rates of procedure-related complications were significantly lower after LITT compared to open surgery (10.8 vs. 29.2%).[17] These general trends for all epilepsy surgeries also hold true for TLE surgery.[9,20] Major complications, as defined by the Society of Interventional Radiology,[36] occurred in 3.8% of cases after SLAH compared to 10.9 and 7.4% of cases after ATL and SAH, respectively.[9] The most common complications associated with SLAH were visual field deficits, followed by transient cranial nerve deficits (such as mild subjective diplopia).
- Unlike open surgery, infection, vascular events, and serious wound problems (such as pseudomeningoceles) were not reported after SLAH.

57.10 Management Pearls

- Epilepsy surgery should be performed in the context of multidisciplinary evaluation at centers that provide comprehensive diagnostic, medical, and surgical care.
- Direct comparisons between SLAH and open temporal lobe surgery are limited by available evidence, which primarily consists of retrospective

case series and case control studies. Prospective randomized controlled trials comparing SLAH with open temporal lobe surgery would be needed to best elucidate the indications for each technique in specific patient subgroups.

- LITT is a safe and effective minimally invasive option for treating MTS and other MTL lesions when noninvasive studies (video EEG, MRI, PET, and neuropsychometry) show concordant results.
- In cases of discordance including nonlesional imaging, an SOZ must be defined by intracranial SEEG prior to treatment with LITT.
- A transoccipital trajectory through the long axis of the anterior hippocampus and terminating in the uncus is required. Additional transoccipital or lateral (transtemporal) trajectories may be used to further optimize ablations of the amygdala, uncus, entorhinal/perirhinal/piriform cortices, or medial temporal pole, especially if implicated by prior SEEG.
- Rates of seizure freedom after SLAH in appropriately selected and treated patients are generally greater than 60%.
- Outcomes with respect to memory, naming, language disturbance, and psychiatric disturbance are superior when compared directly to open surgery, especially in the dominant hemisphere.
- Tract hemorrhages are avoided by use of contrasted volumetric imaging and attention to avoiding vascular structures during careful stereotactic planning and technique. Visual field deficits and cranial neuropathies are avoided by monitoring and minimizing thermal injury near optic tracts, lateral geniculate nucleus, and contiguous CNs III, IV, and V.
- Antiseizure medications should be continued throughout the perioperative period, supplemented as needed, and should only be weaned by an epileptologist after a year or more of seizure freedom.

57.11 Emerging Technologies

- LITT procedures will continue to evolve with advances in robotics, complex multitrajectory capability, MRI guidance/compatibility, computational ablation modeling, and integration with SEEG and SOZ definition. Advances in laser delivery such as wavelength/power control, device/light steerability, and improved 3D thermal monitoring will continue to make LITT more safe, effective, efficient, and accessible.

References

[1] Engel J, Jr, McDermott MP, Wiebe S, et al. Early Randomized Surgical Epilepsy Trial (ERSET) Study Group. Early surgical therapy for drug-resistant temporal lobe epilepsy: a randomized trial. JAMA. 2012; 307(9):922–930

[2] Wiebe S, Blume WT, Girvin JP, Eliasziw M, Effectiveness and Efficiency of Surgery for Temporal Lobe Epilepsy Study Group. A randomized, controlled trial of surgery for temporal-lobe epilepsy. N Engl J Med. 2001; 345(5):311–318

[3] Mohammed HS, Kaufman CB, Limbrick DD, et al. Impact of epilepsy surgery on seizure control and quality of life: a 26-year follow-up study. Epilepsia. 2012; 53(4):712–720

[4] Gleissner U, Helmstaedter C, Schramm J, Elger CE. Memory outcome after selective amygdalohippocampectomy: a study in 140 patients with temporal lobe epilepsy. Epilepsia. 2002; 43(1):87–95

[5] Gleissner U, Helmstaedter C, Schramm J, Elger CE. Memory outcome after selective amygdalohippocampectomy in patients with temporal lobe epilepsy: one-year follow-up. Epilepsia. 2004; 45(8):960–962

[6] Spencer DD, Spencer SS, Mattson RH, Williamson PD, Novelly RA. Access to the posterior medial temporal lobe structures in the surgical treatment of temporal lobe epilepsy. Neurosurgery. 1984; 15(5):667–671

[7] Wieser HG, Yaşargil MG. Selective amygdalohippocampectomy as a surgical treatment of mesiobasal limbic epilepsy. Surg Neurol. 1982; 17(6):445–457

[8] Josephson CB, Dykeman J, Fiest KM, et al. Systematic review and meta-analysis of standard vs selective temporal lobe epilepsy surgery. Neurology. 2013; 80(18):1669–1676

[9] Kohlhase K, Zöllner JP, Tandon N, Strzelczyk A, Rosenow F. Comparison of minimally invasive and traditional surgical approaches for refractory mesial temporal lobe epilepsy: a systematic review and meta-analysis of outcomes. Epilepsia. 2021; 62(4):831–845

[10] Donos C, Breier J, Friedman E, et al. Laser ablation for mesial temporal lobe epilepsy: surgical and cognitive outcomes with and without mesial temporal sclerosis. Epilepsia. 2018; 59(7):1421–1432

[11] Gross RE, Stern MA, Willie JT, et al. Stereotactic laser amygdalohippocampotomy for mesial temporal lobe epilepsy. Ann Neurol. 2018; 83(3):575–587

[12] Jermakowicz WJ, Kanner AM, Sur S, et al. Laser thermal ablation for mesiotemporal epilepsy: analysis of ablation volumes and trajectories. Epilepsia. 2017; 58(5):801–810

[13] Kang JY, Wu C, Tracy J, et al. Laser interstitial thermal therapy for medically intractable mesial temporal lobe epilepsy. Epilepsia. 2016; 57(2):325–334

[14] Le S, Ho AL, Fisher RS, et al. Laser interstitial thermal therapy (LITT): seizure outcomes for refractory mesial temporal lobe epilepsy. Epilepsy Behav. 2018; 89:37–41

[15] Tao JX, Wu S, Lacy M, et al. Stereotactic EEG-guided laser interstitial thermal therapy for mesial temporal lobe epilepsy. J Neurol Neurosurg Psychiatry. 2018; 89(5): 542–548

[16] Waseem H, Osborn KE, Schoenberg MR, et al. Laser ablation therapy: an alternative treatment for medically resistant mesial temporal lobe epilepsy after age 50. Epilepsy Behav. 2015; 51:152–157
[17] Yossofzai O, Stone S, Madsen J, et al. Seizure outcome of pediatric magnetic resonance-guided laser interstitial thermal therapy versus open surgery: a matched noninferiority cohort study. Epilepsia. 2023; 64(1):114–126
[18] Youngerman BE, Oh JY, Anbarasan D, et al. Columbia Comprehensive Epilepsy Center Co-Authors. Laser ablation is effective for temporal lobe epilepsy with and without mesial temporal sclerosis if hippocampal seizure onsets are localized by stereoelectroencephalography. Epilepsia. 2018; 59(3):595–606
[19] Gupta K, Dickey AS, Hu R, Faught E, Willie JT. Robot assisted MRI-guided LITT of the anterior, lateral, and medial temporal lobe for temporal lobe epilepsy. Front Neurol. 2020; 11: 572334
[20] Youngerman BE, Save AV, McKhann GM. Magnetic resonance imaging-guided laser interstitial thermal therapy for epilepsy: systematic review of technique, indications, and outcomes. Neurosurgery. 2020; 86(4):E366–E382
[21] Gleichgerrcht E, Drane DL, Keller SS, et al. Association between anatomical location of surgically induced lesions and postoperative seizure outcome in temporal lobe epilepsy. Neurology. 2022; 98(2):e141–e151
[22] Wu C, Jermakowicz WJ, Chakravorti S, et al. Effects of surgical targeting in laser interstitial thermal therapy for mesial temporal lobe epilepsy: a multicenter study of 234 patients. Epilepsia. 2019; 60(6):1171–1183
[23] Morita-Sherman M, Louis S, Vegh D, et al. Outcomes of resections that spare vs remove an MRI-normal hippocampus. Epilepsia. 2020; 61(11):2545–2557
[24] Satzer D, Tao JX, Warnke PC. Extent of parahippocampal ablation is associated with seizure freedom after laser amygdalohippocampotomy. J Neurosurg. 2021; 135(6): 1742–1751
[25] Liu DD, Lauro PM, Phillips RK, III, et al. Two-trajectory laser amygdalohippocampotomy: anatomic modeling and initial seizure outcomes. Epilepsia. 2021; 62(10):2344–2356
[26] Shields JA, Greven ACM, Shivamurthy VKN, et al. Stereoelectroencephalography-guided radiofrequency ablation of the epileptogenic zone as a treatment and predictor of future success of further surgical intervention. Epilepsia. 2023; 64(8):2081–2093
[27] Michalak AJ, Greenblatt A, Wu S, et al. Seizure onset patterns predict outcome after stereo-electroencephalography-guided laser amygdalohippocampotomy. Epilepsia. 2023; 64(6): 1568–1581
[28] Vakharia VN, Sparks R, Li K, et al. Automated trajectory planning for laser interstitial thermal therapy in mesial temporal lobe epilepsy. Epilepsia. 2018; 59(4):814–824
[29] Cajigas I, Kanner AM, Ribot R, et al. Magnetic resonance-guided laser interstitial thermal therapy for mesial temporal epilepsy: a case series analysis of outcomes and complications at 2-year follow-up. World Neurosurg. 2019; 126:e1121–e1129
[30] Greenway MRF, Lucas JA, Feyissa AM, Grewal S, Wharen RE, Tatum WO. Neuropsychological outcomes following stereotactic laser amygdalohippocampectomy. Epilepsy Behav. 2017; 75:50–55
[31] Grewal SS, Zimmerman RS, Worrell G, et al. Laser ablation for mesial temporal epilepsy: a multi-site, single institutional series. J Neurosurg. 2018; 130(6):2055–2062
[32] Waseem H, Vivas AC, Vale FL. MRI-guided laser interstitial thermal therapy for treatment of medically refractory non-lesional mesial temporal lobe epilepsy: outcomes, complications, and current limitations: a review. J Clin Neurosci. 2017; 38:1–7
[33] Ivanovic J, Larsson PG, Østby Y, et al. Seizure outcomes of temporal lobe epilepsy surgery in patients with normal MRI and without specific histopathology. Acta Neurochir (Wien). 2017; 159(5):757–766
[34] Salvato G, Scarpa P, Francione S, et al. Declarative long-term memory and the mesial temporal lobe: insights from a 5-year postsurgery follow-up study on refractory temporal lobe epilepsy. Epilepsy Behav. 2016; 64 Pt A:102–109
[35] Sheikh S, Thompson N, Bingaman W, Gonzalez-Martinez J, Najm I, Jehi L. (Re)Defining success in epilepsy surgery: the importance of relative seizure reduction in patient-reported quality of life. Epilepsia. 2019; 60(10):2078–2085
[36] Drane DL, Loring DW, Voets NL, et al. Better object recognition and naming outcome with MRI-guided stereotactic laser amygdalohippocampotomy for temporal lobe epilepsy. Epilepsia. 2015; 56(1):101–113
[37] Moritz-Gasser S, Herbet G, Maldonado IL, Duffau H. Lexical access speed is significantly correlated with the return to professional activities after awake surgery for low-grade gliomas. J Neurooncol. 2012; 107(3):633–641
[38] Drane DL, Willie JT, Pedersen NP, et al. Superior verbal memory outcome after stereotactic laser amygdalohippocampotomy. Front Neurol. 2021; 12:779495
[39] Drane DL, Ojemann JG, Phatak V, et al. Famous face identification in temporal lobe epilepsy: support for a multimodal integration model of semantic memory. Cortex. 2013; 49(6):1648–1667
[40] Helmstaedter C, Van Roost D, Clusmann H, Urbach H, Elger CE. Schramm J. Collateral brain damage, a potential source of cognitive impairment after selective surgery for control of mesial temporal lobe epilepsy. J Neurol Neurosurg Psychiatry. 2004; 75(2):323–326
[41] Padda K, Matthews RE, Karakis I, et al. Psychiatric changes after stereotactic laser amygdalohippocampotomy for medial temporal lobe epilepsy. Epilepsy Behav. 2023; 145:109332
[42] Chabardès S, Kahane P, Minotti L, et al. The temporopolar cortex plays a pivotal role in temporal lobe seizures. Brain. 2005; 128(Pt 8):1818–1831
[43] Dupont S, Semah F, Clémenceau S, Adam C, Baulac M, Samson Y. Accurate prediction of postoperative outcome in mesial temporal lobe epilepsy: a study using positron emission tomography with 18fluorodeoxyglucose. Arch Neurol. 2000; 57(9):1331–1336
[44] Schramm J, Kral T, Grunwald T, Blümcke I. Surgical treatment for neocortical temporal lobe epilepsy: clinical and surgical aspects and seizure outcome. J Neurosurg. 2001; 94(1):33–42
[45] Bercovici E, Kumar BS, Mirsattari SM. Neocortical temporal lobe epilepsy. Epilepsy Res Treat. 2012; 2012:103160
[46] Janszky J, Pannek HW, Fogarasi A, et al. Prognostic factors for surgery of neocortical temporal lobe epilepsy. Seizure. 2006; 15(2):125–132
[47] Yun CH, Lee SK, Lee SY, Kim KK, Jeong SW, Chung CK. Prognostic factors in neocortical epilepsy surgery: multivariate analysis. Epilepsia. 2006; 47(3):574–579
[48] Barba C, Rheims S, Minotti L, et al. Temporal plus epilepsy is a major determinant of temporal lobe surgery failures. Brain. 2016; 139(Pt 2):444–451

[49] Hawasli AH, Bandt SK, Hogan RE, Werner N, Leuthardt EC. Laser ablation as treatment strategy for medically refractory dominant insular epilepsy: therapeutic and functional considerations. Stereotact Funct Neurosurg. 2014; 92(6):397–404
[50] Perry MS, Donahue DJ, Malik SI, et al. Magnetic resonance imaging-guided laser interstitial thermal therapy as treatment for intractable insular epilepsy in children. J Neurosurg Pediatr. 2017; 20(6):575–582
[51] Vetkas A, Germann J, Boutet A, et al. Laser interstitial thermal therapy for the treatment of insular lesions: a systematic review. Front Neurol. 2023; 13:1024075
[52] Buraniqi E, Guerin JB, Miller KJ, et al. Temporal encephalocele: a treatable etiology of drug-resistant pediatric temporal lobe epilepsy. Pediatr Neurol. 2023; 142:32–38
[53] Ranjan M, Wilfong AA, Boerwinkle V, Jarrar R, David Adelson P. Temporal encephalocele: a novel indication for magnetic resonance-guided laser interstitial thermal therapy for medically intractable epilepsy. Epileptic Disord. 2019; 21(3):265–270
[54] Willie JT, Laxpati NG, Drane DL, et al. Real-time magnetic resonance-guided stereotactic laser amygdalohippocampotomy for mesial temporal lobe epilepsy. Neurosurgery. 2014; 74(6): 569–584, discussion 584–585
[55] Kwan P, Arzimanoglou A, Berg AT, et al. Definition of drug resistant epilepsy: consensus proposal by the ad hoc Task Force of the ILAE Commission on Therapeutic Strategies. Epilepsia. 2010; 51(6):1069–1077
[56] Pascual MR. Temporal lobe epilepsy: clinical semiology and neurophysiological studies. Semin Ultrasound CT MR. 2007; 28(6):416–423
[57] Baxendale S, Wilson SJ, Baker GA, et al. Indications and expectations for neuropsychological assessment in epilepsy surgery in children and adults. Epileptic Disord. 2019; 21(3): 221–234
[58] Drane DL. Neuropsychological evaluation of the epilepsy surgical candidate. In: Barr WB, Morrison C, eds. Handbook on the Neuropsychology of Epilepsy. New York, NY: Springer; 2015:87–121
[59] Gross RE, Willie JT, Drane DL. The role of stereotactic laser amygdalohippocampotomy in mesial temporal lobe epilepsy. Neurosurg Clin N Am. 2016; 27(1):37–50
[60] Helmstaedter C, Witt JA. How neuropsychology can improve the care of individual patients with epilepsy. Looking back and into the future. Seizure. 2017; 44:113–120
[61] Bonilha L, Kobayashi E, Mattos JP, Honorato DC, Li LM, Cendes F. Value of extent of hippocampal resection in the surgical treatment of temporal lobe epilepsy. Arq Neuropsiquiatr. 2004; 62(1):15–20
[62] Joo EY, Han HJ, Lee EK, et al. Resection extent versus postoperative outcomes of seizure and memory in mesial temporal lobe epilepsy. Seizure. 2005; 14(8):541–551
[63] Silbergeld DL. Extent of medial temporal resection on outcome from anterior temporal lobectomy: a randomized prospective study. Neurosurgery. 1997; 41(1):327–328
[64] Vismer MS, Forcelli PA, Skopin MD, Gale K, Koubeissi MZ. The piriform, perirhinal, and entorhinal cortex in seizure generation. Front Neural Circuits. 2015; 9:27
[65] Haegelen C, Perucca P, Châtillon CE, et al. High-frequency oscillations, extent of surgical resection, and surgical outcome in drug-resistant focal epilepsy. Epilepsia. 2013; 54(5): 848–857
[66] Schramm J. Temporal lobe epilepsy surgery and the quest for optimal extent of resection: a review. Epilepsia. 2008; 49(8): 1296–1307
[67] Bonilha L, Yasuda CL, Rorden C, et al. Does resection of the medial temporal lobe improve the outcome of temporal lobe epilepsy surgery? Epilepsia. 2007; 48(3):571–578
[68] Galovic M, Baudracco I, Wright-Goff E, et al. Association of piriform cortex resection with surgical outcomes in patients with temporal lobe epilepsy. JAMA Neurol. 2019; 76(6):690–700
[69] Sone D, Ahmad M, Thompson PJ, et al. Optimal surgical extent for memory and seizure outcome in temporal lobe epilepsy. Ann Neurol. 2022; 91(1):131–144
[70] Gross RE, Boulis NM, ed. Neurosurgical Operative Atlas. Functional Neurosurgery. New York, NY: Thieme; 2018
[71] Adams JE, Rutkin BB. Treatment of temporal-lobe epilepsy by stereotactic surgery. Confin Neurol. 1969; 31(1):80–85
[72] Schwab RS, Sweet WH, Mark VH, Kjellberg RN, Ervin FR. Treatment of intractable temporal lobe epilepsy by stereotactic amygdala lesions. Trans Am Neurol Assoc. 1965; 90:12–19
[73] Marossero F, Ravagnati L, Sironi VA, et al. Late results of stereotactic radiofrequency lesions in epilepsy. Acta Neurochir Suppl (Wien). 1980; 30:145–149
[74] Liscak R, Malikova H, Kalina M, et al. Stereotactic radiofrequency amygdalohippocampectomy in the treatment of mesial temporal lobe epilepsy. Acta Neurochir (Wien). 2010; 152(8):1291–1298
[75] Vojtěch Z, Malíková H, Krámská L, et al. Long-term seizure outcome after stereotactic amygdalohippocampectomy. Acta Neurochir (Wien). 2014; 156(8):1529–1537

Index

Note: Page numbers set **bold** or *italic* indicate headings or figures, respectively.

D

E

S